THE MILLON INVENTORIES

The Millon Inventories

SECOND EDITION

A Practitioner's Guide to Personalized Clinical Assessment

Edited by

Theodore Millon
Caryl Bloom

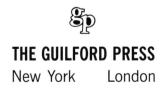

THE GUILFORD PRESS
New York   London

© 2008 The Guilford Press
A Division of Guilford Publications, Inc.
72 Spring Street, New York, NY 10012
www.guilford.com

Printed in the United States of America

This book is printed on acid-free paper.

Last digit is print number: 9 8 7 6 5 4 3 2 1

Library of Congress Cataloging-in-Publication Data

The Millon inventories: a practitioner's guide to personalized clinical assessment / edited by Theodore Millon, Caryl Bloom. — 2nd ed.
   p. ; cm.
   Includes bibliographical references and indexes.
   ISBN 978-1-59385-674-8 (cloth: alk. paper)
   1. Millon inventories (Personality tests)   I. Millon, Theodore.   II. Bloom, Caryl.
   [DNLM: 1. Personality Assessment.   2. Personality Inventory.   3. Mental Disorders—diagnosis.   4. Psychometrics—methods.   WM 145 M656 2008]
   RC554.M55 2008
   155.2′8—dc22

                                                                2007052768

About the Editors

Theodore Millon, PhD, DSc, is Dean and Scientific Director of the Institute for Advanced Studies in Personology and Psychopathology. He was Founding Editor of the *Journal of Personality Disorders* and past president of the International Society for the Study of Personality Disorders. He has held full professorial appointments at Harvard Medical School, the University of Illinois, and the University of Miami. A prolific author, Dr. Millon has written or edited more than 30 books on theory, assessment, and therapy, as well as more than 200 chapters and articles in numerous other books and journals in the field. In August 2008, Dr. Millon will receive the American Psychological Foundation Gold Medal for Life Achievement in the Application of Psychology.

Caryl Bloom, PhD, has served as Assistant Dean of the Institute for Advanced Studies in Personology and Psychopathology and is currently Senior Consultant. She has taught at several graduate psychology programs in California, where she is currently on the faculty at Argosy University. A specialist in family assessment and couple therapy, Dr. Bloom has been in active clinical practice for over 20 years. Currently engaged in research studies on couple compatibility and medical diagnostic studies by nurses and medical paraprofessionals, she has contributed important ideas to the furthering of health assessment.

Contributors

Michael H. Antoni, PhD, Center for Psycho-Oncology Research, University of Miami, Coral Gables, Florida

Caryl Bloom, PhD, Institute for Advanced Studies in Personology and Psychopathology, Coral Gables, Florida

Alyssa Boice, MA, Institute for Advanced Studies in Personology and Psychopathology, Port Jervis, New York

James P. Choca, PhD, Department of Psychology, Roosevelt University, Chicago, Illinois

Jan J. L. Derksen, PhD, Department of Clinical Psychology, Radboud University, Nijmegen, The Netherlands

Stephanie E. Diamond, MA, Counseling Psychology Program, University of Miami, Coral Gables, Florida

Darwin Dorr, PhD, ABPP, Clinical Psychology Program, Wichita State University, Wichita, Kansas

Frank J. Dyer, PhD, ABPP, private practice, Montclair, New Jersey

Ask Elklit, PhD, Department of Psychology, University of Aarhus, Aarhus, Denmark

Seth D. Grossman, PsyD, Institute for Advanced Studies in Personology and Psychopathology, Coral Gables, Florida; Counseling Center, Florida International University, Miami, Florida

Lee Hyer, EdD, ABPP, Georgia Neurosurgical Institute and Department of Psychiatry, Mercer Medical School, Macon, Georgia

John Kamp, PhD, Pearson, Thousand Oaks, California

Jeffrey J. Magnavita, PhD, ABPP, Private Practice, Glastonbury, Connecticut; Department of Clinical Psychology, University of Hartford, West Hartford, Connecticut

Joseph T. McCann, PsyD, JD, UHS Hospitals—Binghamton General Hospital and Upstate Medical University—Clinical Campus, Binghamton, New York

Robert C. McMahon, PhD, Counseling Psychology Program, University of Miami, Coral Gables, Florida

Carrie M. Millon, PhD, Institute for Advanced Studies in Personology and Psychopathology, Coral Gables, Florida

Theodore Millon, PhD, DSc, Institute for Advanced Studies in Personology and Psychopathology, Port Jervis, New York

Whitney L. Mills, BA, School of Aging Studies, University of South Florida, Tampa, Florida

Victor Molinari, PhD, ABPP, Department of Aging and Mental Health, Louis de la Parte Florida Mental Health Institute, University of South Florida, Tampa, Florida

A. Rodney Nurse, PhD, ABPP, Family Psychological Services and Collaborative Divorce Associates, Orinda, California

Gina M. P. Rossi, PhD, Department of Personality and Social Psychology, Faculty of Psychology and Educational Sciences, Vrije Universiteit Brussel, Brussels, Belgium

Edward D. Rossini, PhD, Department of Psychology, Roosevelt University, Chicago, Illinois

Elbert W. Russell, PhD, private practice, Miami, Florida

Sally L. Kolitz Russell, PhD, private practice, Miami, Florida

Erik Simonsen, MD, Psychiatric Research Unit, University of Copenhagen, Zealand Region Psychiatry Roskilde, Roskilde, Denmark

Katherine Sinsabaugh, MA, Institute for Advanced Studies in Personology and Psychopathology, Port Jervis, New York

Hedwig V. Sloore, PhD, Department of Personality and Social Psychology, Faculty of Psychology and Educational Sciences, Vrije Universiteit Brussel, Brussels, Belgium

Mark Stanton, PhD, ABPP, School of Behavioral and Applied Sciences, Azusa Pacific University, Azusa, California

John W. Stoner, PhD, High Security Management Facilities, Colorado Department of Corrections, Cañon City, Colorado

Stephen Strack, PhD, Psychology Service, U.S. Department of Veterans Affairs Ambulatory Care Center, Los Angeles, California

Robert F. Tringone, PhD, Schneider Children's Hospital, Long Island Jewish Hospital, New Hyde Park, New York

Lawrence G. Weiss, PhD, Harcourt Assessments, San Antonio, Texas

Catherine Yeager, PhD, Institute for Mental Health Policy, Research, and Treatment, Essex County Hospital Center, Cedar Grove, New Jersey; Department of Psychiatry, University of Medicine and Dentistry of New Jersey, Piscataway, New Jersey

Preface

Few events are more gratifying to an author or editor than the realization not only that his or her efforts achieved numerous reprintings but that the book was sufficiently well received to justify the updating and expansion of a second edition. And so has it been with *The Millon Inventories*, initially published by The Guilford Press a decade ago. From letters, e-mails, and discussions at conferences, we hear that professional and graduate students found this textbook informative and useful. Instructors reported that it was well organized and easy to teach, as well as providing a more in-depth series of presentations than, for example, the excellent but more introductory *Essentials of Millon Inventories Assessment* (Wiley, 2002) by Stephen Strack, now entering its third edition.

What will the reader find that is new in this edition, sufficient to justify publication beyond that of a simple reprinting? Essentially, three important elements have been added to strengthen and enrich the first edition.

First, our research group has been busily engaged in studies on a score of populations for whom well-constructed self-report inventories may prove clinically useful. Now included in the book is a richly developed chapter on using the Millon Behavioral Medicine Diagnostic (MBMD) (Chapter 19). Chapter 20, which elaborates the Facet Scales of the Millon Adolescent Clinical Inventory (MACI), is also expanded. Notable in this realm is an important new tool, the Millon Pre-Adolescent Clinical Inventory (M-PACI) (Chapter 22). This instrument extends the scope of the MACI to children in the 9- to 12-year-old range; its rapid acceptance these past 2 years has been most gratifying. Newest among our recently developed inventories is the Millon College Counseling Inventory (MCCI) (Chapter 23), a self-report tool whose timeliness has been most appropriate in light of recent tragic events in numerous college settings. The Millon–Grossman Personality Domain Checklist (MG-PDC) (Chapter 24) is an advanced instrument to aid clinicians who wish to integrate the diverse data they have gathered into a coherent diagnostic formulation, especially for purposes of optimizing therapeutic planning.

That brings us to the second major element that is substantially novel in this edition, that of orienting assessment toward therapeutic goals. Several chapters, in addition to Chapter 24, address the rationale and techniques that speak to the issue of how to make assessment maximally useful to clinicians who wish to have a clearer sense of what to do with diagnostic information. Both Chapters 2 and 14 guide the reader in this pragmatic direction.

Third, the book and many of its chapters (e.g., Chapters 1, 2, 3, 24, and 28) have been expanded so that sophisticated clinicians and teaching academics are provided with a philosophical rationale for what assessment is and should be. More specifically, they contend that what we term a "personalized" approach to assessment and therapy should be foremost in our work with patients.

A few words of history about the inventories may be of interest to the reader. The Millon Clinical Multiaxial Inventory (MCMI) originated as a defensive act, a shield against the proliferation of potentially misconceived or poorly designed efforts on the part of well-meaning others to "operationalize" concepts the senior editor had proposed in an earlier publication. Rather than sit back and enjoy the dissemination of his ideas, he began to see this burgeoning of divergent instrument development not only as uncontrolled and possibly misguided, but as a process ultimately endangering the very theoretical notions they were designed to strengthen.

To establish a measure of instrumental uniformity for future investigators, as well as to assure at least a modicum of psychometric quality among tools that ostensibly reflected the theory's constructs, Millon was prompted (perhaps "driven" is a more accurate word) to consider undertaking the test construction task himself. At that time, in early 1971, he fortunately was directing a research supervision group at the universities of Chicago and Illinois composed of psychologists and psychiatrists in training during their internship and residency periods. All of them had read his 1969 *Modern Psychopathology* text and found the suggestion that the group work together to develop instruments to identify and quantify the text's novel personality constructs to be both worthy and challenging.

Naively, the team assumed that the construction task could be completed in about 18 months, a period that would allow most members of the research group to participate on a continuing basis. Despite the fact that the team "postponed" developing a personality-oriented structured interview schedule after an initial effort, the "more limited" task of constructing a self-report inventory took almost 7 years to complete. The framework and preliminary item selections of the inventory were well under way by the end of the first full year of our work; this was described briefly in a book Millon cowrote entitled *Research Methods in Psychopathology* (Wiley, 1972). The initial forms of the clinical instrument were entitled the Millon–Illinois Self-Report Inventory.

Psychodiagnostic assessment procedures in the years preceding the research group's test development work contained a considerable share of mystique. Not only were diagnostic methods often an exercise in oracular craft and intuitive artistry, but they typically were clothed in obscure and esoteric jargon. A change in the character of personality theory and assessment began to brew in the late 1960s. Although these advances progressed slowly, there were clear signs that new ideas would soon emerge. Projective techniques such as the Rorschach began to be analyzed quantitatively and were increasingly anchored to the empirical domain. The so-called objective inventories, such as the Minnesota Multiphasic Personality Inventory (MMPI), were being interpreted increasingly in terms of configural profiles. No longer approached as sets of separate scales, formerly segmented instruments were increasingly analyzed as holistic integrations that possessed clinical significance only as gestalt composites. In addition, the former insistence that diagnostic interpretation be "objective," that is, anchored solely to empirical correlates, gave way to clinical syntheses, including the "dynamics" of the previously maligned projectives. Although part function instruments, oriented toward one expressive form of pathology or another (e.g., the Beck Depression Inventory), are still popular, the newest tools moved increasingly toward composite structures (i.e., "whole" personalities). These personality formulations were not conceived as sets of discrete attributes (i.e., factors) that must be individually deduced and then pieced together, but as integrated configurations from the start. Hence we have seen the development of various tools explicitly designed to diagnose, for example, the "borderline" personality.

The MCMI took a leadership role in fostering this trend toward holistic personality measures. It went one step beyond most techniques by including all of the *Diagnostic and Statistical Manual of Mental Disorders* (DSM) personality disorders in a single inventory. The move to holism was not limited to inventories alone. New structured interview schedules and clinical rating scales were developed to provide another rich source of data. Notable here are the Shedler–Westen Assessment Procedure–200 and the MG-PDC (see Chapter 24, this volume). Not to be overlooked was the sound psychometric manner in which most of these newer tools were constructed, thereby wedding the empirical and quantitative features that were the major strength of the highly structured and objective self-report inventories with the dynamic and integrative qualities that characterized the more intuitive and richly insightful projective techniques.

We should not overlook the very special status assigned to the personality disorders in the DSM. With the third edition of this official classification in 1980, in which this book's senior editor played a substantive role, personality not only gained a place of consequence among psychiatric classifications but became central to its innovative multiaxial schema. The logic for assigning personality (Axis II) its own special status was more than a matter of differentiating syndromes of a more acute and dramatic nature from those of a longstanding and prosaic character. More relevant to this partitioning decision was the assertion that personality can serve usefully as a dynamic substrate from which clinicians can better grasp the significance and meaning of their patients' transient and florid disorders (Axis I). In the DSM, then, personality disorders not only attained a nosological status of prominence in their own right but were assigned a contextual role that made them fundamental to the understanding and interpretation of all other psychopathologies.

As is evident by the variety of "Millon" instruments reported in this book, we opted in favor of focusing an inventory on target rather than broad-based populations; the MCMI is oriented toward matters of import among adult mental health patients, the MAPI and MACI focus on adolescent clinical populations, the M-PACI on preadolescents, the MBHI and the MBMD focus on those whose primary ailments are of a medical or physical nature, the MCCI addresses the issues of college students, and the MIPS-R quantifies traits among nonclinical or so-called normal adults who do not evince discernible psychic pathology.

The senior editor admits, much to both his surprise and pleasure, that the defensively constructed MCMI, as well as its more newly developed sister inventories, quickly matched in acceptance and clinical usage the theory on which they were based. Only the MMPI and Rorschach continue to supersede the Millon inventories as the most widely researched and used of clinically oriented tests. In the past decade, numerous clinicians and researchers have begun to publish books (10 at last count) and articles (approximately a thousand) evaluating the several Millon instruments. The present volume is the second edition of the first book organized and edited by the inventories' primary author, now joined by Caryl Bloom, a senior member of the Institute for Advanced Studies in Personology and Psychopathology staff.

The authors of the books' chapters constitute many of the esteemed lecturers who contributed key seminars at the Institute's decade-long annual conferences. They represent a distinguished group of clinicians and researchers who continue to play a central role in disseminating and illuminating the merits and clinical utility of the inventories.

Special thanks also are owed to the administrative staff of the Institute, namely, Donna Meagher and Alyssa Boice, who organized the various pieces comprising this book, bringing it together into a coherent whole. No less important are several Pearson Assessment staff members, most notably Christine Carlson, Theo Jolosky, John Kamp, Julie Lackaff, and Carol Watson. Equally valuable to us have been the hundreds of fellow professionals and students who offered constructive suggestions that have made this second edition even more useful than the first.

Perhaps the greatest value to this text's readers will be an implicit one, namely, the growing heuristic fertility of the Millon inventories. These inventories are more than another "objective" tool in the diagnostician's assessment kit. They provide clinicians with a theoretical foundation for mastering the realm of clinical and personality pathology and a means for understanding the principles that underlie their patients' functional and dysfunctional behaviors, thoughts, and feelings. Moreover, the openness of the theory not only illuminates the patient's personal life but encourages the clinician to deduce and uncover insights beyond those on which the inventories' interpretive reports have been grounded.

As with the well-received first edition of this book, we believe the second edition will provide professors of psychological assessment courses a comprehensive text for teaching the foundations, development, and personalized clinical applications of each of the several established and new Millon inventories.

THEODORE MILLON
CARYL BLOOM

Contents

PART I. INTRODUCTION

1. The Rationale for Personalized Assessment in Clinical Practice 3
Caryl Bloom and Theodore Millon

2. Relating Personalized Assessment to Personalized Psychotherapy 15
Theodore Millon, Alyssa Boice, and Katherine Sinsabaugh

PART II. A GUIDE TO THE MILLON CLINICAL MULTIAXIAL INVENTORY (MCMI)

3. Scientific Grounding and Validation of the MCMI 49
Theodore Millon and Carrie M. Millon

4. Guidelines for the Contemporary Interpretation of the MCMI-III 83
Edward D. Rossini and James P. Choca

5. A Brief Illustrative MCMI Case Study 96
Caryl Bloom and Theodore Millon

6. The MCMI-III and MACI Grossman Facet Scales 112
Seth D. Grossman

7. Clinical Integration of the MCMI-III
and the Rorschach Comprehensive System 135
Darwin Dorr

8. Studies Relating the MCMI and the MMPI 157
Michael H. Antoni

 9. Using the Millon Inventories in Forensic Psychology   177
    Frank J. Dyer

10. Using the MCMI in Correctional Settings   196
    John W. Stoner

11. Using the MCMI-III in Neuropsychological Evaluations   244
    Sally L. Kolitz Russell and Elbert W. Russell

12. MCMI Applications in Alcohol and Drug Dependence   270
    Robert C. McMahon and Stephanie E. Diamond

13. Personological Assessment and Treatment of Older Adults   296
    Lee Hyer, Victor Molinari, Whitney L. Mills, and Catherine Yeager

14. Using the MCMI in General Treatment Planning   327
    Jeffrey J. Magnavita

15. Using the MCMI in Treating Couples   347
    A. Rodney Nurse and Mark Stanton

16. The Adaptation of the MCMI-III in Two Non-English-Speaking Countries: 369
    State of the Art of the Dutch Language Version
    Gina M. P. Rossi, Hedwig V. Sloore, and Jan J. L. Derksen

17. Experiences in Translating and Validating the MCMI in Denmark   387
    Erik Simonsen and Ask Elklit

18. On the Dimensional Theory, Empirical Support, and Structural Character 405
    of the MCMI-III
    Stephen Strack and Theodore Millon

PART III. A GUIDE TO ASSOCIATED MILLON CLINICAL INVENTORIES

19. Using the Millon Behavioral Medicine Diagnostic (MBMD)   433
    Michael H. Antoni, Carrie M. Millon, and Theodore Millon

20. Using the Millon Adolescent Clinical Inventory (MACI)   494
    and Its Facet Scales
    Joseph T. McCann

21. A Brief Illustrative MACI Case Study   520
    Caryl Bloom

22. Development and Validation of the Millon Pre-Adolescent   528
    Clinical Inventory (M-PACI)
    John Kamp and Robert F. Tringone

23. Using the Millon College Counseling Inventory (MCCI)   548
    in Student Services
    Stephen Strack

24. Using the Millon–Grossman Personality Domains Checklist (MG-PDC)   580
    to Integrate Diverse Clinical Data
    Seth D. Grossman, Robert F. Tringone, and Theodore Millon

PART IV. A GUIDE TO ASSOCIATED MILLON PERSONALITY INVENTORIES

25. Using the Personality Adjective Check List (PACL)   609
to Gauge Normal Personality Styles
Stephen Strack

26. The Millon Index of Personality Styles *Revised* (MIPS *Revised*):   643
Assessing the Dimensions of Normal Personality
Lawrence G. Weiss

27. A Brief MIPS *Revised* Case Study   671
Caryl Bloom

PART V. EPILOGUE

28. Future of the Millon Inventories and Their Scientific Base   679
Theodore Millon and Caryl Bloom

Author Index   697

Subject Index   713

THE MILLON INVENTORIES

PART I

INTRODUCTION

CHAPTER 1

The Rationale for
Personalized Assessment in Clinical Practice

Caryl Bloom
Theodore Millon

Defining "Personalized Assessment"

"Personalized assessment" is not a vague concept or a platitudinous buzzword in our approach, but is instead an explicit commitment to focus on the unique composite of a patient's psychological makeup. That focus should be followed by a precise formulation and specification of techniques to remedy those personal attributes that are assessed as problematic.

Clinicians should take cognizance of the person from the start, for the psychic parts and environmental contexts take on different meanings and call for different responses, depending on the specific person to whom they are anchored. To focus on one social structure or one psychological realm of expression, without understanding its undergirding or reference base, is to engage in potentially misguided, if not random, techniques.

Fledgling clinicians should learn further that the symptoms and disorders they diagnose represent but one or another segment of a complex of organically interwoven psychological elements. The significance of each clinical feature can best be grasped by reviewing a patient's unique psychological experiences and his or her overall psychic pattern or configurational dynamics, of which any one component is but a single part.

Assessments that conceptualize clinical disorders from a single perspective—be it psychodynamic, cognitive, behavioral, or physiological—may be useful and even necessary, but are not sufficient in themselves as a basis for therapy of the patient. The revolution we propose asserts that clinical disorders are not exclusively behavioral or cognitive or unconscious; that is, they are not confined to a particular expressive form. The overall pattern of a person's traits and psychic expressions is systemic and multioperational. No part of the system exists in complete isolation from the others. Every part is directly or indirectly tied to every other, such that there is an emergent synergism that accounts for a disorder's clinical tenacity.

Personality is real; it is a composite of intertwined elements whose totality must be reckoned with in all clinical enterprises. The key to treating each of our patients, therefore, lies in an assessment designed to be as organismically complex as the person him- or herself; this form of assessment should generate more than the sum of its parts. Difficult as this may appear, we hope to demonstrate its ease and utility. If our wish comes true, this book will serve as a revolutionary document—a means of bringing assessment back to the natural reality of patients' lives.

It is our hope that the book will lead all of us back to reality by exploring both the uniqueness and the diversity of the patients we treat. Despite their frequent brilliance, most single-focus clinical schools (e.g., behavioral, psychoanalytic) have become inbred. Of more concern, they persist in narrowing clinicians' attention to just one or another facet of their patients' psychological makeup, thereby wandering ever farther from human reality. They cease to represent the full richness of their patients' lives, considering as significant only one of several psychic spheres: the unconscious, biochemical processes, cognitive schemas, or some other. In effect, what has been taught to most fledgling therapists is an artificial reality—one that may have been formulated in its early stages as an original perspective and insightful methodology, but has drifted increasingly from its moorings over time, no longer anchored to the complex clinical reality from which it was abstracted.

How does our approach differ from others? In essence, we give the patient's unique constellation of personality attributes center stage in the assessment task. Only after a thorough evaluation of the nature and prominence of these personal attributes do we think through which combination and sequence of treatment orientations and methodologies we should employ. It should be noted that a parallel personalized approach to physical treatment has currently achieved recognition in what is called "genomic medicine." Here medical scientists have begun to tinker with a particular patient's DNA so as to decipher and remedy existing, missing, or broken genes, thereby enabling the physician to tailor treatment in a highly personalized manner—that is, specific to the underlying or core genetic defects of that particular patient. Anomalies that are etched into a patient's unique DNA are screened and assessed to determine their source, the vulnerabilities they portend, and the probability of the patient's succumbing to specific manifest diseases.

As detailed later in this book (notably by Grossman, Tringone, & Millon in Chapter 24), we have formulated eight personality components or domains constituting what we might term a "psychic DNA," a framework that conceptually parallels the four chemicals composing biological DNA. Deficiencies, excesses, defects, or dysfunctions in these psychic domains (e.g., mood/temperament, intrapsychic mechanisms) effectively result in a spectrum of 15 manifestly different variants of personality styles and pathology (e.g., avoidant style, borderline disorder), in the same manner as the vulnerabilities in biological DNA result in a variety of different genomically based diseases. The unique constellation of vulnerabilities as expressed in and traceable to one or several of these eight potentially problematic psychic domains is what becomes the object and focus of personalized psychotherapy.

In this book, we attempt to show that all the clinical syndromes constituting Axis I of the *Diagnostic and Statistical Manual of Mental Disorders* (DSM) can be understood more clearly and treated more effectively when conceived as outgrowths of patients' overall personality styles. To say that depression is experienced and expressed differently from one patient to the next is a truism; so general a statement, however, will not suffice for a book such as this. Our task requires much more.

The book provides extensive information and illustrations on how patients with different personality vulnerabilities react to and cope with life's stressors. This body of knowledge should guide therapists to undertake more precise and effective treatment plans. For example, a dependent person will often respond to an impending divorce with feelings of helplessness and hopelessness, whereas a narcissistic individual faced with similar circumstances may respond in a disdainful and cavalier way. Even when a dependent and a narcissistic person exhibit depressive symptoms in common, the precipitant of these symptoms will probably have been quite different; furthermore, treatment—its goals and methods—should likewise differ. In effect, similar symptoms do not call for the same treatment if the patterns of patient vulnerabilities and coping styles differ. In the case of dependent individuals, the emotional turmoil may arise from their feelings of lower self-esteem and their inability to function autonomously; in narcissistic persons, depression may be the outcropping of failed cognitive denials, as well as a consequent collapse of their habitual interpersonal arrogance.

Whether we work with a clinical syndrome's "part functions" as expressed in behavior (social isolation), cognitions (delusional beliefs), affect (depression), or a biological defect (appetite loss), or we address contextual systems that focus on the larger environment, the family, the group, or the socioeconomic and political conditions of life, the crossover point—the place where the varieties of clinical expression are linked to the individual's social context—is the person. The person is the intersection of all functions and systems. Persons, however, are more than just crossover points. They are the only organically integrated systems in the psychological domain, inherently created from birth as natural entities. Moreover, it is the person who lies at the heart of the assessment process: He or she is the substantive being who gives meaning and coherence to symptoms and traits—be they behaviors, affects, or mechanisms—as well as that being, that singular entity, who gives life and expression to family interactions and social processes.

Looking at a patient's totality can present a bewildering if not chaotic array of diagnostic possibilities, potentially driving even the most motivated young clinician to back off into a more manageable and simpler worldview, be it cognitive or pharmacological. But as we contend here, complexity need not be experienced as overwhelming; nor does it mean chaos, if we can bring logic and order to the assessment process. We try to provide such logic and order by illustrating that the systematic integration of an Axis I syndrome into its foundation in an Axis II disorder is not only feasible, but conducive to both briefer and more effective therapy.

Are not all assessments "personalized"? Do not all clinicians concern themselves with the person who is the patient they are treating? What justifies our appropriating the name "personalized" for the approach we espouse? Are we not usurping a universal, laying claim to a label that is commonplace, routinely shared, and employed by most (if not all) therapists? We think not. In fact, we believe that most clinicians only incidentally or secondarily attend to the specific personal qualities of their patients. The majority come to their treatment task with a distinct if implicit bias, a preferred theory or technique they favor—one usually encouraged, sanctioned, and promoted in their early training (be it cognitive, group, family, eclectic, pharmacological, or what have you).

Finally, in personalized assessment we seek to employ customized instruments, such as the Grossman Facet Scales of the Millon Clinical Multiaxial Inventory–III (MCMI-III), to identify the patient's vulnerable psychic domains (e.g., cognitive style, interpersonal conduct). These assessment data furnish a foundation and a guide for implementing the distinctive individualized goals we seek to achieve in personalized psychotherapy (Millon & Grossman, 2007a, 2007b, 2007c; see also Grossman, Chapter 6, this volume).

Our Integrative Model: Natural versus Artificial Theoretical Synthesis

The simplest way to practice clinical psychology is to approach all patients as possessing essentially the same disorder, and then to utilize one standard modality of therapy for their treatment. Many therapists still employ such simplistic models. Yet everything we have learned in the past two or three decades tells us that this approach is only minimally effective and deprives patients of other, more sensitive and effective approaches to treatment. In the past two decades, we have come to recognize that patients differ substantially in their presentations of clinical syndromes and personality disorders. It is clear that not all treatment modalities are equally effective for all patients. The task set before us is to maximize our effectiveness and to outline an integrative model for selective therapeutics. When the selection is based on each patient's personal trait configuration, this integration becomes what we have termed "personalized assessment and psychotherapy."

It is our view that psychopathology itself has structural implications that should determine the form of any assessment one would propose to remedy its constituents. In this book, we present several such implications and propose a new integrative model for action. This model—which, as noted above, is guided by the psychic makeup of a patient's personality, rather than by a preferred theory, modality, or technique—gives promise, we believe, of a new level of efficacy. It is not a ploy to be adopted or dismissed as congruent or incongruent with established preferences or modality styles. Despite its name, we believe that what we have termed a "personalized" approach will be effective not only with Axis II personality disorders, but also with Axis I clinical syndromes.

It is our belief that integrated assessment should be a synthesized system that mirrors the problematic configuration of traits (personality) and symptoms (clinical syndromes) *of the specific patient at hand*. Many in the past have sought to coalesce differing theoretical orientations and treatment modalities. By contrast, those of us adhering to the personalized persuasion bypass the synthesis of theories. Rather, primary attention should be given to the natural synthesis or inherent integration that may be found within patients themselves.

As Arkowitz (1997) has noted, efforts to create a theoretical synthesis are usually not fully integrative, in that most theorists do not draw on component approaches equally. Most are oriented to one particular theory or modality, and then seek to assimilate other strategies and notions to that core approach. Moreover, assimilated theories and techniques are invariably changed by the core model into which they have been imported. In other words, the assimilated orientation or methodology is frequently transformed from its original intent.

By seeking to impose a theoretical synthesis, clinicians may lose the context and thematic logic that each of the standard theoretical approaches (e.g., behavioral, psychoanalytic) has built up over its history. In essence, intrinsically coherent theories are usually disassembled in the effort to recombine their diverse bits and pieces. Such integrative models may be pluralistic, but they reflect separate modalities with varying conceptual networks and their unconnected studies and findings. Therefore, these models do not reflect that which is inherent in nature; instead, they represent schemas for blending what is, in fact, essentially discrete.

Intrinsic unity cannot be invented, but can be discovered in nature by focusing on the intrinsic unity of the person—that is, the full scope of a patient's psychic being. Integration based on the natural order and unity of the person avoids the rather arbitrary efforts at synthesizing disparate and sometimes disjunctive theoretical schemas. Unlike eclecticism, true integration insists on the primacy of an overarching gestalt, provides an interactive framework, and creates an organic order among otherwise discrete units or elements. Whereas theoretical syntheses attempt to provide intellectual bridges across several theories or modalities, personalized integrationists assert that a natural synthesis already exists within the patient. As we better understand the configuration of traits that characterize each patient's psyche, we can better devise a treatment plan that will mirror these traits and, we believe, will provide an optimal therapeutic course and outcome.

Integration is an important concept in considering not only the assessment of the individual case, but also the place of assessment in clinical science. For the treatment of a particular patient to be integrated, the elements of a clinical science—theory, taxonomy, assessment, and therapy—should be integrated as well (Millon & Davis, 1996b). One of the arguments advanced earlier against empirically based eclecticism is that it further insulates assessments from a broad-based clinical science. In contrast to eclecticism, where techniques are justified empirically, personalized assessment should take its shape and character from an integrative theory of human nature. Such a grand theory should be inviting because it attempts to explain all of the natural variations of human behavior, normal or otherwise; moreover, personalized assessment will grow naturally out of such a personalized theory. Theory of this nature will not be disengaged from technique; rather, it will inform and guide it.

Murray (1983) has suggested that the field must develop a new, higher-order theory to help us better understand the interconnections among cognitive, affective, self, and interpersonal psychic systems. This belief is shared by personalized assessment theorists such as ourselves, who claim that interlinked configurations of pathology deduced from such a theory can serve to guide assessments.

The cohesion (or lack thereof) of intrinsically interwoven psychic structures and functions is what distinguishes most complex disorders of psychopathology; likewise, the orchestration of diverse yet synthesized modalities of intervention is what differentiates synergistic from other variants of clinical practice. These two parallel constructs, emerging from different traditions and conceived in different venues, reflect shared philosophical perspectives—one oriented toward the understanding of mental disorders, the other toward effecting their remediation.

Some Philosophical Issues

Before turning to these themes, we would like to comment briefly on some philosophical issues. They bear on our rationale for developing a wide-ranging theory of nature to serve as a basis for both assessment and treatment techniques—that is, universal principles that transcend the merely empirical (e.g., electroconvulsive therapy for patients with depression). It is our conviction that an integrated theoretical foundation of our personological science is essential if we are to succeed in constructing a personalized approach to all aspects of clinical practice.

We believe that several elements characterize all mature clinical sciences: (1) They embody conceptual theories based on universal principles of nature from which their propositional deductions can be derived; (2) these theories provide the basis for coherent taxonomies that specify and characterize the central features of their subject domain (in our case, that of personality and psychopathology, the substantive realm within which scientific psychotherapeutic techniques are applied); (3) these taxonomies are associated with a variety of empirically oriented assessment instruments that can identify and quantify the concepts that constitute their theories (in psychopathology, methods that uncover developmental history and furnish cross-sectional assessments); and (4) in addition to natural theory, clinical taxonomy, and empirically anchored assessment tools, mature clinical sciences possess change-oriented intervention techniques that are therapeutically optimal in modifying the pathological elements of their domain.

Most current clinical schools of thought share a common failure to coordinate these four components. What differentiates them has less to do with their scientific grounding than with the fact that they attend to different levels of data in the natural world (e.g., cognitive processes, neurochemical dysfunctions). It is to the credit of those of an eclectic persuasion that they have recognized, albeit in a fuzzy way, the arbitrary if not illogical character of single-focus positions, as well as the need to bridge schisms among these approaches that have evolved less from philosophical considerations or pragmatic goals than from accidents of history (Millon, 2004). There are numerous other knotty issues with which personalized assessment and therapy must contend (e.g., differing worldviews concerning the essential nature of psychological experience). There is no problem, as we see it, in encouraging active dialectics among these contenders.

However, two important barriers stand in the way of personalized assessment as a philosophy. The first is the DSM. The idea of diagnostic prototypes was a genuine innovation when the DSM-III was published in 1980. The development of diagnostic criteria work groups was intended to provide broad representation of various viewpoints, while preventing any single perspective from foreclosing on the others. Over 25 years later, however, the DSM has not yet officially endorsed an underlying set of principles that would interrelate and differentiate the categories in terms of their deeper principles. Instead, progress proceeds mainly through committee consensus, cloaked by the illusion of empirical research.

The second barrier is the human habit system. The admonition that different clinical approaches should be pursued with different patients and different problems has become almost self-evident. But, given no logical basis for designing effective therapeutic sequences and composites, even the most self-consciously antidogmatic clinician must implicitly lean toward one orientation or another.

It should also be noted that the methodology through which most assessment instruments are created is opposed in spirit to the goal that directs their use. In tapping dimensions of individual differences, we abstract from persons only those dimensions we take as being common to all. Yet, in using such instruments, we seek to build up again as a reconstructive process the very individuality we had previously disassembled, so that the circle completes itself as a kind of synthesis: from rich idiographic individuality, to nomothetic commonalities, and finally to nomothetic individuality. Apparently, we must segment and give up the person first, and then recombine them, if we are ultimately to understand him or her.

Personalized assessment is concerned with the last two links of this process. The fractionated person—the person who has been dispersed across scales and instruments—must be put back together again as the organic whole he or she once was. How is such a venture to be achieved? First, assessment is an eminently theoretical process; indeed, it is an evolutionary process that requires a weighing of this and a disqualifying of that across the idiosyncrasies and commonalities of methods and data sources through multiple iterations of hypothesis generation and testing. The eventual goal, of course, is *the* theory of the patient, wherein every loose end has been tied up in a theory that follows the logic of the patient's own psyche—a theory so compelling that one gets the feeling that things could not be otherwise than they have been supposed to be. Only such an eminently integrative theory allows the referral question to be addressed with confident words and concrete suggestions.

Although we are undoubtedly biased in our appraisal, we believe that no other inventory offers as potentially complete an integrative assessment of problematic personality styles and classical psychiatric disorders as does the MCMI-III. Moreover, perhaps no other instrument is as coordinated with the official DSM taxonomy of personality disorders as is the MCMI-III, or as conceptually consonant with the multiaxial logic that underlies the DSM. In fact, the MCMI-III is but one (essential) link in what has emerged as an integrative schema for conceptualizing both personality and abnormal behavior (Millon, 1969, 1981, 1990).

As noted above, personalized consonance is an ideal worthy not only in the individual assessment case, but within a science as well. Rather than being developed independently as free-standing and uncoordinated structures, a mature clinical science of psychopathology should include the four components we have listed earlier. To restate these a bit differently, such a science should embody explicit (1) *theories*— that is, explanatory and heuristic conceptual schemas that are consistent with established knowledge; (2) a *nosology*—that is, a taxonomic classification of disorders that has been logically derived from the theory, arranged to provide a cohesive organization within which major categories can be grouped and differentiated; (3) *instrumentation*—that is, tools that are empirically grounded and sufficiently sensitive quantitatively to enable the theory's propositions and hypotheses to be adequately investigated and evaluated, and to permit the categories constituting its nosology to be readily identified (diagnosed) and measured (dimensionalized); and (4) *interven-*

tions—that is, strategies and techniques of therapy that are designed in accord with the theory, targeted toward areas specified by the instrumentation, and oriented to modify problematic clinical characteristics (Millon, 1990).

The goals of this book are largely derived from the framework identified in the preceding paragraph. Operating on the assumption that clinicians desire "knowledge why" as much as "knowledge that"—in other words, that clinicians want to know not only what they should do, but also why they should do it—we will try to embed the "how" of the MCMI (and its associated inventories) in the "why." Perhaps test users will then feel that they are doing something more than merely following a flowchart or a chain of stimulus–response bonds to its termination in the clinical report: They must understand the test to understand their clients. And because the test is embedded in a theoretical matrix, they must understand the theory to understand the test. This requires a justification, not merely a dispensation.

Before we begin, we must express a few reservations. In a chapter such as this, which features a particular instrument but nevertheless seeks to illuminate integrative links among the four domains of clinical science, some highly relevant issues must be greatly abbreviated or completely omitted. As a result, what otherwise might appear as a well-worn, incremental theoretical pathway contains abrupt transitions. Most of the more theoretical material presented may be found in *Toward a New Personology: An Evolutionary Model* (Millon, 1990) and *Disorders of Personality: DSM-IV and Beyond* (Millon & Davis, 1996a). Other concerns have been treated at a level of abstraction more gross than their gravity requires. Here must be included the descriptions, developmental pathways (all but omitted), and specific intervention opportunities for each of the personality disorders and their more common two-point variants. Much of this information is available in *Disorders of Personality* (Millon & Davis, 1996a). In an ideal world we should adopt ideal goals, but in a less than ideal world, we must often adopt pragmatic ones.

The Process of Personalized Assessment

The words "integrative" and "personalized" are now used so widely as to be platitudinous: Obviously, given an equivalence of purpose, that which is more integrated is better than that which is less integrated. However, integration neither springs into being fully formed, nor is unveiled or discovered in a single conceptual leap. Instead, integration is perhaps better understood as a dynamic process. Such a conception sees knowledge building as an ongoing activity in which internal inconsistencies are generated and resolved or transcended at successively superordinate levels of conceptualization: While reality is undoubtedly integrated, our ideas about reality must be more or less so. An inquiry into the nature of this process will be worthwhile, because, as we intend to show, essentially the same logic underlies profile interpretation, thus creating another link between theory and instrumentation.

Pepper (1942) formalized the integrative means of knowledge building as a worldview that he called "organicism," one of his four relatively adequate "world hypotheses" or metaphysical worldviews. Pepper described seven categories of organicism, which work in a kind of dialectical interplay between appearance and reality—one that always proceeds in the direction of increasing integration:

These [categories] are (1) *fragments* of experience which appear with (2) *nexuses* or connections or implications, which spontaneously lead as a result of the aggravation of (3) *contradictions*, gaps, oppositions, or counteractions to resolution in (4) an *organic whole*, which is found to have been (5) *implicit* in the fragments, and to (6) *transcend* the previous contradictions by means of a coherent totality, which (7) *economizes*, saves, preserves all the original fragments of experience without any loss. (p. 283; italics in original)

We expand upon this description as follows: (1) Observations (fragments) lead one to (2) form inchoate theoretical propositions (nexuses), which, unfortunately, do not all mesh harmoniously, automatically producing (3) aggravating and ostensibly irreconcilable inconsistencies (contradictions) which are resolved through (4) a unified theory (organic whole), which, upon reflection, is (5) found to have been implicit in the observations (fragments) all along. Thus it (6) transcends the initial, naive inconsistencies among observations by reconceptualizing these observations in terms of a new, coherent theoretical model—one that (7) integrates or accounts for all the evidence (economizes) according to its new terms and relationships.

   Undoubtedly, even this is a lot to digest in a few paragraphs. Extrapolating from the logic presented above, we might say that as a body of implicit theories is formalized, hiatuses are discovered, and the theories inevitably become enmeshed in inconsistencies and contradictions. Eventually, a new theory is formulated that unifies disparate observations and inconsistencies. What was believed to have been contradictory is discovered not to have been so at all, but only to have appeared contradictory, much as special cases are transcended by more general formulations.

   By this account, science cannot exist merely as a descriptive venture that consists of observing, categorizing, and cross-correlating various phenomena at face value. Instead, it proceeds by establishing superordinate theoretical principles that unify the manifestations of a subject domain by explaining why these particular observations or formulations obtain rather than others. The "limit of this series" (Pepper, 1942) is truth itself—what physicists have called the theory of everything, and what philosophers (notably Hegel) have called the absolute. In this ultimate integration, "logical necessity would become identified with ultimate fact" (Pepper, 1942, p. 301). Nothing would remain unassimilated; everything would be harmonized with everything else.

   More than anything else, it is the question "Why this rather than that?" that underlies the force toward integration in this worldview. By answering this question, we escape what is arbitrary and capricious, and move in the direction of necessity. In its most radical form, this argument holds that even if reliable observations of great or even perfect positive predictive power could be made through some infallible methodology, these indicators would stand simply as isolated facts unassimilated as scientific knowledge until unified through some theoretical basis. Predictive power alone does not make a science. Scientific explanations appeal to theoretical principles that operate above the level of superficialities—principles that are sufficient because they predict, and necessary because they explain.

   The process of clinical assessment follows essentially the same logic. Following Pepper (1942), we might say this: The individual scales, instruments, and other data are the (1) fragments. These possess (2) nexuses, implications, or (statistically) intercorrelations both with each other and with other clinical phenomena, leading to inchoate theories about the individual and his or her psychopathology. Inevitably, these theories do not mesh; they cannot be assimilated to each other exactly, leading to (3) contradictions, gaps, or inconsistencies in the assessment thus far. One then steps back, seeking (4) a more integrative theory or organic whole that makes sense of the gaps or inconsistencies. This integrative theory is then found to have been (5) implicit in the scales, observations, and other data (otherwise, an integrative assessment would not be possible at all), and to (6) transcend the foregoing inconsistencies, gaps, or contradictions by means of a coherent totality, which (7) makes sense of all the observations by tying up all loose ends.

In an integrative assessment, one is required to step outside the theoretical fecundity and inevitable contradictions of a morass of scales and data domains to develop a theory of the patient in which all the data somehow make sense. This superordinate theory lies literally at a higher level of formulation than do the individual measures constituting the "raw data" of the assessment. Thus the "loop" from idiographic individuality to nomothetic commonality to nomothetic individuality is brought to closure: Nomothetic individuality explicitly requires the reintegration of the individual, who currently lies fractionated among various scales and dimensions. An integrative assessment, then, does not come into being of its own accord, but is constructed, and its validity is linked to the mode of its construction.

The underlying assumption here is that things do not fit together equally well in all possible combinations. What exists in one personological domain constrains what can exist in another; otherwise, there would be no nexuses or implications across domains. An individual born with an active temperament, for example, is unlikely to possess a phlegmatic phenomenology as an adult; that is, biophysical construction constrains the quality of subjective realities that can evolve in the individual life. The same is true of all the domains of personality: They do not fit together equally well in all combinations. Functional and structural attributes for each of the personality prototypes have been delineated in several prior publications (Millon, 1986, 1990) and are explored in later chapters of this book.

Interestingly, the logic described above presents a point of contrast with that of inventories derived through factor analysis. Orthogonal factors by definition are independent: Scores on one factor do *not* constrain what can exist on any other. The extracted traits do not influence each other in any way. Thus, while factor analysis represents a parsimonious way of looking at a particular area, it implicitly holds that the structure of reality is distinctly unintegrated: There are a few essential underlying dimensions that determine a great variety of appearances, but these dimensions do not constrain each other. It is interesting, then, to speculate whether the methodology of factor-analytic test construction might be inherently inconsistent with the epistemology of test interpretation—indeed, of clinical psychology as a field. The position that fundamental dimensions exist independently runs counter to the clinician's desire to put the patient back together again.

Why should we formulate a personalized assessment approach to psychopathology? The answer may be best grasped if we think of the psychic elements of a person as analogous to the sections of an orchestra, and the trait domains of a patient as a clustering of discordant instruments that exhibit imbalances, deficiencies, or conflicts within these sections. To extend this analogy, a clinician may be seen as the conductor, whose task is to bring forth a harmonious balance among all the sections, as well as their specifically discordant instruments—muting some here, accentuating others there, all to the end of fulfilling the conductor's knowledge of how the composition can best be made consonant. The task is not that of altering one instrument, but of assessing all in concert. What is sought in music, then, is a balanced score, one composed of harmonic counterpoints, rhythmic patterns, and melodic combinations. What is needed in clinical assessment is a likewise balanced program—a coordinated strategy of counterpoised scales and instruments designed to optimize an understanding of the different components that make up the personality as a whole.

If clinical syndromes were anchored exclusively to one particular trait domain (as phobias have been thought to be primarily behavioral in nature), single-scale assessments might be appropriate and desirable. Psychopathology, however, is not exclusively behavioral, cognitive, biological, or intrapsychic—that is, confined to a particular clinical expression. Instead, it is multioperational and systemic. No part of the personality system exists in complete isolation. Instead, every part is directly or indirectly tied to every other, such that a synergism lends the whole a tenacity that makes the full system of pathology "real"—a complex that needs to be fully reckoned with in a comprehensive assessment endeavor. Assessments should mirror the configuration of as many trait and clinical domains as the syndromes and disorders they seek to remedy. If the scope of the assessment is insufficient relative to the scope of the pathology, the clinician will have considerable difficulty fulfilling his or her meliorative and adaptive goals.

Once again, personality and psychopathology are neither exclusively behavioral, exclusively cognitive, nor exclusively interpersonal. Instead, each is a genuine integration of each of its subsidiary domains. Far from overturning established paradigms, such a broad perspective simply allows a given phenomenon to be treated from several angles, so to speak. Even open-minded clinicians with no strong allegiance to any one point of view may avail themselves of a kaleidoscope of assessment tools. By turning the kaleidoscope, by shifting paradigmatic sets, they can view the same phenomenon from any of a variety of internally consistent perspectives. But this can be only a first step toward synthesizing the interacting configuration of each patient's traits and disorders.

An open-minded clinician who makes no move toward such a synthesis is left with several different assessment tools to choose from, each with some utility for understanding a patient's pathology, but no real means of bringing these diverse instruments together in a coherent model of what exactly is the personality as a whole. The clinician's plight is understandable, but not acceptable. For example, assessment techniques considered fundamental in one perspective may not be so regarded in another. The interpersonal model of Lorna Benjamin (1996) and the neurobiological model of Robert Cloninger (1986, 1987) are both structurally strong approaches to understanding personality and psychopathology. Yet their fundamental constructs are different. Rather than adopting the assessment focus of a particular perspective, then, adherents to the theory of the person as a total system should seek some set of tools that can provide a basis for the patient's whole psyche, capitalizing on the natural organic system of the person. The alternative is an uncomfortable eclecticism of unassimilated partial views.

References

Arkowitz, H. (1997). Integrative theories of therapy. In P. L. Wachtel & S. B. Messer (Eds.), *Theories of psychotherapy: Origins and evolution* (pp. 227–288). Washington, DC: American Psychological Association.

Benjamin, L. S. (1996). *Interpersonal diagnosis and treatment of personality disorders* (2nd ed.). New York: Guilford Press.

Cloninger, C. R. (1986). A unified biosocial theory of personality and its role in the development of anxiety states. *Psychiatric Developments, 3,* 167–226.

Cloninger, C. R. (1987). A systematic method for clinical description and classification of personality variants. *Archives of General Psychiatry, 44,* 573–588.

Millon, T. (1969). *Modern psychopathology: A biosocial approach to maladaptive learning and functioning.* Philadelphia: Saunders.

Millon, T. (1981). *Disorders of personality: DSM-III, Axis II.* New York: Wiley-Interscience.

Millon, T. (1986). Personality prototypes and their diagnostic criteria. In T. Millon & G. L. Klerman (Eds.), *Contemporary directions in psychopathology: Toward the DSM-IV* (pp. 671–712). New York: Guilford Press.

Millon, T. (1990). *Toward a new personology: An evolutionary model.* New York: Wiley-Interscience.

Millon, T. (2004). *Masters of the mind: Exploring the stories of mental illness from ancient times to the new millennium.* Hoboken, NJ: Wiley.

Millon, T., & Davis, R. D. (1996a). *Disorders of personality: DSM-IV and beyond.* New York: Wiley.

Millon, T., & Davis, R. D. (1996b). *Personality and psychopathology: Building a clinical science.* New York: Wiley-Interscience..

Millon T., & Grossman, S. D. (2007a). *Resolving difficult clinical syndromes: A personalized psychotherapy approach.* Hoboken, NJ: Wiley.

Millon, T., & Grossman, S. D. (2007b). *Overcoming resistant personality disorders: A personalized psychotherapy approach.* Hoboken, NJ: Wiley.

Millon, T., & Grossman, S. D. (2007c). *Moderating severe personality disorders: A personalized psychotherapy approach.* Hoboken, NJ: Wiley.

Murray, E. J. (1983). Beyond behavioural and dynamic therapy. *British Journal of Clinical Psychology, 22,* 127–128.

Pepper, S. P. (1942). *World hypotheses: A study in evidence.* Berkeley: University of California Press.

CHAPTER 2

Relating Personalized Assessment to Personalized Psychotherapy

Theodore Millon
Alyssa Boice
Katherine Sinsabaugh

Would it not be a great step forward in our field if psychological assessment, following a series of interviews, tests, or laboratory procedures, actually pointed clearly to what a clinician should do in therapy? Would it not be good if evaluations could spell out which specific features of a patient's psychological makeup are fundamentally problematic—biological, cognitive, interpersonal—and therefore deserved primary therapeutic attention? Is it not time for clinicians to recognize that assessment can lead directly to the course of therapy?

A complaint frequently voiced by psychologists and psychiatrists relates to the clinical inutility of the *Diagnostic and Statistical Manual of Mental Disorders* (DSM) classifications. Discontent pervades all venues and institutions—from committees currently drafting revisions of the DSM standards, to clinicians and researchers of diverse (often opposing) schools of thought, down to our graduate training programs (where the complaint is commonly posed as an essay question in the basic psychopathology course). As diverse as the professionals and students discussing the matter are the answers given to the question "What purpose, good or bad, does assessing diagnosis serve?" Answers to such queries vary on a continuum from "Diagnoses are the only true criteria for making sense of human presentation" to "We should do the world a favor and get rid of all diagnoses."

Meritorious arguments could be presented to favor nearly any thoughtful response to these queries, which should make any self-respecting professional stop to contemplate a number of important issues (Barron, 1998). If there is such uncertainty about the utility of this diagnostic tradition, why do we continue to consider assessment, in any form, viable? If it is of such paramount importance to some, how can it

15

be derogated so thoroughly by others? Indeed, there is credibility to some arguments made by adherents of what we might call the "anarchistic" view of assessment—that is, those promoting the view that any attempts at an organizational classification of diagnoses, which orders and names phenomena found in the domain of psychological disturbances, should be abandoned. According to this paradigm's adherents, the diagnostic system merely slaps a label on a person for our "ease of handling," at the tremendous cost of saddling the individual with a bright "neon" insignia pervading any future attempts at health, individuality, or pursuit of a life beyond the therapeutic environment. Furthermore, members of this persuasion are likely to resonate with the belief that a diagnostically driven therapy may flatten any nuance of uniqueness vital to an effective intervention. Perhaps this is true to some extent. If, in fact, we treat every case of specific phobia with a protocol treatment, each case of obsessive–compulsive disorder with the intervention prescribed by the label, and so on, we effectively reduce ourselves to "cookie-cutter" therapy. What, then, is the distinction between the services of the clinician thoroughly versed in individual personality dynamics, and that of the "technician" who "applies" techniques after reading a treatment manual for an intervention "proven" effective in eradicating a given symptom?

On an even more immediate level, it is certainly obvious that psychiatric labels preceding treatment carry expectations for many clinicians—especially for those who are not aware that labels possess potential biases, and hence invite a scripted affective reaction or a blunted receptivity to patient presentations that fall outside of what may be anticipated for any given category. Might we then rightfully question whether or not we are doing a substantial disservice in, as some would have it, "force-fitting" such human-made constructs to individuals? May not the costs considerably outweigh the benefits?

Our immediate reaction to such issues is this: If the central purpose of our diagnostic system was simply to label phenomena for "ease of handling" in the same sense as we organize cargo for economy of space and transit, the concerns just stated would be lent additional credence. As it stands now, the preceding arguments stand firmly on common knowledge of our human tendency to judge and reach conclusions based primarily on expectation and prior knowledge of a construct; in this sense, the anarchists are correct in their concerns. Unfortunately, for all its attempts at inclusiveness and political correctness, the established diagnostic system does little to defend itself against such criticism, despite its imperative to do so. In any science, classification is not an arbitrary extension subject to be summarily and unequivocally dismissed; it is an inextricable component of the very structure of the science. In the absence of a system creating order among its elements, investigators would be completely unable either to advance knowledge or to communicate with each other (Barlow, 1991). Of course, this absence then undermines higher-order "basics"; without a taxonomy, or any sort of benchmark, it is virtually impossible to operationalize, assess, or modify the disparate and chaotic elements and objects that would then be readily apparent (Millon, 1990; Millon & Davis, 1996).

The quandary presented in the previous paragraphs may seem to indict the notion of diagnostic classification in general—and, indeed, this is how many well-intentioned members of our scientific community may view it. However, when we examine the problem more closely, it becomes apparent that the finger pointing may be more than slightly misguided. Certainly, as Westen (1998) indicates, many of the difficulties associated with psychiatric labeling are problems that lie with clinicians and training models. This may be addressed by a concerted effort to become aware of biases and other personal reactions to particular kinds of patients, both in training and in clinical practice. Although it is suggestive of some modifications to our approach, this effort then raises some further unanswered questions. First, while we begin to realize that it may be the established diagnostic system (rather than the notion of classification itself) that is somehow incomplete, we concern ourselves with constructing a more useful means of assessing and identifying variables, compatible with the "industry standard," which will prove pragmatic in our intervention. As we will explain, a mature, scientific approach to therapeutic intervention *must* derive fluidly from the taxonomy. This begins to answer our second question: While aware-ness of personal biases may tell us what *not* to do, and what to watch for in ourselves as clinicians in reaction to certain patients, we must also begin to take a *balanced* and *informed* view of how therapeutic action may be based on a particular presentation, which is manifested in a useful diagnosis.

The current diagnostic system is, by design, descriptive, empirical, and atheo-retical. It purposely avoids assumptions of etiology or therapeutic direction, thereby aiming to accommodate clinicians and researchers of diverse persuasions. In order to be serviceable, and not obstructive, to as many factions as possible, it remains devoid of constructs that are "foreign" to a given persuasion (Blatt & Levy, 1998). Appealing and noble as this approach may sound, there are pronounced problems with this kind of taxonomy. First, if we remove all that is foreign to any school and permit only "empirical" constructs, we leave out the potentially fruitful addition of allowing our conceptualization of the patient and his or her difficulties to inform treatment—which is the intention of diagnosis in the first place. Second, by leaving out theory in this regard, we are encouraging the further splitting between modes of entry to effective therapeutic intervention by disallowing what might rightfully be learned from systems and interactions among data levels (behavioral, cognitive, in-trapsychic, physiological, etc.). Finally, for all its political correctness and good inten-tion, this atheoretical system does not succeed in bringing together these factions. An orthodox behaviorist will not accept personality as a construct, and will therefore not acknowledge Axis II formulations. A staunch psychodynamicist will tend to eschew most diagnostic categories as they exist, and most humanists will ignore all of them, lest they disrupt the perception of the person's individuality via the danger of labeling. In essence, the DSM's theory neutrality makes it irrelevant to those clini-cians who do operate from theory, and the processes of conceptualization and diag-nosis become separate and unrelated entities (Barron, 1998; Westen, 1998). We are then left with many clinicians who begrudge the system, utilizing it essentially for reimbursement purposes.

As Bloom and Millon have noted in Chapter 1, the first of two major barriers standing in the way of integrative diagnostic considerations' being pragmatic for guiding psychotherapy is the DSM itself. The current framework, including such innovations as diagnostic prototypes and broad and diverse viewpoints stemming from work groups intent on preventing any single perspective from dominating the others, dates back to the preparation of 1980's DSM-III. However, over 25 years fol-lowing the DSM-III's publication, the contemporary DSM still cannot interrelate and differentiate its complex constructs without officially endorsing an underlying set of deeper principles. Because the diagnostic criteria have *not* been explicitly constructed to facilitate treatment, the DSM-IV (American Psychiatric Association, 1994) and its text revision, the DSM-IV-TR (American Psychiatric Association, 2000), are relegated to the rather minimalistic function of classifying persons into categories, rather than encouraging an integrative understanding of each patient across all domains in which the person's mental impairments are expressed. The DSM-IV(-TR) criteria are disproportionately weighted across these domains—nonexistent, in fact, in some of them—and therefore cannot perform this function.

The second barrier, as also noted in Chapter 1, is the human habit system. Most therapists, whatever their orientation or mode of treatment, pay minimal attention to the possibility that diagnosis can inform the philosophy and technique they employ. The admonition that different therapeutic approaches should be pursued with different patients and different problems is practically self-evident to the point of being trite, but, given no logical foundation for effective therapeutic sequences and composites, even the most self-consciously antidogmatic clinician must implicitly lean toward one orientation or another. Of little consequence is what the actual syndrome or disorder may be; a family therapist is likely to select and employ a variant of family therapy, a cognitively oriented therapist will find that a cognitive approach will probably "work best," and so on. Even integrative therapists are beginning to become a "school" and join this unfortunate trend of asserting the "truth" that their approach is the most efficacious. In spite of the self-evident admonition against fitting our patients into the proverbial "Procrustean beds" of our therapeutic approaches, it appears that our approaches continue to resonate more with where our training occurred than with the nature of our patients' difficulties.

A diagnostic system—be it categorical, dimensional, or a combination of the two (e.g., the prototypal DSM system as it was intended, or the augmented proposal to follow)—may profitably categorize patients according to presenting personality styles, as well as overt symptomatology. This does not negate the fact that patients, so categorized, will display differences in the presence and constellation of their characteristics. Over a half century ago, the philosopher Grünbaum (1952) stated this thesis:

> Every individual is unique by virtue of being a distinctive assemblage of characteristics not precisely duplicated in any other individual. Nevertheless, it is quite conceivable that the following . . . might hold: If a male child having specifiable characteristics is subjected to maternal hostility and has a strong paternal attachment at a certain stage of his development, he will develop paranoia during adult life. If this . . . holds, then children who are subjected to the stipulated conditions in fact become paranoiacs, however much they may have differed in other respects in childhood and whatever their other differences may be once they are already insane. (p. 672)

The question that must be raised is whether placement in the category impedes or facilitates a variety of clinically relevant objectives. Thus, if this grouping of key characteristics simplifies the task of clinical analysis by alerting a diagnostician to features of the patient's past history and present functioning that he or she has not yet observed, or if it enables clinicians to communicate effectively about their patients, or guides their selection of beneficial therapeutic plans, or assists researchers in the design of experiments, then the existence of these syndromal categories has served many useful purposes. Furthermore, as has been argued here and elsewhere (Millon, 1988, 1999), we must, as a profession, understand that the methodology we utilize should not stem from our particular type of training; rather, it should stem from an informed, organized conception of the nature of each person's problem and, deeper than that, the nature of the person's orientation to the world (i.e., personality).

What has been termed "personalized psychotherapy" (Millon & Grossman, 2007a, 2007b, 2007c) may serve as an example of an integrative, diagnostically informed treatment, as its integrative processes are dictated by the nature of personality itself. The actual content of this synergistic therapy, however, is and must be specified on some other basis. Psychopathology and in particular personality are by definition the patterning of intraindividual variables; nevertheless, the nature of these variables does not follow from the definition, but must be supplied by some principle or on some basis that is superordinate to the construct. In this model, for example, the content of personality and psychopathology are derived from evolutionary theory—a discipline that informs but exists apart from our clinical subject. In and of itself, pathological personality is a structural–functional concept that refers to the intraorganismic patterning of variables; it does not in itself say what these variables are, nor can it.

Why should we formulate a personalized therapeutic approach? The answer may perhaps be best grasped by examining the inherent nature of psychopathology. If clinical syndromes were anchored exclusively to one particular trait domain, a single or modality-bound psychotherapy would always be appropriate and desirable. Psychopathology, however, does not exclusively hold to one or the other modality; rather, it is multioperational and systemic. Every part is tied to every other, so that a holographic synergism lends the whole an integrative tenacity that makes psychic pathology "real"—a complex system of elements to be reckoned with in any therapeutic endeavors. Therapies, then, should mirror the configuration of the many trait and clinical domains of the syndromes and disorders they seek to remedy. If the scope of the therapy is insufficient relative to the scope of the pathology, the treatment system will have considerable difficulty fulfilling its goals of adaptation.

As Bloom and Millon have noted in Chapter 1, it may be useful to compare the psychic elements of a person to the sections of an orchestra, and to think of the trait domains of a patient as a group of discordant instruments exhibiting imbalances, deficiencies, or conflicts within these sections. To extend this analogy, the therapist may be seen as the conductor of the orchestra. The therapist's task is to facilitate a harmonious balance among all the sections, as well as their particular discordant instruments: Some must be muted and others accentuated, with the ultimate goal of fulfilling the conductor's knowledge of how the composition can best be "performed." The task is not that of evaluating and altering one instrument, but of doing so for all *in concert*. What is sought in music, then, is a balance of harmonic counterpoints, rhythmic patterns, and melodic combinations. What is needed in therapy is a similar balance—a coordinated strategy of counterpoised approaches designed to optimize sequential and combinatorial treatment effects.

From Philosophy to Theory

A good theory should allow techniques across many modalities to be dynamically adapted, or integrated as ongoing changes in the patient occur, or utilized as new information comes to light. What has been termed multimodal therapy in the sense of "technical eclecticism" (e.g., Lazarus, 1976) is a quantum leap in terms of opening formerly rigid eyes to the many possibilities of blending data levels from different psychotherapy "camps." However, eclecticism is an insufficient guide to effective personalized therapy. It cannot prescribe the particular forms of those modalities that will remedy the pathologies of persons and their syndromes; it is also too open with regard to content and too imprecise to achieve focused goals. The intrinsically configurational nature of psychopathology, its multioperationism, and the interwoven character of clinical domains simply are not as well integrated into eclecticism as they need to be in treating psychopathology. An open-minded therapist is left, then, with several different modality combinations, each of which may be useful in treating some aspect of the patient's pathology, but no real means of bringing these diverse conceptions together in a coherent model of what exactly to do. Modality techniques considered essential in one perspective may not be so regarded within another; furthermore, their fundamental constructs are different. Rather than endorsing the modality tactics of a particular perspective, then, those looking for a theory of psychotherapy as a total system should seek some set of principles that can be addressed to the patient's whole psyche, thereby capitalizing on the naturally organic system of the person.

Before proceeding to a reasonably detailed outline of assessment and treatment techniques that will foster an informed psychotherapy based on thoughtful, meaningful diagnosis, we would like to emphasize the utility of a theory of the person. Kurt Lewin's (1936) words of more than 70 years ago, that "there is nothing so practical as a good theory," still resonate soundly in this argument. In spite of those who would shun theory for its subjective qualities, it is simply impossible, despite the efforts of empiricists and others who would hold to only "pure" observable phenomena, to remove any theoretical bias. Furthermore, theory is unavoidable if therapists want a system that can be investigated for both its reliability and validity (Carson, 1991; Loevinger, 1957; Millon, 1991). Theory, when properly fashioned, ultimately provides more simplicity and clarity than unintegrated and scattered information. Unrelated knowledge and techniques, especially those based on surface similarities, are signs of a primitive science, as modern philosophers of science have effectively argued (Hempel, 1961; Quine, 1961). The key lies in finding theoretical principles for psychotherapy that fall "beyond" the field of psychology proper. It is necessary, therefore, to go beyond current conceptual boundaries to more established, "adjacent" sciences. Not only may such steps bear new conceptual fruits, but they may provide a foundation that can guide our own discipline's explorations.

Evolution as an Undergirding Framework

Such a search for fundamental principles, we maintain, should begin with human evolution. Just as each person is composed of a total patterning of variables across all domains of human expression, it is the total organism that survives and reproduces, carrying forth both its adaptive and maladaptive potentials into subsequent generations. As the evolutionary success of organisms is dependent on the entire configuration of the organism's characteristics and potentials, so too does psychological fitness derive from the relation of the entire configuration of personal characteristics to the environments in which the person functions.

The evolutionary theory comprises three imperatives, each of which is a necessary aspect of the progression of evolution. First, each organism must survive. Second, it must adapt to its environment. And third, it must reproduce. Each of these imperatives relates to a polarity allowing for its expression in the individual's life. In order to survive, an organism seeks to maximize pleasure (enhance life circumstances) *and* minimize pain (avoid dangerous or threatening stimuli). In order to adapt, an organism must at appropriate times either passively conform to, or actively *re*-form, the surrounding environment's constraints and opportunities. And finally, in order to regenerate, an organism must adopt either a self-oriented or other-oriented strategy, judiciously "choosing" to self-invest or nurture other significant organisms (Millon, 1990). Anywhere in the universe, these are the fundamental evolutionary concerns, and there are none more fundamental.

Polarities—that is, *contrasting* functional directions, representing these three phases (pleasure–pain, passive–active, other–self)—are the basis of the theoretically anchored prototypal classification system of personality styles and clinical disorders (Millon & Davis, 1996), whose interventional utility we will demonstrate. Such bipolar or dimensional schemes are almost universally present throughout the literatures of humankind, as well as in psychology at large (Millon, 1990). The earliest may be traced to ancient Eastern religions, most notably the Chinese *I Ching* texts and the Hebrew *Kabala*. In the life of the individual organism, each individual organism moves through developmental stages that have functional goals related to their respective phases of evolution. Within each stage, every individual acquires character dispositions representing a balance or predilection toward one of the two polarity inclinations; which inclination emerges as dominant over time results from the inextricable and reciprocal interplay of intraorganismic and extraorganismic factors. For example, during early infancy, the primary organismic function is to "continue to exist." Here evolution has supplied mechanisms that orient the infant toward life-enhancing environments (pleasure) and away from life-threatening ones (pain). So-called "normal" individuals exhibit a reasonable balance between each of the polarity pairs. Not all individuals fall at the center, of course. Individual differences in both personality features and overall style will reflect the relative positions and strengths of each polarity component. A particularly "healthy" person, for example, would be one who is high on both ends of the self–other polarity, indicating a solid sense of self-worth, combined with a genuine sensitivity to the needs of others.

The expressions of traits or dispositions acquired in early stages of development may be transformed as later faculties or dispositions develop (Millon, 1969). Temperament is perhaps a classic example. An individual with an active temperament may develop, contingent on contextual factors, into a person with any of several theoretically derived prototypal personality styles (e.g., avoidant or antisocial), the consequences being partly determined by whether the child has a fearful or a fearless temperament when dealt a harsh environment. The transformation of earlier temperamental characteristics takes the form of what has been called "personological bifurcations" (Millon, 1990). Thus if the individual is inclined toward a *passive* orientation and later learns to be self-focused, a prototypal narcissistic style ensues. But if the individual possesses an *active* orientation and later learns to be self-focused, a prototypal antisocial style may ensue. Thus early-developing dispositions may undergo vicissitudes, whereby their meaning in the context of the whole organism is subsequently re-formed into complex personality configurations.

At a slightly more finite level of specification are what we have termed the personality "subtypes." This idea of subtypes recognizes two fundamental facts. The first derives from the chance side of the evolutionary equation, and draws upon the long descriptive tradition in psychology and psychiatry, as perhaps best expressed in the works of the turn-of-the-20th-century nosologist Emil Kraepelin. In the ordinary course of clinical work, we find that every disorder seems to sort itself into ever finer subcategories that rest upon an a priori basis, but instead flow from cultural and social factors and their interaction with biological influences such as constitution, temperament, or perhaps even systematic neurological defects. Accordingly, if society were different, or if the neurotransmitters chosen by evolution to bathe the human brain were different, the subtypes would also be different. Such entities are the pristine products of clinical observation, and however sharply the classification boundaries may be drawn between them, they are in fact unusually blurred.

Although the concepts of prototypes and subtypes allow the natural heterogeneity of persons to be accommodated within a classification system, there are as many ways to fulfill a given diagnosis as there are subsets of the number of diagnostic criteria required at the diagnostic threshold. For example, there are many ways to score five of a total of nine diagnostic criteria, whatever the actual syndrome. In the context of an idealized medical disease model, which Axis I of the DSM approximates, the fact that two different individuals, both of whom are depressed, might possess substantially different sets of depressive symptoms is not really problematic. The symptoms may be expressed somewhat differently, but the underlying pathology process is the same and can be treated in the same way. For example, whereas one person gains weight and wakes early in the morning, and the other loses weight and sleeps long into the day, both may be treated with an antidepressant and cognitive therapy. Personality, however, as represented in Axis II of the DSM, should be seen to follow a fundamentally different conceptual model. Whereas variance from the prototypal ideal is usually considered irrelevant in the Axis I medical model of clinical syndromes, it is the very essence of Axis II. Personality styles or disorders are reified for clinical utility, but are most accurately thought of as variants of personality prototypes—a phrase that communicates their relatively unique clinical "complexion," without conveying the erroneous connotation of a distinct disease entity.

The evolutionary thesis may also be seen to provide a basis for deriving the so-called "clinical syndromes" of Axis I. To illustrate briefly, consider the anxiety disorders. Without explicating its several variants, a low "pain" threshold on the pleasure–pain polarity would dispose such individuals to be sensitive to punishments, which, depending on covariant polarity positions, might result in the acquisition of complex syndromal characteristics such as ease of discouragement, low self-esteem, cautiousness, and social phobia. Similarly, a low "pleasure" threshold on the same polarity might make such individuals prone to experience joy and satisfaction with great ease; again, depending on covariant polarity positions, such persons might be inclined toward impulsiveness and hedonic pursuits, be intolerant of frustration and delay, and (at the clinical level) give evidence of a susceptibility to manic episodes.

To use musical metaphors again, the DSM Axis I clinical syndromes are "composed" essentially of a single theme or subject (e. g., anxiety, depression)—a salient melodic line that may vary in its rhythm and harmony, changing little except in its timing, cadence, and progression. In contrast, the diversely expressed domains that constitute Axis II seem constructed more in accord with the compositional structure known as the fugue, where there is a dovetailing of two or more melodic lines. Framed in the sonata style, the opening exposition in the fugue begins when an introductory theme is announced (or analogously in psychopathology, a series of clinical symptoms become evident), following which a second (and perhaps third), essentially independent set of themes emerges in the form of "answers" to the first (akin to the unfolding expression of underlying personality traits). As the complexity of the fugue is revealed (we now have identified a full-blown personality disorder), variants of the introductory theme (i.e., the initial symptom picture) develop "countersubjects" (less observable, inferred traits), which are interwoven with the preceding in accord with well-known harmonic rules (comparably, mechanisms that regulate intrapsychic dynamics). This matrix of entwined melodic lines progresses over time in an episodic fashion, occasionally augmented, at other times diminished. It is sequenced to follow its evolving contrapuntal structure, unfolding an interlaced tapestry (the development and linkages of several psychological traits). To build this metaphorical elaboration further, not only may personality be viewed much like a fugue, but the melodic lines of its psychological counterpoints consist of the three evolutionary themes presented earlier (i.e., the polarities). Thus some fugues are rhythmically vigorous and rousing (high "active"); others kindle a sweet sentimentality (high "other"); still others evoke a somber and anguished mood (high "pain"); and so on. When the counterpoint of the first three polarities is harmonically balanced, we observe a well-functioning or so-called "normal" person; when deficiencies, imbalances, or conflicts exist among them, we observe one or another variant of the personality disorders.

Creation of a Meaningful Personalized Assessment

The validity of a pragmatic assessment and personalized diagnosis depends on the validity of the system of categorized types and trait dimensions that is brought to bear on the individual case. The prototype construct, which is one of the favorable attributes of the DSM, represents a synthesis of categorical and dimensional models. Prototypal models assume that no necessary or sufficient criteria exist by which syndromes and disorders can be unequivocally diagnosed. The synthetic character of the prototypal model can be seen by comparing what is saved and discarded in the three approaches. The categorical model sacrifices quantitative variation in favor of discrete, binary judgments. The dimensional model sacrifices qualitative distinctions in favor of quantitative scores. Of the three models, the prototypal is the only one that conserves both qualitative and quantitative clinical information.

However, the DSM's personality prototypes represent an approach that is necessary but not sufficient. The DSM simply lists characteristics that have been found to accompany a particular disorder with some regularity and specificity. Although it puts forth several domains in which personality is expressed (notably cognition, affect, interpersonal functioning, and impulse control), these psychological domains are neither comprehensive nor comparable, and this limits the utility of this approach. Because of this, the DSM lacks a basis to organize these structures of personality meaningfully, in a manner amenable to intervention. Furthermore, these problems exist both within and between disorders, so that different disorders evince different content distortions. Finally, theoretically derived prototypes are a good basis for understanding how "real-world" blends of personality style appear, but the DSM does not provide the undergirding for understanding such blends. For example, it is relatively easy to identify a case of "schizoid personality disorder" by "checking off" enough DSM-IV(-TR) criteria for the construct, but it is impossible, by these criteria, to make finer and more useful distinctions as they are more likely to appear outside of textbook-style, theoretically derived prototypes (e.g., what subtype of schizoid personality disorder a particular patient might exhibit), since the criteria to discriminate between subgroups simply do not as yet exist. As will be seen, learning to conceptualize these blends of personality styles is a vital skill in formulating synergistic treatment plans.

Both the nature of the person and the laws of evolution require that the stylistic domains of personality be drawn together in a logical fashion. No domain is an autonomous entity. Instead, the evolution of the structure and content of personality is constrained by the evolutionary imperatives of survival, adaptation, and reproductive success, for it is always the whole organism that is selected and evolves. To synthesize the domains of the person as a coherent unity, we draw on the boundary between organism and environment. What we call "functional" domains relate the organism to the external world, while other domains serve as "structural" substrates for functioning, existing inside the organism.

The preceding issue points to the inadequacy of any approach that links classification to intervention without theoretical guidance. The argument is merely that diagnosis should constrain and guide therapy in a manner consonant with assumptions of the theoretically derived prototypal model; without a philosophical framework, there is no sound basis from which to derive principles that contextualize the person and his or her integrated structures and functions, or a thorough intervention that reflects the complexity of this personality. The scope of the interventions that might be considered appropriate and the form of their application are left unattended. Any set of interventions or techniques might be applied singly or in combination, without regard to the diagnostic complexity of the treated disorder. In the actual practice of therapy, techniques within a particular pathological data level—that is, psychodynamic techniques, behavioral techniques, and so on—are in fact often applied conjointly. Thus systematic desensitization might be followed by *in vivo* exposure, or a patient might keep a diary of his or her thoughts, while at the same time reframing those thoughts in accordance with the therapist's directions when they occur. In these formulations, however, there is no strong a priori reason why any two therapies or techniques should be combined at all. When techniques from different modalities are applied together successfully, it is because the combination mirrors the composition of the individual case, not because it derives its logic from a theory of the personality and the syndrome.

The whole clinical enterprise is thereby changed. The purpose is not to classify individuals into categories, but instead to augment the classification system in a more comprehensive attempt to capture the particular reality that is each person. The purpose is not to put persons into the classification system, but instead to reorient the system with respect to each person by determining how his or her unique, ontological constellation of attributes overflows and exceeds it. The classification thus becomes a point of departure for comparison and contrast, a way station in achieving a total understanding of the complexity of the whole, not a destination in itself. When in the course of an assessment the clinician begins to feel that the subject is understood at a level where ordinary diagnostic labels no longer adequately apply, the classification system is well on its way to being falsified relative to the individual, and a truly idiographic understanding of the person is close at hand, ready to be approached in a comprehensive and systematic way therapeutically.

Much of the confusion that has plagued diagnostic systems in the past can be attributed to the overlapping and changeability of symptom pictures. We argue that greater clarity can be achieved in classification if we focus on the person's basic personality *as a system*, rather than limiting ourselves to the particular dominant symptom the person manifests at any particular time. Moreover, by focusing our attention on enduring personality traits and pervasive clinical domains of expression, we may be able to deduce the cluster of different symptoms the patient is *likely* to display and the sequence of symptoms he or she may exhibit over time. For example, knowing the vulnerabilities and habitual coping strategies of a paranoid person, we would predict that he will evidence (either together or in sequence) both delusions and hostile mania, should he or she become psychotically disordered. Similarly, compulsive personals may be expected to manifest cyclical swings among catatonic rigidity, agitated depression, and manic excitement, should they decompensate into a psychotic state. Focusing on ingrained personality patterns rather than transient symptoms enables us, then, to grasp both each patient's complex syndrome and the symptoms he or she is likely to exhibit, as well as the possible sequence in which they will wax and wane.

Ideally, a diagnosis should function as a means of narrowing the universe of therapeutic techniques to some small set of choices. Within this small set, uniquely personal factors come into play among alternative techniques or the order in which these techniques might be applied. As we have stated, the concept of a system must be brought to the forefront, even when we are discussing simple behavioral reactions and symptoms. Systems function as a whole, but are composed of parts—in this case, the eight structural and functional domains identified in Millon's earlier writings (Millon, 1984, 1986a, 1990, 1999; Millon & Davis, 1996). They serve as a means of classifying the parts or constructs in accord with traditional, historic therapeutic techniques. The nature and intensity of the constraints in each of these domains limit the potential number of states that the system can assume at any moment in time; this total configuration of operative domains results in each patient's distinctive pattern of individuality. Equally significant, this pattern of domain problems serves to construct a model for personalized treatment approaches (Millon & Grossman, 2007a, 2007b, 2007c).

General Clinical Constructs That Inform Personalized Therapy

The evolutionary principles from which we derive our conceptualizations of personality, and the clinical domains that underlie personological structure and function (and in cases of syndromal distress, psychopathology), do, in our judgment, provide a useful framework for identifying both goals and methods of treatment. Before operationally explicating these facets, however, we briefly describe two general clinical constructs that pervade and help structure the blending of treatment techniques in Millon's model. The first relates to the goal of balancing uneven polarities, and the second is the use of techniques to counter thoughts, emotions, and behaviors that perpetuate the patient's difficulties (Millon & Davis, 1996).

As noted above and elsewhere (Millon, 1990), the theoretical basis is developed from the principles of evolution, to which three polarities are considered fundamental: the pain–pleasure, active–passive, and self–other polarities. As a general philosophy, specific treatment techniques are selected as tactics to achieve polarity-oriented balances. Depending on the pathological polarity to be modified, and the integrative treatment sequence one has in mind, the goals of therapy are these, in general: to overcome pleasure deficiencies in persons with schizoid, avoidant, and depressive styles and disorders; to reestablish interpersonally imbalanced polarity disturbances in dependent, histrionic, narcissistic, and antisocial persons; to undo intrapsychic conflicts in sadistic, compulsive, masochistic, and negativistic persons; and, lastly, to reconstruct structural defects in schizotypal, borderline, and paranoid persons (Millon, 1999). These goals are to be achieved by the use of modality tactics that are optimally suited to the clinical domains in which these pathologies are expressed (see the section on "Domain-Oriented Assessment and Treatment," below).

Our second superordinate therapeutic construct relates to continuity in personality and psychopathology, which may be attributed in great measure to the stability of constitutional factors and the deeply ingrained character of early experiential learning. Every behavior, attitude, and feeling that is currently exhibited is a perpetuation—a remnant of the past that persists into the present. Not only do these residues passively shape the present by temporal precedence, if nothing else, but they insidiously distort and transform ongoing life events to make them duplicates of the past. It is this self-perpetuating re-creative process that becomes so problematic in treating psychopathology. In other words, and as Millon (1969, 1981) has said previously, *psychopathology is itself pathogenic.* It sets into motion *new* life experiences that are further pathology-producing. A major goal of therapy, then, is to stop these perpetuating inclinations—that is, to prevent the continued exacerbation and intensification of a patient's established problematic habits and attitudes. Much of what therapists must do is to reverse self-pathogenesis—the intruding into the present of erroneous expectations; the perniciousness of maladaptive interpersonal conduct; and the repetitive establishing of new, self-entrapping "vicious circles," which Horney (1945) has earlier described, and which Wachtel (1973) has referred to as "cyclical psychodynamics."

Complex Syndrome Treatment Goals

Before commencing with an outline of domain-oriented assessment, we would like to make distinctions among three levels of pathogenic processes: "simple reactions," "complex syndromes," and "personality patterns (styles/disorders)" (Millon, 1999). These three levels lie on a continuum. At one extreme are simple reactions, which are essentially straightforward, often dramatic, but essentially singular symptoms, unaffected by other psychosocial traits of which the person as a whole is composed (Millon, 1969). At the other extreme are personality patterns (styles and disorders), which comprise interrelated mixes of psychological traits, such as cognitive attitudes and interpersonal behaviors, as well as biological temperaments and intrapsychic processes. Complex syndromes lie in between—manifestly akin to simple reactions, but deeply interwoven with and mediated by pervasive personality traits and embedded vulnerabilities. It is on this seemingly superficial level, which in fact encompasses many trait domains of personality, that we frequently find many of our most problematic and distressed patients; we focus our attention here within the next section of the chapter.

It should be noted that patients fall at varying levels of severity along the continuum from simple reactions to complex syndromes to personality patterns, and adjustments may have to be made in following a synergistic plan to accommodate possible changes in one's assessment of a case. Cognitive, behavioral, psychodynamic, and interpersonal approaches are *each* likely to demonstrate some level of therapeutic efficacy over waiting-list controls. Even though consistently channeled through a particular bias and directed at a *particular* symptom domain, many interventions will gather enough momentum to eventually change significant portions of the entire person. In cases where the whole complex of psychic processes is reconfigured, it is not likely to be the intervention per se that produces so vast a change, but a synergistic interaction between a syndrome intervention and the personological context in which that intervention takes place. Therefore, it is the interdependent nature of the organismic system that compensates for the inadequacy of a single domain focus. The fact that systems spread the effect of any input throughout its entire infrastructure is likely to be a principal reason why no major school of therapy (i.e., the behavioral, cognitive, interpersonal, intrapsychic, and biological) either has yet to be judged a total failure, or has been able to demonstrate consistent superiority for all disorders.

Domain-Oriented Assessment and Treatment

Several criteria were used to select and develop the trait domains we have included in this section: (1) that they be varied in the features they embody (i.e., not be limited to behaviors or cognitions, but instead encompass a full range of clinically relevant characteristics); (2) that they *parallel*, if not correspond to, many of our profession's current therapeutic modalities (e.g., cognitively oriented techniques for altering dysfunctional beliefs, group treatment procedures for modifying interpersonal conduct); and (3) not only that they be coordinated with the official DSM schema of personality and syndromal prototypes, but also that most syndromes and personality patterns be characterized by a distinctive feature within each clinical domain.

In conducting a domain-oriented assessment, clinicians should be careful to avoid regarding each domain as a concretized, independent entity, and thereby falling into a naïve operationalism. Each domain is a legitimate, but highly contextualized, part of an integrated whole—one absolutely necessary if the integrity of the organism is to be maintained. Nevertheless, individuals differ with respect to which and how many domains of their pathology are expressed. Patients vary not only in the degree to which their domain characteristics approximate a pathological syndrome or personality disorder, but also in the extent to which the influences of each domain shape each patient's overall functioning. Conceptualizing each form of psychopathology as a system, we should recognize that different parts of the system may be salient for different individuals, even where those individuals share a diagnosis.

In the following paragraphs, we provide a more tangible description of our proposed diagnostically informed treatment approach. Herein we outline the eight major clinical domains, which may be manifested singularly, or in complex syndromes, or in personality disorders. No less important, we outline eight covariant and parallel treatment modalities. (See Millon, 1999, for a fuller discussion of what follows.)

Expressive Behaviors

Behavioral Assessment Domain

Expressive behaviors are observable, external patient characteristics, and are usually recorded by noting what the patient does and how the patient acts. Through inference, observations of overt behaviors enable us to deduce either what the patient unknowingly reveals about him- or herself, or, often conversely, what he or she wishes others to think or to know about him or her. The range and character of these expressive behaviors not only are wide and diverse, but convey both distinctive and worthwhile clinical information—from communicating a sense of personal incompetence, to exhibiting general defensiveness, to demonstrating disciplined self-control, and so on. This domain of clinical data is likely to be especially productive in differentiating patients on the passive–active polarity of Millon's (1990) theoretical model. Behavioral methods seem especially suitable to the elimination of problematic behaviors and the creation of more effective adaptations.

Parallel Behavior Therapies

As written previously (Millon, 1999), behaviorists contend that "other" therapeutic approaches are method-oriented rather than problem-oriented. Nonbehaviorists are seen to proceed in a uniform and complicating fashion, regardless of the particular character of a patient's difficulty, utilizing the same "psychoanalytic" or "cognitive" procedure with all forms and varieties of pathology. Not only do behaviorists claim that behavioral approaches are flexible and problem-oriented, but there is no "fixed" technique in pure behavior therapy. As we see it, behavioral techniques are extremely useful in counteracting simple clinical reactions that manifest themselves in overt behaviors. They distinguish the elements of each simple reaction, and then fashion a procedure designed specifically to effect changes only in that problem. For example, if the patient complains of acute anxiety attacks, procedures are designed to eliminate just that symptom, and therapy is completed when it has been removed.

Interpersonal/Relational Conduct

A patient's style of relating to others may be captured in a number of ways, such as the impact of his or her actions on others, intended or otherwise; the attitudes that underlie, prompt, and give shape to these actions; the methods by which he or she engages others to meet his or her needs; or his or her way of coping with social tensions and conflicts. Extrapolating from these observations, the clinician may construct an image of how the patient functions in relation to others, be it antagonistically, respectfully, aversively, secretively, or in other ways.

Interpersonal Assessment Domain

Tenets of interpersonal theory, especially as encoded in the circumplex representation, make this taxonomy a promising one for the assessment of both personality traits/clusters and clinical syndromes. According to its most basic conception, each person constricts the response repertoire of others in order to evoke specifically those responses that confirm his or her perception of the self and world (Kiesler, 1982, 1997). Each party in the interpersonal system is coopted by the other in an effort to elicit validation. Together, the parties must find a stable system state that mutually confirms, and thereby maintains and perpetuates their respective self-concepts. These system states can be based on either reciprocity (on the vertical axis) or correspondence (on the horizontal axis).

While usually presented two-dimensionally, the circumplex can also be visualized as a bivariate distribution, with increasing densification toward the center and increasing sparsity toward the edges. Healthy or flexible interpersonal styles appear as balanced patterns with the circle. Individuals usually possess a full range of styles in which to relate to others, regardless of the kinds of others with whom they find themselves involved. Psychic pathology can be expressed geometrically through distortions of the healthy circular and concentric pattern.

The interpersonal styles of schizoid, avoidant, dependent, histrionic, narcissistic, and antisocial personals seem better assessed by the circumplex than do those of compulsive, borderline, negativistic (passive–aggressive), paranoid, and schizotypal individuals (Pincus & Wiggins, 1989). We would conclude then that any assessment of clinical syndromes and personality that is anchored *only* in the interpersonal domain, while informative, must be regarded as incomplete. Clinicians of an interpersonal bent must balance the increased specificity gained by using an exclusively interpersonally oriented instrument with the knowledge that the paradigm itself is acknowledged to be an incomplete representation of psychic pathology.

Parallel Interpersonal Therapies

Three major variants of treatment focus on the interpersonal domain. The first engages one patient exclusively at a time in a dyadic patient–therapist medium, but centers its attentions primarily on the patient's relationships with others; these techniques are known as "interpersonal psychotherapy." The second set of techniques assembles an assortment of patients together in a group, so that their habitual styles of relating to others can be observed and analyzed as the interactions among the participants unfold; these techniques are known as "group psychotherapy." The third variant is "family therapy," where established and ostensibly problematic relationships are evaluated and treated.

To paraphrase Kiesler (1997), the essential problems of an individual reside in the person's recurrent transactions with significant others. These stem largely from disordered, inappropriate, or inadequate communications, and result from failing to attend to and/or not correcting the unsuccessful and self-defeating nature of these communications. The interpersonal approach centers its attention on the individual's closest relationships—notably current family interactions, relations with the family of origin, past and present love affairs, and friendships, as well as neighborhood and work relations. The patient's habitual interactive and hierarchical roles in these social systems constitute the focus of interpersonal therapy. The dyadic treatment interaction, despite its uniqueness, is seen as paralleling other venues of human communication. The interpersonal therapist becomes sensitized to the intrusions of the patient's habitual styles of interaction by the manner in which he or she "draws out" or "pulls" the therapist's feelings and attitudes. These evocative responses provide a good indication of how the patient continues to relate to others. This transactive process mirrors in many ways what psychoanalysts refer to in their concepts of "transference" and "countertransference." More will be said on these matters later, when we discuss treatment modalities oriented to modifying the patient's "object relationships."

Once assessment of the patient's history has been undertaken and its elements clarified, the task of the interpersonal therapist is to help the patient identify the persons with whom he or she is currently having difficulties, what these difficulties are, and whether there are ways in which they can be resolved or made more satisfactory. Problems in the patient's current environment should be stated explicitly (e.g., being intimidated on the job, arguing over trivia with his or her spouse, missing old friends) and shown to be derivations from past experiences and relationships.

Developed as a comprehensive modality of interpersonal treatment over 60 years ago (e.g., Slavson, 1943), the impact of group psychotherapy in molding and sustaining interpersonal behaviors has been thoroughly explored in recent decades. Clearly, there are several advantages to group and also to family therapies. Perhaps most significant is the fact that the patient acquires new behaviors in a setting that is the same as or similar to his or her "natural" interpersonal world; relating to family or peer group members is a more realistic experience than that of the hierarchical therapist–patient dyad. It is easier to generalize to the extratherapeutic world what one learns in family and peer group settings, since it is closer to "reality" than is the individual treatment setting.

Cognitive Modes

The ways in which the patient focuses and allocates attention, encodes and processes information, organizes thoughts, makes attributions, and communicates reactions and ideas to others represent data at the cognitive level, and are among the most useful indices to the clinician of the patient's distinctive way of functioning. By synthesizing these signs and symptoms, the clinician may be able to identify indications of what may be termed an impoverished style, or distracted thinking, or cognitive flightiness, or constricted thought, and so on.

Cognitive Assessment Domain

Cognitivists place heavy emphasis on internal processes that mediate overt actions. Cognitivists also differ from both behaviorists and intrapsychic therapists with regard to which events and processes they consider central to pathogenesis and treatment. Cognitivists concern themselves with the reorientation of consciously discordant feelings and readily identifiable erroneous beliefs, and not with the modification of narrow behaviors or with disgorging the past and its associated unconscious derivatives.

Parallel Cognitive Therapies

Given their emphasis on conscious attitudes and perceptions, cognitive therapists are inclined to follow an insight-expressive rather than an action-suppressive-treatment process. Both cognitive and intrapsychic therapists employ the insight-expressive approach, but the focus of their explorations differs, at least in theory. Cognitivists attend to dissonant assumptions and expectations, which can be consciously acknowledged by an examination of the patient's everyday relationships and activities. A therapist not only may assume authority for deciding the objectives of treatment, but may confront a patient with the irrationalities of his or her thinking. For example, there is the practice of "exposing" the patient's erroneous or irrational attitudes, and the reworking of his or her belief structures into ones with a more rational and stable composition.

In what he terms "rational–emotive" therapy, Ellis (1967) considers the primary objective of therapy to be countering the patient's tendency to perpetuate his or her difficulties through illogical and negative thinking. The patient, by reiterating these unrealistic and self-defeating beliefs in a self-dialogue, constantly reaffirms their irrationality and aggravates his or her distress. To overcome these implicit but pervasive attitudes, the therapist confronts the patient with them and induces him or her to think about them consciously and concertedly and to "attack them" forcefully and unequivocally until they no longer influence the patient's behavior. By revealing and assailing these beliefs, and by "commanding" the patient to engage in activities that run counter to them, the therapist helps the patient to break their hold on his or her life, and new directions become possible.

The other highly regarded cognitive approach has been developed by Beck and his associates (Beck, Freeman, Davis, & Associates, 2004). Central to Beck's approach is the concept of "schemas"—that is, sets of specific rules that govern information processing and behavior. To Beck, the disentangling and clarification of these schemas lies at the heart of therapeutic work with psychopathology. They persist despite their dysfunctional consequences, owing largely to the fact that they enable the patient to find ways to extract short-term benefits from them, thereby diverting the patient from pursuing more effective, long-term solutions. As other sophisticated therapists do, Beck emphasizes the therapist–patient relationship as a central element in the therapeutic process. As he notes further, considerable "artistry" is involved in unraveling the origins of the patient's beliefs and in exploring the meaning of significant past events.

Self-Image

One major configuration emerges during development to impose a measure of sameness on an otherwise fluid environment: the perception of self as object—a distinct, ever-present, and identifiable "I" or "me."

Self-Image Assessment Domain

Self-identity stems largely from conceptions formed at a cognitive level. The self is especially significant, in that it provides a stable anchor to serve as a guidepost and to give continuity to changing experience. Most persons have an implicit sense of who they are, but differ greatly in the clarity, accuracy, and complexity (Millon, 1986b) of their self-introspections.

The character and valuation of the self-image are often problematic, as seen in the avoidant person's feeling of being alienated, the depressive person's image of worthlessness, or the negativistic individual's sense of self-discontent. On the other hand, the schizoid person's self-image is one of complacence, the histrionic individual's is one of being gregarious, and the narcissistic person's is one of being admirable. Thus self-image, despite the many particulars of a patient's character, appears to be predominantly of either a positive or a negative quality.

Parallel Self-Image Therapies

Self-actualization or humanistic therapists are those whose orientation is to "free" patients to develop a more positive and confident image of their self-worth. Liberated in this manner, the patients ostensibly learn to act in ways that are "right" for them, and thereby enable them to "actualize" their inherent potentials. To promote these objectives, the therapist views events from each patient's frame of reference and conveys both a caring attitude and a genuine respect for the patient's worth as a human being. According to Carl Rogers (1942, 1951, 1961, 1967), patient "growth" is a product neither of special treatment procedures nor of professional know-how; rather, it emerges from the quality and character of the therapeutic relationship. More specifically, it occurs as a consequence of attitudes expressed by the therapist, notably genuineness and unconditional positive regard.

Also suitable for those who have experienced the anguish of a chronically troubled life are the philosophies and techniques of modern-day "existential therapists"—those who seek to enable patients to deal with their unhappiness realistically, yet in a constructive and positive manner. The existential school possesses a less sanguine view of human fate than do Rogerians, believing that people must struggle to find a valued meaning to life; therapy, then, attempts to strengthen patients' capacity to choose an "authentic" existence. Self-actualizing therapists of this latter persuasion are committed to the view that people must confront and accept the inevitable dilemmas of life if they are to achieve a measure of "authentic" self-realization. Mutual acceptance and self-revelation enable patients to find an authentic meaning to their existence, despite the profound and inescapable contradictions that life presents. These existentially oriented self-image therapies may be especially suitable for psychopathologies in which life has been a series of alienations and unhappiness (e.g., avoidant and depressive personality styles). By contrast, the underlying assumption of the more humanistically oriented self-actualizing therapies, including client-centered, experiential, and Gestalt, is that people may have been too harsh with themselves, tending to blame themselves and judge their actions more severely than is necessary.

Intrapsychic Objects, Mechanisms, and Morphology

As noted previously, significant experiences from the past leave an inner imprint—a structural residue composed of memories, attitudes, and affects that serve as a substrate of dispositions for perceiving and reacting to life's ongoing events.

Intrapsychic Assessment Domains

OBJECT RELATIONS

Analogous to the various organ systems of which the body is composed, both the character and substance of these internalized representations of significant figures and relationships of the past can be differentiated and analyzed for clinical purposes. Variations in the nature and content of this inner world can be associated with one or another complex syndrome or personality pattern, and lead us to employ descriptive terms to represent them, such as "shallow," "vexatious," "undifferentiated," "concealed," and "irreconcilable."

REGULATORY MECHANISMS

Although "mechanisms" of self-protection, need gratification, and conflict resolution are consciously recognized at times, they represent data derived primarily from intrapsychic sources. Because regulatory mechanisms are also internal processes, they are even more difficult to discern and describe than processes that are anchored a bit more firmly in the observable world. As such, they are not directly amenable to assessment by self-reflective appraisal in pure form, but only as derivatives many levels removed from their core conflicts and their dynamic regulation. By definition, dynamic regulatory mechanisms coopt and transform both internal and external realities before they can enter conscious awareness in a robust and unaltered form. When chronically enacted, they often perpetuate a sequence of events that intensifies the very problems they were intended to circumvent.

   Great care must be taken not to challenge or undo these intrapsychic mechanisms that regulate and balance the inner psychic system of a patient. Therapists must appraise the character of these regulatory functions, so they can be quickly identified and handled in as beneficial a manner as possible. Moreover, these regulatory/defensive mechanisms may restrict patients from dealing with their difficulties in a rational and honest fashion.

   Although the measurement of defense mechanisms, historically a troublesome and inconsistent procedure, has improved through content objectification and specification, current procedures still leave something to be desired. Because the size of the correlation coefficient that can be achieved between measures is limited by their reliabilities, it is likely that the external validity of defensive measures will remain more difficult to establish than that of self-report inventories.

MORPHOLOGICAL ORGANIZATION

The overall architecture that serves as a framework for an individual's psychic interior may display weakness in its structural cohesion; exhibit deficient coordination among its components; and possess few mechanisms to maintain balance and harmony, regulate internal conflicts, or mediate external pressures. The concept of "morphological organization" refers to the structural strength, interior congruity, and functional efficacy of the overall personality system. "Organization" of the mind is a concept almost exclusively derived from inferences at the intrapsychic level of analysis—one akin to and employed in conjunction with current psychoanalytic notions, such as borderline and psychotic levels—but this usage tends to be limited, relating essentially to quantitative degrees of integrative pathology, not to qualitative variations in either integrative structure or configuration. "Stylistic" variants of this structural attribute may be employed to characterize each of the complex syndromes or personality disorder prototypes; their distinctive organizational attributes are represented with descriptors such as "inchoate," "disjoined," and "compartmentalized."

Morphological structures represent deeply embedded and relatively enduring templates of imprinted memories, attitudes, needs, fears, conflicts, and so on, which guide experience and transform the nature of ongoing life events. Psychic structures are architectural in form. Moreover, they have an orienting and preemptive effect, in that they alter the character of action and the impact of subsequent experiences in line with preformed inclinations and expectancies. By selectively lowering thresholds for transactions that are consonant with either constitutional proclivities or early learnings, future events are often experienced as variations of the past. Of course, the residues of the past do more than passively contribute their share to the present. By temporal precedence, if nothing else, they guide, shape, or distort the character of current events and objective realities.

For purposes of definition, morphological organization represents structural domains that can be conceived as substrates and action dispositions of a quasi-permanent nature. Possessing a network of interconnecting pathways, this organization constitutes a framework in which the internalized residues of the past are cast. These structures often serve to close the organism off to novel interpretations of the world, and tend to limit the possibilities of expression to those that have already become prepotent. Their preemptive and channeling character plays an important role in perpetuating the maladaptive behavior and vicious circles of pathology.

Parallel Intrapsychic Therapies

Readers are likely to have discussed both frequently and at length the history, rationale, and considerable heterogeneity of intrapsychic theory (Millon, 1990). Despite inevitable controversies and divergences in emphasis, often appearing more divisive upon first than later examination, intrapsychic therapists do share certain beliefs and goals in common that are worthy of note and distinguish them from other modality orientations; two are noted here.

First, all intrapsychic therapists focus on internal mediating processes (e.g., regulatory mechanisms) and structures (object representations) that ostensibly "underlie" and give rise to overt behavior. In contrast to cognitivists, however, their attention is directed to those mediating events that operate at the unconscious rather than the conscious level. To them, overt behaviors and cognitive reports are merely "surface" expressions of dynamically orchestrated but deeply repressed emotions and associated defensive strategies (Magnavita, 1997), all framed in a distinctive structural morphology (Kernberg, 1984). Since these unconscious processes and structures are essentially impervious to "surface" maneuvers, techniques of behavior modification are seen as mere palliatives, and methods of cognitive reorientation are thought to resolve only those difficulties that are so trivial or painless as to be tolerated consciously. "True" therapy occurs only when these deeply ingrained elements of the unconscious are fully unearthed and analyzed. The tasks of intrapsychic therapy, then, are to circumvent or pierce resistances that shield these insidious structures and processes, to bring them into consciousness, and to rework them into more constructive forms.

Second, intrapsychic therapists see as their goal the *reconstruction* of the patient's complex syndrome or personality pattern—not the repair or removal of a single domain syndrome, or the reframing of a "superficial" cognitive attitude. Disentangling the underlying structure of complex syndromes or personality pathology, forged of many interlocking elements that build into a network of pervasive strategies and mechanisms, is the object of their therapy. They set for themselves the laborious task of rebuilding those functions (regulatory mechanisms) and structures (morphological organization) that constitute the substance of the patient's psychic world, not merely its "facade." Treatment approaches designed "merely" to modify behavioral conduct and cognitive complaints fail to deal with the root source of pathology and are bound therefore to be of short-lived efficacy. As they view it, therapy must reconstruct the inner structures and processes that underlie overt behaviors and beliefs. It does not sacrifice the goal of syndromal or personality reconstruction for short-term behavioral or cognitive relief. Reworking the source of the problem, rather than controlling its effects, is what distinguishes intrapsychic therapies as treatment procedures.

Mood/Temperament

Mood/Temperament Assessment Domain

Few observables are clinically more relevant from the biophysical level of data analysis than the predominant character of an individual's affect and the intensity and frequency with which he or she expresses it. The "meaning" of extreme emotions is easy to decode. This is not so with the more subtle moods and feelings that insidiously and repetitively pervade the patient's ongoing relationships and experiences. Not only are the expressive features of mood and drive conveyed by terms such as "distraught," "labile," "fickle," or "hostile" communicated via self-report; they are revealed as well, albeit indirectly, in the patient's level of activity, speech quality, and physical appearance.

Parallel Mood/Temperament Therapies

Although the direct action of pharmacological medications is chemical, and their effects are formulable in terms of altered neurophysiological relationships, there are those who believe that the crucial variable is not chemical or neurophysiological, but psychological. To them, the factors that determine a patient's response are not molecular events or processes, but the patient's prior psychological state and the environment within which he or she currently functions. According to this view, biophysical changes induced by medications take on a "meaning" to the patient, and it is this meaning that determines his or her "final" clinical response.

Theorists of this persuasion pay less attention to specifying the mechanisms and pathways of biophysical change than to the impact of these changes on the patient's self-image, coping competencies, social relationships, and the like. To support their thesis, they note that barbiturates, which typically produce sedative reactions, often produce excitement and hyperactivity. Similarly, many persons exhibit a cheerful state of intoxication when given sodium amytal in a congenial social setting, but succumb to a hypnotic state when the drug is administered to them in a therapeutic environment.

Of even greater significance than social factors, according to this view, is the patient's awareness of the energy and temperamental changes that have taken place within him or her as a consequence of drug action. Freyhan (1959), discussing the effect of "tranquilizers" in reducing mobility and drive, stated that patients with compulsive traits, who need intensified activity to control their anxiety, may react unfavorably to their loss of initiative, resulting thereby in an upsurge rather than a decrement in anxiety. Other patients—such as those with avoidant traits, who are comforted by feelings of reduced activity and energy—may view such a drug's tranquilizing effect as a welcome relief. Thus, even if a drug produced a uniform biophysical effect on all patients, its psychological impact would differ from patient to patient, depending on the meaning these changes have in the larger context of each patient's needs, attitudes, and coping strategies.

If a drug facilitates the control of disturbing impulses, or if it activates a new sense of competence and adequacy, then it may be spoken of as beneficial. Conversely, if the effect is to weaken the patient's defenses and upset his or her self-image, it may prove detrimental. The key to a drug's effectiveness, then, is not only its chemical impact, but the significance of the psychological changes it activates.

Personalized Assessment in a Therapeutic Context

If no one subset of DSM-IV(-TR) diagnostic criteria is necessary or sufficient for membership in a diagnostic class, and if the structure of the taxonomy and the planning and practice of therapy are to be linked in a meaningful way, it seems likely that no one therapy or technique can be regarded as a necessary or sufficient remediation as well. Diagnostic heterogeneity–therapeutic heterogeneity is a more intrinsically agreeable pairing than diagnostic heterogeneity–therapeutic homogeneity, which treats every person with a particular diagnosis the same way, ignoring individual differences. The argument is one of parallelism: *The palette of methods and techniques available to the therapist must be commensurate with the idiographic heterogeneity of the patient for whom the methods and techniques are intended.*

When translated into psychological terms, a theory of psychopathology should be able to generate answers to a number of key questions. For example, how do its essential constructs interrelate and combine to form specific syndromes and disorders? And, if it is to meet the criteria of an integrative or unifying schema, can it help derive all forms of personality and syndrome with the same set of constructs (i.e., not employ one set of explanatory concepts for a borderline personality style, another for a somatoform style, a third for a depressive style, etc.)? If we may recall, one of the great appeals of early analytic theory was its ability to explain several "character types" from a single developmental model of psychosexual stages. Can the same be said for other, more encompassing theories? Moreover, can these theories provide a structure and serve as a guide for planning psychotherapy with all varieties of psychopathologies?

A major point about treatment recorded earlier in the chapter is that the polarity schemas and the clinical assessment domains can serve as useful points of focus for corresponding modalities of therapy. It would be ideal, of course, if patients exhibited "pure" prototypes, and if all expressive psychic domains were prototypal and invariably present. Were this so, each diagnosis would automatically match a particular polarity configuration and corresponding therapeutic mode. Unfortunately, "real" patients rarely exhibit pure textbook prototypes; most by far are characterized by complex mixtures. Examples include, the deficient pain *and* pleasure polarities that typify the schizoid prototype, the interpersonal conduct and cognitive style features of the avoidant prototype, and the self-image qualities of the schizotypal prototype. Furthermore, the polarity configurations and their expressive domains are not likely to be of equal clinical relevance or prominence in a particular case; for instance, interpersonal characteristics may be especially troublesome, whereas cognitive processes, though problematic, may be of lesser significance. Answering the question of which domains and which polarities should be selected for therapeutic intervention requires a comprehensive assessment—one that not only appraises the overall configuration of polarities and domains, but differentiates their balance and degrees of salience.

The task of the therapist is to identify domain dysfunctions and to provide matching treatment modalities that derive logically from the theory of that particular person. That is, the therapist puts together a combination of treatment modalities that mirror the different domains in which the specific patient's pathology is expressed and configured. When techniques drawn from different modalities are applied together, it should be because that combination reflects the domains of the individual person's characteristics, not because it is required by the logic of one or another theory or technological preference. The orchestration of diverse yet synthesized techniques of intervention is what differentiates personalized synergism from other variants of psychotherapy. These two parallel constructs, emerging from different traditions and conceived in different venues, reflect shared philosophical perspectives—one oriented toward the understanding of complex psychopathologies, the other toward effecting their remediation. It is the very interwoven nature of the patient's problematic domains that defines his or her syndromes and personality traits, and that makes a multifaceted and integrated approach a necessity.

Potentiated Pairings and Catalytic Sequences

As the great neurological surgeon/psychologist Kurt Goldstein (1940) stated, patients whose brains have been altered to remedy a major neurological disorder do not simply lose the function that the disturbed or extirpated area subserved. Rather, such patients restructure and reorganize their brain capacities so that they can maintain an integrated sense of self. In a similar way, when one or another major domain of a patient's habitual psychological makeup is removed or diminished (e.g., depression), the patient must reorganize him- or herself—not only to compensate for the loss, but also to formulate a new, reconstructed self.

There is a separateness among eclectically designed techniques, reflecting each individual therapist's selection of what works best. In synergistic therapy, by contrast, there are psychologically designed composites and progressions among diverse techniques. Millon (1988, 1999) has used such terms as "catalytic sequences" and "potentiating pairings" to represent the nature and intent of these polarity- and domain-oriented treatment plans. In essence, these comprise therapeutic arrangements and timing series that will resolve polarity imbalances and effect clinical domain changes, which would not occur with the use of several essentially uncoordinated techniques.

The first of the personalized procedures we recommend (Millon, 1988, 1999) has been termed "potentiated pairings." These consist of treatment methods that are combined simultaneously to overcome problematic characteristics that might be refractory to each technique if they were administered separately. These composites pull and push for change on many different fronts, so that the therapy becomes as multioperational and as tenacious as the disorder itself. A popular illustration of these treatment pairings is cognitive-behavioral therapy, perhaps the first of the synergistic therapies (Craighead, Craighead, Kazdin, & Mahoney, 1994).

In the second personalized procedure, termed "catalytic sequences," a therapist might seek first to alter a patient's humiliating and painful stuttering via behavior modification procedures; if this is successful, it may facilitate the use of cognitive or self-actualizing methods to produce changes in self-confidence, which may in turn foster the use of interpersonal techniques to effect improvements in relationships with others. Catalytic sequences are timing series intended to maximize the impact of changes that would be less effective if the sequential combination were otherwise arranged.

Of course, there are no discrete boundaries between potentiating pairings and catalytic sequences, just as there is no line between their respective pathological analogues, adaptive inflexibility and vicious circles (Millon, 1969). Nor should therapists be concerned about when to use one rather than another. Instead, they are intrinsically interdependent phenomena whose application is intended to foster increased flexibility and (ideally) a beneficent rather than a vicious circle. Potentiated pairings and catalytic sequences represent but the first level of therapeutic synergism. The idea of a "potentiated sequence" or a "catalytic pairing" recognizes that these logical composites may be built on each other in proportion to what the tenacity of the disorder requires.

One question we may want to ask concerns the limits to which the content of synergistic therapy can be specified in advance at a tactical level—that is, the extent to which specific potentiating pairings and catalytic sequences can be identified for each of the complex syndromes and personality disorders. To the extent that each patient's presentation is prototypal, the potentiating pairings and catalytic sequences that are actually used should derive from modality tactics oriented to alter several of the more problematic domains. This statement, however, probably represents the limit to which theory can guide practice in an abstract sense—that is, without any knowledge about the history and characteristics of the *specific* individual case to which the theory is to be applied. Just as individuality is ultimately so rich that it cannot be exhausted by any taxonomic schema, synergistic therapy, ideally performed, is full of specificities that cannot readily be resolved by generalities. Potentiating pairings, catalytic sequences, and whatever other higher-order composites that therapists may evolve are conducted at an idiographic rather than at a diagnostic level. Accordingly, their precise content is specified as much by the logic of each individual case as by the logic of a syndrome or disorder itself. At an idiographic level, each of us must ultimately be "artful" and open-minded therapists, using simultaneous or alternately focused methods. The synergism and enhancement produced by catalytic and potentiating processes are the characteristics of genuinely innovative treatment strategies.

Polarity-Oriented Goals

As stated earlier, we should select our specific treatment techniques as tactics to achieve the evolution-theory-based polarity-oriented goals. Depending on the pathological polarity, the domains to be modified, and the overall treatment sequence one has in mind, the goals of therapy should be oriented toward the improvement of imbalanced or deficient polarities by the use of techniques that are optimally suited to modify their expression in the patient's problematic clinical domains.

Therapeutic responses to problems in the pain–pleasure polarity would, for example, have as their essential aim the enhancement of pleasure among schizoid, avoidant, and depressive personalities (+ pleasure). Given the probability of intrinsic deficits in this area, schizoid patients may require the use of pharmacological agents designed to activate their "flat" mood/temperament. Increments in pleasure for avoidant individuals, however, are likely to depend more on cognitive techniques designed to alter their "alienated" self-image, and behavioral methods oriented to counter their "aversive" interpersonal inclination. Equally important for avoidant patients is reducing their hypersensitivities, especially to social rejection (– pain); this may be achieved by coordinating the use of anxiolytic medications for their characteristic "anguished" mood/temperament with cognitive-behavioral methods geared to desensitization. In the passive–active polarity, increasing patients' capacity and skills to take a less reactive and more proactive role in dealing with the affairs of their lives (– passive; + active) would be a major goal of treatment for schizoid, depressive, dependent, narcissistic, masochistic, and compulsive individuals. In the other–self polarity, imbalances found among narcissistic and antisocial persons, for example, suggest that a major aim of their treatment would be a reduction in their predominant self-focus, and a corresponding augmentation of their sensitivity to the needs of others (+ other; – self).

Making unbalanced or deficient polarities the primary aim of therapy is a new approach, and the goal has been only modestly tested. In contrast, the clinical domains in which problems are expressed lend themselves to a wide variety of therapeutic techniques, the efficacy of which must, of course, continue to be gauged by ongoing experience and future systematic research. Nevertheless, our repertoire here is a rich one. For example, numerous cognitive-behavioral techniques (Bandura, 1969; Goldfried & Davison, 1976; Craighead et al., 1994), such as assertiveness training, may fruitfully be employed to establish a greater sense of self-autonomy or an active rather than a passive stance with regard to life. Similarly, pharmaceuticals are notably efficacious in reducing the intensity of pain (anxiety, depression) when the pleasure–pain polarity is in marked imbalance.

Domain Tactics

Turning to the specific domains in which clinical problems exhibit themselves, we can address dysfunctions in the realm of interpersonal/relational conduct by employing any number of family (Gurman & Kniskern, 1991; Gurman & Jacobson, 2002) or group (Yalom, 2005) therapeutic methods, as well as a series of explicitly formulated interpersonal techniques (Benjamin, 1996; Kiesler, 1997). Methods of classical analysis or its more contemporary schools may be especially suited to the realms of object representations and morphological organization. The cognitively oriented methods of Beck (1976; Beck et al., 2004) and Ellis (1970; Ellis & MacLauren, 1998) would be well chosen to modify difficulties of cognitive beliefs and self-image.

"Tactics" and "strategies" keep in balance the two conceptual ingredients of therapy; the first refers to what goes on with a particular focused intervention, while the second refers to the overall plan or design that characterizes the entire course of therapy. Both are required. Having tactical specificity without strategic goals implies doing particular things without knowing why in the big picture; having strategic goals without tactical specificity implies knowing where to go, but having no way to get there. Obviously, one uses short-term modality tactics to accomplish higher-level strategies or goals over the long term.

System Transactions

The distinction between "interaction" and "transaction" points to an important element in the practice of personalized psychotherapy. Because the goal of therapy is personality and clinical change, patient and therapist cannot be satisfied merely to interact like casual acquaintances and emerge from therapy unchanged. Instead, we must invent modes of therapy that maximize the transactive potential of the therapeutic process. Because of its lack of structure and feedback, traditional psychotherapy may go on around essentially indefinitely, without ever reaching termination. In fact, since patient and therapist may not have previously determined what constitutes success, it is not inconceivable that an appropriate point of termination might be reached without either the therapist's or patient's ever realizing it, only for new issues to be raised and the process to begin again.

Pessimistically speaking, we must remember that the primary function of any system is homeostasis. In an earlier conceptualization (Millon, 1981), personality was likened to an immune system for the psyche, such that stability, constancy, and internal equilibrium become the "goals" of a personality. Obviously, these run directly in opposition to the explicit goal of therapy, which is change. Usually, the dialogue between patient and therapist is not so directly confrontational that it is experienced as particularly threatening. In these cases, the personality system functions for the patient as a form of passive resistance, albeit one that may be experienced as a positive force (or trait) by the therapist. In fact, by their very nature, self-image and object representations are so preemptive and confirmation-seeking that the true meaning of the therapist's comments may never reach the level of conscious processing. Alternately, even if a patient's equilibrium is initially up-ended by a particular interpretation, his or her defensive mechanisms may kick in to ensure that a therapist's comments are somehow distorted, misunderstood, interpreted in a less threatening manner, or even ignored. The first is a passive form of resistance; the second is an active form. No wonder then, that effective therapy is often considered anxiety-provoking, for it is in situations where the patient really has no effective response—where the functioning of the immune system is temporarily suppressed—

that the scope of his or her response repertoire is most likely to be broadened. Personality "goes with what it knows," and it is with the "unknown" that learning is most possible. Arguing essentially the same point, Kiesler (1966, 1997) has stated that the therapist is obliged to make the "asocial" response—one other than that which the patient is specifically trying to evoke.

If the psychic makeup of a person is regarded as a system, then the question becomes this: How can the characteristics that define systems be coopted to facilitate rather than retard transactive change? A coordinated schema of strategic goals and tactical modalities to accomplish these ends is what we mean by "synergistic psychotherapy." Through various coordinated approaches that mirror the system-based structure of pathology, an effort is made to select domain-focused tactics that will fulfill the strategic goals of treatment.

If interventions are unfocused, rambling, and diffuse, the patient will merely "lean forward a little," passively resisting change by using his or her own "weight"— that is, habitual characteristics already intrinsic to the system. Although creating rapport is always important, nothing happens unless the system is eventually "shook up" in some way. Therapists should not always be toiling to expose their patients' defenses, but sooner or later, something must happen that the patients cannot readily deal with by habitual processes—something that they will often experience as uncomfortable or even threatening.

In fact, personalized therapy appears in many ways to be like a "punctuated equilibrium" (Eldridge & Gould, 1972) rather than a slow and continuous process. The systems model argues for periods of rapid growth during which the psychic system reconfigures itself into a new gestalt, alternating with periods of relative constancy. The purpose of therapists' keeping to a domain or tactical focus, or knowing clearly what they are doing and why they are doing it, is to keep the whole of psychotherapy from becoming diffused. The person-focused systems model runs counter to the deterministic universe-as-machine model of the late 19th century, which features slow but incremental gains. In a standard systems model, diffuse interventions are experienced simply as more inputs to be discharged homeostatically, producing zero change. In the machine model, in which conservation laws play a prominent role, diffuse interventions produce small increments of change, with the promise that therapeutic goals will be reached, given enough time and effort. In contrast, in the personalized synergistic model, few therapeutic goals may be reached at all unless something unusual is planned that has genuine transformational potential. This potential is optimized through what we have termed "potentiated pairings" and "catalytic sequences."

Tactical specificity is required in part because the psychic level at which therapy is practiced is fairly explicit. Most often, the in-session dialogue between patient and therapist is dominated by a discussion of specific behaviors, specific feelings, and specific events, not by a broad discussion of personality traits or clinical syndromes. When the latter are discussed, they are often perceived by the patient as ego-alien or intrusive characterizations. A statement such as "You have a troublesome personality" conceives the patient as a vessel filled by some noxious substance. Under these conditions, the professional is expected to empty and refill the vessel with something more desirable; the patient has relinquished control and responsibility, and simply waits passively for the therapist to perform some mystical ritual. This is one of the worst assumptive sets in which to carry out psychotherapy. Whatever the physical substrates and dynamic forces involved in creating and sustaining particular traits, trait terms are evoked as inferences from particular constituent behaviors. Behaviors can be changed; traits have a more permanent connotation.

Modality Selections

Despite the foregoing, viewing traits in an explicit way—that is, by anchoring them to "real" and "objective" events—is beneficial to both patients and therapists. Knowing what behaviors are descriptively linked to particular traits helps patients understand how others perceive them, and that these behaviors should not be repeated. Additionally, if patients are led to understand that their personality traits are, or are derived from, their concrete behaviors, there is hope, since behavior is more easily controlled and changed than is a clinical diagnosis. In this latter sense, the diagnosis or trait ascription itself may become the enemy. There is, after all, a difference between what is practically impossible because it is at the limits of one's endurance or ability, and what is logically impossible. With support and courage, human beings can be coaxed into transcending their limitations—into doing what was before considered practically impossible. No one, however, can do what is logically impossible. When clinical syndromes and personality disorders are framed through the medical model, change is paradigmatically impossible. Individuals who see themselves as vessels for a diseased syndrome or personality should be disabused of this notion.

For the therapist, operationalizing traits as clusters of behavioral acts or cognitive expectancies can be especially beneficial in selecting tactical modalities. First, some behaviors are linked to multiple traits, and some of these traits are more desirable than others, so that some play exists in the interpretation or spin put on any particular behavior at the trait level. This play can be utilized by the therapist in order to reframe patient attributions about self and others in more positive ways. For example, the avoidant person's social withdrawal can be seen as having enough pride in him- or herself to leave a humiliating situation, while the dependent person's clinging to a significant other can be seen as having the strength to devote him- or herself to another's care. Of course, these reframes will not be sufficient in and of themselves to produce change. They do, however, seek to create a bond with the patient by way of making positive attributions and thereby raising self-esteem, while simultaneously working to disconfirm or make the patient reexamine beliefs that lower esteem and function to keep the person closed off from trying on new roles and behaviors.

Second, understanding traits as clusters of behaviors and/or cognitions is just as beneficial for the therapist as for the patient when it comes to overturning the medical model of syndromal and personality pathology and replacing it with a synergistic systems model. One of the problems faced by adherents to a medical model of complex syndromes and personality disorders is that their range of attributions and perceptions is too narrow to characterize the richness that in fact exists in patients and their social environments. As a result, such therapists often end up perpetuating old problems by interpreting even innocuous behaviors and events as noxious. The belief that personality pathologies are medical diseases, monolithically fixed and beyond remediation, should itself be viewed as a form of paradigmatic pathology.

As has been outlined previously, there are the "strategic goals" of therapy, that is, those that endure across numerous sessions and against which progress is measured. Second, there are the specific "domain modality tactics" by which these goals are pursued. Ideally, strategies and tactics should be integrated, with the tactics chosen to accomplish strategic goals, and the strategies chosen on the basis of what tactics might actually achieve, given other constraints (such as the number of therapy sessions and the nature of the problem). To illustrate, intrapsychic therapies are highly strategic, but tactically impoverished; pure behavioral therapies are highly tactical, but strategically narrow and inflexible. There are in fact many different ways that strategies might be operationalized. Just as diagnostic criteria are neither necessary nor sufficient for membership in a given class, it is likely that no technique is an inevitable consequence of a given clinical strategy. Subtle variations in technique and the ingenuity of individual therapists to invent techniques ad hoc assure an almost infinite number of ways to operationalize or put into action a given clinical strategy.

Ideally, in a truly integrated clinical science, the theoretical basis that lends complex syndromes and personality disorders their content—that is, the basis on which its taxonomy is generated and patients are assessed and classified—will also provide the basis for the goals and modalities of therapy. Without such a basis, anarchy will ensue, for we will have no rationale by which to select from an almost infinite number of specific domain tactics that can be used, except for the dogmas of past traditions. The "truth" is what will work in the end—a pragmatism based on what we term a "synergistic integrationism."

Concluding Comment

The system we have termed "personalized therapy" or "synergistic therapy" may have raised concerns about whether any one therapist can be sufficiently skilled, not only in employing a wide variety of therapeutic approaches, but also in synthesizing them and planning their sequence. As Millon was asked at a conference some years ago, "Can a highly competent behavioral therapist employ cognitive techniques with any measure of efficacy, and can he [or she] prove able, when necessary, to function as an insightful intrapsychic therapist? Can we find people who are strongly self-actualizing in their orientation, [but] who can, at other times, be cognitively confronting?" Is there any wisdom in selecting different modalities for treating a patient if the therapist has not been trained diversely or is not particularly competent in more than one or two therapeutic modalities?

It is our belief that the majority of therapists have the ability to break out of their single-minded or loosely eclectic frameworks, to overcome their prior limitations, and to acquire a solid working knowledge of diverse treatment modalities. Developing a measure of expertise with the widest possible range of modalities is highly likely to increase treatment efficacy, and thus to help therapist achieve the primary goal of his or her professional career—that of helping patients and clients overcome their mental health difficulties.

References

American Psychiatric Association. (1980). *Diagnostic and statistical manual of mental disorders* (3rd ed.). Washington, DC: Author.

American Psychiatric Association. (1994). *Diagnostic and statistical manual of mental disorders* (4th ed.). Washington, DC: Author.

American Psychiatric Association. (2000). *Diagnostic and statistical manual of mental disorders* (4th ed., text rev.). Washington, DC: Author.

Bandura, A. (1969). *Principles of behavior modification.* New York: Holt, Rinehart & Winston.

Barlow, D. H. (1991). Introduction to the special issues on diagnoses, dimensions, and DSM-IV: The science of classification. *Journal of Abnormal Psychology, 100,* 243–244.

Barron, J. W. (Ed.). (1998). *Making diagnosis meaningful: Enhancing evaluation and treatment of psychological disorders.* Washington, DC: American Psychological Association.

Beck, A. T. (1976). *Cognitive therapy and the emotional disorders.* New York: International Universities Press.

Beck, A. T., Freeman, A., Davis, D. D., & Associates (2004). *Cognitive therapy of personality disorders* (2nd ed.). New York: Guilford Press.

Benjamin, L. S. (1996). *Interpersonal diagnosis and treatment of personality disorders* (2nd ed.). New York: Guilford Press.

Blatt, S. J., & Levy, K. N. (1998). A psychodynamic approach to the diagnosis of psychopathology. In J. W. Barron, (Ed.), *Making diagnosis meaningful: Enhancing evaluation and treatment of psychological disorders* (pp. 73–110). Washington, DC: American Psychological Association.

Carson, R. C. (1991). Dilemmas in the pathway of the DSM-IV. *Journal of Abnormal Psychology, 100,* 302–307.

Craighead, L. W., Craighead, W. E., Kazdin, A. E., & Mahoney, M. J. (Eds.). (1994). *Cognitive and behavioral interventions: An empirical approach to mental health problems.* Boston: Allyn & Bacon.

Eldridge, N., & Gould, S. (1972). Punctuated equilibria: An alternative to phyletic gradualism. In T. Schopf (Ed.), *Models in paleobiology.* San Francisco: Freeman.

Ellis, A. (1967). *A guide to rational living.* Englewood Cliffs, NJ: Prentice-Hall.

Ellis, A. (1970). *The essence of rational psychotherapy: A comprehensive approach to treatment.* New York: Institute for Rational Living.

Ellis, A., & MacLauren, C. (1998). *Rational emotive behavior therapy: A therapist's guide.* Atascadero, CA: Impact.

Freyhan, F. A. (1959). Clinical and integrative aspects. In N. S. Kline (Ed.), *Psychopharmacology frontiers.* Boston: Little, Brown.

Goldfried, M. R., & Davison, G. C. (1976). *Clinical behavior therapy.* New York: Holt, Rinehart & Winston.

Goldstein, K. (1940). *Human nature in the light of psychopathology.* Cambridge, MA: Harvard University Press.

Grünbaum, A. (1952). Causality and the science of human behavior. *American Scientist, 26,* 665–676.

Gurman, A. S., & Jacobson, N. S. (Eds.). (2002). *Clinical handbook of couple therapy* (3rd ed.). New York: Guilford Press.

Gurman, A. S., & Kniskern, K. (Eds.). (1991). *Handbook of family therapy* (Vol. 2). New York: Brunner/Mazel.

Hempel, C. G. (1961). Introduction to problems of taxonomy. In J. Zubin (Ed.), *Field studies in the mental disorders.* New York: Grune & Stratton.

Horney, K. (1945). *Our inner conflicts: A constructive theory of neurosis.* New York: Norton.

Kernberg, O. F. (1984). *Severe personality disorders.* New Haven, CT: Yale University Press.

Kiesler, D. J. (1966). Some myths of psychotherapy research and the search for a paradigm. *Psychological Bulletin, 65,* 110–136.

Kiesler, D. J. (1982). The 1982 interpersonal circle: A taxonomy for complementarity in human transactions. *Psychological Review*, 90, 185–214.

Kiesler, D. J. (1997). *Contemporary interpersonal theory and research*. New York: Wiley.

Lazarus, A. A. (1976). *Multimodal behavior therapy*. New York: Springer.

Lewin, K. (1936). *Principles of topographical psychology*. New York: McGraw-Hill.

Loevinger, J. (1957). Objective tests on measurements of psychological theory. *Psychological Reports*, 3, 635–694.

Magnavita, J. J. (1997). *Restructuring personality disorders: A short-term dynamic approach*. New York: Guilford Press.

Millon, T. (1969). *Modern psychopathology: A biosocial approach to maladaptive learning and functioning*. Philadelphia: Saunders.

Millon, T. (1981). *Disorders of personality: DSM-III, Axis II*. New York: Wiley-Interscience.

Millon, T. (1984). On the renaissance of personality assessment and personality theory. *Journal of Personality Assessment*, 48, 450–466.

Millon, T. (1986a). Personality prototypes and their diagnostic criteria. In T. Millon & G. L. Klerman (Eds.), *Contemporary directions in psychopathology: Toward the DSM-IV* (pp. 671-712). New York: Guilford Press.

Millon, T. (1986b). A theoretical derivation of pathological personalities. In T. Millon & G. L. Klerman (Eds.), *Contemporary directions in psychopathology: Toward the DSM-IV* (pp. 639–669). New York: Guilford Press.

Millon, T. (1988). Personologic psychotherapy: Ten commandments for a post-eclectic approach to integrative treatment. *Psychotherapy*, 25, 209–219.

Millon, T. (1990). *Toward a new personology: An evolutionary model*. New York: Wiley.

Millon, T. (1991). Classification in psychopathology: Rationale, alternative, and standards. *Journal of Abnormal Psychology*, 100, 245–261.

Millon, T., & Davis, R. D. (1996). *Disorders of personality: DSM-IV and beyond*. New York: Wiley.

Millon, T., & Grossman, S. D. (2007a). *Resolving difficult clinical syndromes: A personalized psychotherapy approach*. Hoboken, NJ: Wiley.

Millon, T., & Grossman, S. D. (2007b). *Overcoming resistant personality disorders: A personalized psychotherapy approach*. Hoboken, NJ: Wiley.

Millon, T., & Grossman, S. D. (2007c). *Moderating severe personality disorders: A personalized psychotherapy approach*. Hoboken, NJ: Wiley.

Millon, T. (with Grossman, S., Meagher, S., Millon, C., & Everly, G.). (1999). *Personality-guided therapy*. New York: Wiley.

Quine, W. V. O. (1961). *From a logical point of view* (2nd ed.). New York: Harper/Row.

Pincus, A. L., & Wiggins, J. S. (1989). Conceptions of personality disorders and dimensions of personality. *Psychological Assessment*, 1, 305–316.

Rogers, C. R. (1942). *Counseling and psychotherapy*. Boston: Houghton Mifflin.

Rogers, C. R. (1951). *Client-centered therapy*. Boston: Houghton Mifflin.

Rogers, C. R. (1961). *On becoming a person*. Boston: Houghton Mifflin.

Rogers, C. R. (1967). *The therapeutic relationship and its impact*. Madison: University of Wisconsin Press.

Slavson, S. R. (1943). *An introduction to group therapy*. New York: Commonwealth Fund.

Wachtel, P. L. (1973). Psychodynamics, behavior therapy and the implacable experimenter: An inquiry into the consistency of personality. *Journal of Abnormal Psychology*, 82, 324–334.

Westen, D. (1998). Case formulation and personality diagnosis: Two processes or one? In J. W. Barron (Ed.), *Making diagnosis meaningful: Enhancing evaluation and treatment of psychological disorders* (pp. 111–138). Washington, DC: American Psychological Association.

Yalom, I. D. (with Leszcz, M.). (2005). *The theory and practice of group psychotherapy* (5th ed.). New York: Basic Books.

PART II

A GUIDE TO THE MILLON CLINICAL MULTIAXIAL INVENTORY (MCMI)

Scientific Grounding and Validation of the MCMI

Theodore Millon
Carrie M. Millon

This chapter is intended for readers who wish to explore the scientific grounding and validation of the Millon Clinical Multiaxial Inventory (MCMI) throughout its history (Millon, 1977, 1987, 1994). While the logic and rationale presented here may be more abstract than in other sections of this text, the discussion furnishes our perspective on how the constructs were derived and why we believe them to be consonant with recent developments in the field of personology.

As we have noted elsewhere (e.g., Millon, 1990), this is a time of rapid scientific and clinical advances—a time that seems optimal for ventures designed to generate new ideas and syntheses. The territory where "personality" and "psychopathology" intersect is an area of significant academic activity and clinical responsibility. Providing theoretical formulations that bridge these intersections would alone represent a major intellectual step, but we want to do more. To limit our focus to contemporary research models that address these junctions directly might lead us to overlook the solid footings provided by our field's historic thinkers (such as Freud and Jung), as well as our more mature sciences (such as physics and evolutionary biology). If we fail to coordinate propositions and constructs with principles and laws established by these intellectual giants and advanced disciplines, the different domains constituting our subject will remain unconnected to other realms of nature, and hence will require that we return to the important task of synthesis another day. Therefore, in this chapter we go beyond current conceptual and research boundaries in personology and incorporate the contributions of past theorists, as well as those of our more firmly grounded "adjacent" sciences. Not only may such steps bear new conceptual fruits, but they also may provide a foundation to guide our own discipline's explorations.

Much of psychology as a whole remains divorced from broader spheres of scientific knowledge, isolated from deeper and more fundamental (if not universal) principles. As the history of psychology amply illustrates, the propositions of our science are not in themselves sufficient to orient its development in a consistent and focused fashion. Consequently, psychology has become a patchwork quilt of dissonant concepts and diverse data domains. Preoccupied with but our own small portions of the quilt, or fearing accusations of reductionism, we psychologists have failed to draw on the rich possibilities that may be found in both historical and adjacent realms of scholarly pursuit. With few exceptions, cohering concepts that would connect current topics to those of the past have not been developed. We seem repeatedly trapped in (obsessed with?) contemporary fads and horizontal refinements.

A search for integrative schemas and constructs that will link us to relevant observations and laws in other fields of contemporary "science" is also needed. The goal, admittedly a rather grandiose one, is to refashion our patchwork quilt into a well-patterned and cohesive tapestry that interweaves the diverse forms in which nature expresses itself. There is no better sphere within the psychological sciences to undertake such a synthesis than the subject matter of personology—the study of persons. The individual person is the only organically integrated system in the psychological domain, evolved through the millennia and basically created from birth as a natural entity. The individual person is not simply a culture-bound and experience-derived gestalt. The intrinsic cohesion of the person is not a rhetorical construction, but an authentic substantive unity. Personological features may be differentiated into "normal" or "pathological," and may be partitioned conceptually for pragmatic or scientific purposes, but they are segments of an inseparable biopsychosocial entity.

Historical Traditions in Personology

The study of personality may be approached from either of two great historical traditions, the "nomothetic" or the "idiographic," both of which go back at least to the time of the ancient Greeks. The nomothetic approach is focused primarily on constructs and the theoretical propositions that relate them, and not on any one individual. In contrast, the idiographic approach is primarily clinical, and thus is focused on understanding the individual person. Although their purposes are obviously different, these perspectives are not necessarily antagonistic. In fact, we argue that they are complementary, not by accident or intent, but by necessity: The success of theoretical propositions can be judged only in terms of the extent to which they facilitate idiographic or clinical goals; conversely, if idiographic propositions are to possess a validity that is distinctly psychological, as opposed to being merely descriptive (however elegantly done), this requires that case conceptualization proceed from some theoretical basis—an assessment should meet certain criteria of scientific respectability. This section of the chapter is devoted to tracking these conceptual reciprocities and their implications for theory building and clinical work.

The Nomothetic Perspective: Seeking Universal Principles

The first of the two traditions to be discussed, the nomothetic or construct-centered (Allport, 1937) approach, is concerned with personality in an abstract sense and not with any one individual. The emphasis is on discovering how certain constructs tend to relate to or cohere with others and why. Most often the focus is on constructs subsidiary to personality as an integrated phenomenon, such as needs, motives, mechanisms, traits, schemas, and defenses—that is, on part functions. Questions grounded in this approach include "What is the relationship of locus of control to depression?" and "How does the continuum of self-schema complexity relate to stress vulnerability?" Nowhere is mention made of the individual person.

The nomothetic approach is inherently taxonomy-seeking. Although strongly nomothetically oriented psychologists do not deny the existence of individuality, they do believe that once the fundamental units of personality are isolated it will be possible to express each particular personality in terms of these units, with little or no "residual variance," or relevant information, left over. Individuals are simply different combinations of different levels of the same variables. This attitude, inherited from the worldview of determinism or mechanism, holds that as science advances, the shrouds of mystery will recede indefinitely, and that every fact (no matter how small, trivial, or individual) will be accounted for in some scientific context. Experimental error or residual variance is seen as reflecting our ignorance of important independent variables that, when accounted for, will render what is yet to be explained vanishingly small. In classical psychometric terms, personality is described along many dimensions in terms of the deviation of each individual score from the group mean. In modern psychometric terms, the individual's score may be described in terms of sample-free logits. Either way, the subject's profile or code type is regarded as the complete representation of his or her personality.

An expression of these characteristics is seen in taxonomies constructed using factor-analytic methods. Here numerous scales representing a broad selection of personality traits are factor-analyzed for latent patterns of covariation—the dimensions that, according to its proponents, underlie the true or fundamental structure of personality. Variance not accounted for by the factor model is rejected as irrelevant (i.e., as being due to measurement error). The derived factors are then accorded causal primacy in the specification of other, more circumscribed traits or facets of personality, and ultimately these factors become the axes of a nomothetic hyperspace in which any particular personality may be plotted. Parsimony is paramount; thousands of traits may be telescoped into a handful of dimensions. Whether this approach can sustain important challenges to the auxiliary assumptions required to support it (e.g., whether the linear nature of the methodology distorts the structure of the subject domain in its inexorable extraction of a purely dimensional model) is, of course, another matter completely. Nevertheless, it embodies important characteristics of the nomothetic ideal.

The advantage of the nomothetic perspective is that it serves the needs of science. Because science thrives on generalizability, a science of personality cannot afford to be limited to the discovery and explication of laws of behavior specific to one person, or at most to a very small group of persons. If science is the discovery and explanation of invariances across instances, the instances cannot be singular. Instead, science must show the applicability of its theories to realms of manifest phenomena not heretofore seen, approached, or understood. To locate such universal propositions about behavior, personality psychologists look for regularities or covariations that hold across many different people, rather than merely within one person. Allport (1937, p. 4) compared the nomothetic approach to "finding a single thread running from individual nature to individual nature, visible only through the magical spectacles of a special, theoretic attitude."

The Idiographic Perspective: Particular Truths about Particular Persons

Whereas the nomothetic perspective emphasizes commonalities among people—that is, regularities consistent across a class of objects—the idiographic perspective emphasizes the individuality, complexity, and uniqueness of each person or object. Obviously, people have different personalities; otherwise, assessment would need not exist at all. Were everyone the same, were there no variation between persons, then personality as a construct would be entirely unnecessary. The idiographic perspective reminds us that just as personality is not only that which makes each individual what he or she is, it is also that which makes each person different from others, and potentially different from *all* others. At the extreme end, it may even be held that there is something ineffable about each of us—something that cannot be gotten wholly into any symbolic system of description. The psychodynamic idea that personality consists of a series of layers of defense and compromise, through which the impulses of sex and aggression may be transformed in circuitous and unexpected ways, begins to approximate this complexity.

Perhaps the most important point of this perspective is the idea that individuality is the result of a unique history of transactions between biological factors (e.g., temperament and genetic constitution) and contextual factors (e.g., the mother's womb, the family environment, social roles to which the child is exposed, culture, and socioeconomic status)—a history that has never existed before and will never be repeated. Because each personality is such a singular product, it cannot be understood either through the application of universal laws or through dimensions of individual differences. Instead, understanding personality requires a developmental approach, one whose descriptive potential is as rich as the person's own history—so rich, in fact, that ultimately it might only be called biographical. According to Henry Murray (1938, p. 604), originator of the term "personology," "the history of personality *is* the personality." Whereas the nomothetic approach asks about the "what" of personality, the idiographic perspective asks about the "how" and the "why." The question is this: How has the person become the unique creature he or she is? Accordingly, the focus in this perspective shifts from the description of each individual personality as a positive phenomenon—that is, from the classification of a person as "antisocial" (or the dimensionalization of the person as a code type in some nomothetic space)—to the view that personality is a richly contextualized and intrinsically transactional phenomenon that emerges with stochastic indeterminateness from a nearly infinite ground of possibilities. In this view, cross-sectional descriptions or personality diagnoses are only the beginning points. Scientific explanation requires discovering why each individual has evolved into just exactly who he or she has become, rather than into someone else. Personology, then, is an exercise in elucidating the developmentally necessary and sufficient conditions through which the particular individual as a distinct entity was "culled" from an infinite universe of possibilities. Given the antithesis of this perspective to universal laws, it is not impossible that these constraints might include such "softer" concepts as free will and chance.

Linking the Nomothetic and Idiographic Approaches

The nomothetic–idiographic duality is a classic and inevitable problem, and one for which no easy solution is forthcoming. One way out is reductionism: simply reducing one pole of the duality to the other, and effectively ignoring the existence of contrary views. Thus strongly nomothetically oriented psychologists typically maintain that variance unaccounted for by their pet dimensions consists wholly of error and nothing more. Any other admission impugns the completeness of the preferred model by acknowledging the omission of relevant and substantive content, and thus begs for supplementary constructs or dimensions that may not easily fit with an author's theoretical preconceptions. Any theorist may argue that his or her set of dimensions is fundamental, of course; however, such rationales are particularly apparent in factor-analytically derived schemes, which always extract a small number of dimensions, followed by so-called "error factors."

Where the idiographic pole is emphasized, each person may be regarded as an entity so ineffably complex that any form of description simplifies, and so trivializes, the totality of the individual's unique "existential situation." Psychodynamically "deep" case analyses, which emphasize the circuitous transformations of drives and impulses through multiple latent layers of character formation, begin to approximate the hermeneutic potential of the idiographic perspective. As this potential increases— that is, as the interpretive thread is spun more and more finely to reflect the mutually intercontextualized and developmentally transactional nature of the individual personality—the approach itself becomes less objective and therefore seemingly antiscientific, if only because the individual has been specified to the point of existing *sui generis.* Clearly, reductionism is not a solution. How then are we to reconcile these two approaches?

Building a Clinical Science

Clinical science may be said to consist of four intercontextualized domains: "theory," "taxonomy," "assessment," and "intervention." All the activities of clinical scientists are oriented toward one or more of these clinical domains. Theory may be said to consist of a corpus of propositions that relate various constructs in personality and psychopathology to observed clinical realities; taxonomy refers to the categories into, or dimensions along which, pathologies and personalities may be classified or appraised. Assessment is concerned with the description, measurement, and explanation of individual pathology, while intervention seeks to address and remedy this pathology. The first two domains are more construct-centered, reflecting psychopathology and personality considered as a pure science that focuses on clinical "diseases" (Axis I), such as anxiety and depression, and their relationships to other traits (Axis II), physical characteristics (Axis III), and environmental factors (Axis IV). The second two domains are focused more on the individual, reflecting clinical science as it exists in its applied form—focused on the person who must be understood as the particular being who actually has the so-called disease, and for whom help must be found.

If the nomothetic–idiographic issue is linked to clinical science in this way (one that frames the duality as complementary rather than antagonistic), then each domain places constraints on the structure of the others and so acts as a check on the validity of the science as a whole. The conceptual opposite is a disconnected science consisting of the same four domains—each independent of the others, built on its own specific principles, evolved exclusively out of itself, and content in the cognizance of its own internal consistency. In such an unintegrated science, theory exists as a self-perpetuating, unverifiable mass; taxonomy consists of categories of convenience; instrumentation is informed only by history and tradition; and interventions rely mainly on placebo effects and nonspecific factors and tend to multiply without bounds. Unfortunately, the state of clinical science today, fueled in part by the distinction between academicians and clinicians, largely favors the independence of domains rather than their integration.

Although it is obvious that the clinical domains are, and should be, interrelated, the history of clinical science bears out what intuition knows to be true. As genuinely interdependent parts of a single science, developments in each domain influence the form of the others and of the science as a whole. Thus, with the publication of the third edition of the *Diagnostic and Statistical Manual of Mental Disorders* (DSM-III) in 1980, the psychodynamic foundation of much of psychopathology was officially overthrown; the result was that the value and relevance of instruments oriented toward constructs no longer officially sanctioned, such as the Rorschach and the Thematic Apperception Test (TAT), became more limited. With the evolution of managed care, assessment has become more integral to intervention. Patients may now start down the so-called "clinical pathways" depending upon testing results, for which a particular intervention may be operationalized in great detail. These essentially historical facts illustrate the interdependence of taxonomy and assessment. Other examples could easily be given for any given pair of domains.

The fundamental thesis, however, is that the integration of clinical domains is not merely historical—in the way, for example, that the Eiffel Tower is integrated into the cultural history of Paris—but also logically necessary. The ideal of an integrated science leads us to require certain relationships among the various domains, which, if we were unaware of the ideal of integration, or if in fact we were to regard the domains as independent, we most definitely would not propose. *In general, idiographic formulations must be held to scientific standards; conversely, nomothetic propositions must be tested against clinical realities.* It may be said, for example, that while interventions guided by the intuition of a seasoned professional are often admirably effective, they are not truly scientific in a strict sense unless guided by clinical theory; that while taxonomy should ultimately be based in theory, clinical observation may suggest additional categories or subcategories of pathology for the investigation and elaboration of theory; that case conceptualization is dependent upon theory if it is to be genuinely explanatory, rather than merely descriptive; and so on. Many such propositions might be enumerated. Each domain is connected to, constrained according to, or informed by the others. These constraints or informational pathways are grouped into two kinds: those oriented toward theory and taxonomy, which tend to be nomothetic in nature; and those oriented toward assessment and intervention, which tend to be more idiographic. Grouping the constraints in this way not only brings the reciprocity between traditionally academic or theoretical work and traditionally clinical or applied work into the foreground, but also allows them to be discussed in reciprocal pairs. For example, the question "How does psychological theory constrain psychological assessment?" can easily and legitimately be turned around to read "How do the results of psychological assessment constrain psychological theory?"

In this chapter, we are interested only in those constraints that impinge upon assessment and those that issue from it. These form a set of necessary (but probably not sufficient) criteria that must be met if assessment is to be fully integrated into clinical science.

Theory and the Assessment of the Individual

As long as science remains incomplete, there will always be a certain reciprocity between scientific theory and observation, for observation, which in its more rigorous forms consists of empirical experimentation, is needed to test theory. This is also true for theories of the individual.

Nomothetic Proposition: Theory Provides the Only Point of Departure for a Genuinely Scientific Assessment of the Individual

What prescriptions does the nomothetic approach make for assessment? Recall that this perspective is concerned with personality in the abstract and with the theoretical linkages among its constructs. Any psychological assessment must then, in Allport's (1937, p. 4) words, pay homage to the "theoretic thread that runs from individual to individual." To possess a validity that is distinctly psychological, as opposed to what might be termed "Theophrastean" (after Theophrastus, the ancient Greek writer who provided vivid portrayals of certain commonly seen personality types), the constructs used to appraise personality should possess a genuine explanatory power.

To do so, they must somehow be more "fundamental" than terms taken from that store of descriptors usually referred to as the "common lexicon." Scientific languages differ from the natural language not only because they serve a different purpose, but also because they have been refined of theoretical ambiguities and surface similarities present in the terms of the natural language. In its beginning stages, science is mainly concerned with the questions "What is there?" and "What is it like?"—a strategy of inventory and description. The philosopher of science Carl Hempel (1965) noted:

> The development of a scientific discipline may often be said to proceed from an initial "natural history" stage . . . to subsequent more and more theoretical stages. . . . The vocabulary required in the early stages of this development will be largely observational. . . . The shift toward theoretical systematization is marked by the introduction of new, "theoretical" terms . . . more or less removed from the level of directly observable

things and events. . . . These terms have a distinct meaning and function only in the context of a corresponding theory. (pp. 39–140)

Even at this natural history stage, however, knowledge is never theory-neutral or paradigm-free. Surplus meanings are inevitable. Even what we term as "facts" are not objective statements about the natural world. They are, rather, statements whose assumptive context has become so consensual that it need not be explicitly stated in order to communicate. Such assumptions are neither conscious nor preconscious, but unconscious—so much so, in fact, that their elucidation often becomes the stuff of philosophical and scientific revolutions. Consider gravity: In Newton's world, gravity was understood as a force. No less a genius than Einstein was required for gravity to be understood as a curvature of space. After relativity, our experience of gravity as a force could be seen as an artifact of our own perceptual mechanisms.

In the area of personality disorders, for example, the term "disorders" brings to the assessment enterprise a set of assumptions that are paradigmatically inappropriate. Personality disorders are not illnesses for which some discrete pathogen can be found, or for which there exists some underlying unitary cause, either past or present. The use of such language as "disorder" is indeed unfortunate, for personality pathologies are not disorders at all in the medical sense. Instead, personality disorders are best conceptualized as disorders of the entire matrix of the person. Hence we prefer the terms "pattern" or "style" rather than the intrinsically reifying "disorder." This misconception is more paradigmatic than diagnostic, but it leads to subsequent distortions in multiaxial logic—encouraging the view that classical clinical syndromes and personality disorders exist alongside each other in a horizontal relationship, when in fact clinical symptoms are best viewed as being embedded in the context of a personality pattern.

A second sense in which theory is relevant to assessment concerns not content, but process: How are we to get from clinical theory to case conceptualization? The fractionated person—the person who has been dispersed across scales, instruments, and interviews—must be put back together again as an organic whole. How is this to be achieved? As Bloom and Millon have argued in Chapter 1, assessment is an eminently theoretical process that requires a weighing of this and a disqualifying of that across the differences and similarities of methods and data sources through multiple rounds of hypothesis generation and testing. The ideal result is *the* "theory of the patient"—a theory in which every loose end has been tied up in a logic so compelling that it seems to follow from the logic of the patient's own psyche. It is so convincing that one gets the feeling that things could not be otherwise.

To achieve this ideal insofar as is possible, theories of the person should pay homage to the same virtues as do other scientific theories. For one thing, they should be made as internally consistent (i.e., as free of internal contradictions) as possible. Individuals cannot possess both psychopathic indifference to suffering and altruistic sacrifice for others as cardinal traits, for example. Where contradictions are indicated by the data, they may often be resolved by invoking the dynamic idea of conflict, and by inspecting the data for objects around which the conflict is expressed. In addition, a good theory of the patient should be as complete as possible; that is, it is should avail itself of as many data, in as many domains, as can be expeditiously gathered—a fact that makes sense both psychometrically and personologically. Psychometrically, confidence is increased when aggregated data converge toward a single result. Personologically, information within a particular domain speaks more strongly about that domain than does other data. For example, although we might expect someone who is interpersonally dramatic and gregarious to be cognitively scattered as well, evidence directly relevant to the ideational process is preferred for such a conclusion. Directly relevant data not only allow us to have higher confidence in our conclusions, but also allow the theory to be as specific as possible.

Idiographic Proposition: The Ultimate Purpose of Clinical Assessment Must Be to Understand the Person

From an extreme idiographic perspective, taxonomy is only a point of departure used in understanding individuals. Individuality is ultimately too complex to be organized into classes or placed along dimensions of individual differences. If taxonomies are used at all, they must be used self-consciously as contrivances that facilitate the investigation of individuality, not as clinical endpoints. As clinical heuristics, they are guidelines to be replaced and reformulated as necessary; it is the unique instantiation of the construct or trait in the particular individual that is of immediate clinical interest. Any personality construct, any literary metaphor, is fair game if it is relevant and effective in conceptualizing and communicating clinically relevant matters.

Even widely consensual and officially sanctioned taxonomies of personality and personality disorders are limited in their explanatory power and clinical utility. Not only is the DSM not an exhaustive listing of personality constructs that might be relevant to any particular individual; it does not even begin to scratch the surface. Nomothetic propositions and diagnostic labels are mere superficialities to be overcome and replaced by more complete hypotheses as test results and other data are gathered and understanding is gained. To clinicians, who might justifiably be called "scientists of the individual," the categories of DSM represent a kind of natural history stage—a gross, cross-sectional description of pathology that must be augmented with biographical data before the individual can be understood and treated. Questions to be answered include these: Why does the patient have this particular personality style rather than some other? What are the developmental antecedents of his or her defensive mechanisms? How is the patient's personality related to symptom production? What psychosocial forces undermine the adequacy of the patient's coping mechanisms?

Whereas from a nomothetic perspective it is constructs that are viewed as open concepts, from an idiographic perspective it is individuality that is to be pinned down and understood to the degree that it can be brought to closure through links with scientific constructs. Individuals may be viewed as open concepts as well. In fact, we might identify a continuum of interpretive openness running from very incomplete to extremely idiographic. At the first level would be a score on a single dimension. Here the individual is spoken of as being self-conscious or extraverted, for example. To the extent that this dimension is indeed the organizing principle of the whole personality—what Allport (1937) referred to as an individual's "cardinal trait"—it describes how the person will behave in a given situation, and in fact functions as a rather good inductive summary for the entire matrix of the individual.

Unfortunately, very few subjects are pure prototypes of any particular construct; cardinal traits are rare. The second level of interpretation is configural and hierarchical, but remains cross-sectional. Here "configural" simply means that the scores on particular traits or dimensions are not interpreted in and of themselves, but in relation to one another. At a bare minimum, two dimensions are involved in the clinician's configural efforts—as, for example, with the interpersonal circle, which features love–hate and dominance–submission. As the number of dimensions increases, profile interpretation becomes successively more nuanced as the meaning of each trait is transformed by virtue of its existence in the context of the others. Thus, for example, a high Narcissistic score may be considered in conjunction with a secondary Antisocial elevation. Such individuals are likely to be grandiose and entitled, and to act out when their self-esteem is deflated, or to become explosive if their entitlement is not honored by others. If yet a third elevation is added (say, Masochistic), we would be required to integrate certain aspects of this prototype into our formulation. We might conclude that such individuals are likely to realize their errors at a later date and attempt to undo their transgressions through some form of self-torment. Note that nowhere in these formulations is developmental information explicitly considered. Accordingly, interpretations produced at this level lie somewhere between description and explanation: They are descriptive in the sense that they cannot explain the origins of the particular personality, and explanatory in that they are nevertheless formulated in terms that are theoretically anchored.

The deepest level of interpretation is distinctly biographical, asking, "How has this person come to be as he or she is?" Here the substance of the individual's personality is subjected to developmental inquiry, in the context of developmental theory and the individual's unique biography. If the clinical interview reveals, for example, rigid, compulsive parents, we might conclude that the Narcissistic elevation is in fact a defense against highly critical introjects, and that the person's grandiosity allows him or her to transcend these disparaging internal voices and keeps him or her compensated.

Theory and Instrument Construction

Just as the understanding of any physical phenomenon is limited by the paradigms available, so also is the validity of the individual assessment. In fact, the availability of theory is a primary constraint on the validity of the assessment (just as the experience of the clinician is another constraint). No assessment can be stronger than its limiting conditions. Just as water cannot rise higher than its source, no case conceptualization can be more valid than the perspectives brought to bear in its formulation. Although this principle holds for any diagnostic syndrome, it is even more relevant to the personality disorders, which are, as disorders of the entire matrix of the individual, anchored to multiple domains of structure and functioning—behavioral, phenomenological, intrapsychic, and biophysical. The clinician must draw from these perspectives to discover the relationship between the symptom and the larger matrix. It is the intent to draw upon deeper and more precise principles that distinguishes this activity as genuinely scientific and sets it apart from more common-sense ascriptions. Interpretive accuracy, however, requires valid instrumentation.

Nomothetic Proposition: Assessment Instruments Should Be Constructed on the Basis of Theory

Assessment instruments in psychological science tend to endure. A comparison of the top 20 instruments of 20 years ago with those of today shows little change. The Rorschach has been with us for almost 90 years, the Minnesota Multiphasic Personality Inventory (MMPI) for more than 60 years. These instruments are somewhat like the character armor of our field. Their existence ritualizes clinical assessment activities, assures us that the more difficult and essentially philosophical questions have already been answered, and so encourages us to put aside these truly troublesome quandaries and get on with our work. And as with good defensive armor, their future use is set, even if their relevance and utility are questionable.

Whatever the current state of clinical knowledge, it is the generation of theory that suggests not only the latent structure of a subject domain, but also those gauges that might be shown upon further empirical research to be optimally suited to the assessment of this structure. If a researcher wishes to construct a self-report scale to measure narcissistic personality disorder, the researcher's theory of the disorder becomes a major guiding force in shaping the character of the items written for the initial pool; they are not simply a random selection of stimulus materials. Unfortunately, a review of the most frequently used projective and objective tests, the Rorschach and the MMPI, shows their structure and content to be much less theoretically grounded than might at first be believed. As a field, we appear to be far more concerned with retrofitting modern psychological innovations (whether theoretical or taxonomic) to old instruments than with revising and optimizing the instruments themselves.

When Hermann Rorschach began to explore the use of inkblots in his studies with schizophrenic individuals, for example, he originally used about 40 cards (Exner, 1986). From these he selected 15 that, from his own empirical experience, were most clinically useful. Unfortunately, even 15 proved too expensive to reproduce, given the technology of the times, so he rewrote his classic *Psychodiagnostik* (Rorschach, 1921) to feature only the 10 blots he used most often. If the reader has ever watched the Mel Brooks film *History of the World, Part I*, there is a point in the movie when Moses, having descended from his mountaintop conference with God, stands dramatically on a rocky ledge before the Hebrew people, holding three stone tablets on which are inscribed 15 commandments. Just as Moses is presenting the law of God, he loses his grasp on one of the tablets, and it drops to the ground and shatters on the earth below. A long moment of anticlimactic silence follows, during which Moses quickly and cleverly conceives a means of concealing his awkwardness: "I give you these 15 . . . (*crash*) . . . No, 10 . . . 10 commandments!" The effect upon the audience is a mix of humor, amazement, and curiosity. What did the five lost commandments say? Is this one clumsy error the reason the world has been screwed up ever since? How might things be different if the lost commandments had survived?

Given the rather desultory development of the final Rorschach plates, we are entitled to ask the same questions of Hermann Rorschach (though, in fairness, Rorschach expired before he could develop the inkblot technique more fully). The point is this: Although there was some selection of stimulus materials through Rorschach's own research and personal experience, it is by no means clear that this set of plates was optimal for the nosological categories of the 1920s, much less for use with the DSM-IV-TR today. Were modern clinicians to attempt the construction of a new set of plates, optimized to the structure and content of modern DSMs with the idea of providing meaningful information for Axes I, II, and IV, the resulting set of stimulus materials would probably bear little resemblance to the Rorschach. Yet there is also little doubt that the same 10 plates will be with us 80 years in the future, if only because these plates were what set the whole enterprise in motion and have served as the basis for thousands of research studies. For assessment instruments, the importance of continuity with the past cannot be underestimated.

A similar case may be made with regard to the clinical scales of the MMPI. At the time of the MMPI's construction, an exclusively empirical approach to inventory construction seemed worthwhile. The philosophy of science known as "logical positivism" was in its ascendancy, and psychological theory was considered as yet too weak to inform inventory construction. If items of ostensibly unrelated content were found to differentiate psychiatric groups, then this could simply be considered a point of departure for scientific interest that might be explored at some future date.

Unfortunately, the original MMPI scales proved unsatisfactory. First, the clinical scales proved difficult to interpret. Not only were the latent elements important to particular elevations and profile patterns difficult to resolve, but also the same elevation or profile pattern might mean different things for different patients. The Harris–Lingoes subscales (Harris & Lingoes, 1955, 1968), which group items of each MMPI scale into rationally coherent subgroups, were constructed to address these considerations. Clusters of item endorsements could now be examined to explain profile patterns at a more molecular level. Later, Wiggins (1969) would construct his own content scales, grouping together items from the entire pool. And today we have the MMPI-2 content scales, constructed as part of the restandardization project itself, as well as the MMPI-2 restructured clinical scales.

In the larger picture, however, the reason why the initial MMPI clinical scales proved disappointing was that clinical taxonomy evolved out from underneath them. Unlike the MMPI, the categories of mental illness on which the instrument was based did not endure. Had this psychiatric nosology in fact "carved nature at its joints," the criterion groups method of instrument construction might still be with us today. The item selection statistics would almost certainly be revved up, but the essential idea that items can be chosen and be diagnostically effective while being ostensibly unrelated to their diagnostic criterion would be sound, from a practical viewpoint. After all, if nature exists in categories, then predicting these categories is all that is important.

In turn, the categories of the 1940s evolved because they lacked the kind of generative power about which Hempel (1965) has written. Fortunately, the MMPI has survived by recombining its items in ways more fruitful than those of the clinical scales—for example, the content scales of the MMPI-2. The lesson is that it is extremely difficult, if not impossible, to get more out of an assessment than what is afforded by the generativity of the underlying constructs on which an instrument is based. Earlier we have argued that theory forms the only scientific point of departure for an assessment. Scientific theories are always in a state of evolution. However, the validity of the case conceptualization stands upon the generation of theoretical propositions. The upper bounds of precision and explanatory power for the assessment are the precision and explanatory power of the propositions of the underlying science.

Idiographic Proposition: The Results of Clinical Observation Must Inform the Content and Structure of Clinical Instruments

For nosologists, the inexact fit between patient and diagnosis is a nagging and noisome reminder of individuality—one that has continued to fuel the development of modern psychiatric taxonomies. Ideally, a diagnosis alone should be both necessary and sufficient to begin treatment, and should be all the clinician needs to know. Were ideals realities, individuals would fit their diagnostic categories perfectly with pristinely prototypal presentations. Yet such a thing seldom occurs. An early developmental theorist argued that development always proceeds from the global to the more differentiated. The monotypic categories of earlier DSMs may be seen as the global beginnings of later specifications and accommodations. In the initial phases of its development, a diagnostic taxonomy consists generally of entities of broad bandwidth, but little specificity. Inevitably, some diagnostic categories begin to be viewed as invalid and are simply discarded. As theoretical knowledge and empirical studies accrue, however, broad diagnostic taxons begin to be broken down into multiple, narrow taxons of greater specificity and descriptive value. As the process continues, an interesting structural change occurs: The taxonomy begins to take on a hierarchical structure—one that allows it to accommodate to the contextualism which exists in the world at large. Coverage increases as big taxons are broken down into little taxons. The big taxons are now merely what the little taxons have in common, as anxiety is for panic disorder, agoraphobia, and posttraumatic stress disorder, among others.

The same kind of hierarchical evolution is now occurring on Axis II. Whenever kinds of schizoid or antisocial or borderline patients are discussed, a hierarchical conception is implicit. Subvarieties of the Axis II constructs have been abstracted from historical works to provide further refinement, sharper distinctions, and greater descriptive power within these diagnostic entities (Millon & Davis, 1996). In addition, Millon (1986a, 1990) has articulated each of the Axis II prototypes as integrative personality patterns that are expressed in a variety of functional and structural clinical domains (see Grossman, Tringone, & Millon, Chapter 24, this volume). Among assessment instruments, which are much more easily constructed and altered than are official nosologies, the emergence of contextualism is even more clear. Despite its metatheoretical weaknesses, one strength of the lexical approach is its assertion that personality traits are hierarchically organized. Personality descriptors are broad but somewhat inaccurate near the top of the hierarchy, becoming increasingly narrow but more precise as one moves down into regions of lower traits and ultimately into behavioral acts. The NEO Personality Inventory— Revised (NEO-PI-R; Costa & McCrae, 1992), for example, includes facet scales for each of its five broad-band factors. The MMPI-2 content scales have been broken up into experimental content component scales (Butcher, Graham, Williams, & Ben-Porath, 1990). Content subscales have been developed for the Millon family of instruments as well (see Grossman, Chapter 6, this volume).

Utilizing Assessment for Therapeutic Planning

The form of therapy and its content are the two principal considerations in setting forth a logical model for assessing of personality disorders. The ideal form of therapy should be implicit in the structural properties of the assessment process itself. Unfortunately, many therapies are often practiced in a "linear" format, which assumes that a simple additivity of the same therapeutic method will be sufficient to deal with the problems at hand. Thus many mental health professionals continue to apply the same therapeutic modality—exclusively cognitive therapy, exclusively behavior therapy, exclusively pharmacological therapy, exclusively family therapy, and so on—to every patient they encounter. If personality disorders were anchored exclusively to one of these domains, such single-minded approaches would be both appropriate and desirable. Personality disorders, however, are not exclusively behavioral or cognitive or intrapsychic constructs. Instead, they are multioperational and systemic. No part of the system exists in complete isolation. Instead, every part is directly or indirectly tied to every other. An emergent synergism lends the whole a clinical tenacity that makes personality a "real" thing to be reckoned with in any therapeutic endeavor.

As Millon, Boice, and Sinsabaugh have described in Chapter 2, Millon has put forward two integrative procedures for treating the personality disorders. In the first of these, called "potentiated pairings," two or more treatment methods oriented to different clinical domains (e.g., interpersonal, cognitive) are combined simultaneously to overcome problematic characteristics that might be refractory to each focused technique if they were administered separately. These composites pull and push for change on many different fronts, so that the therapy becomes as multioperational and as tenacious as the disorder itself. The term "catalytic sequences" has been proposed to represent procedures whose intent is to plan the order in which several coordinated treatments are executed. They comprise timing series chosen to maximize the impact of changes that would be less effective if the sequential combination were otherwise arranged.

Nomothetic Proposition: The Therapeutic Plan Should Be Developed from Prototypes as Assessed in Terms of the Individual's Personality Style

Although we may know that personality disorders require a fundamentally different kind of therapy than do the Axis I disorders, this does not in itself tell us what to do when confronted with an actual patient unless assessment has guided our treatment thinking. The integrative forms of personalized therapy are dictated by the nature of the personality construct (Millon & Grossman, 2007a, 2007b, 2007c). The content of personalized therapy, however, must be specified on some other basis. Personality is by definition the patterning of intraindividual variables, but the nature of these variables does not follow from the definition, and must be supplied by some assessment technique or on some basis "outside" the personality construct itself. "Personality" is a structural–functional concept that refers to the intraorganismic patterning of variables; it does not in itself say what these variables are, nor can it be expected to, just as the generic idea of personality cannot be expected to tell us anything particular about the personality of a specific individual.

To ask the question "How do I address the personality pathologies of the patient who sits before me?" is once again to ask about the fundamental assessment tool that serves to identify the elements that give rise to, or combine to form, the personality disorders. As a construct, personality seeks to capture the entire matrix of the person, to distill from the major currents and subtle eddies of the behavioral stream some set of underlying, logical, organizing principles which capture precisely individual functioning. Personality clinical assessment asks us not to look at behaviors, cognitions, and so forth one at a time—as if each were simply the next on the list, or next in a sequence relevant to and yet isolated from the larger whole—but rather to examine psychic components in connection with one another, so as to infer some underlying theme or unity of purpose to which each aspect of the whole is somehow accountable. As a construct, clinical personality assessment begs us to dive beneath the surface, to make inferences, and to integrate manifest diversities according to latent logical principles. As clinical assessors, we are called upon not merely to record this or that psychic domain, but to explain it.

In Millon's model, for example, the content of personality is derived from evolutionary theory—a discipline that informs and serves as a basis for, but exists apart from, personology. By comparing and contrasting the specific person against the personality prototypes deduced from the theory, an assessment approach to a therapeutic plan can be formed that provides a basis for approaching the individual's pathologies in terms of the fundamental "forces" of which personality is composed.

Idiographic Proposition: The Therapeutic Plan Must Assess Idiographic Specificities That Fit Only Partially into Any One Clinical Prototype

In the DSM, the personality disorders are operationalized as singular prototypes. Each prototype consists of a variety of diagnostic attributes. Possessing a threshold number of these attributes qualifies one for a particular personality diagnosis. For example, if five of nine are required, then a patient positive for any five of the nine will be diagnosed with the disorder. Although every pair of patients will inevitably have at least two attributes in common, no one particular criterion is either necessary or sufficient for the diagnosis. The resemblance of an individual to the prototype is necessarily a qualitative as well as a quantitative affair. That is, by its heuristic nature, the prototype asks both how and how much the individual resembles the ideal; implicitly, it looks beyond the one-disorder, one-cause, one-therapy perspective implicit in the current diagnostic system. Heterogeneity, then, is seen not as an epistemic problem reflecting our ignorance of an individual's true diagnostic disposition, but rather as a substantive part of the diagnostic landscape that must be considered *in addition* to whatever diagnoses are made.

Thus classifying a patient into a particular set of prototypes does not represent a stopping point, but is instead a point of departure for creating a much longer narrative that conceptualizes the individual's distinctive personality. On what basis will this narrative be generated? Currently, there are two directions within Millon's model in which the clinician can proceed. In the first, the clinical prototypes are operationalized in terms of their manifestations in eight functional–structural domains of personality. These domains suggest additional and more specific characteristics that may be inquired to derive rich and relatively complete conceptions of a patient's personality structure and functioning. Assume, for example, that an individual, upon completing the MCMI, obtains a Narcissistic–Dependent profile. Specific domain attributes can then be examined in conjunction with auxiliary evidence to generate more detailed, idiographically valid portrayals of personality (Grossman et al., Chapter 24, this volume).

As a second means of deriving more idiographic conceptions of individual personality, the clinician may wish to inspect what are being called the "adult subtypes" of the personality disorders (Millon & Davis, 1996). Whereas the major prototypes represent "inevitable deductions" from the evolutionary theory, the subtypes represent instead what are believed, on the basis of clinical experience and a reading of the historical literature for personality, to be the more common manifestations of the major clinical variants in our particular time and culture. Often they represent the convergence of the major types with organizing principles from particular domains of personality—for example, the idea of the "compensating narcissistic" type. And often they represent commonly found fusions of the major types—for example, the histrionic and borderline types. Nevertheless, although the increased specificity of the subtypes relative to the major prototypes promises an increase in the fit of actual patients to the diagnostic system, the subtypes should be viewed again as proto-subtypes, rather than taxonomic endpoints. They simply constitute another way station or frame of reference that clinicians may avail themselves of on the way to a narrative formulation of high "fit" with the individual—that is, one that brings the person as open concept to closure in terms of constructs anchored within a schema that is genuinely explanatory, rather than descriptive.

Obviously, a tremendous amount of knowledge—both about the nature of the patient's disorders and about diverse modes of intervention—is required to perform personalized assessment and therapy planning. To maximize this synergism requires the therapist to be a little like a jazz soloist. Not only should the professional be fully versed in the various musical keys (i.e., in techniques of psychotherapy that span all personological domains), but he or she should also be prepared to respond to subtle fluctuations in the patient's thoughts, actions, and emotions, any of which could take the composition in a wide variety of directions, and integrate these with the overall plan of therapy as it evolves. After the assessment instruments and therapeutic history has been packed away and "the band" has gone home, a retrospective account on the entire assessment and therapeutic process should reveal a level of thematic continuity and logical order commensurate with that which would have existed, had all relevant constraints been known in advance.

The Role of the MCMI in Assessment History

It may be of interest to record a few words regarding the origin and sequential development of the various forms of the MCMI. A year or two after the publication of *Modern Psychopathology* (Millon, 1969), Theodore Millon began with some regularity to receive letters and phone calls from graduate students who had read the book and thought it provided ideas that could aid them in formulating their dissertations. Most inquired about the availability of an "operational" measure they could use to assess or diagnose the pathologies of personality that were generated by the text's theoretical model. Regrettably, no such tool was available. Nevertheless, they were encouraged to pursue whatever lines of interest they might have in the subject. Some were sufficiently motivated to state that they would attempt to develop their own "Millon" instrument as part of the dissertation enterprise.

When the number of these potential "Millon" inventories grew into the teens, however, concern grew proportionately about both the diversity and the adequacy of these representations of the theory. As described in the Preface to the first edition of this book, Millon began to consider undertaking the test construction task himself in order to establish some degree of instrumental uniformity for future investigators, as well as to assure at least a measure of psychometric quality among tools that ostensibly reflected the theory's constructs. At that time, in early 1971, Millon was directing a research supervision group composed of psychologists and psychiatrists in training. All of them had read *Modern Psychopathology* and found the proposal of helping to develop instruments that would identify and quantify the text's personality constructs to be both worthy and challenging.

The initial task was that of exploring alternate methods for gathering relevant clinical data. About 11 or 12 persons were involved in that early phase. Some were asked to analyze the possibilities of identifying new indices from well-established projective tests, such as the Rorschach and the TAT; others were to investigate whether we could compose relevant scales from existing objective inventories, such as the Sixteen Personality Factor Questionnaire (16PF) and the MMPI. Another group examined the potential inherent in developing a new and original structured interview. After 4 or 5 months of weekly discussions, the group concluded that an entirely new instrument would be required if we were to represent the full scope of the theory, especially its diverse and then-novel "pathological" personality patterns (our work, it should be recalled, preceded by several years the effort undertaken by the DSM-III Task Force). It was judged further that we would attempt to construct both a self-report inventory and a semistructured interview schedule.

Naively, it was assumed that both construction tasks could be completed in about 18 months—a time period that would allow several members of the research group to participate on a continuing basis. Despite the fact that we "postponed" developing the interview schedule after a brief initial period, the "more limited" task of the inventory took almost 7 years to complete. The framework and preliminary item selections of the inventory were well underway, however, by the end of the first full year of our work, and these were described briefly in *Research Methods in Psychopathology* (Millon & Diesenhaus, 1972). The initial forms of the clinical instrument were entitled the Millon–Illinois Self-Report Inventory (MI-SRI).

Millon became involved thereafter in the development of the DSM-III (American Psychiatric Association, 1980), playing a major role in formulating both the constructs and the criteria that were to characterize its Axis II personality disorders. Although the MI-SRI was regularly refined and strengthened on the basis of theoretical logic and research data, an effort was made during this period to coordinate both its items and scales with the forthcoming syndromes of DSM-III. Once it was so modified, its name was changed to the Millon Clinical Multiaxial Inventory (MCMI; Millon, 1977), and it was published by National Computer Systems, Inc. (NCS).

In the ensuing 10-year period, numerous refinements of the inventory were introduced (e.g., corrections for response-distorting tendencies such as current emotional state), and expansions were made to incorporate theoretical extensions and the newly published DSM-III-R (e.g., the addition of the Self-Defeating and Sadistic Personality Disorder scales; American Psychiatric Association, 1987). The MCMI-II (Millon, 1987) reflected these changes and additions. Ongoing investigations, further refinements in its undergirding theory, and modifications in the anticipated DSM-IV personality disorders criteria served as the primary impetus to refashion the inventory into the MCMI-III (Millon, 1994), designed to reflect its theory optimally and to maximize its consonance with the most recent and empirically grounded official classification system.

Theoretical Basis of the MCMI

Philosophers of science agree that theory provides the conceptual glue that binds a nosology together. Moreover, a good theory not only summarizes and incorporates extant knowledge; it also possesses systematic import, in that it originates and develops new observations and new methods. In a theory of personality prototypes, what is desired is not merely a *descriptive* list of disorders and their correlated attributes, but also an *explanatory* derivation based on theoretical principles. Again, the question of interest is this: "Why these particular personality disorders rather than others?"

To address this question, a taxonomy must seek a theoretical schema that "carves nature at its joints," so to speak. Carl Hempel (1965) clearly distinguished between natural and artificial classification systems. The difference, according to Hempel, is that natural classifications possess "systematic import." Hempel wrote:

> Distinctions between "natural" and "artificial" classifications may well be explicated as referring to the difference between classifications that are scientifically fruitful and those that are not: in a classification of the former kind, those characteristics of the elements which serve as criteria of membership in a given class are associated, universally or with high-probability, with more or less extensive clusters of other characteristics. . . . A classification of this sort should be viewed as somehow having objective existence in nature, as "carving nature at the joints." (pp. 146–147)

The biological sexes (male and female) and the periodic table of elements are both examples of classification schemes that can be viewed as possessing "objective" existence in nature. The items we seek to classify are not sexes or chemical elements, however, but persons. In so doing, we seek the ideal of a classification scheme or taxonomy that is "natural"—one that "inheres" in the subject domain and is not "imposed" on it.

Again, to achieve such an end, the system of kinds that undergirds any domain of inquiry must itself be answerable to the question that forms the very point of departure for the scientific enterprise: "Why does nature take this particular form rather than some other?" The goal of science is to explain the objects and events we find in the world, and among the objects we find in the world are classification systems for objects themselves. Applied to a taxonomy, the question is thus rephrased: "Why this particular system of kinds rather than some other?" Accordingly, a taxonomic scheme must be justified, and to be justified scientifically it must be justified theoretically. Consonant with integrative principles, then, theory and taxonomy are intimately intertwined. Rather than remaining an uncoordinated and free-floating fragment, each taxon finds its true nexus with others in transcending theoretical principles through which the entire taxonomy can be deduced as an organic whole: The validity of a taxonomy is linked to its theoretical construction. Quine (1977) makes a parallel case:

> One's sense of similarity or one's system of kinds develops and changes . . . as one matures. . . . And at length standards of similarity set in which are geared to theoretical science. The development is away from the immediate, subjective, animal sense of similarity to the remoter objectivity of a similarity determined by scientific hypotheses . . . and constructs. Things are similar in the later or theoretical sense to the degree that they are . . . revealed by science. (p. 171)

This "remoter sense of objectivity" is essentially what is sought in the assessment process—most obviously in terms of the referral question, but also in terms of the intermediate constructs required to address the referral question, such as personality style. The purpose of personalized assessment is to develop a theory of the unique patient. That anyone would want to develop a theory of the person without a proportionally integrative theory of the constructs used to explain the person is somewhat puzzling, if not amazing. But when theory is ignored in favor of exclusively empirical inductions or factor-analytically derived orthogonal dimensions, that is essentially what is being done.

Does this mean that one has to buy into the MCMI's underlying theory to buy into the test itself? Not at all. While no other instrument is as coordinated with the official DSM taxonomy of personality disorders as is the MCMI, the official position of the DSM with regard to all taxonomic categories, including personality prototypes, is atheoretical. Moreover, the MCMI was designed from the beginning to function as an explicitly clinical inventory. It is not set in stone. As substantive advances in knowledge take place, whether as the result of compelling empirical research or well-justified theoretical deduction, the MCMI will be upgraded and refined as well. Minor elaborations and modifications have been introduced since the original MCMI's formal publication over 30 years ago; these fine-tunings will continue regularly as our understanding of the MCMI's strengths, limits, and potentials develops further.

We must add, however, that to jettison the theory would be to sell the MCMI short. In the absence of a theoretical foundation, the outline of this chapter could be effectively abbreviated to read something like the following: "These are the disorders, and this is the test, and this is how to give the test, and this is what to watch out for, and this is what to expect when such and such shows up." No "why?," just "that." In contrast, a theoretical perspective embodies well-ordered and codified links among constructs, providing a *generative* basis for making clinical inferences founded on a small number of fundamental principles. We now turn to these principles.

One goal of this chapter is to connect the conceptual structure of personality to its foundations in the natural world, which also was an aim of both Freud and Jung. The formulation presented here is akin to Freud's (1895/1966) abandoned "Project for a Scientific Psychology." Freud was endeavoring to advance our understanding of human nature by exploring interconnections among disciplines that evolved from ostensibly unrelated bodies of research and that used manifestly dissimilar languages. The approach here is also akin to Jung's effort to explicate personality functions with reference to the balancing of deeply rooted bipolarities—a theory most clearly formulated in his book *Psychological Types* (Jung, 1921/1971).

Contemporary formulations by psychologists likewise have set forth the potential and analyzed the problems involved in combining evolutionary notions with theories of individual differences and personality traits (e.g., Buss, 1990). The common goal among these proposals is not only to apply analogous principles across diverse scientific realms, but also to reduce the enormous range of psychological concepts that have proliferated throughout history; this might be achieved by exploring the power of evolutionary theory to simplify and order previously disparate personality features.

For example, all organisms seek to avoid injury, find nourishment, and reproduce their kind if they are to survive and maintain their populations. Each species is marked by commonalities in its adaptive or survival style among all members. Within each species, however, there are differences in style and in the success with which various members adapt to the diverse and changing environments they face. On this basic level, "personality" would be employed as a term to represent the more or less distinctive style of adaptive functioning that a particular member of a species exhibits as it relates to its typical range of habitats or environments. "Normal personality," so conceived, would reflect a species member's specific modes of adaptation that are effective in "average" or "expectable" environments. "Disorders of personality," in this context, would represent different styles of maladaptive functioning that can be traced to deficiencies, imbalances, or conflicts in a member's capacity to relate to the environments it faces.

A few more words should be said concerning comparisons made between evolution and ecology on the one hand, and normal and abnormal personality on the other. During its life history, an organism develops an assemblage of traits that contributes to its individual survival and reproductive success—the two essential components of fitness formulated by Darwin. Such assemblages, termed "complex adaptations and strategies" in the literature of evolutionary ecology, may be conceptualized as the biological equivalents of personality styles in the mental health literature. Biological explanations of an organism's lifetime strategy of adaptations refer primarily to variations among constituent biogenetic traits, their overall covariance structure, and the nature and ratio of favorable to unfavorable ecological resources that have been available for purposes of extending longevity and optimizing reproduction. Such explanations are not appreciably different from those used to account for the development of normal and pathological personality styles.

A relevant and intriguing parallel may be drawn between the phylogenetic evolution of a species' genetic composition and the ontogenetic development of an individual organism's adaptive strategies (i.e., its "personality style"). At any point in time, a species will possess a limited set of genes that serve as trait potentials. Over succeeding generations, the frequency distributions of these genes are likely to change in their relative proportions, depending on how well the traits they undergird contribute to the species' "fittedness" within its varying ecological habitats.

In a similar fashion, individual organisms begin life with a limited subset of their species' genes and the trait potentials they subserve. Over time, the salience of these trait potentials—not the proportions of the genes themselves—will become differentially prominent as the organism interacts with its environments. It "learns" from these experiences which of its traits "fit" best—that is, which are optimally suited to its ecosystem. In phylogenesis, then, actual gene frequencies change during the generation-to-generation adaptive process; in ontogenesis, the salience or prominence of gene-based traits is what changes as adaptive learning takes place. Parallel evolutionary processes occur, both within the life of a species and within the life of a member organism, respectively.

What is seen in the individual organism is a shaping of latent potentialities into adaptive and manifest styles of perceiving, feeling, thinking, and acting. It is our view that these distinctive modes of adaptation, engendered by the interaction of biological endowment and social experience, constitute the elements of what are termed "personality styles," whether normal or abnormal. There is a formative process over the course of a single individual's lifetime that parallels gene redistributions within a whole species during its entire evolutionary history.

The Personality Polarity Model

The theoretical model that follows is grounded in evolutionary theory (Millon, 1990; Millon & Davis, 1996). In essence, it seeks to explicate the structure and styles of personality with reference to deficient, imbalanced, or conflicted modes of ecological adaptation and reproductive strategy. The proposition that the development and functions of personological traits may be usefully explored through the lens of evolutionary principles has a long, if yet unfulfilled, tradition. Spencer (1870) and Huxley (1870) offered suggestions of this nature shortly after Darwin's seminal *Origin of Species* was published. In more recent times, we have seen the emergence of sociobiology, an interdisciplinary science that explores the interface between human social functioning and evolutionary biology (Wilson, 1975, 1978).

Four periods or phases in which evolutionary principles are demonstrated are labeled as "existence," "adaptation," "replication," and "abstraction." The first, existence, relates the serendipitous transformation of random or less organized states into those possessing distinct structures of greater organization and survivability; the second, adaptation, refers to homeostatic processes employed to sustain survival in open ecosystems; the third, replication, pertains to reproductive styles that maximize the diversification and selection of ecologically effective attributes; and the fourth, abstraction, concerns the emergence of competencies that foster anticipatory planning and reasoned decision making. Polarities derived from the first three phases (pleasure–pain, passive–active, and other–self) are used to construct a theoretically embedded classification system of personality disorders.

These polarities have forerunners in psychological theory that may be traced as far back as the early 1900s. A number of pre-World War I theorists, including Freud, proposed sets of three polarities that were used time and again as the raw materials for constructing psychological processes. Aspects of these polarities were "discovered" and employed by theorists in France, Germany, Russia, and other European nations, as well as the United States (Millon, 1990). In addition, the work of several later scholars has illuminated aspects of these polar dimensions, including Eysenck (1957, 1967), Gray (1973), Buss and Plomin (1975, 1984), Russell (1980), Tellegen (1985), and Cloninger (1986, 1987).

Much as Godel (1931) argued that the consistency of a system cannot be proven at the same level as that system, disputations between "subdisciplines" cannot be resolved by means of imperial ambitions and internecine battles; they can only be transcended at a superordinate level of integration in metatheory. Interested readers should consult Millon (1990) for an explication of these relationships.

1. The first period, "existence," concerns the maintenance of integrative phenomena—whether nuclear particles, viruses, or human beings—against the background of entropic decompensation. Evolutionary mechanisms derived from this phase regard life enhancement and life preservation. The former are concerned with orienting individuals toward improvement in the quality of life, and the latter with orienting individuals away from actions or environments that decrease the quality of life or even jeopardize existence itself. These may be called "existential aims." At the highest level of abstraction, such mechanisms form, phenomenologically or metaphorically expressed, a pleasure–pain polarity. Some individuals are conflicted in regard to these existential aims (e.g., sadistic persons), while others possess deficits in these crucial substrates (e.g., schizoid individuals). In terms of neuropsychological growth stages (Millon, 1969, 1981; Millon & Davis, 1996), the pleasure–pain polarity is recapitulated in a "sensory/attachment" phase, the purpose of which is the largely innate and rather mechanical discrimination of pleasure and pain signals (close physical warmth vs. harsh sounds, rough handling).

2. Existence, however, is but an initial phase. Once an integrative structure exists, it must maintain its existence through exchanges of energy and information with its environment. The second evolutionary phase relates to what are termed the "modes of adaptation." It too is framed as a two-part polarity: a passive orientation (i.e., a tendency to accommodate to one's ecological niche) versus an active orientation (i.e., a tendency to modify or intervene in one's surroundings). These "modes of adaptation" differ from the first phase of evolution in that they regard how that which exists endures. In terms of neuropsychological growth stages, these modes are recapitulated in a "sensorimotor/autonomy" stage, during which the child either progresses to an active orientation toward his or her physical and social context, or perpetuates the passive and dependent mode of earlier prenatal and infantile existence.

3. Although organisms may be well adapted to their environments, the existence of any life form is time-limited. To circumvent this limitation, organisms have developed "replicatory strategies" by which to generate progeny. These strategies regard what biologists have referred to as a "self-propagating strategy," at one polar extreme, and an "other-nurturing strategy," at the opposite extreme. Psychologically, the former strategy is disposed toward actions that are egotistic, insensitive, inconsiderate, and uncaring, whereas the latter is disposed toward actions that are affiliative, intimate, protective, and solicitous (Gilligan, 1982; Rushton, 1985; Wilson, 1978). Like the pleasure–pain, this self–other polarity is often deficient or conflicted. Some personality types are ambivalent on this polarity, such as the compulsive and passive-aggressive types. In terms of neuropsychological growth stages, an individual's orientation toward self and/or others is recapitulated in the pubertal gender identity stage (Millon & Davis, 1996).

Discussion of the fourth or "abstract" phase of development may be found in a number of Millon's publications (e.g., Millon, 1990).

Validation of the MCMI

According to Loevinger (1957) and Jackson (1970), validation should be an ongoing process involved in all phases of test construction, rather than a procedure for corroborating the instrument's effectiveness after its completion. With this principle in mind, validation of the MCMI, MCMI-II, and MCMI-III became an integral element at each step of development, rather than an afterthought.

Once a commitment was made to this strategy, the question remained as to what validation procedures should be used to make the final product as efficient as possible in achieving the goals of differential diagnostic and clinical interpretive utility. In her highly illuminating monograph, Loevinger (1957) proposed that development validation possesses three sequential components: "substantive," "structural," and "external." Each of these is a necessary component in construction, but not a sufficient one. Where feasible, steps should be taken to progress from the first stage through the third. A validation sequence such as this departs from procedures employed in the construction of most clinical inventories. A brief introduction to the rationale and methods of each of these three components may be a useful précis of the procedures followed in developing the MCMI, MCMI-II, and MCMI-III.

The first validation step, relabeled "theoretical/substantive validation" and termed the "deductive approach" by Burisch (1984), examines the extent to which the items constituting the instrument derive their content from an explicit theoretical framework. Such a theory has been developed (Millon, 1969, 1981, 1986b, 1990). In the MCMIs, it provides a series of clinically relevant constructs for personality trait and syndrome definition to be used as a guide in writing relevant scale items. Moreover, because both clear boundaries and anticipated relationships between syndromes can be established on rational grounds, the test can be constructed with either distinct or interrelated scales at the initial stage of development.

The second step, "internal/structural validation," refers to the model (i.e., the purity of the separate scales or the character of their expected relationships) to which the instruments' items are expected to conform. For example, each scale may be constructed as a measure of an independent trait in accord with a factorial model. In another model, each scale may be designed to possess a high degree of internal consistency and also expected to display considerable overlap with other specific scales. In the internal/structural stage, items that have already been substantively validated are administered to appropriate populations. For the MCMI, MCMI-II, and MCMI-III, the items that survived this second stage were those that maximized scale homogeneity, displayed a measure of overlap with other theoretically congruent scales, and demonstrated satisfactory levels of endorsement frequency and temporal stability.

The third step, described here as "external/criterion validation," includes only those items and scales that have met the requirements of both the substantive and the structural steps of development. It pertains to the empirical correspondence between each test scale and various nonscale measures of the trait or syndrome under study. This third step entails correlating results obtained on preliminary forms of the inventory with relevant clinical behaviors. When performed in conjunction with other assessment methods and employing diverse external criteria, this procedure may also establish each scale's convergent and discriminant validity (Campbell & Fiske, 1959).

In a classic article, Hase and Goldberg (1967) compared alternative construction strategies and found that each displayed equivalent levels of validity across a set of diverse criteria. After reviewing several subsequent parallel studies, Burisch (1984) concluded that these findings of method equivalence continued to be supported. It would seem, nevertheless, that a sequential validation strategy employing all three of these approaches would at the very least prove equal to and perhaps enjoy a measure of superiority over any single method alone. With this untested assumption in mind, developmental validation studies were begun on the MCMI. It was hoped that each stage would produce increasingly refined and accurate forms of the inventory.

Theoretical/Substantive Validation

Some of the major principles and aims that guided the development of the MCMI are presented in this section. The steps taken to generate the preliminary items of the MCMI are also presented.

Reflecting on her years of experience in test construction and evaluation, Loevinger (1972) concludes:

> If I were to draw a single conclusion from my own studies of personality measurement, it would be this: I consider it exceedingly unlikely that either by accident or by automation one will discover a measure of a major personality variable. There is no substitute for having a psychologist in charge who has at least a first-approximation conception of the trait he wishes to measure, always open to revision, of course, as data demand. Theory has always been the mark of a mature science. The time is overdue for psychology, in general, and personality measurement, in particular, to come of age. (p. 56)

Commenting on the development of the MMPI, Norman (1972) noted that criterion keying was the only recourse possible, as no adequate theory or body of established empirical data was available as an alternative. Meehl (1954), the most persuasive exponent of the criterion-keying approach, shifted from an earlier antitheoretical position to one in which a guiding theory is seen as a valuable test development tool (Meehl, 1972). In his usual insightful fashion, Meehl (1972) stated:

> One reason for the difficulties of psychometric personology, a reason I did not appreciate in my "dustbowl empiricist" paper of 1945, is the sad state of psychological theory . . .
>
> I now think that at all stages in personality test development, from initial phase of item pool construction to a late-stage optimized clinical interpretive procedure for the fully developed and "validated" instrument, theory—and by this I mean all sorts of theory, including trait theory, developmental theory, learning theory, psychodynamics, and behavior genetics—should play an important role. . . .
>
> I believe that psychology can no longer afford to adopt psychometric procedures whose methodology proceeds with almost zero reference to what bets it is reasonable to lay upon substantive personological horses. The "theory" . . . may be only weakly corroborated but I think we have to make do with it anyway. (pp. 149–151)
>
> . . . the preliminary item pool should be constructed in reliance upon all of the facts and theories bearing upon the test. Even one who advocates a relatively atheoretical

"blind empirical criterion keying" . . . need not deprive himself of whatever theoretical insight is available at the item construction stage. . . . I now believe (as I did not formerly) that an item ought to make theoretical sense. (p. 155)

Although Meehl maintained his strong commitment to the critical role played by external validation, his recognition of the guiding value of a theoretical model served significantly to reinforce the strategy undertaken in developing the MCMI, MCMI-II, and MCMI-III. Together with Loevinger, Meehl's growing appreciation of the use of theory strengthened the belief that such a course would prove both wise and fruitful.

Internal/Structural Validation

As described and elaborated by Loevinger (1957), the structural component of validity refers to an instrument's fidelity to its underlying model. Thus relationships found among the test's items and scales should correspond to the structural pattern of the instrument's theory. For example, assume that a theory posits the existence of personality characteristics formulated as independent or "pure" traits. In this case, the instrument should be designed with a factorial structure; that is, the items constituting each scale should intercorrelate positively with one another and negatively with all other scales of the instrument. The test would then exhibit fidelity to its guiding theory. Despite its use in many distinguished instruments (e.g., the Eysenck Personality Inventory [Eysenck, 1957] and the 16PF [Cattell, 1946]), a factorial model is not universally applicable, as many personality theories do not accept the notion of trait independence (Allport, 1937, 1950).

The MCMI was constructed in accord with a "polythetic" structural model, which stresses internal scale consistency but does not require the scale independence that characterizes factorial approaches. To accord with the underlying "prototypal" model of its guiding theory and its polythetic syndromal structure (Cantor, Smith, French, & Mezzich, 1980; Horowitz, Wright, Lowenstein, & Parad, 1981; Millon, 1986a, 1987b; Rosch, 1978), the scales of the MCMI should possess a high level of internal consistency, yet at the same time display selective overlap and a high degree of correlation with other theoretically related scales. For example, according to the theory, the basic personality pattern assessed by the Avoidant scale is viewed as a less severe precursor of the pathological personality disorder assessed by the Schizotypal scale. Because they represent relatively coherent clinical syndromes, each scale should exhibit reasonably strong evidence of internal consistency. At the same time, because of their polythetic structure, and hence the inherent commonalities between these two syndromes, many items on both scales should overlap, resulting in substantial interscale correlations. When high interscale correlations of this sort occur, it is often suggested that one scale could be readily substituted for the other. For a variety of reasons beyond their polythetic nature, not the least of which are the different prevalence base rates for these scale syndromes, this contention is neither logical nor pragmatic in terms of clinical theory.

In contrast to the MMPI, for which scale overlap through joint item keying evolved strictly as a result of empirically derived commonalities in diagnostic efficiency (Wakefield, Bradley, Doughtie, & Kraft, 1975), item overlap is both anticipated and guided by the polythetic structural model and the dynamic features of its underlying theory. In addition, as stated by Dahlstrom, Welsh, and Dahlstrom (1972, p. 23), "If the syndrome used in developing a given scale is relatively complex and is characterized by a wide variety of symptoms, then the scale, reflecting this behavioral heterogeneity, is likely to show important relationships with some other scales in the profile."

Dahlstrom (1969), a distinguished and active MMPI researcher, provided an articulate rationale for scale redundancy. Reflecting on whether two scales showing a high level of intercorrelation are really two measures or one, Dahlstrom recounted the experience of McKinley and Hathaway (1944), who found a substantial overlap between the MMPI's Hysteria and Hypochondriasis scales. Dahlstrom wrote:

> These investigators indicated that their initial temptation was to drop one or the other of these scales on general psychiatric cases because the two scales correlated .71. Yet careful examination of the clinical contributions of each of these scales led McKinley and Hathaway to retain both scales. . . . Several kinds of evidence were used (such as the fact that 32% of the cases of conversion hysteria had scores beyond the arbitrary cutting score on Hysteria, while being missed by the Hypochondriasis scale), but the most compelling reasons for retaining both scales lay in their configural relationships. The way these scales related to each other and the third scale in the neurotic triad, the Depression scale, provided useful data in psychodiagnostic evaluations of anxiety, depression, and somatic reactions. Information provided by such indices as hit rates or summarized in nonlinear combinations of test scales is not adequately represented in tables of intercorrelations nor accurately preserved in factor solutions . . . [which do] serious injustice to clinical assessment formulations that operate outside a narrow, geometrical view of human personality. (pp. 23–24)

Dahlstrom's suggestion for revising the MMPI consisted largely of devising separate scales for personological predispositions (personality pattern scales) and for psychopathological states (clinical syndrome scales)—precisely the distinction developed in constructing the MCMIs. And, in accord with these instruments' underlying theory, Dahlstrom commented that a separation of scales along these lines would enable researchers to test the thesis that specific ties exist between particular personality types and the clinical disorders that persons of each type will exhibit under stress, as well as the specific kinds of disorders to which each type is most susceptible. The underlying theory of the MCMI, MCMI-II, and MCMI-III can contribute most usefully in formulating these hypothesized relationships.

External/Criterion Validation

The central idea behind using external/criterion validation is quite straightforward: The items constituting a test scale should be selected on the basis of their empirically verified association with a significant and relevant criterion measure (Millon, 1994). The procedure by which this association is gauged is also direct. Preliminary items should be administered to two groups of subjects who differ on the criterion measure. The "criterion" group exhibits the trait with which the item is to be associated; the "comparison" group does not. After the test is administered, the "true" and "false" endorsement frequencies for both groups on every item are calculated. Items that statistically differentiate the criterion group from the comparison group are judged "externally valid." To ensure that these item discriminations are not spurious or do not occur merely by chance, they should be reassessed through additional studies with new cross-validation samples.

The prime virtue of the external/criterion method is that it verifies, in fact, what is only intuitively, structurally, or theoretically assumed to be an item–criterion relationship. Moreover, the method may uncover associations that are neither obvious nor readily deduced on consistency or theoretical grounds. Among the incidental advantages that may accrue from the criterion method is the identification of subtle or indirect items that subjects would have difficulty falsifying or dissembling.

There are several disadvantages to test development procedures that depend exclusively on external validation methods. These are especially problematic when diverse cross-validation follow-up studies have not been done. The items this method produces may stem from chance relationships that characterize the particular population sample used for item selections. Significant item discriminations that emerge with the construction sample, particularly those that are surprising in terms of clinical "logic," often fail to hold up when reevaluated with an apparently similar, but new, cross-validation sample.

One of the merits of the MCMI construction procedure is that all items survived the criteria of theoretical/substantive and internal/structural validity before being subjected to external validation. Hence those that survived this final stage are not likely to be judged either "surprising" or logically "inconsistent."

Accepting the rationale of external/criterion validation still leaves two additional problems. First, there is the question of the nature of the criteria to be chosen for external reference. Second, a decision must be made about which comparison groups would be most relevant for contrast with the criterion groups.

The use of practical or pragmatic criteria for external validation reference has been a subject of much debate for many years (Cattell, 1946; Lord, 1955; Loevinger, 1957; Gough, 1965). The issue is whether the criteria chosen should be composed of real clinical functions and decisions for which the test will be a substitute gauge, or whether the criteria should be less specific and reflect more generalized functions, traits, and purposes.

Lord (1955) wrote that the goal of generalized, nonpragmatic validity is neither feasible nor relevant. Rather, the true measure of validation is the instrument's discriminating power for specific decision problems. Similarly, Gough (1965) argued that the ultimate standard for validation should be the setting within which the test will be used; that is, the instrument should be evaluated by its predictive or descriptive use in a real-world, functional setting. This pragmatic philosophy for external criteria, successfully applied in validating the Strong Vocational Blank, the MMPI, and the California Psychological Inventory (CPI), achieves its greatest value by ensuring that an instrument is directly relevant to the operational services it is intended to perform.

Applying the pragmatic model to the MCMIs suggests that its use would be best gauged by its ability to predict what clinicians are likely to say in describing their patients' personality characteristics and symptom disorders. Because the items of the MCMIs had already been screened in accord with theoretical/substantive and internal/structural validation procedures, the instrument fulfilled the goals of those espousing less pragmatic and more generalizable criteria. Enhancing the practical use of the MCMIs seemed to be fully justified for the ensuing external state of validation. A careful selection of pragmatic criteria would not only refine the MCMIs by providing additional validation data, but would also help make them maximally useful to clinicians who employ them primarily for differential diagnostic and interpretive purposes.

There are numerous methods by which useful data can be gathered about patients. The most direct and clinically relevant approach would be to obtain assessments by mental health professionals who are well acquainted with the specific psychological traits and disorders of particular patients. Diagnostic appraisals by experienced psychologists, psychiatrists, and psychiatric social workers, in contrast to those of nonprofessional relatives and acquaintances, would discriminate psychologically subtle as well as gross differences among patients. Thus operational criteria composed of professional clinical assessments would not only be pertinent and practical, but would also furnish those more precise discriminations necessary to make the instrument an efficient differential diagnostic tool.

Guidelines for Use of the MCMI-III

Like its predecessors, the MCMI-III is not a general personality instrument to be used for "normal" populations or for purposes other than diagnostic screening or clinical assessment. Hence it contrasts with other, more broadly applied inventories whose presumed utility for diverse populations may not be as suitable as is often thought.

Normative data and transformation scores for the MCMI-III are based entirely on clinical samples and are applicable only to persons who evidence psychological symptoms or are engaged in a program of professional psychotherapy or psychodiagnostic evaluation. Although its use as an operational measure of relevant theoretical constructs is fully justified, the samples employed for such purposes are best drawn only from comparable clinical populations. To administer the MCMI-III to a wider range of problems or class of subjects (such as those found in business and industry), or to identify neurological lesions, or to use it for the assessment of general personality traits among college students is to apply the instrument to settings and samples for which it is neither intended nor appropriate.

Clinicians working with physically ill, behavioral medicine, or rehabilitation patients are directed to one of the MCMI-III's associated inventories, the Millon Behavioral Medicine Diagnostic (MBMD; Millon, Antoni, Millon, Minor, & Grossman, 2001). Similarly, when the population to be assessed is composed of psychologically troubled teenagers at the junior or senior high school or beginning college levels, the clinician is advised to employ the Millon Adolescent Clinical Inventory (MACI; Millon, 1993). Both of these instruments are available through Pearson Assessments, as the MCMI-III itself now is. Those who wish to appraise the psychological attributes and traits of nonclinical (i.e., "normal") adults may wish to utilize the Millon Index of Personality Styles *Revised* (MIPS *Revised*; Millon, 2003). This latter inventory is especially suitable as a gauge of the broader theory's constructs.

The MCMI-III provides in-depth clinical reports that can be transmitted via U.S. mail, on-site software programs, or electronic teleprocessing methods with instant turnaround. Several principles should be followed to protect confidentiality and to assure appropriate professional standards among those who use the instrument or who avail themselves of its associated computer scoring and interpretive services (Zachary & Pope, 1984). To maintain anonymity, the use of code numbers rather than names is recommended in completing answer sheets; furthermore, only the mental health professional responsible for each case should possess the code for patient identification. This recommendation is especially warranted when the automated interpretive report is used.

In general, those who use the instrument and its associated reports or those who supervise its use should have a sufficient background in test logic, psychometric methods, and clinical practice theory to understand test manuals (Skinner & Pakula, 1986). Those who use the MCMI-III and its reports should have at a minimum a master's degree in clinical or counseling psychology or psychiatric social work, or should have internship or psychiatric residency status. With the exception of graduate school training or research situations (in which supervision should be mandatory), the use of the automated scoring and interpretive services should be limited to clinicians who meet full membership qualifications for the American Psychological Association, the American Psychiatric Association, the American Medical Association, the American Association for Marriage and Family Therapy, or the National Association of Social Workers. In short, the reading of a computerized report is no substitute for clinical judgment. Only those trained in the limits of psychological tests should make use of them.

Because the automated interpretive report service is considered a professional-to-professional consultation, it is the responsibility of the consultee to view the report as only one facet of a total patient evaluation, and to recognize that the information it contains is a series of tentative judgments rather than a set of definitive statements. The integration of selected features of the report into ongoing management and treatment decisions with patients is fully appropriate, but the direct sharing of the report's explicit content with either patients or their relatives is strongly discouraged.

The paragraphs that precede all MCMI-III interpretive reports state that the narrative text "should be evaluated in conjunction with additional clinical data." Such data include current life circumstances, observed behavior, biographical history, interview responses, and information from other tests. The accuracy and richness of any self-report measure's results are enhanced when these findings are appraised in the context of other clinical sources. Not only does the combination of various gauges from diverse settings provide the data aggregates (Epstein, 1979, 1983) that increase the likelihood of drawing correct inferences; multimethod approaches (Campbell & Fiske, 1959) provide both the experienced and the novice clinician with an optimal base for deciphering those special, if not unique, features that characterize each patient.

No less important than the insights provided by non-self-report sources of clinical data is the interpretive guidance furnished by various nonclinical demographic indices (e.g., age, sex, marital status, vocation, ethnicity, socioeconomic factors, educational level). Although higher or lower MCMI-III scale elevations associated with these population characteristics often reflect "real" differences in prevalence rates (e.g., male police officers score higher on certain scales than do male teachers, and do so in a manner consistent with nontest personality data), it is important for clinicians to have a reasonable notion of what is typical for patients of particular demographic backgrounds. Special scoring norms are being developed for ethnicity to accommodate this major variable. Similarly, a number of scale "modifiers" are utilized in the MCMI-III to compensate for differences among patients in their distortion tendencies, notably candor and exaggeration. Whatever the efficacy of these corrections may be, it behooves the clinician to consider carefully the impact of important demographics—not only to compensate for their effects, but for the insights they may furnish and for their ability to individualize and enrich the meaning of the MCMI-III's clinical data.

Important implications for evaluating MCMI-III results stem from the fact that certain personality scales are sensitive to the current affective state of a patient. All self-report inventory scales, be they personality-oriented (Axis II) or syndrome-oriented (Axis I), reflect in varying degrees both "traits" and "states." Despite methodological and psychometric procedures to tease the enduring characteristics of personality apart from clinical features of a more transient quality, every scale reflects a mix of predisposing and generalizing attributes, as well as those of a more situational or acute nature. Noteworthy are the partial blurring effects of current depressive and anxiety states upon specific personality scales (Hirschfeld et al., 1983). These results stem in part from shared scale items (Wiggins, 1982), but the level of covariation is appreciably greater than can be accounted for by item overlap alone. Experience with earlier versions of the MCMI indicates that dysthymic and anxious states accentuate scores on certain MCMI personality scales while unduly diminishing those obtained on others—a view consistent with research by such investigators as Shea, Glass, Pilkonis, Watkins, and Docherty (1987).

Compensatory efforts have been made to counter the effect of other potentially distorting effects by rephrasing MCMI-III items so as to separate clinical and state phenomena more clearly from those of a more long-standing or trait nature, as well as to build in scoring adjustments that automatically correct for the influences of marked or acute affective states. Nevertheless, clinicians should bear in mind the possibility of occasional personality disorder misrenderings when scores on the Anxiety and Dysthymia scales appear unusually or unexpectedly high or low, in light of other sources of clinical evidence.

Users of computer-based interpretive reports register high levels of satisfaction, both in the overall quality of these reports and in their correspondence with independently derived clinical observations and judgments (Green, 1982; Craig, 1993). Encouraging as studies such as these may be in affirming "customer satisfaction," they may prove spurious in failing to recognize the so-called "Barnum effect"—that is, the tendency of recipients of personality characterizations to conclude that such reports are accurate, not because they are, but because they present attributes of such high generality or commonality as to be applicable to almost all individuals. Moreover, the mysterious and seemingly mythic powers of computer technologies have no doubt imbued its reports, at least for some, with an undue measure of scientific merit and clinical acumen.

Users of diagnostic characterizations provided via computer systems should be wary lest they find themselves lulled over time into an uncritical acceptance of computer-based reports; they should routinely compare the interpretive statements contained in such reports against independently generated clinical evidence.

However—and notwithstanding the preceding caution—the findings of investigations into the validity of MCMI interpretive reports provided strong evidence that ratings of that inventory's accuracy were higher than could be accounted for by either the Barnum effect or the computer-generated format (Moreland & Onstad, 1987; Sandberg, 1987; Craig, 1993).

As should be evident, there are distinct boundaries to the accuracy of the self-report method of clinical data collection; by no means is it a perfect data source. The inherent psychometric limits of the tool, the tendency of similar patients to interpret questions differently, the effect of current affective states on trait measures, and the efforts of patients to effect certain false appearances and impressions all reduce the upper boundaries of this method's potential accuracy. However, when a self-report instrument is constructed in line with accepted techniques of validation (Loevinger, 1957), the inventory should begin to approach these upper boundaries. Given that it progressed through such a developmental background, we found that MCMI reports proved to be on the mark in about 55% to 65% of patients to whom it was administered; it was appraised as both useful and generally valid, although with partial misjudgments, in about another 25% to 30% of cases; and they appeared off target (i.e., appreciably in error) about 10% to 15% of the time. These positive figures, we should note, were in the quantitative range of five to six times greater than chance.

Although accuracy levels vary from setting to setting, these differences largely reflect difficulties in decoding the presence of a disorder at the time it is being appraised (e.g., identifying histrionic personality disorder during a patient's depression). Also problematic is the disorder's prevalence or base rate; on purely mathematical grounds, diagnostic groups with notably low (e.g., suicide) or high (e.g., dysthymia) base rates prove statistically troublesome, in that even the most optimal of selected cutoffs often produce hit rates that are only marginally superior to chance (Meehl & Rosen, 1955; Rorer & Dawes, 1982).

A point related to the preceding is that the MCMI-III's diagnostic scale cutoffs and profile interpretations are oriented to the majority of patients who take the inventory—that is, to those displaying psychic disturbances in the midranges of severity, rather than to those whose difficulties are either close to "normal" (e.g., workers' compensation litigants, spouses of patients in marital therapy) or of manifest clinical severity (e.g., patients with acute psychoses or chronic schizophrenia). To maximize both diagnostic and interpretive validity, narratives have been written to focus on moderate levels of pathology; this results in a slightly diminished degree of diagnostic and interpretive accuracy among patients in both the least and the most severe ranges of psychological disturbance—a fact that users of the interpretive reports should bear in mind. Narrative analyses of patients experiencing ordinary life difficulties or minor adjustment disorders will tend to be construed as more troubled than they are; conversely, those with the most serious pathologies will often be considered as less severely disturbed than they are.

In summary, this discussion has stressed the importance of having the results of the MCMI-III evaluated concurrently with a variety of other clinical data, and of having this endeavor undertaken by properly trained clinicians who know the limitations both of the self-report modality in general and of the MCMI-III in particular.

References

Allport, G. W. (1937). *Personality: A psychological interpretation.* New York: Holt.

Allport, G. W. (1950). *The nature of personality: Selected papers.* Cambridge, MA: Addison-Wesley.

American Psychiatric Association. (1980). *Diagnostic and statistical manual of mental disorders* (3rd ed.). Washington, DC: Author.

American Psychiatric Association. (1987). *Diagnostic and statistical manual of mental disorders* (3rd ed., rev.). Washington, DC: Author.

Burisch, M. (1984). Approaches to personality inventory construction: A comparison of merits. *American Psychologist, 39,* 214–227.

Buss, A., & Plomin, R. (1975). *A temperament theory of personality development.* New York: Wiley.

Buss, A., & Plomin, R. (1984). *Temperament: Early developing personality traits.* Hillsdale, NJ: Erlbaum.

Buss, D. (1990). Biological foundations of personality. *Journal of Personality, 58,* 1–34.

Butcher, J. N., Graham, J. R., Williams, C. L., & Ben-Porath, Y. S. (1990). *Development and use of the MMPI-2 content scales.* Minneapolis: University of Minnesota Press.

Campbell, D. T., & Fiske, D. W. (1959). Convergent and discriminant validation by the multitrait-multimethod matrix. *Psychological Bulletin, 56,* 81–105.

Cantor, N., Smith, E. E., French, R. D., & Mezzich, J. (1980). Psychiatric diagnosis as prototype categorization. *Journal of Abnormal Psychology, 89,* 181–193.

Cattell, R. B. (1946). *Description and measurement of personality.* Yonkers, NY: World Book.

Cloninger, C. R. (1986). A unified biosocial theory of personality and its role in the development of anxiety states. *Psychiatric Developments, 3,* 167–226.

Cloninger, C. R. (1987). A systematic method for clinical description and classification of personality variants. *Archives of General Psychiatry, 44,* 573–588.

Costa, P. T., & McCrae, R. R. (1992). *The NEO Personality Inventory—Revised manual.* Odessa, FL: Psychological Assessment Resources.

Craig, R. J. (Ed.). (1993). *The Millon Clinical Multiaxial Inventory: A clinical research information synthesis.* Hillsdale, NJ: Erlbaum.

Dahlstrom, W. G. (1969). Recurrent issues in the development of the MMPI. In J. N. Butcher (Ed.), *MMPI: Research developments and clinical applications* (pp. 1–40). New York: McGraw-Hill.

Dahlstrom, W. G., Welsh, G. S., & Dahlstrom, L. E. (1972). *An MMPI handbook* (Vol. 1). Minneapolis: University of Minnesota Press.

Epstein, S. (1979). The stability of behavior: 1. On predicting most of the people much of the time. *Journal of Personality and Social Psychology, 37,* 1097–1126.

Epstein, S. (1983). Aggregation and beyond: Some basic issues on the prediction of behavior. *Journal of Personality, 51,* 360–392.

Exner, J. E., Jr. (1986). *The Rorschach: A comprehensive system.* New York: Wiley Interscience.

Eysenck, H. J. (1957). *The dynamics of anxiety and hysteria.* London: Routledge & Kegan Paul.

Eysenck, H. J. (1967). *The biological basis of personality.* Springfield, IL: Thomas.

Freud, S. (1966). Project for a scientific psychology. In J. Strachey (Ed. & Trans.), *The standard edition of the complete psychological works of Sigmund Freud* (Vol. 1, pp. 281–397). London: Hogarth Press. (Original work composed 1895)

Gilligan, C. (1982). *In a different voice.* Cambridge, MA: Harvard University Press.

Godel, K. (1931). *On formally undecidable propositions of principia mathematica and related systems.* Unpublished doctoral dissertation, University of Vienna.

Gough, H. G. (1965). *Some thoughts on test usage and test development.* Paper presented at the annual meeting of the American Personnel and Guidance Association, Los Angeles.

Gray, J. A. (1973). Causal theories of personalities and how to test them. In J. R. Royce (Ed.), *Multivariate analysis and psychological theory.* New York: Academic Press.

Green, C. J. (1982). The diagnostic accuracy and utility of MMPI and MCMI computer interpretive reports. *Journal of Personality Assessment, 46,* 359–365.

Harris, R. E., & Lingoes, J. C. (1955, 1968). *Subscales for the MMPI: An aid to profile interpretation.* Unpublished manuscripts, Langley–Porter Neuropsychiatric Institute.

Hase, H. E., & Goldberg, L. R. (1967). Comparative validity of different strategies of devising personality inventory scales. *Psychological Bulletin, 67,* 231–248.

Hempel, C. (1965). *Aspects of scientific explanation.* New York: Free Press.

Hirschfeld, R. M., Klerman, G. L., Clayton, P. J., Keller, M. P., McDonald-Scott, M. A., & Larkin, B. H. (1983). Assessing personality: Effects of the depressive state on trait measurement. *American Journal of Psychiatry, 140,* 695–699.

Horowitz, L. M., Wright, J. C., Lowenstein, E., & Parad, H. W. (1981). The prototype as a construct in abnormal psychology: 1. A method for deriving prototypes. *Journal of Abnormal Psychology, 90,* 568–574.

Huxley, T. H. (1870). Mr. Darwin's critics. *Contemporary Review, 18,* 443–476.

Jackson, D. N. (1970). A sequential system for personality scale development. In C. D. Spielberger (Ed.), *Current topics in clinical and community psychology* (Vol. 2, pp. 61–92). New York: Academic Press.

Jung, C. (1971). *Psychological types.* Zurich: Rasher Verlag. (Original work published 1921)

Loevinger, J. (1957). Objective tests as instruments of psychological theory. *Psychological Reports, 3,* 635–694.

Loevinger, J. (1972). Some limitations of objective personality tests. In J. N. Butcher (Ed.), *Objective personality assessment* (pp. 45–58). New York: Academic Press.

Lord, F. M. (1955). Some perspectives on "The alternation paradox in test theory." *Psychological Bulletin, 52,* 505–510.

McKinley, J. C., & Hathaway, S. R. (1944). The Minnesota Multiphasic Personality Inventory: V. Hysteria, Hypomania, and Psychopathic Deviate. *Journal of Applied Psychology, 28,* 153–174.

Meehl, P. E. (1954). *Clinical versus statistical prediction.* Minneapolis: University of Minnesota Press.

Meehl, P. E. (1972). Specific genetic etiology, psychodynamics, and therapeutic nihilism. *International Journal of Mental Health, 1,* 10–27.

Meehl, P. E., & Rosen, A. (1955). Antecedent probability and the efficiency of psychometric signs, patterns, or cutting scores. *Psychological Bulletin, 52,* 194–216.

Millon, T. (1969). *Modern psychopathology: A biosocial approach to maladaptive learning and functioning.* Philadelphia: Saunders.

Millon, T. (1977). *Millon Clinical Multiaxial Inventory manual.* Minneapolis, MN: National Computer Systems.

Millon, T. (1981). *Disorders of personality: DSM-III, Axis II.* New York: Wiley-Interscience.

Millon, T. (1986a). Personality prototypes and their diagnostic criteria. In T. Millon & G. L. Klerman (Eds.), *Contemporary directions in psychopathology: Toward the DSM-IV* (pp. 571–712). New York: Guilford Press.

Millon, T. (1986b). A theoretical derivation of pathological personalities. In T. Millon & G. L. Klerman (Eds.), *Contemporary directions in psychopathology: Toward the DSM-IV* (pp. 639–669). New York: Guilford Press.

Millon, T. (1987). *Manual for the MCMI-II.* Minneapolis, MN: National Computer Systems.

Millon, T. (1990). *Toward a new personology: An evolutionary model.* New York: Wiley-Interscience.

Millon, T. (2003). *Millon Index of Personality Styles Revised.* Minneapolis, MN: Pearson Assessments.

Millon, T., Antoni, M. H., Millon, C., Minor, S., & Grossman, S. D. (2001). *Millon Behavioral Medicine Diagnostic (MBMD).* Minneapolis, MN: Pearson Assessments.

Millon, T., & Davis, R. (1996). *Disorders of personality: DSM-IV and beyond.* New York: Wiley.

Millon, T., & Diesenhaus, H. (1972). *Research methods in psychopathology.* New York: Wiley.

Millon, T., & Grossman, S. D. (2007a). *Resolving difficult clinical syndromes: A personalized psychotherapy approach.* Hoboken, NJ: Wiley.

Millon, T., & Grossman, S. D. (2007b). *Overcoming resistant personality disorders: A personalized psychotherapy approach.* Hoboken, NJ: Wiley.

Millon, T., & Grossman, S. D. (2007c). *Moderating severe personality disorders: A personalized psychotherapy approach.* Hoboken, NJ: Wiley.

Millon, T. (with Millon, C., & Davis, R.). (1993). *Millon Adolescent Clinical Inventory.* Minneapolis, MN: National Computer Systems.

Millon, T. (with Millon, C., & Davis, R.). (1994). *Millon Clinical Multiaxial Inventory–III manual.* Minneapolis, MN: National Computer Systems.

Moreland, K. L., & Onstad, J. A. (1987). Validity of Millon's computerized interpretation system for the MCMI: A controlled study. *Journal of Consulting and Clinical Psychology, 55,* 113–114.

Murray, H. A. (Ed.). (1938). *Explorations in personality.* New York: Oxford University Press.

Norman, W. T. (1972). Psychometric considerations for a revision of the MMPI. In J. N. Butcher (Ed.), *Objective personality assessment* (pp. 59–84). New York: Academic Press.

Quine, W. V. O. (1977). Natural kinds. In S. P. Schwartz (Ed.), *Naming, necessity, and natural groups.* Ithaca, NY: Cornell University Press.

Rorer, L. G., & Dawes, R. M. (1982). A base-rate bootstrap. *Journal of Consulting and Clinical Psychology, 50,* 419–425.

Rorschach, H. (1921). *Psychodiagnostik.* Bern, Switzerland: Bircher.

Rosch, E. (1978). Principles of categorization. In E. Rosch & D. B. Lloyds (Eds.), *Cognition and categorization.* Hillsdale, NJ: Erlbaum.

Rushton, J. P. (1985). Differential K theory: The sociobiology of individual and group differences. *Personality and Individual Differences, 6,* 441–452.

Russell, J. A. (1980). A circumplex model of affect. *Journal of Personality and Social Psychology, 39*(1), 1611–1678.

Sandberg, M. L. (1987). Is the ostensive accuracy of computer interpretive reports a result of the Barnum effect?: A study of the MCMI. In C. Green (Ed.), *Conference on the Millon clinical inventories (MCMI, MBHI, MAPI)* (pp. 155–164). Minneapolis: National Computer Systems.

Shea, M. T., Glass, D. R., Pilkonis, P. A., Watkins, J., & Docherty, J. P. (1987). Frequency and complications of personality disorders in a sample of depressed outpatients. *Journal of Personality Disorders, 1,* 27–42.

Skinner, H. A., & Pakula, A. (1986). Challenge of computers in psychological assessment. *Professional Psychology: Research and Practice, 17,* 44–50.

Spencer, H. (1870). *The principles of psychology.* London: Williams & Norgate.

Tellegen, A. (1985). Structures of mood and personality and relevance to assessing anxiety with an emphasis on self-report. In A. H. Tuma & J. Maser (Eds.), *Anxiety and the anxiety disorders.* Hillsdale, NJ: Erlbaum.

Wakefield, J. A., Bradley, P. E., Doughtie, E. B., & Kraft, I. A. (1975). Influence of overlapping and nonoverlapping items on the theoretical interrelationships of MMPI scales. *Journal of Consulting and Clinical Psychology, 43,* 851–857.

Wiggins, J. (1982). Circumplex models of interpersonal behavior in clinical psychology. In P. Kendall & J. N. Butcher (Eds.), *Handbook of research methods in clinical psychology* (pp. 183–222). New York: Wiley.

Wiggins, J. S. (1969). Content dimensions in the MMPI. In J. N. Butcher (Ed.), *MMPI: Research developments and clinical applications* (pp. 129–180). New York: McGraw-Hill.

Wilson, E. O. (1975). *Sociobiology: The new synthesis.* Cambridge, MA: Harvard University Press.

Wilson, E. O. (1978). *On human nature.* Cambridge, MA: Harvard University Press.

Zachary, R. A., & Pope, K. S. (1984). Legal and ethical issues in the clinical use of computerized testing. In M. D. Schwartz (Ed.), *Using computers in clinical practice* (pp. 212–238). New York: Haworth Press.

CHAPTER 4

Guidelines for the Contemporary Interpretation of the MCMI-III

Edward D. Rossini
James P. Choca

Over 30 years after the publication of the initial version, the Millon Clinical Multiaxial Inventory–III (MCMI-III; Millon, 1994) has met the millennium and is firmly established as the briefest and yet most distinctive of the "Big Three" comprehensive psychometric inventories measuring adult personality traits and adult psychopathology. The others are obviously the substantially longer Minnesota Multiphasic Personality Inventory–2 (MMPI-2; Butcher, Dahlstrom, Graham, Tellegen, & Kaemmer, 1989) and, to a lesser extent, the Personality Assessment Inventory (Morey, 1991). The latter two have considerable practical and conceptual limitations, despite their widespread use. However, surveys of psychological test usage consistently rate the MCMI-III and its companion inventories as quite popular across evaluation and treatment settings, with increasing popularity noted over the 1990s (Belter & Piotrowski, 2001).

The clinical utility of the MCMI-III is evident from the growing library of supplemental books now available. These range from basic descriptive textbooks for psychology graduate students and beginning MCMI-III assessors (e.g., Jankowski, 2002; Strack, 2002), to more sophisticated interpretive guides for seasoned clinicians who are familiar both with Millon's evolving personality theories and with the unique psychometric characteristics of the test itself (Choca, 2004; Craig, 1993). There are more specialized volumes for traditional psychotherapists using the MCMI-III in case formulation and treatment planning (Retzlaff, 1995), as well as for clinicians treating substance abuse/chemical dependence (Craig, 2005a). Finally, there is now a comprehensive handbook for research-based MCMI-III clinicians (Craig, 2005b).

This chapter presents our method of interpreting MCMI-III profiles. This approach is presented in depth in Chapter 10 of the textbook published by the American Psychological Association (Choca, 2004). Although other MCMI-III interpretive strategies and guidelines are available and potentially useful in assessment situations, we have found the logical seven-step, sequential process we describe in this chapter to be especially helpful for understanding *patients as people*. This means developing a more dynamic understanding of the patients' basic or premorbid personality style, their level of personality organization, and the likelihood of their being diagnosed with a personality disorder, in addition to the standard psychometric task of measuring their subtle or obvious psychiatric symptoms.

The MCMI-III was explicitly designed as a stand-alone comprehensive personality inventory to measure both major psychiatric disorders and the full range of character psychopathology. One unique aspect of the MCMI-III is its ability to detect and rank-order the traditional personality disorders. Millon's conceptualizations of the number and description of personality disorders and their subtypes (Millon, Grossman, Millon, Meagher, & Ramnath, 2004) derive from his theories of personality and are not necessarily isomorphic with the official psychiatric nomenclature of Axis II personality disorders found in the current version (fourth edition, text revision) of the *Diagnostic and Statistical Manual of Mental Disorders* (DSM-IV-TR; American Psychiatric Association, 2000).

A comprehensive MCMI-III interpretation model will also provide guidelines for refining basic diagnostic inferences (e.g., standard diagnoses), as well as for linking patients with more specific forms of individual or group psychotherapy, or even recommending for or against such common self-help programs as Alcoholics Anonymous/Narcotics Anonymous. One unique feature of our approach is using the MCMI-III profile to identify potential personality-based problems in establishing (or deepening) a working therapeutic alliance, as well as possibly providing the treating clinician with a roadmap for treatment planning by predicting likely treatment problems. Millon's personality-based psychotherapy textbook (Millon, 1999) and the series of treatment books inspired by his theoretical model (e.g., Craig, 2005c) are based on this element of our model. Improvements in MCMI-III interpretation are largely due to the availability of these alternate clinical–psychometric perspectives, each developed by front-line clinical psychologists.

Careful, ongoing use of the MCMI-III—ideally, with patients with whom professionals are well acquainted—will help users at all levels of experience to best understand and utilize this deceptively complex instrument. But, as in all psychodiagnostic practice, close initial supervision and ongoing consultation constitute the other avenue to developing MCMI-III expertise. Guidelines for using the MCMI-III in report writing are also available (Kvaal, Choca, & Groth-Marnat, 2003). Little prerequisite knowledge is needed for using and interpreting the MCMI-III beyond a graduate-level understanding of psychometrics, familiarity with the principles of clinical assessment practice, and a more in-depth knowledge of the test itself. Because it is linked to the standard psychiatric diagnostic system, using the MCMI-III requires a professional-level knowledge of DSM-IV-TR (American Psychiatric Association, 2000). In addition, familiarity with the recently published *Psychodynamic Diagnostic Manual* (PDM Task Force, 2006), a psychodynamic and dimensional nosology of lifespan mental disorders, is also recommended—especially for more psychoanalytic clinicians and for psychotherapists using the MCMI-III in an interactive therapeutic assessment model, as is done with the Psychodynamic Character Inventory (Glickhauf-Hughes & Wells, 1997).

Our interpretive approach has seven logical steps:

1. Understand the test-taking approach of the patient, and amend one's interpretation of the MCMI-III profile accordingly.
2. Review for any critical individual items.
3. Define the patient's basic personality *style*, using the best-fitting of the 80 common MCMI-III code types presented in Choca (2004).
4. Assess the level of personality organization or adaptive functioning, using both MCMI-III and known case history; consider formal Axis II diagnoses.
5. Determine the nature and severity of the Axis I symptom pattern reported.
6. Review all of the information to posit a holistic diagnostic formulation, again focused on the *patient as person*.
7. Make focal treatment or other aftercare recommendations based on that holistic formulation, rather than by using mechanistic psychiatric guidelines based exclusively on Axis I diagnoses.

A Descriptive Précis of the MCMI-III

Our goal in this chapter is not just to provide another scale-by-scale description of the MCMI-III. This essential information is presented in detail in the MCMI-III manual (Millon, 1994, 1997, 2006), and there are now many useful, thoughtful chapter-length descriptive treatments (e.g., Van Denburg & Choca, 1997; Groth-Marnat, 2003; Retzlaff & Dunn, 2003). Rather, we hope to provide a brief, engaging version of the comprehensive interpretive system presented in Choca (2004)—the coherent approach to integrating the divergent patterns that often emerge on this complex test, once the structural essential elements are reviewed.

Most readers know the basic structure of the test. The MCMI-III has 175 dichotomous (true–false) questions that are scored on 28 scales. The scales are divided into 4 Modifying/Validity Indices, 11 Moderate Personality Disorder Scales or Clinical Personality Patterns, 3 Severe Personality Pathology Scales, and 10 Moderate or Severe Clinical Syndrome Scales. Our system somewhat rearranges the personality scales, so that 3 of the current Moderate Personality Disorder scales/Clinical Personality Patterns are considered along with the Severe Personality Pathology canon.

All but 2 of the MCMI-III scales use the base rate metric rather than the more commonly used standard scaled scores (*T*-scores). A failure to understand base rate scores is a principal and enduring source of confusion regarding all of the Millon tests. Base rates are initially complex to appreciate, but are essentially ordinal-level classifications of trait/style/syndrome severity. Base rates are numbered on an arbitrary scale ranging from 0 to 115. The most relevant diagnostic base rate anchor points are 0, 75, and 85. Most clinicians accept 75 as the base rate or anchor point to infer the definite presence of the specific trait or syndrome being measured. It is the "critical cutoff" score used to make a dichotomous normal-or-abnormal decision. Any MCMI-III base rate score lower than 75 is generally considered to be a nonclinical elevation. From a more conceptual perspective, understanding the meanings of the base rate score 35 (the median score for nonclinical populations) and 60 (the median score for psychiatric patients) is also useful for locating a person in a conceptual distribution of psychopathology. In contrast to other comprehensive personality tests, low base rate scores do not imply low (or the absence of) psychopathology.

Again, a MCMI-III base rate score is considered elevated or is interpreted as in the "clinical" range only if it is at least 75. The initial decision rule is dichotomous: whether a scale is "clinical" or "nonclinical" in elevation. A base rate score of 75 on any scale means that the patient has a clinically interesting amount or degree of the syndrome or personality style. The second decision is to assign its level of severity within the "clinical" classification. A base rate score of 85 is the traditional anchor point for inferring that a patient has the strongest possibility of manifesting a serious amount/degree of the relevant scale. The higher the base rate score, the more severe the diagnostic inference.

Profile Validity

One of the hallmarks of comprehensive psychometric tests—inventories as contrasted with simple single-score psychiatric rating scales—is the embedding of items useful in detecting the test taker's attitude toward self-disclosure. These are usually called "validity scales," and they can help the evaluator decide whether or not to discard a profile. The MCMI-III has one Validity scale (V). This scale has three items that virtually no person could affirmatively endorse (e.g., "I have not seen a car in the last ten years" [item 157]). If any of these three items is endorsed, the clinician needs to reassess the client's reading level, check his or her ability to sustain attention, or inquire about obvious dissimulation. The Pearson Assessments readout flags these critical items, and when two or more are endorsed, the profile is considered truly invalid (discardable). Many patients freely report that they found the "trick" questions and responded appropriately.

However, it is a false dichotomy to view a MCMI-III profile as either valid (interpretable) or invalid (uninterpretable). Such a simple view misses the rich interpretive potential for understanding a person on the initial basis of his or her response style. In routine clinical practice, exceedingly few MCMI-III profiles are truly invalid (i.e., inferentially useless and thereby discardable). These rare instances inevitably occur in forensic evaluations or other involuntary evaluations with clients who are openly hostile to the assessment process. Such rare patients either are so acutely impaired that any psychometric evaluation is impossible, or are not paying attention to the items of the test (e.g., all true profiles). We have also seen obvious attempts at oppositional humor as well (e.g., coding curse words or "happy faces" onto the answer sheet).

Beyond simple validity, the MCMI-III has three other relevant scales referred to as Modifying Indices: Disclosure, Desirability, and Debasement. Aberrant scores on these scales are used to modify the base rate score and the interpretation of the clinical and personality scales. As the MCMI-III is a self-report inventory, the initial step in the interpretive process is to assess the person's candor and/or self-presentational persona: How does this individual portray him- or herself? Understanding the Modifying Indices provides an insight into a patient's self-presentation and is especially useful for crafting psychodynamic case formulations beyond DSM-IV-TR diagnoses (Perry, Cooper, & Michels, 1987; Ivey, 2006).

The three Modifying Indices can be interpreted in the following manner. The Debasement index (Z) is used to understand whether a patient is presenting him- or herself in a harshly self-critical or pathological manner. Elevations on this index are roughly analogous to elevations on the basic F scale of the MMPI-2. However, this level of polysymptomatic presentation may be authentic or feigned for secondary gain purposes. To use another MMPI-2 analogy, this scale can be seen as measuring self-presented psychological pain (Trimboli & Kilgore, 1983). The Desirability index (Y) is the converse. This index offers insight into positive self-representation, especially useful for inferring "flight-into-health" presentations or frank denial of an obvious clinical syndrome.

The Disclosure index (X) is not a true psychometric scale, but a composite score computed from items across the personality scales. It can be interpreted as an index of candid self-disclosure or, conversely, a measure of self-reporting defensiveness.

Clinical Syndrome Scales

Some of the 10 Clinical Syndrome Scales have direct relevance to any assessment situation (e.g., Anxiety, Dysthymia), whereas others reflect more specialized assessment (e.g., Somatoform). Many referrals are received for patients with known Axis I disorders, in which case elevated scores on these scales merely serve to corroborate what is already known, or to update the currency of the presenting symptoms. The interpretation of these scales is fairly straightforward.

However, several authors have described some of the Clinical Syndrome Scales as relatively weak or problematic, including Somatoform, Alcohol Dependence, Drug Dependence, and Post-Traumatic Stress Disorder. For example, Retzlaff and Dunn (2003) have recommended that the Somatoform scale be cautiously interpreted at best, especially among medical patients. The others have been criticized for their overt (face valid) statements, which can be readily denied. Any comprehensive personality measure must measure the range of common psychiatric symptoms, but the uniqueness of the MCMI-III and its increasing use are largely due to its focus on personality traits and Axis II disorders.

Scales for Personality Styles/Disorders

In our view, 8 of the 11 current Moderate Personality Disorder Scales/Clinical Personality Patterns constitute the beginning point of any truly idiographic understanding of the person who has completed the MCMI-III. To interpret these scales, the clinician needs to (1) select the appropriate elevated scales though to be of clinical relevance; (2) integrate the different, often divergent, aspects of the elevated scales into a cohesive description, rather than a string of concurrent validity statements;

and (3) reach an understanding about the developmental level of organization (e.g., Acklin, 1992, 1993), or the severity of dysfunctionality, of the individual's personality.

The first task of selecting which of these basic personality scales to interpret is not as straightforward as it would appear at first glance. Some profiles have a single high-point elevation, whereas most clinical profiles have multiple clinical elevations. As Millon (2004) has noted in another context, even seemingly discrete personality disorder prototypes usually have important, if subtle, subtypes.

One strategy, that of interpreting the single highest scale ("spike"), is appealing in its diagnostic simplicity; however, it does not do justice either to the inherent complexity of most people, or to the psychometric discriminating power of the test itself. This approach reinforces the common, if pejorative, clinical practice of referring to people as diagnostic prototypes (e.g., "I just saw another borderline"). This approach misses the continuity of even dominant personality styles from mild to severe, as well as the well-known fact that few people actually match their putative focal DSM-IV-TR prototypal descriptions. The use of the single high score distributes individuals into neat categorical classes at the expense of idiosyncratic understanding of their complexity. However, such an approach may be useful in clinical research, where discrete nominal-level groups may be needed. Moreover, the single-high-point approach may indeed be useful clinically if only one personality scale score is elevated, and no other score is close. Some people do report themselves in a manner consistent with a single prototypal portrait, such as that of the dependent personality (e.g., Bornstein, 2005).

A more sophisticated approach is to interpret in an integrative fashion several personality scales if more than one of these is elevated. A common practice is to consider up to three personality scale elevations. Clinical judgment may be necessary for determining which elevations to interpret. If there are two very highly elevated scales, for instance, and the score on the third scale is substantially lower, the examiner may decide only to consider the top two scales.

One major difference between our approach and the canonical interpretation is our focus on Millon's eight original basic personality scales: Schizoid, Avoidant, Dependent, Histrionic, Narcissistic, Antisocial, Compulsive, and Negativistic. As was proposed in Millon's (1969) original book, milder forms of these personality styles are often found in relatively healthy individuals. Having any one of these styles gives the individual some advantages in coping with the interpersonal environment, as well as some disadvantages. An individual's success may take place in part as a result of having a particular personality style rather than in spite of that style.

Viewing these scales as measuring personality styles leads to an interpretive approach that differs in two ways from the more conventional approach. First, we do not interpret elevations on these scales as de facto indices of personality disorders. The defining personality traits can range from relatively mild to very strong, and from adaptive to maladaptive. We posit that a clinical-level elevation on one of these scales does not necessarily imply Axis II psychopathology.

Second, we emphasize a distinction between the interpretation of these eight basic personality style scales and the rest of the personality scales, which we see as intrinsically psychopathological. Choca's (2004) current volume, and earlier editions of his textbook (Choca, Shanley, & Van Denburg, 1992; Choca & Van Denburg, 1996), provide a comprehensive coding/mapping system for understanding MCMI-III profiles based on up to three high points (elevations), using the original eight scales. Taking all possible permutations of the eight basic scales results in an inordinately large number of personality styles (336). However, in actual clinical practice, relatively few of these possible combinations are found (Craig, 1995; Retzlaff, Ofman, Hyer, & Matheson, 1994).

Choca (2004) advocates narrowing the volume of possible MCMI-III profiles to approximately 80. He provides detailed interpretive narratives for each of these 80 MCMI-III code type patterns. This system advocates using the narrative that approximates a particular profile, even if it does not exactly fit the required base rate elevations that the patient has reported (i.e., use of the base rate score of 75 as the hard-and-fast rule is somewhat flexible). A simple coding scheme is used: The first number represents the highest elevation above the cutoff base rate, usually 75. The second number represents the second such clinical elevation, and the third number represents the third such elevation. A 0 (zero) denotes that no scale is elevated above the cutoff, so that a 1–2A–0 code type 12A0 means that the Schizoid scale is the highest elevation, the Avoidant scale is also elevated, and no other scales are elevated into the clinical range. The narratives were based on actual individual patients and were constructed by using three methods: theoretical understanding of the personality characteristics and inferred dynamics; an item-metric analysis, using the specific behaviors acknowledged; and, finally, an actuarial approach, using actual case history, demographic information, and other psychometric test scores or projective technique inferences. These 80 interpretive narratives provide an alternative model to the computer-generated diagnostic inferences provided by the Pearson Assessments reports. Clinical judgment determines which, if any, of the narrative text applies to a specific patient.

In contrast to the way we view the original eight basic personality scales, the remaining Moderate Personality Disorder Scales/Clinical Personality Patterns (Depressive, Sadistic, Masochistic) as well as the standard Severe Personality Pathology Scales (Borderline, Paranoid, Schizotypal) are interpreted as having few, if any, adaptive aspects in real life. These scales represent the frank character deficits that define character psychopathology. In our view, these scales are pathognomonic of their respective disordered traits and reflect severe psychopathology with inevitable chronic implications. These scales are best interpreted as indications of frank Axis II psychopathology at the severe topological level suggested by Kernberg (1977), or at the "more difficult to treat" to "untreatable" end of the character pathology continuum posited by Stone (2006).

When any of the six nonbasic personality scales is elevated, our narrative case reports often begin with an unequivocal statement such as this: "Ms. Smith is a severely disturbed woman. Her MCMI-III profile is at the severe range of self-reported adult character psychopathology." Nearly all reviewers of the MCMI-III acknowledge that it is by far the best psychometric test for diagnosing personality disorders, and we concur that the six nonbasic personality scales are the most sensitive for that inference.

Case Example

The following actual case seen by one of us (Choca) allows for the sequential posing and refining of diagnostic and characterological inferences about a person with a not uncommon, but complex or "floating," MCMI-III profile (i.e., one with many clinical elevations).

Table 4.1 shows the MCMI-III scores of a 61-year-old Hispanic woman. Mrs. Fernández (her pseudonym in this chapter) became convinced that she was pregnant and could not be persuaded to the contrary. Neither the repeated negative pregnancy tests nor her husband's argument that she was well past menopause had any impact on her thinking. The patient had a long history of mild psychotic symptomatology. For instance, she was always seeing "shadows" of people with whom she held conversations; she spoke to the "spirits" of deceased relatives; and there had always been a certain oddity about Mrs. Fernández that was well recognized by all of the family members. She suffered from headaches and fainting attacks for which no medical explanation was ever found. From the time she was a child, she was never very connected to others, typically remaining by herself and not having much to say when she was with others. Nevertheless, she was happily married, had five children with her husband, and had always been able to function (at least at a marginal way) in her very simple domestic environment. She was a homemaker and had never worked outside the home.

Mrs. Fernández continued to believe her delusion through the 9 months of her "pregnancy." At times she would wear a pillow and would actually appear pregnant. The patient had a cousin who also believed that Mrs. Fernández was pregnant. The rest of the extended family did not share her delusion, but eventually gave up trying to convince her of her fallacy. Thus the family accepted the delusion as one of those oddities of the patient and thought that it would eventually go away.

Shortly after her "due date," Mrs. Fernández was apprehended while trying to abduct a newborn baby waiting to be placed in the parents' car for the trip home. She was arrested for attempted kidnapping, a serious felony. The patient was seen for evaluation in the jail at the request of her assigned public defender. She had become very anxious, was dysphoric/depressed, and was voicing suicidal ideation, seemingly as a result of her incarceration. She was being closely monitored and medicated with both an antidepressant and a major tranquilizer.

In order to evaluate the MCMI-III profile, we will start by noting that the Validity Index score is 0, so that the protocol is broadly valid. Both the Disclosure and Debasement Indices are elevated. Again, these indices are often elevated when a patient acknowledges a variety of relatively severe psychiatric symptoms. These elevations pose a difficult diagnostic problem, especially in a forensic case where the patient has an obvious incentive to "look bad" in the testing. The decision of whether the results are to be trusted has to be made on the basis of how well the scores fit what is known about the patient. In this case, we have decided that the protocol is interpretable, since (as will be seen) the elevations portray Mrs. Fernández in a way consistent with the presenting symptoms and her history.

Next we look at the basic personality scales to find that Mrs. Fernández has an Avoidant–Dependent personality style. This profile, the 2A–3–0 profile, is fairly prevalent and can be described as follows:

> Persons with similar scores usually do not have close friends and tend to remain detached and isolated. These individuals often view themselves as weak, inadequate, inferior, and unattractive. However, strongly wishing to be liked and accepted by others, they nevertheless have a great fear of rejection. This concern tends to put them on guard and make them uncomfortable, so that social

TABLE 4.1. MCMI-III Scores of a 61-Year-Old Hispanic Woman with a Delusional Pregnancy

Scales	Scores	
	Raw	Base rate
Basic Personality Style Scales		
1 Schizoid	13	63
2A Avoidant	21	86**
3 Dependent	18	78*
4 Histrionic	5	6
5 Narcissistic	16	54
6A Antisocial	11	54
7 Compulsive	11	27
8A Negativistic (Passive–Aggressive)	19	74
Severe Personality Scales		
2B Depressive	21	86**
6B Sadistic (Aggressive)	18	67
8B Masochistic (Self-Defeating)	18	77*
S Schizotypal	23	93**
C Borderline	14	63
P Paranoid	11	69
Clinical Syndrome Scales		
A Anxiety	17	95**
H Somatoform	15	91**
N Bipolar: Manic	13	71
D Dysthymia	20	106***
B Alcohol Dependence	10	66
T Drug Dependence	3	53
R Post-Traumatic Stress Disorder	21	106***
SS Thought Disorder	19	76*
CC Major Depression	22	103***
PP Delusional Disorder	11	96**
Modifying Indices		
X Disclosure	166	96**
Y Desirability	4	20
Z Debasement	30	95**
V Validity	0	

No asterisk: Base rate score is below 75 (not elevated).
*Base rate score elevation is between 75 and 84 (mildly elevated).
**Base rate score elevation is between 85 and 99 (moderately elevated).
***Base rate score elevation is above 99 (highly elevated).

situations are experienced with distaste. They seem apprehensive when relating to others and shy and nervous in social situations. Relating to others is a difficult and threatening experience that this type of person tries to avoid. In so doing, however, Mrs. Fernández gives up the support and affection that the avoided relationship could have brought. Thus life is experienced as a conflict between taking a risk and accepting the discomfort of forming a relationship or retreating to the unfulfilling safety of her isolation. These individuals are usually sensitive, compassionate, and emotionally responsive. However, they are often nervous, awkward, mistrustful, and isolated. (Adapted from Choca, 2004, pp. 120–121)

In evaluating the functionality of her personality structure, we are helped by the fact that the Schizotypal scale is very significantly elevated. Consistent with the history, the findings point to the presence of a frank personality disorder. The Schizotypal scale elevation characterizes the patient as follows:

Judging from the test results, Mrs. Fernández prefers a life of isolation with few strong interpersonal relationships. Some such people are uncomfortable in social situations. They retreat into their own fantasy world partly to avoid their social anxiety. There may be a tendency to be eccentric in appearance, thinking, or verbal expression, and the person may have habits that others find peculiar. At times the emotional reactions may seem odd or inappropriate. Neutral events can be misinterpreted as actions that relate in a very specific way to the individual, or that have some sort of special meaning. This individual may report unusual perceptions or experiences, and may express strange beliefs. For instance, Mrs. Fernández may have feelings of depersonalization, emptiness, or meaninglessness. Finally, she may seamlessly mix her own personal idiosyncrasies with other more conventional material in her conversations. (p. 28)

At this point we are ready to focus on the clinical syndrome. The MCMI-III shows Mrs. Fernández to be seriously anxious and depressed. Her depression is pervasive and documented by the fact that all three of the MCMI-III depression scales (the Depressive personality scale and the Dysthymia and Major Depression clinical scales) are clinically elevated. Based on this finding, the patient may be described as follows:

According to the MCMI-III, Mrs. Fernández has been sad, and has demonstrated a dysphoric or melancholic mood. Similar people show diminished interest in their daily activities, and cannot derive much pleasure from their current involvements. Life may become a burden, an unwanted task that has little personal meaning. Making decisions, even about minor matters, may be difficult, with the individual being encumbered by indecisiveness. At times Mrs. Fernández may have crying spells. Most troubling, suicide ideation may be present for extended periods of time even if not overtly expressed. Low self-esteem and feelings of worthlessness may be accompanied by guilt about past actions. Individuals with similar test profiles typically experience vegetative symptoms, such as a loss of appetite, sleep difficulties, fatigue, or a low energy level. They may move at a slow pace, or become anxious and agitated.

In fact, the indications are that Mrs. Fernández has been experiencing a significant amount of chronic anxiety. Similar individuals worry a great deal about different aspects of their lives and feel a high level of distress. Often such people have episodes of intense anxiety, during which they may become unable to function—sick with the worry that a dreadful event is about to happen. The experience of this incendiary anxiety has undoubtedly been a significant problem for her. (p. 30)

Judging from the history, the patient's depression and anxiety have been produced, or at least markedly exacerbated, by her incarceration and legal problems. The MCMI-III analysis reminds us, however, of the longer-standing problem of her headaches and fainting spells. The elevation of the Somatoform scale describes an individual who is preoccupied with somatic complaints. Similar individuals worry excessively about possible problems with their bodily functions. Typically they do not restrict their concerns to one area of functioning, but, rather, complain about a variety of different issues or pains. They become increasingly limited in the activities in which they are able or willing to participate. Secondary benefits may also play a role, as the individual is able to obtain attention or special considerations as a result of her medical condition. Anxiety, irritability, or sadness may arise as emotional repercussions of the somatic concerns. Finally, similar individuals feel they have no control over their medical problems and are pessimistic or even hopeless about the prospect of improvement. (p. 31)

The elevation of the Post-Traumatic Stress Disorder scale is not expected, since Mrs. Fernández previously acknowledged no instances of trauma or interpersonal abuse. (In speaking to her after she had taken the test, however, it became clear that she found her arrest and incarceration to be itself traumatizing, and was referring to those near-term experiences when she endorsed the Post-Traumatic Stress Disorder scale items.)

Probably the most important MCMI-III findings in this case are represented by the scales that remain to be addressed. In the elevated Thought Disorder and Delusional Disorder scales, Mrs. Fernández has given evidence of the irrational thinking process and the delusional state that led to her downfall. These elevations characterize an individual whose

> thinking is typically disorganized. Similar individuals may jump from one topic to the next and explain themselves poorly, so that they cannot be clearly understood. Judging from the MCMI-III, Mrs. Fernández suffers from delusions or hallucinations. She may be prone to misinterpreting the statements or actions of others, believing these communications or observations to mean something different than what they meant. She may also act in peculiar or odd ways. (p. 30)

Once we have understood the MCMI-III findings in a sequential but "piecemeal" fashion, we are ready to integrate it in a way that conceptualizes the individual in an insightful and effective manner—again, the *patient as person*.

In Mrs. Fernández's case, we would start by talking about a woman who arrived at her adult life with an already flawed psychological makeup, a defective personality structure that carried the marks of various defects in ego functioning, and likely deficits in parental input that left her "to face life's tasks with a stunted array of tools and with painful subjective states" (Pine, 2006, p. 2). From the beginning, she was an odd, peculiar individual who could only relate superficially and in a stereotypical, immature manner with a few significant others. In marriage, she typically assumed a submissive position, waiting for her husband to take the leadership role.

Although the patient's thinking and behavior often bordered on psychotic, her delusions had been mostly benign and even domesticated. They had never been a threat or even a great inconvenience to her family system or to others. Consequently, she had been able to live a simple, conventional life, despite manifesting fairly serious psychopathology in a textbook sense. We suspect that the sometimes idealized role of wife/mother in a Hispanic subculture partially obviated her underlying chronic dependency conflicts, providing her with a safe, structured environment and some elements of self-esteem. Her delusion of an older-age pregnancy could have remained just another benign delusion, except that the action she took was one that her community could not tolerate. In her frantic attempt to prove her pregnancy, she could only access her dominant and lifelong way of adaptive problem solving, using severely schizotypal ideation to "solve a problem." Attempted kidnapping—the abduction of an infant to raise, and thereby restore her previous lifestyle—was a psychotic solution to a severe internalized set of conflicts and personality deficits. In supporting the history, the MCMI-III has helped us conceptualize the case of Mrs. Fernández in a way that would not have been possible without the test findings.

References

Acklin, M. W. (1992). Psychodiagnosis of personality structure: Psychotic personality organization. *Journal of Personality Assessment, 58,* 454–463.

Acklin, M. W. (1993). Psychodiagnosis of personality structure II: Borderline personality organization. *Journal of Personality Assessment, 61,* 329–341.

American Psychiatric Association. (2000). *Diagnostic and statistical manual of mental disorders* (4th ed., text rev.). Washington, DC: Author.

Belter, R. W., & Piotrowski, C. (2001). Current status of doctoral-level training in psychological testing. *Journal of Clinical Psychology, 57,* 717–726.

Bornstein, R. F. (2005). The dependent patient: Diagnosis, assessment, and treatment. *Professional Psychology: Research and Practice, 36,* 82–89.

Butcher, J. N., Dahlstrom, W. G., Graham, J. R., Tellegen, A., & Kaemmer, B. (1989). *MMPI-2: Minnesota Multiphasic Personality Inventory–2: Manual for administration and scoring.* Minneapolis: University of Minnesota Press.

Choca, J., Shanley, L. A., & Van Denburg, E. (1992). *Interpretive guide to the Millon Clinical Multiaxial Inventory.* Washington, DC: American Psychological Association.

Choca, J. P. (2004). *Interpretive guide to the Millon Clinical Multiaxial Inventory* (3rd ed.). Washington, DC: American Psychological Association.

Choca, J. P., & Van Denberg, E. (1997). *Interpretative guide to the Millon Clinical Multiaxial Inventory* (2nd ed.). Washington, DC: American Psychological Association.

Craig, R. J. (1993). *Psychological assessment with the Millon Clinical Multiaxial Inventory (II): An interpretative guide.* Odessa, FL: Psychological Assessment Resources.

Craig, R. J. (1995). Clinical diagnoses and MCMI codetypes. *Journal of Clinical Psychology, 51,* 352–360.

Craig, R. J. (2005a). *Assessing substance abusers with the Millon Clinical Multiaxial Inventory (MCMI).* Springfield, IL: Thomas.

Craig, R. J. (Ed.). (2005b). *New directions in interpreting the Millon Clinical Multiaxial Inventory–III (MCMI-III).* Hoboken, NJ: Wiley.

Craig, R. J. (2005c). *Personality-guided forensic psychotherapy.* Washington, DC: American Psychological Association.

Glickauf-Hughes, C., & Wells, M. (1997). *Object relations psychotherapy: An individualized and interactive approach to diagnosis and treatment.* Northvale, NJ: Aronson.

Groth-Marnat, G. (2003). *Handbook of psychological assessment* (4th ed.). Hoboken, NJ: Wiley.

Ivey, G. (2006). A method of teaching psychodynamic case formulation. *Psychotherapy: Theory, Research, Practice, Training, 43,* 322–336.

Jankowski, D. (2002). *A beginner's guide to the MCMI-III.* Washington, DC: American Psychological Association.

Kernberg, O. F. (1977). The structural diagnosis of borderline personality organization. In P. Hartocoulis (Ed.), *Borderline personality disorder* (pp. 87–121). Madison, CT: International Universities Press.

Kvaal, S. A., Choca, J. P., & Groth-Marnat, G. (2003). The integrated psychological report. In L. E. Beutler & G. Groth-Marnat (Eds.), *Integrative assessment of adult personality* (2nd ed., pp. 398–433). New York: Guilford Press.

Millon, T. (1969). *Modern psychopathology: A biosocial approach to maladaptive learning and functioning.* Philadelphia: Saunders.

Millon, T. (with Grossman, S., Meagher, S., Millon, C., & Everly, G). (1999). *Personality-guided therapy.* New York: Wiley.

Millon, T., Grossman, S., Millon, C., Meagher, S., & Ramnath, R. (2004). *Personality disorders in modern life* (2nd ed.) Hoboken, NJ: Wiley.

Millon, T. (with Millon, C., & Davis, R.). (1994). *Manual for the Millon Clinical Multiaxial inventory–III.* Minneapolis, MN: National Computer Systems.

Millon, T. (with Millon, C., & Davis, R.). (1997). *Manual for the Millon Clinical Multiaxial Inventory–III* (2nd ed.). Minneapolis, MN: National Computer Systems.

Millon, T. (with Millon, C., Davis, R., & Grossman, S.). (2006). *Manual for the Millon Clinical Multiaxial Inventory–III* (3rd ed.). Minneapolis, MN: Pearson Assessments.

Morey, L. C. (1991). *Personality Assessment Inventory professional manual.* Odessa, FL: Psychological Assessment Resources.

PDM Task Force. (2006). *Psychodynamic diagnostic manual.* Silver Spring, MD: Alliance of Psychoanalytic Organizations.

Perry, S., Cooper, A. M., & Michels, R. (1987). The psychodynamic formulation: Its purpose, structure, and clinical application. *American Journal of Psychiatry, 144,* 543–550.

Pine, F. (2006). If I knew then what I know now: Theme and variation. *Psychoanalytic Psychology, 23,* 1–7.

Retzlaff, P. (Ed.). (1995). *Tactical psychotherapy of the personality disorders: An MCMI-III based approach.* Needham Heights, MA: Allyn & Bacon.

Retzlaff, P. D., & Dunn, T. (2003). The Millon Clinical Multiaxial Inventory–III. In L. E. Beutler & G. Groth-Marnat (Eds.), *Integrative assessment of adult personality* (2nd ed., pp. 192–227). New York: Guilford Press.

Retzlaff, P. D., Ofman, P., Hyer, L., & Matheson, S. (1994). MCMI-II high-point codes: Severe personality disorder and clinical syndrome extensions. *Journal of Clinical Psychology, 50,* 228–234.

Stone, M. H. (2006). *Personality-disordered patients: Treatable and untreatable.* Washington, DC: American Psychiatric Publishing.

Strack, S. (2002). *Essentials of Millon inventories assessment* (2nd ed.). New York: Wiley.

Trimboli, F., & Kilgore, R. B. (1983). A psychodynamic approach to MMPI interpretation. *Journal of Personality Assessment, 47,* 614–626.

Van Denburg, E., & Choca, J. P. (1997). Interpretation of the MCMI-III. In T. Millon (Ed.), *The Millon inventories* (pp. 41–58). New York: Guilford Press.

CHAPTER 5

A Brief Illustrative MCMI Case Study

Caryl Bloom
Theodore Millon

Levels of Interpretation with the MCMI

The Millon Clinical Multiaxial Inventory–III (Millon, 1994), which we refer to as simply the MCMI in this chapter's discussion, offers several layers or levels of interpretation. Consistent with integrative logic, each level subsumes the previous one in an exploratory hierarchy, demanding a higher order of complexity and integration. At the first level, an evaluator merely examines the personality and clinical syndrome scales for single-scale elevations. If these scales are sufficiently elevated, certain diagnoses may (or may not) be warranted. At the second level, the interpretive process branches to follow one of two pathways, depending upon whether any of the Severe Personality Pathology Scales are elevated, or whether elevations are confined to the less severe basic personality scales (currently referred to as the Moderate Personality Disorder Scales or the Clinical Personality Patterns). Regardless of which branch the interpretive process follows, the goal at the second layer is to obtain an integrated picture of the patient's Axis II personality disorders and Axis I clinical syndromes according to multiaxial logic. In this chapter, we address each of these levels in turn, and follow this discussion with a case illustration. We refrain from making statements about the strengths and weaknesses of particular scales, and instead concentrate on the general interpretive logic of the instrument.

When self-report instruments consist of multiple scales, the results are usually presented in the form of a profile. At the first layer of interpretation, again, we are only interested in determining which scales are elevated and their importance for making diagnostic decisions. For two reasons, this must be viewed as the most basic level of interpretation. First, this layer looks only at single scales rather than at the profile as a whole. Second, it collapses continuous data down to a dichotomous level; information is first ignored, and then it is actively discarded.

For MCMI neophytes, perhaps the first thing to notice is a difference from other instruments: The elevation of each scale of the profile is given in terms of a base rate (BR) score, rather than the more familiar *T*-score or percentile rank. Each is a transformation of the raw scores, and each has the purpose of putting the raw scores on a common metric. Unlike *T*-scores or percentile ranks, however, the BR scores are created so that the percentage of the clinical population deemed diagnosable with a particular disorder falls (1) either at or above a common threshold (clinical scales), or (2) at a particular rank order in the profile (personality scales). Thus, if 5% of the clinical population is deemed to possess a schizoid pattern as its primary personality style, and another 2% of the population has the schizoid pattern as a secondary feature, then the raw scores have been transformed so that the normative sample reflects these prevalence rates or BRs.

Obviously, the BR score implies that we are not so much interested in the "absolute quantity" of a particular trait as we are in the implications of that quantity for psychological functioning. For example, while a certain level of narcissism is considered healthy in our society, the same level of antisocial behavior may not be; we might want to treat the second, but not the first. Thus the BR concept permits us to acknowledge that *equal quantities of a trait or characteristic have different pathological implications*. Such scales have been equated in terms of the implications of a particular quantity for psychological functioning. The BR score simply represents the most direct way of getting at such considerations. BR scores are superior to *T*-scores, which implicitly assume the converse—that pathology varies directly with deviation from the average of one's normative group.

The BR score thus suggests likely characteristics of psychopathology. In Pepper's (1942) terms, it represents something of a fragment, in that it makes a prediction in and of itself without appealing to anything immediately outside itself (such as auxiliary evidence for corroboration). Consequently, there is a possibility of interpretive error in always diagnosing a personality disorder—or, worse, multiple personality disorders—whenever BR scores equal or exceed a particular threshold. Although it has become traditional to view BR = 75 and BR = 85 as indicating the presence of pathological personality traits or disorders, there are always "false positives" and "false negatives," as with every test. In a false-positive result, the test indicates the presence of pathology where pathology does not exist. In a *false negative* result, the test indicates the absence of pathology where pathology in fact exists. As with most tests, false positives and false negatives derive principally from the insensitivity of a measurement procedure, whether self-report, interview, or physiological. In this chapter's featured case, several personality scales are diagnostic candidates, and we have no reason to believe that other Axis II disorders might be applicable. As we need not worry about false negatives, our attitude in the dichotomous world of diagnostic judgments is one of culling the true positives from the set of several positives.

To elaborate on this problem, let us consider some definitions of personality pathology. Personality disorders are defined as clinical syndromes composed of intrinsic, deeply embedded, and pervasive ways of functioning (Millon, 1969; Millon & Davis, 1996). The *Diagnostic and Statistical Manual of Mental Disorders*, fourth edition, text revision (DSM-IV-TR; American Psychiatric Association, 2000, p. 689) states that it is only when *personality traits* are inflexible and maladaptive and cause either significant functional impairment or subjective distress that they constitute *personality disorders*. Thus the principal problem faced here is to separate scale elevations that have become inflexible or pervasive from those that have not. However, the degree to which a trait is problematic is not a direct function of the quality of the trait, but instead is a function of (1) its interaction with other characteristics of the organism in which the trait is embedded, and (2) the interaction between the organism and the context in which it is embedded. That is, not one but two interactions separate the quantity of a trait and its flexibility or pervasiveness. Thus scale elevations that are problematic for one individual may not be pathological for another. Schizoid individuals, for example, are notable for their lack of emotional reactivity. Such individuals not only function well in, but actively seek out, environments that make few interpersonal demands. An accountant whose job requires long hours of tedious work may be well served by such characteristics. If this individual were suddenly thrust into a management position, would difficulties ensue? Quite possibly. Nevertheless, what exists can only be said to represent a vulnerability to contextual change, not a disorder per se.

This prefigures a second way of falling into error: that of viewing personality disorders as medical illnesses for which some discrete pathogen can be found, or for which there exists some underlying unitary cause, either past or present. As Millon and Millon have noted in Chapter 3, the use of such language as "disorder" is regrettable, for personality disorders are not disorders at all in the medical sense. Instead, they are best conceptualized as disorders of the entire matrix of the person. Accordingly, we would prefer the terms "pattern" or "style" rather than the reifying label "disorder." This problem is more conceptual than diagnostic, but it leads to subsequent flaws in multiaxial logic; in particular, it encourages the view that classical clinical syndromes and personality disorders exist in a horizontal relationship, rather than in a vertical one (where clinical symptoms are embedded in personality patterns). What threatens to undermine the interpretive process will surely undermine the intervention as well.

As noted, the quality of information that can be deduced from the profile analysis of a test is a function of several factors, including the adequacy and generativity of the theory that provides the logic underlying its various scales, the overall empirical validity of the inventory, and its internal consistency and scale generalizability. An interpretation that in fact mirrors the patient's characteristic style of functioning as well as his or her current problems depends ultimately on the clinician's skill in weighing the degree to which numerous trait variables interact to corroborate, moderate, or even disqualify straightforward hypotheses, as well as to suggest ones that are more subtle. As noted by many clinicians and researchers, even the best inventory is only as good as the clinician interpreting it. Perfect construct validity and generalizability will not make up for inadequate knowledge of the theory undergirding an inventory, or for ignorance of fundamental principles of pathology.

Although examining the elevations of single scales may be useful for making diagnostic assignments, their interpretive value is greatly amplified when viewed in the context of the remaining profile of scales. Why? The explanation of this obvious and widely accepted tenet of test interpretation can be traced back to the metatheoretical assumptions of integrative logic. The short answer is that the process of profile interpretation is similar to that of knowledge building in the integrative worldview. We are working our way toward an integrative conception of the patient—what we have called "nomothetic individuality." In doing so, we put ourselves at a distance from the individual scales and diagnoses to reconstruct the personality as an organic whole. In the context of the entire profile, the meaning of each scale becomes something other than it would have been, had that scale alone been available for interpretation. Thus we want to know more than just whether a person is "avoidant" or "paranoid," as in the case of Cho Seung-Hui, the perpetrator of the massacre at Virginia Tech in April 2007. In Pepper's (1942) more metaphysical terminology, each scale and even each diagnosis becomes a mere fragment to be transcended by successively more integrative formulations, the limit of the series being reality itself. From the superordinate vista of this final product, it is little wonder that diagnosis, such as it often is, seems pathetic, inadequate, and usually next to useless.

In each case, test results suggest several diagnoses and other characteristics, each being a hypothesis about the nature of the patient's pathology. True to Pepper's (1942) model, however, some of these diagnoses may already be enmeshed in contradictions. For example, when we consult the various theory-derived personality prototype descriptions given by Millon and Davis (1996), an elevated MCMI Schizoid scale (BR = 89) argues for a patient's having an apathetic attitude and an absence of emotionality, suggesting that the patient may function as a passive observer detached from the rewards and affections as well as from the demands of human relationships. Additional elevations of the Avoidant (BR = 87) and Paranoid (BR = 85) scales on the MCMI profile, however, argues against such a procrustean first-order interpretive logic, as would multiple elevations of MMPI-2 scales 2, 7, and 8. The schizoid hypothesis might perhaps find some corroboration in the elevation of the MMPI-2 Social Introversion scale. However, social introversion is a trait more narrow in scope than a MCMI Schizoid personality score—and, what is worse, useless without references to the patient's Avoidant and Paranoid personality scores. The undergirding theory of the MCMI holds that the patient's personality may be a detached type, with the schizoid part passive, and the other components more active and more severely pathological. How, then, does one make sense of these ostensibly disparate findings? One means is to conceptualize the individual's personality as a mixed type with features of the schizoid, avoidant, and paranoid prototypes (as seen in the case of Cho Seung-Hui).

Such integrative configural logic is inherently nonlinear or nonmechanistic. It asks for a level of sophistication that breaks the pattern of labeling patients and fitting them to discrete diagnostic categories: It conceptualizes diagnostic constructs as the beginning points of an assessment rather than its endpoints. An Avoidant–Paranoid pattern on the MCMI, for example, is somewhat different from either the purely prototypal Avoidant pattern or the purely prototypal Paranoid pattern. Although the "two-point" pattern in part resembles these focal constructs (nomothetic commonality), it is also more than either of these two patterns added together (nomothetic individuality) by virtue of the synergism of these elements. An Avoidant–Paranoid pattern indicates something more than avoidant plus paranoid behavior; it is referred to as an "insular paranoid subtype," a distinctive and special variant in the Millon classification schema (Millon & Davis, 1996), again as seen in the case of Cho Seung-Hui.

In making configural personality interpretations, a separation should be made between those MCMI scales pertaining to the *basic* Clinical Personality Patterns (1–

8B) and the Severe Personality Pathology Scales: the Borderline (C), Schizotypal (S), and Paranoid (P) scales. These structural pathologies differ from the Clinical Personality Patterns by several criteria—notably, deficits in social competence and frequent (but usually reversible) psychotic episodes. Less integrated in terms of their personality organization and less effective in coping than their more mildly affected counterparts, individuals with such pathologies are especially vulnerable to decompensation when confronted with the strains of everyday life.

In terms of the theoretical model, these more severe patterns are significantly less adaptable in the face of ecological vicissitudes. They are dysfunctional variants of the more moderately pathological patterns—a feature that leads to several predictions concerning these MCMI patterns and profiles. First, we have noted earlier that at least two interactions mediate the role of a single personality trait for psychological functioning, and that for this reason the quantity of that trait constrains but does not determine the level of personality pathology. The elevation of S, C, and/or P may be used as a rough index of the degree to which a patient's basic personality pattern has become structurally compromised. If, for example, a patient receives BR = 105 on the Narcissistic scale, but S, C, and P scores are low, then structurally the personality appears to be fundamentally intact, despite the elevated BR score. If, on the other hand, a patient receives BR = 80 on the Narcissistic scale, but scale P is also at BR = 80, this suggests a basic narcissistic pattern with paranoid tendencies—possibly an incipient structural pathology.

The Case Example

We have selected the following case for presentation because it clearly illustrates clinically useful interpretive strategies.

Eva is a 44-year-old divorced female, highly intelligent and facile in her expressive abilities. She is a large woman who is loud in both voice and appearance, overly assertive and abrasive. In her first session, she appeared guarded and defensive; however, she asked if the therapist was likely to cry because her problems had made her previous therapist cry. She added that she was disappointed and angry with her former therapist for not being sufficiently accessible to her.

Eva reported difficulties in sustaining her positions as a computer programmer/analyst. Although she established contracts with various companies for 6- to 24-month periods, she never completed any of these commitments. Feelings of depression had suddenly increased following the loss of her most recent contract. In her first therapeutic session, she also reported feeling dejected and spoke of experiencing self-defeating behaviors throughout most of her life. As she saw it, people inevitably came to dislike her when they "really" learned the kind of person she is. Usually isolated at her jobs, she believed that her coworkers invariably began to make fun of her. She decided to begin working alone, so she would be safer and less likely to be judged or criticized. Feelings of anger and worthlessness were expressed about her recent job loss. Unable to deal with these feelings, however, she had recently begun to spend her time drinking excessively and smoking pot.

Eva routinely voiced concerns about her social life, making derogatory remarks about the men she dated, insisting that they mistreated and took advantage of her. These relationships were based on online dating contacts. She generally fabricated her history and sent touched-up and out-of-date photos. Her need for closeness led her to be intimate on her first dates. Her offer of sexual favors exacerbated her feelings of having been debased and dependent, leading often to angry feelings and outbursts when she was "abandoned" (i.e., when she failed to be invited for a second date). Chronically lonely or depressed, she quickly attached herself to any person on whom she might depend. She had recently put her eggs in one basket—a newly designated "loved one," to whom she became very attached. As in the past, this attachment did not prove secure. He was an unreliable anchor, putting her psychic equilibrium in constant jeopardy. Deprived of the attention she sought from him, she intensified her characteristic strategy of seductiveness, and began to stalk him daily. Such repetitive social failures and insecurities precipitated new distress and conflicts—turning life itself into an empty burden, so to speak. During these periods she occasionally returned to her family, but experienced increasing depression there, as well as feelings of uselessness and infantile dependency. She would act out there—exhibiting brief outbursts of angry resentment, verbally attacking others for having exploited or abused her, and berating them for failing to see how desperately needy she was for love and attention.

Eva's pattern of feeling insecure and rejected probably arose in her family of origin. She was the middle child, with an older and a younger brother. Her parents were either indifferent toward or critical of her. Her father was dependent on alcohol; he also demanded perfection, as did her mother, who was a highly successful executive in her work. Eva was seen as never good enough. Most significantly, she was sexually abused by both her father and older brother. She felt strong resentment and anger toward them for having sexually coerced and then betrayed her. These feelings often erupted into an angry surge of fury—directed almost randomly at times toward coworkers and friends, but especially toward so-called romantic partners. These impulsive and erratic outbursts created new conflicts and intense tension in her work settings. Her anger and fury was often directed toward the very persons upon whom she depended. As a consequence of provoking their wrath, she was repeatedly rejected and deserted. At times, Eva tried to counter these abusive impulses; she would become overly constrained and turn her angry feelings inward. A growing sense of unworthiness and guilt led her to begin to plan suicide acts as a means of self-punishment.

As soon as each of her previous therapists offered to interpret her erratic and self-defeating emotions, Eva would argue that these hypotheses could not be accurate. To "prove" her arguments, she often produced contradictory biographical information that had been previously withheld. She would become agitated and blame the therapist, stating that the therapist did not understand her any better than anyone else. It was when she had reached that point with her most recent therapist that Eva decided to engage her current therapist, who then sought to have her take the MCMI-III to guide the clinical work with Eva. Figure 5.1 (pp. 102–111) presents Eva's MCMI-III Profile and Interpretive Report.

References

American Psychiatric Association. (2000). *Diagnostic and statistical manual of mental disorders* (4th ed., text rev.). Washington, DC: Author.

Millon, T. (1969). *Modern psychopathology: A biosocial approach to maladaptive learning and functioning.* Philadelphia: Saunders.

Millon, T., & Davis, R. D. (1996). *Disorders of personality: DSM-IV and beyond.* New York: Wiley.

Millon, T. (with Millon, C., & Davis, R. D.). (1994). *Millon Clinical Multiaxial Inventory–III manual.* Minneapolis, MN: National Computer Systems.

Pepper, S. P. (1942). *World hypotheses: A study in evidence.* Berkeley: University of California Press.

CAPSULE SUMMARY

MCMI-III reports are normed on patients who were in the early phases of assessment or psychotherapy for emotional discomfort or social difficulties. Respondents who do not fit this normative population or who have inappropriately taken the MCMI-III for nonclinical purposes may have inaccurate reports. The MCMI-III report cannot be considered definitive. It should be evaluated in conjunction with additional clinical data, The report should be evaluated by a mental health clinician trained in the use of psychological tests. The report should not be shown to patients or their relatives.

Interpretive Considerations

The client is a 44-year-old divorced white female. She is currently being seen as an outpatient, and she did not identify specific problems and difficulties of an Axis I nature in the demographic portion of this test.

This patient's response style may indicate a tendency to magnify illness, an inclination to complain, or feelings of extreme vulnerability associated with a current episode of acute turmoil. The patient's scale scores may be somewhat exaggerated; and the interpretations should be read with this in mind.

Profile Severity

On the basis of the test data, it may be assumed that the patient is experiencing a severe mental disorder; further professional observation and inpatient care may be appropriate. The text of the following interpretive report may need to be modulated upward given this probable level of severity.

Possible Diagnoses

She appears to fit the following Axis II classifications best: Negativistic (Passive-Aggressive) Personality Disorder, and Borderline Personality Disorder with Dependent Personality Traits and Depressive Personality Traits.

Axis I clinical syndromes are suggested by the client's MCMI-III profile in the areas of Major Depression (recurrent, severe, without psychotic features), Generalized Anxiety Disorder, and Psychoactive Substance Abuse NOS.

Therapeutic Considerations

Inconsistent and pessimistic, this patient may expect to be mishandled, if not harmed, even by well-intentioned therapists. Sensitive to messages of disapproval and lack of interest, she may complain excessively and be irritable and erratic in her relations with therapists. Straightforward and consistent communication may moderate her dependent/negativistic attitude. Focused, brief treatment approaches are likely to overcome her initial oppositional outlook.

FIGURE 5.1. MCMI-III Profile and Interpretive Report for Eva *(p. 1 of 10)*.

MILLON CLINICAL MULTIAXIAL INVENTORY - III
CONFIDENTIAL INFORMATION FOR PROFESSIONAL USE ONLY

FACET SCORES FOR HIGHEST PERSONALITY SCALES BR 65 OR HIGHER

HIGHEST PERSONALITY SCALE BR 65 OR HIGHER: SCALE 8A Negativistic (Passive-Aggressive)

SCALE	RAW	BR	PROFILE OF BR SCORES	FACET SCALES
8A.1	8	83		Temperamentally Irritable
8A.2	6	88		Expressively Resentful
8A.3	5	81		Discontented Self-Image

SECOND HIGHEST PERSONALITY SCALE BR 65 OR HIGHER: SCALE C Borderline

SCALE	RAW	BR	PROFILE OF BR SCORES	FACET SCALES
C.1	9	95		Temperamentally Labile
C.2	8	94		Interpersonally Paradoxical
C.3	5	66		Uncertain Self-Image

THIRD HIGHEST PERSONALITY SCALE BR 65 OR HIGHER: SCALE 3 Dependent

SCALE	RAW	BR	PROFILE OF SR SCORES	FACET SCALES
3.1	8	97		Inept Self-Image
3.2	7	95		Interpersonally Submissive
3.3	4	77		Immature Representations

FIGURE 5.1. *(p. 2 of 10)*

MILLON CLINICAL MULTIAXIAL INVENTORY - III
CONFIDENTIAL INFORMATION FOR PROFESSIONAL USE ONLY

COMPLETE LISTING OF MCMI-III GROSSMAN FACET SCALE SCORES

		RAW	BR			RAW	BR
1	**Schizoid**			**6B**	**Sadistic**		
1.1	Temperamentally Apathetic	6	79	68.1	Temperamentally Hostile	6	92
1.2	Interpersonally Unengaged	6	74	68.2	Eruptive Organization	5	87
1.3	Expressively Impassive	5	83	68.3	Pernicious Representations	5	80
2A	**Avoidant**			**7**	**Compulsive**		
2A.1	Interpersonally Aversive	7	87	7.1	Cognitively Constricted	4	40
2A.2	Alienated Self-Image	8	86	7.2	Interpersonally Respectful	2	37
2A.3	Vexatious Representations	4	63	7.3	Reliable Self-Image	3	34
2B	**Depressive**			**8A**	**Negativistic**		
2B.1	Temperamentally Woeful	7	99	8A.1	Temperamentally Irritable	8	83
2B.2	Worthless Self-Image	5	71	8A.2	Expressively Resentful	6	88
2B.3	Cognitively Fatalistic	7	83	8A.3	Discontented Self-Image	5	81
3	**Dependent**			**8B**	**Masochistic**		
3.1	Inept Self-Image	8	97	8B.1	Discredited Representations	7	90
3.2	Interpersonally Submissive	7	95	8B.2	Cognitively Diffident	7	84
3.3	Immature Representations	4	77	8B.3	Undeserving Self-Image	6	76
4	**Histrionic**			**S**	**Schizotypal**		
4.1	Gregarious Self-Image	2	27	S.1	Estranged Self-Image	9	92
4.2	Interpersonally Attention-Seeking	5	62	S.2	Cognitively Autistic	5	81
4.3	Expressively Dramatic	0	0	S.3	Chaotic Representations	7	89
5	**Narcissistic**			**C**	**Borderline**		
5.1	Admirable Self-Image	2	17	C.1	Temperamentally Labile	9	95
5.2	Cognitively Expansive	2	45	C.2	Interpersonally Paradoxical	8	94
5.3	Interpersonally Exploitive	6	92	C.3	Uncertain Self-Image	5	66
6A	**Antisocial**			**P**	**Paranoid**		
6A.1	Expressively Impulsive	5	74	P.1	Cognitlvely Mistrustful	2	60
6A.2	Acting-Out Mechanism	5	87	P.2	Expressively Defensive	3	72
6A.3	Interpersonally Irresponsible	6	96	P.3	Projection Mechanism	8	98

For each of the Clinical Personality Patterns and Severe Personality Pathology scales (the scale names shown in **bold**), scores on the three facet scales are shown beneath the scale name.

FIGURE 5.1. *(p. 3 of 10)*

MILLON CLINICAL MULTIAXIAL INVENTORY - III
CONFIDENTIAL INFORMATION FOR PROFESSIONAL USE ONLY

Valid Profile

PERSONALITY CODE: 8A 3 2B 2A ** - * 8B 6A 1 + 6B 5 " 4 7 ' ' // C ** - * //

SYNDROME CODE: A ** T H D R * // CC ** - * //

DEMOGRAPHIC: 12566/ON/F/44/W/D/-/--/--/-----/--/-----/

CATEGORY		SCORE		PROFILE OF SR SCORES				DIAGNOSTIC SCALES
		RAW	BR 0	60	75	85	115	
MODIFYING INDICES	X	163	93					DISCLOSURE
	Y	4	20					DESIRABILITY
	Z	28	91					DEBASEMENT
CLINICAL PERSONALITY PATTERNS	1	13	64					SCHIZOID
	2A	20	86					AVOIDANT
	2B	20	87					DEPRESSIVE
	3	22	88					DEPENDENT
	4	7	16					HISTRIONIC
	5	12	46					NARCISSISTIC
	6A	14	66					ANTISOCIAL
	6B	14	56					SADISTIC
	7	8	16					COMPULSIVE
	8A	24	98					NEGATIVISTIC
	8B	13	71					MASOCHISTIC
SEVERE PERSONALITY PATHOLOGY	S	16	64					SCHIZOTYPAL
	C	23	95					BORDERLINE
	P	15	70					PARANOID
CLINICAL SYNDROMES	A	17	95					ANXIETY
	H	13	76					SOMATOFORM
	N	11	63					BIPOLAR: MANIC
	D	17	76					DYSTHYMIA
	B	8	61					ALCOHOL DEPENDENCE
	T	14	82					DRUG DEPENDENCE
	R	18	76					POST-TRAUMATIC STRESS
SEVERE CLINICAL SYNDROMES	SS	17	66					THOUGHT DISORDER
	CC	21	99					MAJOR DEPRESSION
	PP	7	66					DELUSIONAL DISORDER

FIGURE 5.1. *(p. 4 of 10)*

RESPONSE TENDENCIES

This patient's response style may indicate a broad tendency to magnify the level of experienced illness or a characterological inclination to complain or to be self-pitying, On the other hand, the response style may convey feelings of extreme vulnerability that are associated with a current episode of acute turmoil. Whatever the impetus for the response style, the patient's scale scores, particularly those on Axis I, may be somewhat exaggerated, and the interpretation of this profile should be made with this consideration in mind.

The BR scores reported for this individual have been modified to account for the high self-revealing inclinations indicated by the high raw score on scale X (Disclosure) and the psychic tension and dejection indicated by the elevations on scale A (Anxiety) and scale D (Dysthymia).

AXIS II: PERSONALITY PATTERNS

The following paragraphs refer to those enduring and pervasive personality traits that underlie this woman's emotional, cognitive, and interpersonal difficulties. Rather than focus on the largely transitory symptoms that make up Axis I clinical syndromes, this section concentrates on her more habitual and maladaptive methods of relating, behaving, thinking, and feeling.

There is reason to believe that at least a moderate level of pathology characterizes the overall personality organization of this woman. Defective psychic structures suggest a failure to develop adequate internal cohesion and a less than satisfactory hierarchy of coping strategies. This woman's foundation for effective intrapsychic regulation and socially acceptable interpersonal conduct appears deficient or incompetent. She is subjected to the flux of her own enigmatic attitudes and contradictory behavior, and her sense of psychic coherence is often precarious. She has probably had a checkered history of disappointments in her personal and family relationships. Deficits in her social attainments may also be notable, as well as a tendency to precipitate self-defeating vicious circles. Earlier aspirations may have resulted in frustrating setbacks, and efforts to achieve a consistent niche in life may have failed. Although she is usually able to function on a satisfactory basis, she may experience periods of marked emotional, cognitive, or behavioral dysfunction.

The MCMI-III profile of this woman suggests her marked dependency needs, deep and variable moods, and impulsive, angry outbursts. She may anxiously seek reassurance from others and is especially vulnerable to fear of separation from those who provide support, despite her frequent attempts to undo their efforts to be helpful. Dependency fears may compel her to be alternately overly compliant, profoundly gloomy, and irrationally argumentative and negativistic. Almost seeking to court undeserved blame and criticism, she may appear to find circumstances to anchor her feeling that she deserves to suffer.

She strives at times to be submissive and cooperative, but her behavior has become increasingly unpredictable, irritable) and pessimistic. She often seeks to induce guilt in others for failing her, as she sees it. Repeatedly struggling to express attitudes contrary to her feelings, she may exhibit conflicting emotions simultaneously toward others and herself, most notably love, rage, and guilt. Also notable may be her confusion over her self-image, her highly variable energy levels, easy fatigability, and her irregular sleep-wake cycle.

She is particularly sensitive to external pressure and demands, and she may vacillate among being socially agreeable, sullen, self-pitying, irritably aggressive, and contrite. She may make irrational and bitter complaints about the lack of care expressed by others and about being treated unfairly. This behavior keeps others on edge, never knowing if she will react to them in a cooperative or a sulky manner. Although she may make efforts to be obliging and submissive to others, she has learned to anticipate disillusioning relationships, and she often creates the expected disappointment by constantly questioning and doubting the genuine interest and support shown by others. Self-destructive acts and suicidal gestures may be employed to gain attention. These irritable testing

FIGURE 5.1. *(p. 5 of 10)*

maneuvers may exasperate and alienate those on whom she depends. When threatened by separation and disapproval, she may express guilt, remorse, and self-condemnation in the hope of regaining support, reassurance, and sympathy.

Beyond her helplessness and clinging behavior, she may exhibit an irritable argumentativeness. Recognizing that others may have grown weary of this behavior, she may alternate between voicing gloomy self-deprecation, being apologetic and repentant, and being petulant and bitter. A struggle between dependent acquiescence and assertive independence constantly intrudes into most relationships. Her inability to regulate her emotional controls, her feeling of being misunderstood, and her erratic moodiness contribute to innumerable wrangles and conflicts with others and to persistent tension, resentfulness, and depression.

GROSSMAN PERSONALITY FACET SCALES

The Grossman Facet Scales are designed to aid in the interpretation of elevations on the Clinical Personality Patterns and Severe Personality Pathology Scales by helping to pinpoint the specific personality processes (e.g., self-image, interpersonal relations) that underlie overall scale elevations. A careful analysis of this patient's facet scale scores suggests that the following characteristics are among her most prominent personality features.

Most notable is her view of herself as weak, fragile, and inadequate to meet life's tasks competently or with ease—a generalized deficit in self-confidence that is aggravated by the habit of belittling her own abilities. Much of this self-belittling has little basis in reality. Clinically, this pattern of self-deprecation may best be conceived as a strategy by which she elicits assurances that she is worthy and loved. Hence it serves as an instrument for evoking praise and support.

Also salient is her pattern of changing moods that shift erratically from normality to depression to excitement, with chronic feelings of dejection and apathy interspersed with brief spells of anger, euphoria, and anxiety. The intensity of her affect and the changeability of her actions are striking. She generally fails to accord her unstable mood levels with external reality. She may exhibit a single, dominant outlook or temperament, such as a self-ingratiating depressive tone, which periodically gives way to anxious agitation or impulsive outbursts of anger or resentment. She may engage in self-destructive behavior, but she usually realizes later that her behavior was irrational and foolish.

Also worthy of attention is her inclination to subordinate her own wishes to a stronger and (she hopes) nurturing person, resulting in the habit of being conciliatory, deferential, and self-sacrificing. She probably believes that it is best to abdicate responsibility, to leave matters to others, and to place her fate in others' hands. In her view, other people are much better equipped to shoulder responsibility, to navigate the intricacies of a complex world, and to discover and achieve the pleasures to be found in the competitions of life.

Early treatment efforts are likely to produce optimal results if they are oriented toward modifying the personality features just described.

AXIS I: CLINICAL SYNDROMES

The features and dynamics of the following Axis I clinical syndromes appear worthy of description and analysis. They may arise in response to external precipitants, but are likely to reflect and accentuate several of the more enduring and pervasive aspects of this woman's basic personality makeup.

Testy and demanding, this woman evinces an agitated, major depression that can be noted by her daily moodiness and vacillation. She is likely to display a rapidly shifting mix of disparaging com-

FIGURE 5.1. *(p. 6 of 10)*

ments about herself, anxiously expressed suicidal thoughts, and outbursts of bitter resentment inter-woven with a demanding irritability toward others. Feeling trapped by constraints imposed by her circumstances and upset by emotions and thoughts she can neither understand nor control, she has turned her reservoir of anger inward, periodically voicing severe self-recrimination and self-loathing. These signs of contrition may serve to induce guilt in others—an effective manipulation in which she can give a measure of retribution without further jeopardizing what she sees as her currently precarious, if not hopeless, situation.

Failing to keep deep and powerful sources of inner conflict from overwhelming her controls, this characteristically difficult and conflicted woman may be experiencing the clinical signs of an anxiety disorder. She is unable to rid herself of preoccupations with her tension, fearful presentiments, recurring headaches, fatigue, and insomnia, and she is upset by their uncharacteristic presence in her life. Feeling at the mercy of unknown and upsetting forces that seem to well up within her, she is at a loss as to how to counteract them, but she may exploit them to manipulate others or to complain at great length.

Abuse of either legal or street drugs or both is indicated in the MCMI-III protocol of this woman, who is often erratic, irritable, and negativistic. Her use of drugs may be both a statement of resentful independence from the constraints of conventional life and a means of disjoining her conflicts and liberating her uncharitable impulses toward others. An act of assertive defiance that has undertones of self-destruction, her drug abuse may be employed with a careless indifference to its consequences.

Related to but beyond her characteristic level of emotional responsivity, this woman appears to have been confronted with an event or events in which she was exposed to a severe threat to her life—a traumatic experience that precipitated intense fear or horror on her part. Currently the residuals of this event appear to be persistently reexperienced with recurrent and distressing recollections, such as in cues that resemble or symbolize an aspect of the traumatic event. Where possible, she seeks to avoid such cues and recollections. Where they cannot be anticipated and actively avoided, as in dreams or nightmares, she may become terrified, exhibiting a number of symptoms of intense anxiety. Other signs of distress might include difficulty falling asleep, outbursts of anger, panic attacks, hypervigilance, exaggerated startle response, or a subjective sense of numbing and detachment.

This moody and conflicted woman's bodily preoccupations and concerns are likely to be produced by both physical and psychological factors, resulting in a syndrome of features suggestive of a somatoform disorder. Enmeshed in an erratic pattern of resentment and brittle emotions, her anxious concerns about her somatic state aggravate her characteristic sullenness, leading her to demand attention and special treatment. Not only does she exploit her ailments to control the lives of others, but she is also likely to complain of her discomfort in ways that induce others to feel guilty.

NOTEWORTHY RESPONSES

The client answered the following statements in the direction noted in parentheses. These items suggest specific problem areas that the clinician may wish to investigate.

Health Preoccupation

1. Lately, my strength seems to be draining out of me, even in the morning. (True)
4. I feel weak and tired much of the time. (True)
55. In recent weeks I feel worn out for no special reason. (True)
74. I can't seem to sleep, and wake up just as tired as when I went to bed. (True)
75. Lately, I've been sweating a great deal and feel very tense. (True)

FIGURE 5.1. *(p. 7 of 10)*

107. I have completely lost my appetite and have trouble sleeping most nights. (True)
130. I don't have the energy to concentrate on my everyday responsibilities anymore. (True)
149. I feel shaky and have difficulty falling asleep because painful memories of a past event keep running through my mind. (True)

Interpersonal Alienation

10. What few feelings I seem to have I rarely show to the outside world. (True)
18. I'm afraid to get really close to another person because it may end up with my being ridiculed or shamed. (True)
27. When I have a choice, I prefer to do things alone. (True)
48. A long time ago, I decided it's best to have little to do with people. (True)
69. I avoid most social situations because I expect people to criticize or reject me. (True)
99. In social groups I am almost always very self-conscious and tense. (True)
161. I seem to create situations with others in which I get hurt or feel rejected. (True)
165. Other than my family, I have no close friends. (True)
174. Although I'm afraid to make friendships, I wish I had more than I do. (True)

Emotional Dyscontrol

14. Sometimes I can be pretty rough and mean in my relations with my family. (True)
22. I'm a very erratic person, changing my mind and feelings all the time. (True)
30. Lately, I have begun to feel like smashing things. (True)
34. Lately, I have gone all to pieces. (True)
83. My moods seem to change a great deal from one day to the next. (True)
96. People have said in the past that I became too interested and too excited about too many things. (True)
97. I sometimes feel crazy-like or unreal when things start to go badly in my life. (True)

Self-Destructive Potential

44. I feel terribly depressed and sad much of the time now. (True)
112. I have been downhearted and sad much of my life since I was quite young. (True) 128. I feel deeply depressed for no reason I can figure out. (True)
142. I frequently feel there's nothing inside me, like I'm empty and hollow. (True)
150. Looking ahead as each day begins makes me feel terribly depressed. (True)
151. I've never been able to shake the feeling that I'm worthless to others. (True)
171. I have given serious thought recently to doing away with myself. (True)

Childhood Abuse

132. I hate to think about some of the ways I was abused as a child. (True)

Eating Disorder

No items endorsed.

POSSIBLE DSM-IV-TR® MULTIAXIAL DIAGNOSES

The following diagnostic assignments should be considered judgments of personality and clinical prototypes that correspond conceptually to formal diagnostic categories. The diagnostic criteria and items used in the MCMI-III differ somewhat from those in the DSM-IV-TR, but there are sufficient parallels in the MCMI-III items to recommend consideration of the following assignments. It should be noted that several DSM-IV-TR Axis I syndromes are not assessed in the MCMI-III. Definitive

FIGURE 5.1. *(p. 8 of 10)*

diagnoses must draw on biographical, observational, and interview data in addition to self-report inventories such as the MCMI-III.

Axis I: Clinical Syndromes

The major complaints and behaviors of the patient parallel the following Axis 1 diagnoses, listed in order of their clinical significance and salience.

296.33	Major Depression (recurrent, severe, without psychotic features)
300.02	Generalized Anxiety Disorder
305.90	Psychoactive Substance Abuse NOS

Axis II: Personality Disorders

Deeply ingrained and pervasive patterns of maladaptive functioning underlie Axis I clinical syndromal pictures. The following personality prototypes correspond to the most probable DSM-IV-TR Axis II diagnoses (disorders, traits, features) that characterize this patient.

Personality configuration composed of the following:

301.90	Negativistic (Passive-Aggressive) Personality Disorder
301.83	Borderline Personality Disorder
	with Dependent Personality Traits
	and Depressive Personality Traits

Course: The major personality features described previously reflect long-term or chronic traits that are likely to have persisted for several years prior to the present assessment.
The clinical syndromes described previously tend to be relatively transient, waxing and waning in their prominence and intensity depending on the presence of environmental stress.

Axis IV: Psychosocial and Environmental Problems

In completing the MCMI~III, this individual identified the following problems that may be complicating or exacerbating her present emotional state. They are listed in order of importance as indicated by the client. This information should be viewed as a guide for further investigation by the clinician.

    None identified

TREATMENT GUIDE

If additional clinical data are supportive of the MCMI-III's hypotheses, it is likely that this patient's difficulties can be managed with either brief or extended therapeutic methods. The following guide to treatment planning is oriented toward issues and techniques of a short-term character, focusing on matters that might call for immediate attention, followed by time-limited procedures designed to reduce the likelihood of repeated relapses.

As a first step, it would appear advisable to implement methods to ameliorate this patient's current state of clinical anxiety, depressive hopelessness, or pathological personality functioning by the rapid implementation of supportive psychotherapeutic measures. With appropriate consultation, targeted psychopharmacological medications may also be useful at this initial stage.

Worthy of note is the possibility of a troublesome alcohol and/or other substance-use disorder. If verified, appropriate short-term behavioral management or group therapy programs should be rapidly implemented.

FIGURE 5.1. *(p. 9 of 10)*

Once this patient's more pressing or acute difficulties are adequately stabilized, attention should be directed toward goals that would aid in preventing a recurrence of problems, focusing on circumscribed issues and employing delimited methods such as those discussed in the following paragraphs.

A primary short-term goal of treatment with this patient is to aid her in reducing her intense ambivalence and growing resentment of others. With an empathic and brief focus, it should be possible to sustain a productive, therapeutic relationship. With a therapist who can convey genuine caring and firmness, she may be able to overcome her tendency to employ maneuvers to test the sincerity and motives of the therapist. Although she will be slow to reveal her resentment because she dislikes being viewed as an angry person, it can be brought into the open, if advisable, and dealt with in a kind and understanding way. She is not inclined to face her ambivalence, but her mixed feelings and attitudes must be a major focus of treatment. To prevent her from trying to terminate treatment before improvement occurs or to forestall relapses, the therapist should employ brief and circumscribed techniques to counter the patient's expectation that supportive figures will ultimately prove disillusioning.

Circumscribed interpersonal approaches (e.g., Benjamin, Kiesler) may be used to deal with the seesaw struggle enacted by the patient in her relationship with her therapist. She may alternately exhibit ingratiating submissiveness and a taunting and demanding attitude, Similarly, she may solicit the therapist's affections, but when these are expressed, she may reject them, voicing doubt about the genuineness of the therapist's feelings. The therapist may use cognitive procedures to point out these contradictory attitudes. It is important to keep these inconsistencies in focus or the patient may appreciate the therapist's perceptiveness verbally but not alter her attitudes. Involved in an unconscious repetition compulsion in which she recreates disillusioning experiences that parallel those of the past, the patient must not only come to recognize the expectations cognitively, but may be taught to deal with their enactment interpersonally.

Despite her ambivalence and pessimistic outlook, there is good reason to operate on the premise that the patient can overcome past disappointments. To capture the love and attention only modestly gained in childhood cannot be achieved, although habits that preclude partial satisfaction can be altered in the here and now. Toward that end, the therapist must help her disentangle needs that are in opposition to one another. For example, she both wants and does not want the love of those upon whom she depends. Despite this ambivalence, she enters new relationships, such as in therapy, as if an idyllic state could be achieved. She goes through the act of seeking a consistent and true source of love—one that will not betray her as she believes her parents and others did in the past. Despite this optimism, she remains unsure of the trust she can place in others. Mindful of past betrayals and disappointments, she begins to test her new relationships to see if they are loyal and faithful. In a parallel manner, she may attempt to irritate and frustrate the therapist to check whether he or she will prove to be as fickle and insubstantial as others have in the past. It is here that the therapist's warm support and firmness can play a significant short-term role in reframing the patient's erroneous expectations and in exhibiting consistency in relationship behavior.

Although the rooted character of these attitudes and behavior will complicate the ease with which these therapeutic procedures will progress, short-term and circumscribed cognitive and interpersonal therapy techniques may be quite successful. A thorough reconstruction of personality may not be necessary to alter the patient's problematic pattern. In this regard, family treatment methods focusing on the network of relationships that often sustain her problems may prove to be a useful technique. Group methods may also be fruitfully employed to help the patient acquire self-control and consistency in close relationships.

It is advisable that the therapist not set goals too high, because the patient may not be able to tolerate demands or expectations well. Brief therapeutic efforts should be directed to build the patient's trust, to focus on positive traits, and to enhance her confidence and self-esteem.

FIGURE 5.1. *(p. 10 of 10)*

CHAPTER 6

The MCMI-III and MACI
Grossman Facet Scales

Seth D. Grossman

The Millon Clinical Multiaxial Inventory–III (MCMI-III) and Millon Adolescent Clinical Inventory (MACI) have been, throughout their respective histories, instruments intended for maximum clinical utility; they thus operationalize the third (assessment) component of Millon's five-pillar architecture for a coherent science of clinical personology (Millon & Grossman, 2006). One of several recent studies (Grossman & del Rio, 2005) aimed at refinements leading to the most recent edition of the MCMI-III (Millon, 2006a) examined the MCMI-III for its capacity to support facet subscales intrinsically tied to Millon's (1990) evolutionary theory, which provides the instrument's foundation. Rational examination of the 14 personality scales sought to have the most salient of the theory's eight functional and structural domains of personality emerge from the extant item pools. In accordance with the theory, each basic prototypal personality pattern is expected to present most saliently within two to three of these eight personological domains; the initial study produced 35 subscales ("Facet scales") for the MCMI-III that corresponded with personological domains predicted by the theory (Grossman & del Rio, 2005). This preliminary exploration demonstrated sufficient internal consistency and construct validity that the decision was made to "fine-tune" this structure further for the creation of supportive, clinical-hypothesis-building subscales—first for the revised MCMI-III, and then for the revision of the MACI (Millon, 2006b), which follows the same theoretical framework. This chapter examines the resultant Grossman Facet Scales for both of these instruments' recent revisions, and discusses implications for their use in personality assessment, treatment planning, and intervention.

The impetus for the creation of the Grossman Facet Scales follows a tradition set forth by the parallel development of content subscales for other instruments, such as the various sets of subscales for the Minnesota Multiphasic Personality Inventory (MMPI) (e.g., Harris & Lingoes, 1955, 1968). In general, these subscales have as their central purpose the further breakdown of extant assessment information derived from their primary measure, and the Grossman Facet Scales are no exception. Where the intent of the Facet Scales differs, however, is in clinical utility, as they are designed to adhere to Millon's aforementioned five-component philosophy of intervention progression (Millon & Grossman, 2006), supporting targeted and evidence-based treatment efforts. In following the theoretical model, the Facet Scales illuminate the theory's specifications of the expression of personality at the trait level, and this trait level directly coordinates with established therapeutic modalities. Current demands in service delivery aimed at intervention economy and evidence-based practice are oriented toward such targeted intervention strategies, and these Facet Scales intend to help direct treatment toward both symptom and personality levels simultaneously.

The personality scales of the various Millon inventories may be described as multifaceted psychological constructs representing Millon's (1990) evolutionary theoretical taxonomy, demonstrating both construct and content validity consonant not only with the overarching theory, but with *Diagnostic and Statistical Manual of Mental Disorders*, fourth edition, text revision (DSM-IV-TR; American Psychiatric Association, 2000) criteria. In itself, the instruments provide for valuable focused treatment suggestions at the personological level; the finer distinctions of the taxonomic system are present within the instrument. Millon and Davis (1997), in commenting on historical and future developments of the MCMI and other Millon instruments, have encouraged researchers and clinicians to view the instruments as constantly evolving entities that will continue to undergo revisions and development as the field's knowledge base is expanded and modified. Furthermore, they lament that while these instruments in fact are capable of discriminating subtypes (admixtures of personality styles), the current categorical approach of the DSM limits their ability to do this cleanly, often yielding a confusing array of elevated scales. It remains their hope that future DSMs will yield more of a dimensional approach congruent with the intent of Millon's evolutionary theory, and that future versions of the instruments will further reflect this. Congruent with their call to further explore the instrument's more molecular elements, the Facet Scales seek to reflect fundamental facets of personality in the clinical inventories that may be clinically useful.

Indeed, working on a more molecular level than the instrument's original scales (which in most cases are construct scales), content subscales allow test administrators to examine underlying dimensions and latent facets at a level of detail beyond the scope of the original test design. Also, content subscales are developed from the original test's item pool in a post hoc manner; as a consequence, the development of such scales presents a substantial opportunity for clinical gain without detracting in any manner from the original instrument's design.

Deductive Methodology and the Millon Inventories

Millon's personality theory was first presented as a biosocial–learning theory (Millon, 1969); in more recent decades, it has become a more comprehensive ecological–motivational theory closely related to evolutionary biology, sharing ubiquitous principles of the physical sciences (Millon, 1990; Millon & Davis, 1996; Millon & Grossman, 2006). The theory has at its core three polarity structures representative of universal motivating aims shared in the animal and plant kingdoms, and connected to principles found in studies of particle physics, chemistry, and cosmogony, among other natural sciences. These are a pain–pleasure (survival) polarity, an active–passive (adaptation) polarity, and a self–other (replication) polarity. These structures form the basis for the combined categorical–dimensional approach to personality known as the "prototypal" approach. Millon posits that few if any real-life individuals' personalities will represent direct matches with prototypes derived from the theory, but that all persons, whether or not they are "disordered," may be compared to these theoretical models, which represent the general manner in which most personality constellations cluster. Dimensionally speaking, then, all persons will exhibit variants of these prototypal constructs—more or less rigidly or fluidly, depending on their relative pathology or health.

From these dimensions, further divisions may be made into functional and structural domains of personality (Millon & Davis, 1996), each of which is represented within the individual personality styles or disorders. These eight domains are as follows: expressive behaviors (functional), interpersonal conduct (functional), cognitive style (functional), self-image (structural), object representations (structural), regulatory mechanisms (structural), morphologic organization (structural), and mood/temperament (structural). The characteristics of the prototypal personality styles/disorders are then deduced (Choca, 1998), with prototypal features within these domains, although in reality admixtures of two or more personality styles are likely to occur (e.g., antisocial personality with schizoid features). Such admixtures are referred to as "subtypes." From here, it is possible, after assessment, to deduce the subtype structure of an individual's personality and to address salient therapeutic concerns from a personality-guided conceptualization of the individual (Davis, 1999; Dorr, 1999; Millon, 2000); the most recent explications of these focused therapeutic models are three volumes on what is now called "personalized psychotherapy" (Millon & Grossman, 2007a, 2007b, 2007c). The items constituting the Millon inventories, then, are based on the polarity scheme, and expressed via these prototypal functional and structural domains.

Content Scales and Subscales: A History

Content scales are challenging to define operationally, owing to the lack of clear distinction between the terms "content" and "construct." In practice, these ideas overlap considerably, and their fine distinction may lack usefulness beyond basic pedagogical purposes. However, their direct comparison, at specific points, may help delineate differences that are central to differentiating the use and definition of content scales and subscales from those of the "primary" or construct scales in any given objective psychometric instrument. The "main" scales of any given psychological inventory (i.e., those constructed by the test authors at the time of the original test's development) are generally construct scales. Inherent in this definition is the fact that constructs are based in specific psychological theory (Cronbach & Meehl, 1955). As they represent conceptions and distinctions created and authored by humans, rather than simply existing in nature, they must be held to greater scientific rigor: They must demonstrate not only content validity, but construct validity as well.

Constructs usually bridge naturally occurring phenomena that seem unrelated at first glance but, according to the particular framework in question, are bound together via some scientific methodology such as theoretical deduction, correlation, or criterion grouping. As such, the connections among the items of a construct scale may not be immediately apparent to those unfamiliar with the given framework from which the construct is derived. For example, the MMPI-2's scale 4, Psychopathic Deviate, contains subject matter dealing with family dysfunction, directed by an assumed concordance between strained family relations and individual psychopathology—a connection provided by the overarching "construct" of deviance. This MMPI-2 scale, then, demonstrates construct validity, delineating the relationship between these two subject areas. Constructs, then, must be consonant with the framework and methodology of the scale's construction, but they do not necessarily demonstrate "face validity" (i.e., the self-evidence of these connections to laypersons).

The preceding example is but one of the many assessment anomalies making the case for more rudimentary breakdown in psychological measurement. Although constructs are certainly useful in generating hypotheses regarding the nature of presenting clinical phenomena in relation to what has been "established" in psychology and mental health, it is also necessary to gain a more elucidated, contextual picture of the patient and his or her multifaceted presentation. It is hardly enough for a clinician to describe an individual's presentation by giving it an Axis II label with symptoms of an Axis I condition such as major depression. It is much more useful to inspect the many elements of the individual's multifaceted personality style, noting especially the differences between this person's presentation and what may be surmised from "typical" diagnostic presentation.

As the previous example illuminates, it is possible that specific elements are shared by separate theoretical constructs, and nowhere is this more evident than in the systemic, intricate area of personality and its assessment. Although this polythetic quality is consonant with basic assumptions about personality (Millon, 2006a, 2006b), the astute clinician must be able to make these important distinctions between disparate contents—a function made more reliable with the use of content scales. Family dysfunction is not an element unique to the construct measured by the Psychopathic Deviate scale, as it is certainly possible that an individual whose profile falls outside the description of a "psychopathic deviate" may acknowledge such an item. Such a response would be represented more accurately within a more specific content subscale—for instance, the MMPI Harris–Lingoes subscale known as Family Discord (Harris & Lingoes, 1955, 1968).

The purpose of content scales has always been rooted in a desire to make more targeted and focused distinctions than those that are possible with an extant instrument. The most famous and historic examples of such endeavors began with the original MMPI scales (Hathaway & McKinley, 1943), which were originally designed simply to predict group diagnostic membership. Clinicians using the original instrument sometimes found the underlying dimensions of each scale inconsistent, and many scale elevations and profiles seen in practice remained mysterious and ill defined (Graham, 2000). Fortunately, the large and diverse item pool inherent in the MMPI served well for the development of a number of content scales, the most famous of which are those developed by Harris and Lingoes (1955, 1968). The widely used and comprehensive Harris–Lingoes subscales represented the first systematic effort to analyze the heterogeneous content of many of the major MMPI scales. Six of the 10 standard clinical scales considered to be most heterogeneous underwent factor analysis, yielding between three and six underlying factors for each of these six scales.

The MMPI has been investigated for its underlying structure many times over the past 60 years. Several other content scales have achieved widespread use for this instrument, including those developed by Wiggins (1966, 1969), as well as those developed as part of the MMPI-2 restandardization project, known simply as the MMPI-2 "content scales" (Butcher, Graham, Williams, & Ben-Porath, 1990) and "content component scales" (Ben-Porath & Sherwood, 1993). Moreover, many "supplementary scales" have been developed, perhaps most notably Morey, Waugh, and Blashfield's (1985) MMPI DSM-III personality disorder scales. Other supplementary scales (e.g., the MacAndrew Alcoholism scale; MacAndrew, 1965) tend to focus on a single construct, whereas the scales by Morey et al. (1985) seem to capture more of the underlying content of the overall instrument. These content scales and subscales have demonstrated significant clinical contribution beyond the scope of the original instruments' design. In a study of the MMPI-2 content scales in an outpatient mental health environment, Barthlow, Graham, Ben-Porath, and McNulty (1999) found that many of these scales demonstrated incremental validity in predicting therapists' ratings of clients' behavior and personality characteristics, with seven scales for men and three scales for women adding to the information and interpretive power provided by the instrument's primary clinical scales. Similar results were obtained in an earlier study examining incremental validity with the MMPI-2 content scales in a psychiatric sample (Archer, Aiduk, Griffin, & Elkins, 1996).

Specific mental health problems further reveal the clinical utility of examining personality dimensions on a more molecular level than allotted by the principal scales. Interpretation of the MMPI-2 content scales has been found particularly valuable in identifying distressing symptomatology among patients with traumatic brain injury within rehabilitation settings (Palav, Ortega, & McCaffrey, 2001), and in significantly discriminating particular aspects of subjective distress in a population of patients with chronic pain. In more traditional mental health settings, these factorially derived scales have been instrumental in identifying serious pathology and patient risk factors. Specific content scales and Harris–Lingoes subscales of the MMPI-A have been shown to predict suicide probability differentially in boys and girls, to an extent beyond what is provided by the clinical scales (Kopper, Osman, Osman, & Hoffman, 1998). Among adults, Kopper, Osman, and Barrios (2001) found that two of the MMPI-2 content scales, Anger (for women) and Type A (for men), contributed significantly to the predictability of suicidal behavior. In other studies, another two MMPI-2 content scales—namely, the Depression (DEP) and Bizarre Mentation (BIZ) scales—have contributed significantly to differential diagnosis and predictive utility beyond that afforded by the primary clinical scale 2 (Depression) in the affective and psychotic spectra. Boone (1994) noted that within a group of 62 psychiatric inpatients with diagnoses ranging from adjustment reaction with depressed mood to schizophrenia, the DEP content scale not only correctly identified DSM-IV aspects of depression, but was a significant suicidal behavior predictor as well. Both the DEP and BIZ content scales (in conjunction with the primary clinical scales) have demonstrated incremental contribution to differentiating the often confusing realm of schizophrenic spectrum disorders (with their frequently comorbid affective features) from that of affective spectrum disorders (with their sometimes comorbid psychoses) (Ben-Porath, Butcher, & Graham, 1991)—a finding replicated in similar studies (e.g., Munley, Busby, & Jaynes, 1997).

The Millon Instruments: Factorial Structure

The Grossman Facet Scales do not represent the first factorial exploration of the MCMI-III or other Millon instruments, as several previous researchers have explored the factorial structure of Millon's theory and instrumentation. However, few studies have explored subsets of within-scale factors; that is, few have attempted to identify the latent composition of MCMI-III's individual personality construct scales. One study (Choca, Retzlaff, Strack, & Mouton, 1996) attempted to demonstrate the factorial structure of test items for each of the personality scales. A primary consideration for determining the number of factors was concurrence with what was theoretically expected. Five of the eight domains specified by the theory emerged in the analysis of the factors' content, with the three domains not represented in the factor structure being domains concerned with intrapsychic and psychodynamically oriented constructs. Another (Petrocelli, Glaser, Calhoun, & Campbell, 2001) was more successful in demonstrating convergence with all eight domains of personality. This study identified the eight domains, plus one "core belief" composite, as relating directly to a cluster analysis of the instrument's scales identifying five cognitive schemas.

Several unpublished subscales were developed for the MCMI (Millon, 1977) and MCMI-II (Millon, 1987) over the years, but no special effort was made to uncover underlying "facets" within construct scales specifically for use as content subscales until the most recent editions of the chief instruments were developed. Davis (1993) was the first to develop such a set of facet subscales for the MACI (Millon, 1993), utilizing a combined statistical–rational approach and factor analyzing each of the primary scales in isolation; this study yielded content scales that hierarchically fit under each of the primary scales in a manner similar to the Harris–Lingoes subscales of the MMPI (Harris & Lingoes, 1955, 1968), but with sounder psychometric qualities. This earlier study served as a guide for the structure of the Grossman Facet Scales as subscales of the primary constructs, but did not investigate the possibility of linking the facets with the established theory.

Methodological Traditions in Instrument and Scale Development

When possible development strategies for the Grossman Facet Scales were examined, it was necessary to review similar developments and examine how other subscale developers addressed the question of how their methodology might tie in with the spirit and intent of the original instrument. Traditionally, content scales have been derived in a manner compatible with the primary personality scales of a given instrument. Burisch (1984) described three prototypical methods historically utilized for personality scale construction that are consonant with Loevinger's (1957) paradigm for item-driven test development: (1) external (criterion group); (2) inductive (internal consistency or itemic); and (3) deductive (rational, theoretical). These three methods are reviewed briefly here to help elucidate choices for the Grossman Facet Scales.

MMPI instrumentation is a product of the external (criterion group) method of construction, and is a prime example of the need for content scales. Congruent with the external methodology of "dustbowl empiricism" (Meehl, 1945), the original MMPI items were retained on their ability to distinguish criterion groups from "normal" subjects. Of secondary concern were several important clinical and statistical concerns, such as internal consistency or item content. To externalists, who consider themselves scientific realists, the world exists in categories (such as diagnoses), with groupings such as "hypochondriasis," "psychasthenia," and "depression" composing the palette of human existence. In this form of scale construction, a very large item pool is developed and given to a large number of diagnosed subjects and "normal" controls. The resulting scales contain highly disparate sources of variation, a generally moderate Cronbach's alpha measure, and little explanation concerning how or why an individual is placed in a category. Such questions of causality or context, in general, were addressed by those who pursued some inductive methodology with the instruments—that is, those who then developed factor or content scales.

The inductive tradition represents a second pathway in scientific instrumentation. Those subscribing to this paradigm believe that personality has some latent dimensional structure that is accessible primarily via statistical measures, such as factor analysis. The inductivist, like the externalist, does not approach scientific problems with any preconceived notions regarding overarching theory; for this reason, the inductive approach relies heavily on a representative sampling of the content domain. This methodology's most famous example is the Cattell, Eber, and Tatsuoka (1970) Sixteen Personality Factor Inventory (16PF). It is also represented contemporarily by the NEO inventories representing the five-factor model of personality (Costa & McCrae, 1992; Costa & Widiger, 1994), as well as Goldberg's (1990) "Big Five" lexical model, and the models for personality disorders proposed by Livesley, Jackson, and Schroeder (1989), and Clark (1993). This approach does yield the most internally consistent, statistically sound measures of personality based on ostensibly real traits, but there is a real danger that the methodology and sampling procedure may serve as a magnifying lens that distorts appearances. Davis and Millon (1993) have presented a further important argument questioning the validity of the inductivists' claim that their methodology is a true reflection of underlying personality structure. That is, these approaches are based in a lexical tradition, yet new constructs are introduced as latent theoretical constructs, as opposed to surface, manifest constructs. By definition, however, the lexical approach begins with words based in the natural lexicon. This raises the question of whether the distillation of terms in the natural language can serve as the basis of a science. Such a methodology seems prone to distortion by virtue of this lexical assumption. Davis and Millon (1993) state that inductive methods of theory building achieve simplicity mechanically, essentially by projecting data into some geometric space. If one is willing to go to the next step, to assume that the axes of this geometric space drive behavior, then one has only to name the axes to feel that something of fundamental importance has been discovered. . . . Far from selecting and discarding on some theoretical basis, the claim of [such] models rests on the representative sampling of content domains. (p. 107)

The third tradition, the deductive (rational) approach, seeks to address many of the shortcomings found in the expression of the first two methods. In contrast with inductivists, deductivists believe that the structure of personality may be accessed most pragmatically via theoretical grounds. An inventory is prepared that incorporates core constructs selected by the theorist in accordance with his or her theory, and items are written to represent operational definitions of those chosen constructs. After construction, the theory and inventory are statistically and psychometrically evaluated. Of the three methodologies discussed, this is the one most congruent with the decisive and now historic discussion by Cronbach and Meehl (1955) regarding construct validity, in which they explicitly called for a theoretical basis for any given construct. Rather than making the often quantum leap from observation to theory (in this case, from content to construct validity), as is seen with the inductive approach, the deductive theoretician begins his or her study with theory. The MCMI-III is derived deductively via theoretical means, as all Millon instruments are. So, too, may the entire DSM taxonomy of personality disorders be derived, and this overlap of the objective, empirical standard of the DSM with the theoretically deduced instrument and taxonomy demonstrates convergent validity highly pragmatic for the purposes of achieving clinical economy and accuracy. The weakness in this or any deductive approach, however, is simply that of theories in general: Virtually any theory is possible (if not plausible), and some are simply better than others.

MCMI-III Facet Scales: Development Schema and Procedural Considerations

A schema for developing content scales from the items of an established instrument requires an investigator to make several choices. Burisch's (1984) taxonomy, discussed earlier, applied primarily to original scale development, when the item pool has not been written or the boundaries of constructs are extremely fluid; such a taxonomy, although it is a good overarching theoretical guideline to the development of content scales, does not fully explicate specific methodology for the task. A schema that is specific to post hoc scales, in addition to the obvious task of helping the scale developer to structure his or her choices, should ideally serve two additional roles: First, it should possess some logical basis allowing it to serve as a means of categorizing sets of content scales that have already been developed. Second, it should be generative with respect to ways that content scales might be developed in the future. In constructing the MACI content scales, Davis (1993) suggested a model that serves this purpose. His schema involved two elemental choices to be made by content scale developers, each represented in a bipolar axis. The first axis involves the method of scale development—rationally initiated and statistically refined versus statistically initiated and rationally defined. The second involves the level at which the post hoc scales are designed—whether the entire inventory or some logical subset of the inventory's scales is used as an item pool.

The first-axis choice is whether to construct the candidate content scales with rational or statistical means as the initial consideration. An investigator choosing a rational route is likely to have in mind a functional need the scale will meet. The methodology here invariably fits existing items to some set of concepts. The researcher choosing a statistically initiated route will develop content scales through some multivariate technique such as factor or cluster analysis, in order to identify domains of communality or clusters of items. These investigators typically believe that the statistical methodology is sufficient to permit latent dimensions to emerge from an existing item pool. Here the definition of candidate content scales is left to methodological formalities, rather than the researcher's theoretical orientation or utilitarian desire. Functionality is generally determined after the construction has taken place.

The second-axis decision is whether the established inventory's entire item pool may serve as the raw material for the candidate content scales, or whether some extant logical boundaries exist that may be retained within the development process. Advantages and liabilities exist with either choice, as they do with the first pair of choices regarding methodological initiation. For the Millon inventories, owing to their multiaxial framework, this decision was further divided into subset decisions; that is, some items represent Axis I constructs, while others represent Axis II constructs (although some overlap is common). In this case, the first consideration was whether the focus should be on classic psychiatric symptomatology or personality characteristics.

When the focus for the initial facet scale study (Grossman & del Rio, 2005) was considered, further questions resided in what sublevel of inquiry would be most meaningful and desirable in terms of clinical efficacy and consonance with the parent instrument. Several possible delineations existed within the theory. One possibility was Millon's (1990; Millon & Davis, 1996) distinction among four groups of personalities: the "pleasure-deficient," the "interpersonally imbalanced," the "intrapsychically conflicted," and the "structurally defective." Items from these scales could be pooled in an effort to seek out organizational and structural elements of personality. A second possibility was to conduct an analysis to explore the three polarities (existence, adaptation, replication), in an attempt to illuminate motivational patterns from the core of the theory.

The most molecular choice was the possibility of utilizing the items of each principal scale as its own separate, small item pool. At this level of analysis, the size of the pools is minimized, while the logical meaningfulness of potential content scales, by virtue of the theory that deduces these personalities, is maximized. The content scales then became aptly termed "facet scales," because each represented a facet of a prototypal personality (as measured by the principal Axis II construct scales). A further utilitarian purpose to such a design was the ability to examine the divergence of elevations between the primary scales, as well as their associated subscales, for purposes of treatment planning. Knowing from a clinical interview that a person is likely to be diagnosed with histrionic personality disorder, for example, the clinician would be in a position, after assessment, to determine what *subtype* (or admixture of personality prototypes) of histrionic expression this individual would present, and within that, what *traits* at the domain level would be most salient. The deductive methodology of the Millon inventories, along with the nature of the intended subscales' intended use, suggested that the most empirically sound, theoretically logical, and clinically effective framework for facet scale development, stated in terms of Davis's (1993) model, would be to develop subscales for each prototypal personality pattern of the MCMI-III (working within logical boundaries of the extant scales); this would best be achieved by utilizing a combined rational–empirical approach, with the initial generation of the subscales grounded in the overarching theory (i.e., initiated via rational means).

A first consideration was to identify a pragmatic level of the theory on which to base predictions. Two choices were obvious: The first was the evolutionary dimension level (i.e., survival, modification, adaptation), and the second was the functional–structural personological domain level (i.e., expressive behaviors, interpersonal conduct, and the other six domains). However, neither of these possibilities was seen to be generative of theoretical or empirical promise for subscales. The first represented the derivation of personality styles *across* logical domains, and would have been more appropriate for an analysis that had as its goal the construction of content scales seeking basic motivations of persons across prototypal constructs. The latter would be an attempt to extract precisely eight factors for each individual, small item pool. This would be unwieldy at best in terms of clinical utility, and would also be highly unlikely to be psychometrically sound, given the properties of available statistical procedures. Beyond these possibilities, two other logical options for this breakdown emerged as delineations predicted by the overarching theory, which then appeared to be the most viable alternatives.

Two logical means of organization for the domain expression of the personality styles were described by Millon and Davis (1996). First, the eight personological domains may be grouped together into four logical classes representing the gestalt of personality, as follows: (1) behavioral (subsuming expressive behaviors and interpersonal conduct); (2) phenomenological (subsuming cognitive style, self-image, and object representations); (3) intrapsychic (subsuming regulatory mechanisms and morphological organization); and (4) biophysical (subsuming mood/temperament). These categories appeared highly convenient in terms of clinical use, as they correspond to contemporary treatment modalities, and four similar subscales for each personality scale would have certainly proven useful. In essence, all other things being equal, this would have been the structure of choice in terms of parsimony and comprehensiveness. Although this option represented the basic prototypal structure of each personality style on which the primary scales are based, each prototypal pattern in reality emphasizes different domains; that is, some of the eight domains in a prototype will be accented and prominent, while others of those eight may be quite subtle. The Millon inventories, owing to their deductive test construction methodology, reflect these relative compositions. In other words, it concentrates items as the theory predicts for prototypal presentation.

The other possibility is a manifestation of the foregoing, and is represented in the theory as the salience of personological domains. For each personality style, Millon (1990; Millon & Davis, 1996) posits that two to three of the personological domains will be most salient for a given prototype; one to three others will probably be of moderate (supportive) importance; and the remaining domains will be present, but often subtle. Which domain presents as the most salient, according to prototypal structure, varies among personality styles. For example, the histrionic personality prototype is primarily identified by interpersonal conduct and mood/temperament, with expressive behaviors and cognitive style playing a secondary but important role. In contrast, for the depressive prototype, cognitive style and mood/temperament are the most salient features, with three other domains presenting as significant but more moderate. Successful statistical analyses conducted within each item pool would then provide further support for these theoretical notions, and would be consistent with the ultimate objective of constructing subscales under each primary scale.

This level of the theory, then, appeared to be the most congruent and stable starting point to guide examination of the items contained in each of the 14 item pools of the MCMI-III personality scales. The investigation began with predictions about the most salient domains contained in each primary scale, many of which were predicted to match the most salient domains of the theory. Preliminary choices at this stage determined which and how many domains would best capture extant item content, guided by salience predictions of the overarching theory, as well as rational examination of each item pool. Table 6.1 delineates the functional and structural domains of each of the prototypal personality patterns.

The following stage involved a choice of statistical methodology to support these predictions. The data pool to be used consisted of item responses from the original MCMI-III standardization sample. Subjects consisted of 600 subjects used for the development of the clinical scales, and 393 individuals used for cross-validation purposes, who were administered an MCMI-III research form. As has been the case with most content scales or subscales in the past, the most logical choices for empirical substantiation of the subscales would be factor-analytic methods. However, because of the enigmatic scale construction utilizing single items on multiple primary scales, the brevity of each item pool, and the high covariance expected due to the polythetic nature of the theory, most statistical methods would not be expected to yield highly parsimonious results (Choca, 1998).

Given the theoretical nature of the task, one might argue that a sound choice would have been to employ one of several confirmatory factor-analytic (CFA) methods now available (Goldberg & Digman, 1994). However, CFA, by its nature, assumes a normal distribution of the data under consideration. The Millon inventories do not follow this assumption. Rather, its normative data are based on estimates of prevalence rates of clinical patterns known *not* to be normally distributed (Millon, 2006a, 2006b). Hence, as other researchers considering CFA in analyzing Millon instrumentation have noted (e.g., Derksen & Sloore, 2005), CFA is inappropriate for applications involving the MCMI-III, whereas exploratory factor analysis (EFA) options remain viable.

The best choice for this procedure, then, became alpha method factor analysis, as it maximizes internal consistency of the extracted factors; it differs from principal components analysis, a more widely utilized method, in that it extracts factors specifically with this end in mind. This affords the researcher a degree of freedom to concentrate on distal concerns, such as the rational refinement of the resultant factors, without as much concomitant concern with deleting items manually in order to max-

TABLE 6.1. Personality Pattern Attributes by Functional–Structural Domain

	Expressive behaviors	Interpersonal conduct	Cognitive style	Self-image	Object representations	Regulatory mechanisms	Morphological organization	Mood/ temperament
Schizoid	Impassive	Unengaged	Impoverished	Complacent	Meager	Intellectualization	Undifferentiated	Apathetic
Avoidant	Fretful	Aversive	Distracted	Alienated	Vexatious	Fantasy	Fragile	Anguished
Depressive	Disconsolate	Defenseless	Pessimistic	Worthless	Forsaken	Asceticism	Depleted	Melancholic
Dependent	Incompetent	Submissive	Naive	Inept	Immature	Introjection	Inchoate	Pacific
Histrionic	Dramatic	Attention-seeking	Flighty	Gregarious	Shallow	Dissociation	Disjointed	Fickle
Narcissistic	Haughty	Exploitive	Expansive	Admirable	Contrived	Rationalization	Spurious	Insouciant
Antisocial	Impulsive	Irresponsible	Deviant	Autonomous	Debased	Acting out	Unruly	Callous
Sadistic	Precipitate	Abrasive	Dogmatic	Combative	Pernicious	Isolation	Eruptive	Hostile
Compulsive	Disciplined	Respectful	Constricted	Conscientious	Concealed	Reaction formation	Compartmentalized	Solemn
Negativistic	Resentful	Contrary	Skeptical	Discontented	Vacillating	Displacement	Divergent	Irritable
Masochistic	Abstinent	Deferential	Diffident	Undeserving	Discredited	Exaggeration	Inverted	Dysphoric
Schizotypal	Eccentric	Secretive	Autistic	Estranged	Chaotic	Undoing	Fragmented	Distraught or insentient
Borderline	Spasmodic	Paradoxical	Capricious	Uncertain	Incompatible	Regression	Split	Labile
Paranoid	Defensive	Provocative	Suspicious	Inviolable	Unalterable	Projection	Inelastic	Irascible

123

imize coefficient alphas (Davis, 1993). In addition, an oblique rotation method was employed, allowing for correlated factors consonant with the polythetic model that undergirds the DSM personality disorders. Of the available choices for oblique rotations, promax rotation was the best choice, given the large size of the data set and its endorsement by previous investigators of polythetic personality attributes (e.g., Goldberg & Digman, 1994).

Owing to the first rational step, a factor-analytic procedure to help substantiate theoretical predictions required some rationale for extracting the appropriate number of factors likely to differ from common approaches, such as Kaiser's (1960) stopping rule related to eigenvectors over 1.00, or Cattell's (1966) graphical scree test procedure. Hair, Anderson, Tatham, and Black (1992) have suggested an alternative, a priori criterion, useful for researchers motivated by a predetermined theory that specifies an appropriate number of factors. This procedure was followed, using the first-stage predictions as a guide for specifying factor solutions.

Following the aforementioned factor-analytic stage, the factors that emerged were subjected to a rational refinement stage. Results of the factor analysis were scrutinized for their concordance with the predicted personological domains, and adjustments were made on the basis of content and relative factor loadings. The next stage involved calculating alphas for the proposed subscales. Given the predicted brevity of many of the subscales, and the polythetic nature of personality constructs, a moderate alpha (in this early stage, .50) was deemed acceptable.

The final preparation stage, incorporation of the proposed facet subscales as a supplementary MCMI-III interpretive tool, involved further scrutiny of various elements of the emerged factor structure. Intercorrelations, as predicted by the polythetic model, were anticipated to be moderately high; those scales demonstrating more orthogonal qualities were scrutinized closely for their concordance with the theory. Also, personality measures demonstrating an unacceptably high level of skewness would lack appropriate sensitivity at the higher end of the scale where clinical distinction is most important. These required further adjustment in item composition.

As this final stage neared completion, it became apparent that the instruments would benefit from augmentation of items with those outside the original 14 distinct item pools. Although this broke with the original idea of working within scale, it stayed with the sprit of this approach; the original study (Grossman & del Rio, 2005) offered support to the notion that trends in the data would empirically support rationally divided content along theoretical lines. To bolster the statistical properties of this content, and to "flesh out" the domains identified via the original study, Theodore Millon suggested the use of supportive items, mostly derived from the MCMI-III Clinical Syndrome Scales (Axis I), that followed the face intent of the identified domains (e.g., items from the Dysthymia scale worked well to augment and complete Depressive personality facet scales such as Temperamentally Woeful and Cognitively Pessimistic. Experimentation with these additions, as appropriate with the polythetic nature of these personality constructs, served not only to strengthen extant scales, but to round out the full set of Grossman Facet Scales to three subscales per primary scale—a development thought to expand clinical utility. Base rate (BR) scores for the final facet scales were then calculated, the augmented scales were reassessed for alpha coefficient consistency, and skewness was analyzed.

In the final preparatory stage, the Grossman Facet Scales adopted BR conversions reflecting those for each of the "parent" scales, but did not retain the weighted point system. It was also decided—owing to the MCMI-III system of shared items between primary scales, as well as clinical utility considerations—that a general threshold for interpretability would be established at BR = 65. This consideration is consistent with the tradition set by the Harris–Lingoes subscales of the MMPI (Harris & Lingoes, 1955, 1968). It is useful to interpret some Facet scales without a clinically significant elevation on the corresponding primary scale (i.e., BR = 75), as this can denote domain/traits that are worthy of clinical consideration; however, limitations needed to be set in order to increase clarity and diminish "false positives" on less relevant facets. As clinical experience with these facets grows, it is anticipated that clinicians may benefit from examining Facet Scale elevations on nonelevated primary scales, in conjunction with sound clinical judgment that takes into account the full context of the presenting picture. In the recent revision of the manual, profile,

TABLE 6.2. The MCMI-III Grossman Facet Scales

Schizoid
1.1: Temperamentally Apathetic
1.2: Interpersonally Unengaged
1.3: Expressively Impassive

Avoidant
2A.1: Interpersonally Aversive
2A.2: Alienated Self-Image
2A.3: Vexatious Representations

Depressive
2B.1: Temperamentally Woeful
2B.2: Worthless Self-Image
2B.3: Cognitively Fatalistic

Dependent
3.1: Inept Self-Image
3.2: Interpersonally Submissive
3.3: Immature Representations

Histrionic
4.1: Gregarious Self-Image
4.2: Interpersonally Attention-Seeking
4.3: Expressively Dramatic

Narcissistic
5.1: Admirable Self-Image
5.2: Cognitively Expansive
5.3: Interpersonally Exploitive

Antisocial
6A.1: Expressively Impulsive
6A.2: Acting-Out Mechanism
6A.3: Interpersonally Irresponsible

Sadistic
6B.1: Temperamentally Hostile
6B.2: Eruptive Organization
6B.3: Pernicious Representations

Compulsive
7.1: Cognitively Constricted
7.2: Interpersonally Respectful
7.3: Reliable Self-Image

Negativistic
8A.1: Temperamentally Irritable
8A.2: Expressively Resentful
8A.3: Discontented Self-Image

Masochistic
8B.1: Discredited Representations
8B.2: Cognitively Diffident
8B.3: Undeserving Self-Image

Schizotypal
S.1: Estranged Self-Image
S.2: Cognitively Autistic
S.3: Chaotic Representations

Borderline
C.1: Temperamentally Labile
C.2: Interpersonally Paradoxical
C.3: Uncertain Self-Image

Paranoid
P.1: Cognitively Mistrustful
P.2: Expressively Defensive
P.3: Projection Mechanism

and interpretive report, however, only those Facet Scales of the top three primary scale elevations over BR = 65 are graphically portrayed on a second profile page; all Facet Scale scores are listed on the page immediately following.

The MCMI-III Grossman Facet Scales are presented in Table 6.2.

MACI Grossman Facet Scales

Consistent with the rationale for the MCMI-III Grossman Facet Scales (Millon, 2006a), the decision was subsequently made to create a similar set of Facet Scales for the manual and report revisions of the MACI (Millon, 2006b). A different starting point was utilized, however: The factor structure of Davis's (1993) earlier formulation for MACI content subscales was assessed for its concordance with the overarching theory. As Davis had taken a path initiated by empirical study and followed by rational refinement that drew more on the factor-analytic (i.e., inductive) tradition, these initial content scales were deemed a strong basis for the new study, and they eventually demonstrated a reasonable overlap with the new rational framework. However, certain clear differences in structure and intent were noted, and Millon and

---

TABLE 6.3. The MACI Grossman Facet Scales

Introversive	Unruly
1.1: Expressively Impassive	6A.1: Expressively Impulsive
1.2: Temperamentally Apathetic	6A.2: Acting-Out Mechanism
1.3: Interpersonally Unengaged	6A.3: Interpersonally Irresponsible
Inhibited	Forceful
2A.1: Expressively Fretful	6B.1: Interpersonally Abrasive
2A.2: Interpersonally Aversive	6B.2: Expressively Precipitate
2A.3: Alienated Self-Image	6B.3: Isolation Mechanism
Doleful	Conforming
2B.1: Temperamentally Woeful	7.1: Expressively Disciplined
2B.2: Expressively Disconsolate	7.2: Interpersonally Respectful
2B.3: Cognitively Fatalistic	7.3: Conscientious Self-Image
Submissive	Oppositional
3.1: Interpersonally Docile	8A.1: Discontented Self-Image
3.2: Temperamentally Pacific	8A.2: Expressively Resentful
3.3: Expressively Incompetent	8A.3: Interpersonally Contrary
Dramatizing	Self-Demeaning
4.1: Interpersonally Attention-Seeking	8B.1: Cognitively Diffident
4.2: Gregarious Self-Image	8B.2: Undeserving Self-Image
4.3: Cognitively Flighty	8B.3: Temperamentally Dysphoric
Egotistic	Borderline Tendency
5.1: Admirable Self-Image	9.1: Temperamentally Labile
5.2: Cognitively Expansive	9.2: Cognitively Capricious
5.3: Interpersonally Exploitive	9.3: Uncertain Self-Image

I decided to apply what had been explored only as was reasonable to the newer concept that was used for the MCMI-III Facet Scales.

As with the MCMI-III, then, reconstruction of the MACI subscales began with rational examination of each MACI personality scale item pool, and with initial assignments to corroborate with the eight functional and structural domains of personality, partially guided by the work of Davis (1993); the intent was the construction of three facet scales for each of the MACI's 12 primary personality scales, utilizing theoretical predictions for most salient domains. Many of these domains were similar to the adult salient domains represented in the MCMI-III, but some age-related differences were found. Again as with the MCMI-III, the scales were then analyzed for internal consistency, skewness, and rational reflection of theoretical concepts. Some items from syndromal scales were added to these scales, as was done with the MCMI-III Facet Scales, and final alpha calculations and BR scoring were conducted to reflect age–gender groups and trends from the original MACI sample.

Table 6.3 lists the final MACI Grossman Facet Scales.

Facet Scales in Context with Assessment

Personality is composed of facets that, taken individually, are neither necessary nor sufficient conditions for a diagnosis of a personality disorder. Both Millon's evolutionary theory (Millon, 1990; Millon & Davis, 1996) and the DSM-IV-TR (American Psychiatric Association, 2000) demonstrate this concept. For example, the DSM specifies nine criteria for narcissistic personality disorder, but only five are required for a diagnosis. In the evolutionary theory, eight domains are listed as core components of the prototypal narcissistic personality pattern (as is the case with all prototypal patterns derived from this theory) but, as stated previously, there are very few truly prototypal personalities. Instead, most clinical presentations involve admixtures of personality patterns, probably involving parallel domains from other prototypes in the spectrum of personological patterns. In other words, two people with the same DSM Axis II diagnosis are almost guaranteed to differ in their clinical presentation, and this divergence is very likely to be clinically significant. Regardless of whether an assessment clinician is oriented toward one or the other (or possibly both) of these paradigms, simply stating that a person falls under one or more of the established diagnostic categories is not sufficient for real clinical utility. The real world demonstrates that divergence between the diagnosis and possession of its defining features is the "norm," not the exception, and that considerable heterogeneity is probable within the established diagnostic system.

The Grossman Facet Scales address these assessment shortcomings on several levels. The first level speaks to distinctions that are now illuminated within each primary scale. Two individuals diagnosed with the same Axis II syndrome may be expected to demonstrate markedly different problematic domains within that diagnostic category. The addition of the Facet scales allows for a more molecular view of the primary diagnosis, highlighting important dimensions of personological function at a more discriminating level than can be achieved via categorical labels. In other words, clinicians may now note the most important functional and structural domains of a person's Axis II diagnosis.

A second level relates to individuals who present with significant personality features, but who do not qualify for an Axis II diagnosis. The DSM multiaxial system does allow personality features to be noted on Axis II, in order to allow clinicians to conceptualize how "personality traits" may be affecting an Axis I presentation. However, this system does not allow for much specificity other than noting either that the person presents with nonspecific traits of a given category, or that a particular coping mechanism is used (American Psychiatric Association, 2000). The Facet Scales are designed so as not to require a full elevation of a primary scale in order to hold interpretive value; rather, the threshold for interpretability is at a set BR point (generally, BR = 65) *below* clinical likelihood of a given Axis II disorder. In this capacity, the clinician may then make note of problematic functional and structural domains with a greater degree of specificity.

A further consideration goes well beyond within-category distinctions to a much more focused, cross-sectional level of personality functioning, in that the Facet Scales are able to draw attention to specific elevations *across* primary scales. As noted earlier in this chapter, Millon's evolutionary theory predicts that most personality presentations are admixtures of two or more personality patterns that form "subtypes" (e.g., narcissistic with antisocial features, dependent with avoidant features, etc.). Sixty-one subtype patterns have been identified in Millon's writings of the past decade or so (Millon, 1999a; Millon & Davis, 1996; Millon, Grossman, Millon, Meagher, & Ramnath, 2004); further combinations appear regularly in clinical presentations. As the Facet Scales are tied to the eight functional and structural domains consistent across all primary patterns, it is possible that a subtype pattern may be detected by the primary scales, and that specific comparable facets may be identified by the corresponding subscales. As an example, an individual's primary MCMI-III score may suggest a subtype of antisocial with histrionic features (identified by the theory as "risk-taking antisocial"); while the subscales may then identify "impulsive expressive behavior" (from the Antisocial facets) and "attention-seeking interpersonal conduct" (from the Histrionic facets). A clearer, more detailed clinical picture emerges with this greater level of specificity.

Beyond Assessment:
Implications for Treatment Planning and Intervention

In a mature science, a theory is posited that serves as the generative source for a system of classifying the phenomena found within the domain of the subject matter at hand, as well as a method for measuring and substantiating the content of the classification system. What makes such a science clinical in nature, however, is the additional ability to manipulate and modify those phenomena (Millon, 1990). Clinical psychology, of course, is no exception to this rule; the definitive function that makes this subject domain a clinical science is the ability to intervene in a manner most consonant with beneficial change. The ultimate goal of the MCMI-III Facet Scales is to promote such intervention.

The Grossman Facet Scales, being aligned with evolutionary theory domains that are aligned in turn with the various "schools of thought" in psychotherapy (cognitive, psychodynamic, pharmacological, etc.), may be employed to help identify and target those constructs on which established, evidence-based treatments are likely to focus. Furthermore, although purists and strict adherents to the various unilateral schools of psychotherapy are not likely to accept the myriad of choices from competing therapeutic paradigms, the growing numbers of integrative and eclectic approaches to treatment in both traditional and "short-term" modalities may benefit from this new focus. For example, combinations of cognitive and pharmacological modalities, as well as cognitive and behavioral modalities (e.g., Beck, Freeman, Davis, & Associates, 2004; Young, 1990), are now widely utilized strategies for the treatment of personality and mood disorders. Generally speaking, these models seek not only to ascertain an individual's cognitive schemas (relating to subscales oriented to cognitive style and self-image), but also to understand and modify mood difficulties and behavioral tendencies (relating to subscales oriented to mood/temperament, expressive behaviors, and interpersonal conduct). In these and other contemporary examples, the greater specificity afforded by the addition of personality facet subscales will enhance therapists' efforts at efficient and pragmatic intervention.

The personalized psychotherapy paradigm (Millon & Grossman, 2007a, 2007b, 2007c) is a direct outgrowth of the same theory that has guided the development of the Facet Scales. This paradigm is integrative in nature, recognizing the eight personological domains employed by the subscales as key guides to appropriate therapeutic strategies. Taken together, they constitute the complex, interwoven system of the individual's personality, which may be viewed as the "psychic immune system." Any given personality pattern will have certain vulnerabilities that may, given environmental and constitutional conditions, result in problematic psychological functioning. By intervening pragmatically at the personality level (i.e., choosing strategies from the various available therapeutic modalities aligned with personological domains), while tactically orienting treatment toward balancing and/or restructuring the "motivating aims" as represented by the evolutionary polarities (i.e., pain–pleasure, passive–active, self–other), a therapist employing this system of psychotherapy can work toward bolstering an individual's personological functioning, rather than simply treating the person's symptoms alone and out of context. A brief case example may serve to illustrate the type of efficient, targeted intervention possible with the introduction of the Grossman Facet Scales.

Presenting Picture

Hector Q., 24, was considered a "bookworm" in high school. He was routinely picked up and dropped off by his mother, spoke to no one in school, and was harassed venomously by school bullies. On evenings and weekends, he spent his time asocially, generally either studying or writing poetry extolling the virtues of traditional family values. Prior to entering college, he attempted suicide and was thereafter held at home by his mother for several years, until, as he put it, "she unshackled me." Feeling awkward and still devoid of social experience, Hector entered college while still living in the family's home; he was usually chauffeured to campus by his mother, as he had never learned to drive and was now fearful to start learning. Now in his second year, he had attempted to join some clubs but was, according to his report, "shunned" by most people even when he tried to participate. He admitted that he was developing a kind of arrogance toward others in defense of his perception of rejection, and that the only place he felt "safe" to express his frustration was in his writing, wherein he began creating "morally righteous" characters who punished anyone straying from traditional values. However, he admitted that he was extremely lonely, and wanted to "just be a normal guy and fit in."

Initial Impressions

Although he was insightful into his difficulties during more lucid, comfortable moments, Hector usually presented as highly constricted and fearful, uncertain even of his "right" to state his own introspections. More so than usual, rapport building required an emphasis on acceptance while being grounded in credibility and objectivity, even when genuine reflections veered toward stark and direct statements of intent in terms of his treatment. For example, one early exchange involved Hector's admitting that he felt safe by eliciting pity from others (usually family members), to which the therapist replied, "I do feel for you; the circumstances that have brought you here—be they your perceptions, your outward experiences, and maybe even your biological temperament—those are truly unfortunate. But I'm not about to pity you, and that's going to feel pretty uncomfortable for a while." From the start, this set the tone that although Hector could consider therapy a safe environment, this environment would not be subject to "usual" safety tactics. In essence, there was a here-and-now opportunity to depict safety, an integral part of his pain-avoidant personality framework (which vacillated between activity and passivity in its adaptive process), in a different light. Early interactions in this regard were intense, sometimes painful to the point of causing anguish, but representative of a different level of self-exposure in which Hector nevertheless remained safe. Still, this would prove difficult to generalize to his overall environment.

Domain Analysis

In an early therapeutic session, Hector was administered the MCMI-III with the Grossman Facet Scales, along with a projective measure and several brief symptom measures. For purposes of illustration, our discussion here is limited to the MCMI-III and Grossman Facet Scale scores. Hector's MCMI-III results indicated very high (above BR = 85) scores on both scales 2A (Avoidant) and 2B (Depressive), with a significant (above BR = 75) score on scale 3 (Dependent). Several other scales showed significant elevations (e.g., Schizoid, Masochistic), which added some depth to the overall portrait. Taken together, the overall picture suggested a primary motivating emphasis on "playing it safe," actively limiting his exposure to the world, while succumbing to feelings that there is no escaping perceived pain and torment. One of Hector's primary defenses, as mentioned before, was to play "inept" or "pitiful," in order to solicit protectiveness from close family members. However, in situations where he was forced to socialize, Hector appeared to elicit a kind of subordination that invited trouble in the form of being either rejected or publicly humiliated or abused.

Several Facet Scale scores proved enlightening for purposes of treatment planning. Self-image constructs were highly elevated on all three of the highest scales (2A, 2B, 3); Hector described himself on these scales as alienated, worthless, and inept, respectively, all as reflected in BR scores higher than 95. This combination suggested that Hector faulted himself as being unable to fit in, overemphasizing his lack of social acumen, and fusing this with a degraded sense of self-worth. These self-reflections were further bolstered by significant elevations in social-behavioral and interpersonal constructs such as Vexatious Representations and Immature Representations (from the Avoidant and Dependent scales, respectively) and Interpersonally Submissive (from the Dependent scale). This combination reflected Hector's limited worldview of people who are inherently troublesome, who take precedence over his needs, but who are represented in his perceptions only by these almost caricaturish and larger-than-life qualities. Finally, Hector scored very high on the Depressive subscale Temperamentally Woe-ful, illustrating the pervasive melancholic and gloomy quality of his affective state, which undoubtedly cast his worries into states of helplessness and served to fuel his self-image and interpersonal difficulties.

Treatment Course

This case illustrates the compounding and interrelated nature of some of these personological domains. Initial explorations served primarily to dispel the troublesome nature of interrela-tionships by using the therapeutic relationship as a form of "reparenting," in which Hector could begin to put ideas together that were previously incompatible. By accepting him, while not accepting his perceptions of ineptitude, the therapist began fostering positive change by means of a progressively challenging relationship, where Hector was able to recognize the dif-ference between conflict and threat. The first domains to be tackled were Hector's inept self-image and vexatious/immature representations. Gaining a respect for the multifaceted presen-tation offered by the therapist, Hector began self-challenges to his belief structure about the world as a ubiquitously harmful place and started to take minor risks in social communica-tions, alleviating some of his feelings of alienation as well as his "safe zone" of acting submis-sive. Because of Hector's refusal of pharmacotherapy, special attention needed to be paid to his pervasive woefulness; cognitive reframing, effectively placed throughout this largely brief dynamic intervention, served to challenge his worries and perpetual downheartedness, but this procedure would have been augmented and catalyzed by appropriate use of medication. Com-bining these cognitive methods with continued supportive–existential initiatives began to break up Hector's deeply entrenched beliefs of worthlessness enough for him, as he became ready, to prove himself "wrong." At the time of writing, Hector had made considerable social strides, but continued to hold himself back from some basic competencies (e.g., learning to drive); in this way, he was holding onto his ineptness to assure a modicum of safety by assur-ing himself that he would continue to be cared for. Further therapeutic efforts will be made, on supportive and behavioral levels, to address these concerns while continuing to bolster Hector's gradually improving but still troubled self-image beliefs.

Concluding Comments

The Grossman Facet Scales of the MCMI-III and MACI are strong supportive clinical tools that may be most adequately utilized as clinical-hypothesis-building measures, rather than as "absolutes" in terms of identifying precise personological constructs. No single psychometric measure should be used alone, and the Facet Scales are not exempt from this caveat. Fortunately, although subscales respecting logical bound-aries at the personality construct level (i.e., primary personality scales) retain the dis-advantages of their parent scale, they also inherit their advantages. As content areas reflective of the parent construct, they retain qualities such as validity and theoretical consonance, and may be substantiated beyond their own internal consistency by vir-tue of this overarching theory and its primary personality patterns. However, they must be taken in context with the presenting clinical picture, and their measures can be sustained only insofar as the evidence external to the measure itself (inclusive of primary scales, other assessment data, and ongoing clinical observation) remains consistent with its findings.

References

American Psychiatric Association. (2000). *Diagnostic and statistical manual of mental disorders* (4th ed., text rev.). Washington, DC: Author.

Archer, R. P., Aiduk, R., Griffin, R., & Elkins, D. E. (1996). Incremental validity of the MMPI-2 content scales in a psychiatric sample. *Assessment, 3,* 79–90.

Barthlow, D. L., Graham, J. R., Ben-Porath, Y. S., & McNulty, J. L. (1999). Incremental validity of the MMPI-2 content scales in an outpatient mental heath setting. *Psychological Assessment, 11,* 39–47.

Beck, A. T., Freeman, A., Davis, D. D., & Associates. (2004). *Cognitive therapy of personality disorders* (2nd ed.). New York: Guilford Press.

Ben-Porath, Y. S., Butcher, J. N., & Graham, J. R. (1991). Contribution of the MMPI-2 content scales to the differential diagnosis of schizophrenia and major depression. *Psychological Assessment, 3,* 634–640.

Ben-Porath, Y. S., & Sherwood, N. E. (1993). *The MMPI-2 content component scales: Development, psychometric characteristics, and clinical application.* Minneapolis: University of Minnesota Press.

Boone, D. E. (1994). Validity of the MMPI-2 Depression content scale with psychiatric inpatients. *Psychological Reports, 74,* 159–162.

Burisch, M. (1984). Approaches to personality inventory construction. *American Psychologist, 39,* 214–227.

Butcher, J. N., Graham, J. R., Williams, C. L., & Ben-Porath, Y. S. (1990). *Development and use of the MMPI-2 content scales.* Minneapolis: University of Minnesota Press.

Cattell, R. B. (1966). The meaning and strategic use of factor analysis. In R. B. Cattell (Ed.), *Handbook of multivariate experimental psychology* (pp. 174–243). Chicago: Rand McNally.

Cattell, R. B., Eber, H. W., & Tatsuoka, M. M. (1970). *Handbook for the Sixteen Personality Factor Questionnaire (16PF).* Champaign, IL: Institute for Personality and Ability Testing.

Choca, J., Retzlaff, P., Strack, S., & Mouton, A. (1996). Factorial elements in Millon's personality theory. *Journal of Personality Disorders, 10,* 377–383.

Choca, J. P. (1998). [Review of the Millon Index of Personality Styles]. In J. C. Impara & B. S. Plake (Eds.), *The thirteenth mental measurements yearbook.* (See Test Number 202). Lincoln, NE: Buros Institute of Mental Measurements.

Clark, L. A. (1993). *Schedule for Nonadaptive and Adaptive Personality (SNAP) manual.* Minneapolis: University of Minnesota Press.

Costa, P. T., & McCrae, R. R. (1992). *Revised NEO Personality Inventory (NEO-PI-R) and NEO Five Factor Inventory (NEO-FFI) professional manual.* Odessa, FL: Psychological Assessment Resources.

Costa, P. T., & Widiger, T. A. (Eds.). (1994). *Personality disorders and the five-factor model of personality.* Washington, DC: American Psychological Association.

Cronbach, L. J., & Meehl, P. E. (1955). Construct validity in psychological tests. *Psychological Bulletin, 52,* 281–302.

Davis, R. D. (1993). *Development of content scales for the Millon Adolescent Clinical Inventory.* Unpublished master's thesis, University of Miami.

Davis, R. D. (1999). Millon: Essentials of his science, theory, classification, assessment, and therapy. *Journal of Personality Assessment, 72,* 330–353.

Davis, R. D., & Millon, T. (1993). The five-factor model for personality disorders: Apt or misguided? *Psychological Inquiry, 4,* 104–109.

Derksen, J., & Sloore, H. (2005). Issues in the international use of psychological tests. In S. Strack (Ed.), *Handbook of personology and psychopathology: Essays in honor of Theodore Millon.* Hoboken, NJ: Wiley.

Dorr, D. (1999). Approaching psychotherapy of the personality disorders from the Millon perspective. *Journal of Personality Assessment, 72,* 407–426.

Goldberg, L. R. (1990). An alternative "description of personality": The Big-Five factor structure. *Journal of Personality and Social Psychology, 59*, 1216–1229.

Goldberg, L. R., & Digman, J. M. (1994). Revealing structure in the data: Principles of exploratory factor analysis. In S. Strack (Ed.), *Differentiating normal and abnormal personality* (pp. 216–242). New York: Springer.

Graham, J. R. (2000). *MMPI-2: Assessing personality and psychopathology* (3rd ed.). New York: Oxford University Press.

Grossman, S. D., & del Rio, C. (2005). [ch 1]. In R. J. Craig (Ed.), *New directions on interpreting the MCMI-III*. Hoboken, NJ: Wiley.

Hair, J. F., Anderson, R. E., Tatham, R. L., & Black, W. C. (1992). *Multivariate data analysis with readings* (3rd ed.). New York: Macmillan.

Harris, R., & Lingoes, J. (1955). *Subscales for the Minnesota Multiphasic Personality Inventory.* Unpublished manuscript, Langley Porter Neuropsychiatric Institute.

Harris, R., & Lingoes, J. (1968). *Subscales for the Minnesota Multiphasic Personality Inventory.* Unpublished manuscript, Langley–Porter Neuropsychiatric Institute.

Hathaway, S. R., & McKinley, J. C. (1943). *Minnesota Multiphasic Personality Inventory (MMPI).* Minneapolis: University of Minnesota Press.

Kaiser, H. F. (1960). The application of electronic computers to factor analysis. *Educational and Psychological Measurement, 20*, 141–151.

Kopper, B. A., Osman, A., & Barrios, F. X. (2001). Assessment of suicidal ideation in young men and women: The incremental validity of the MMPI-2 content scales. *Death Studies 25*, 593–607.

Kopper, B. A., Osman, A., Osman, J. R., & Hoffman, J. (1998). Clinical utility of the MMPI-A content scales and Harris–Lingoes subscales in the assessment of suicidal risk factors in psychiatric adolescents. *Journal of Clinical Psychology, 54*, 191–200.

Livesley, W. J., Jackson, D. N., & Schroeder, M. L. (1989). A study of the factorial structure of personality pathology. *Journal of Personality Disorders, 3*, 292–306.

Loevinger, J. (1957). Objective tests as instruments of psychological theory. *Psychological Reports, 3*, 635–694.

MacAndrew, C. (1965). The differentiation of male alcoholic out-patients from nonalcoholic psychiatric patients by means of the MMPI. *Quarterly Journal of Studies on Alcohol, 26*, 238–246.

Meehl, P. E. (1945). The dynamics of "structured" personality tests. *Journal of Clinical Psychology, 1*, 296–303.

Millon, T. (1969). *Modern psychopathology: A biosocial approach to maladaptive learning and functioning.* Philadelphia: Saunders.

Millon, T. (1977). *Millon Clinical Multiaxial Inventory (MCMI) manual.* Minneapolis, MN: National Computer Systems.

Millon, T. (1987). *Millon Clinical Multiaxial Inventory–II (MCMI-II) manual.* Minneapolis, MN: National Computer Systems.

Millon, T. (1990). *Toward a new personology: An evolutionary model.* New York: Wiley.

Millon, T. (1999). Reflections on psychosynergy: A model for integrating science, theory, classification, assessment, and therapy. *Journal of Personality Assessment, 72*, 437–457.

Millon, T., & Davis, R. D. (1996). *Disorders of personality: DSM-IV and beyond.* New York: Wiley.

Millon, T., & Davis, R. D. (1997). The MCMI-III: Present and future directions. *Journal of Personality Assessment, 68*, 69–85.

Millon, T., & Grossman, S. D. (2006). Millon's evolutionary model for unifying the study of normal and abnormal personality. In S. Strack (Ed.), *Differentiating normal and abnormal personality* (2nd ed., pp.). New York: Springer.

Millon, T., & Grossman, S. D. (2007a). *Resolving difficult clinical syndromes: A personalized psychotherapy approach.* Hoboken, NJ: Wiley.

Millon, T., & Grossman, S. D. (2007b). *Overcoming resistant personality disorders: A personalized psychotherapy approach*. Hoboken, NJ: Wiley.

Millon, T., & Grossman, S. D. (2007c). *Moderating severe personality disorders: A personalized psychotherapy approach*. Hoboken, NJ: Wiley.

Millon, T., Grossman, S. D., Millon, C., Meagher, S., & Ramnath, R. (2004). *Personality disorders in modern life* (2nd ed.). Hoboken, NJ: Wiley.

Millon, T. (with Millon, C., & Davis, R. D.). (1993). *Millon Adolescent Clinical Inventory*. Minneapolis, MN: National Computer Systems.

Millon, T. (with Millon, C., Davis, R. D., & Grossman, S. D.). (2006a). *Millon Clinical Multiaxial Inventory–III (MCMI-III) manual* (3rd ed.). Minneapolis, MN: Pearson Assessments.

Millon, T. (with Millon, C., Davis, R. D., & Grossman, S. D.). (2006b). *Millon Adolescent Clinical Inventory (MACI) manual* (2nd ed.). Minneapolis, MN: Pearson Assessments.

Morey, L. C., Waugh, M. H., & Blashfield, R. K. (1985). MMPI scales for DSM-III personality disorders: Their derivation and correlates. *Journal of Personality Assessment, 49,* 245–256.

Munley, P. H., Busby, R. M., & Jaynes, G. (1997). MMPI-2 findings in schizophrenia and depression. *Psychological Assessment, 9,* 508–511.

Palav, A., Ortega, A., & McCaffrey, R. J. (2001). Incremental validity of the MMPI-2 content scales: A preliminary study with brain-injured patients. *Journal of Head Trauma Rehabilitation, 16,* 275–283.

Petrocelli, J. V., Glaser, B. A., Calhoun, G. B., & Campbell, L. F. (2001). Early maladaptive schemas of personality disorder subtypes. *Journal of Personality Disorders, 15,* 546–559.

Wiggins, J. S. (1966). Substantive dimensions of self-report in the MMPI item pool. *Psychological Monographs, 80*(22, Whole No. 630).

Wiggins, J. S. (1969). Content dimensions in the MMPI. In J. N. Butcher (Ed.), *MMPI: Research developments and clinical applications* (pp. 127–180). New York: McGraw-Hill.

Young, J. E. (1990). *Cognitive therapy for personality disorders: A schema-focused approach*. Sarasota, FL: Professional Resource Exchange.

CHAPTER 7

Clinical Integration of the MCMI-III and the Rorschach Comprehensive System

Darwin Dorr

This chapter examines the clinical use of the Millon Clinical Multiaxial Inventory–III (MCMI-III; Millon, 1994) with the Rorschach Comprehensive System (Exner, 2003). It represents a revision of a similar chapter (Dorr, 1997) in the first edition of *The Millon Inventories*. Where possible, the relevant literature has been updated; issues relevant to interpretation, test comparison, and integration are addressed; and there is a discussion of the few examples of integrative models of interpretation. In the final part of the chapter, case studies are reviewed to illustrate the advantages and difficulties of using these two instruments together clinically.

Assumptions Regarding Psychometric Properties of the Instruments

One assumption of this chapter is that both of the instruments being discussed are psychometrically sound. This is emphasized because projective tests do not generally correlate highly with self-report measures (Archer & Krishnamurthy, 1993a, 1993b), and because some writers assume that the "fault" for this lack of correlation must lie with the Rorschach. Attacks from some quarters on the Rorschach have been relentless (e.g., Wood, Nezworski, Lilienfeld, & Garb, 2003). Indeed, the criticism of the Rorschach by some authors had became so strident that there were calls to ban the clinical use of the Rorschach and to prohibit teaching it in graduate programs! Such hyperbole led the Board of Trustees of the Society of Personality Assessment (SPA) to undertake an intensive reexamination of the Rorschach's extant technical properties. The results of this major review are summarized in an official statement (SPA, 2005).

Studies and meta-analytic reviews examined by the authors of this statement included those by Bornstein (1999); Gronnerod (2004); Hiller, Rosenthal, Bornstein, Berry, and Brunell-Neulieb (1999); Jorgensen, Andersen, and Dam (2000, 2001); Meyer (2000); Meyer and Archer (2001); Meyer and Handler (1997, 2000); Rosenthal, Hiller, Bornstein, Berry and Brunell-Neulieb (2001); Meyer (2004); and Meyer et al. (2002). The Meyer et al. (2002) article is one of the most extensive reviews in the literature and served to place the validity of psychological assessment with the Rorschach in context relative to the use of other measures throughout the health sciences. It presented the findings of 125 meta-analyses and 800 multimethod assessment studies, and found that psychological assessment with the Rorschach performed as well as a variety of common medical tests (electrocardiograms, mammography, magnetic resonance imaging, etc.). Other studies and meta-analytic reviews examined by the SPA board included those by Gronnerod (2003); Roberts and DelVecchio (2001); Viglione and Hilsenroth (2001); and Meyer, Mihura, and Smith (2005). On the basis of its review of these and yet other studies and meta-analyses, the SPA (2005) concluded that the "Rorschach possesses documented reliability and validity similar to other generally accepted test instruments used in the assessment of personality and psychopathology and that its responsible use in personality assessment is appropriate and justified" (p. 221). Clearly, the preponderance of scientific evidence provides strong support for the psychometric properties of the Rorschach. Hence I proceed with this chapter confident that the Rorschach, properly used, is psychometrically sound. Since this volume contains multiple chapters on the technical value of the MCMI-III in clinical and research assessment, I do not review this literature herein.

Research on the Relationship of the Millon Inventories and MMPI to the Rorschach

In my initial search for empirical or clinical studies on the relationship between Rorschach variables and any of the Millon instruments (Dorr, 1997), I found very little. The few that were found reported modest to nil relationships. A similar search for the present chapter has yielded the same result. This should not be too surprising, in view of the findings in the literature on patterns of covariation between the Rorschach and another widely used self-report measure, the Minnesota Multiphasic Personality Inventory (MMPI2). Archer and Krishnamurthy (1993b) reviewed about 50 studies explicitly examining relationships between the MMPI and Rorschach. They concluded that, taken as an aggregate, 73% of the studies revealed either no statistically related significance or minimal associations between Rorschach and MMPI variables in these adult samples. Among the remaining 27% of the studies, most yielded moderate associations, with Pearson product–moment correlations in the range of $r \geq .24$ to $r \leq .34$. The authors noted that these findings were similar to those examining the relationship of Rorschach to MMPI patterns in adolescents (Archer & Krishnamurthy, 1993a). At the basic construct level, these authors concluded that "variables given similar labels on both instruments may, in fact, represent independent and largely non-overlapping constructs" (Archer & Krishnamurthy, 1993b, p. 284). They clearly discounted the possibility that either the MMPI or the Rorschach might have limited reliability or validity, citing the general reliability coefficients of $r = .84$ for the Rorschach and $r = .86$ for the MMPI. The comparable convergent validity coefficients ($r = .46$ and $r = .41$, respectively) were also cited. In sum, both measures enjoy a reasonable degree of reliability and validity, while apparently measuring different aspects of the personality.

In view of the low covariation between the MMPI and Rorschach, one might conclude that it would be fruitless to examine the ways in which the Rorschach and the Millon instruments might complement each other. However, additional points of view regarding test integration suggest that it may be clinically and scientifically reasonable to consider ways in which these instruments may be integrated to enrich our understanding of our patients, as well as to design and articulate specific treatment interventions.

The Nature and Purpose of the MCMI-III and the Rorschach

Ganellen (1996a) reported on a comparison of the diagnostic efficiency of the MMPI, MCMI-II, and Rorschach. Among other things, Ganellen found that the Rorschach was more sensitive and specific to psychotic disorders than either the MMPI or MCMI-II. He suggested that clinicians should include the Rorschach when the major purpose of an assessment is to determine if a patient presents with a psychotic disorder of some kind.

In his book on integrating the Rorschach with the MMPI-2, Ganellen (1996b) addressed the issue of divergent findings with these two instruments. He began by commenting that "Resolving conflicting findings in data obtained during a psychological evaluation is a major challenge for clinicians" (p. 70). He then addressed the questions each test actually measures. Indeed, these two venerable instruments differ considerably, and it may be unwise to assume that they work in the same way. Indeed, if they did, we would not need to use them both for most applications. Ganellen also discussed what the clinician is to do when the two instruments may differ. Both Ganellen and Weiner (1993) emphasize that contradictions between the Rorschach and MMPI-2 are not necessarily invalidating. Weiner makes the point that seeming contradictions may be generative instead. The same may be true in the case of the Rorschach and MCMI-III. So let us take a brief look at the latter two instruments.

According to Weiner (2000), the Rorschach is a complex procedure that can be conceptualized in at least four ways, and each of these conceptualizations identifies critical building blocks of good interpretation. He points out that the Rorschach can be understood to be a perceptual task in which subjects observe inkblots and report what they see (and censor other things that they also see), and answer open-ended and even vague questions to help the examiner identify locations and determinant. At this level, the inkblots are primarily perceptual stimuli. The procedure may also be seen as an associational task. We do not ask our clients, "What does this remind you of?", but clients often in fact offer fantasy associations to the stimuli. Third, Weiner (2000) reminds us that the process is an interpersonal task in which subtle social cues may influence the response given. For example, it is generally considered unwise for an examiner to administer a Rorschach to someone he or she knows very well, as the typical censoring that takes place in most testing situations is relaxed, thus disturbing the norms. Finally, the Rorschach consists of a sequential task in which a client may respond to subsequent stimuli based on their inherent qualities (color shock?) or reactions to his or her own responses. Because several processes are going on at once, the Rorschach is thought to tap multiple levels of awareness and consciousness. It might also be noted that McClelland (1989) made the argument that the projective Thematic Apperception Test (TAT) procedure and direct questionnaire measures reflected two fundamentally different motive systems—one unconscious or "implicit," the other conscious and self-attributed. The same could be said of the Rorschach and the MCMI-III.

It might also be worth emphasizing that Eugen Bleuler was one of Hermann Rorschach's professors in medical school, and he directed Rorschach's doctoral dissertation, which concerned hallucinations. Bleuler coined the term "schizophrenia." The psychiatric community was intrigued by Bleuler's concepts, and this interest led to concerns about how to differentiate patients with schizophrenia from patients with other forms of psychosis. Rorschach himself was impressed that patients identified as schizophrenic responded quite differently to the Klecksographie game (precursor of the Rorschach cards) than did other persons. Rorschach continued to develop his diagnostic system, and by mid-1919 he believed that the analyses of his data were sufficient to demonstrate that the method he had devised offered considerable diagnostic utility, especially in identifying schizophrenia. In investigating clusterings of various responses, he also came to the conclusion that his method also shed some light on ingrained psychological and behavioral characteristics—qualities that today we would refer to "personality traits," "habits," or "personality styles." Hence, from the very beginning, Rorschach found that his method was useful in the diagnosis of psychosis as well as some other personal characteristics. Finally, the Rorschach method itself is very indirect, even arcane, and highly complex. It is very difficult to learn to administer and interpret skillfully, and it may be described as a labor-intensive but high-yielding assessment instrument. And for these reasons it is expensive in terms of the time needed to learn, administer, score, and interpret it, and these expenses must be factored into the cost of the instrument. In this day of rationed mental health care, few clinicians are turning out Rorschachs by the hundreds each year. It might also be important to mention that although some fine psychoanalytic theory has been woven into Rorschach administration and interpretation, it is fundamentally not a theory-based instrument.

Now if we contrast this brief description of the Rorschach with that of the MCMI-III, we see enormous differences. The MCMI-III was designed to be a rapid, relatively inexpensive self-report measure. It was intentionally constructed in such a way that it assessed the middle range of psychopathology. Indeed, earlier editions of the MCMI manuals pointed out that because the instrument was designed to assess middle-range pathology, potential test items that were endorsed by fewer of the subjects in the tryout pool were eliminated. This eliminated most of the "infrequency" items, but it also effectively ridded the item pool of those items that tapped the most severe psychopathology. For these reasons, clinicians familiar with the MCMI-III know that the Clinical Syndrome Scales that assess more severe Axis I psychopathology are not as sensitive as its other scales. It is generally believed that a client who gets clinically significant elevations on these scales probably has severe pathology.

However, if they are not elevated, a clinician should be cautious in ruling out pathology. Indeed, the Millon scales were primarily designed to assess Axis II pathology, and the MCMI-III does this very well.

Unlike the Rorschach, which was not founded on a theoretical base, all the Millon instruments rest on Theodore Millon's remarkably rich and extensive theory of personality and psychopathology. The fusing of theory and psychometric technology was highly intentional. The theory was built in from the beginning. Indeed, Millon believed that since his assessment method was tightly woven around theory, it was not necessary to design an unnecessarily lengthy test to accomplish the measurement goals. As a result, the MCMI-III is brief in comparison to, say, the MMPI-2 or even the 240-item NEO Personality Inventory—Revised (NEO-PI-R). Yet it does its work well.

Finally, Millon argued that since dimensions of psychopathology are not normally distributed, the metric of the scales need not assume a normal curve. Instead, he asserted that scale cutoffs be made to approximate the base rate (BR) of each disorder or syndrome in clinical nature. Hence he offered the innovation of the BR score, which improved sensitivity and specificity.

So, then, these two instruments differ considerably in design, method, theoretical foundations, measurement intent, and statistical expression. We should not be surprised that the few studies of them used together do not find high test–test correlations. But the fact remains that both methods of assessment have a good psychometric track record.

It would seem that clinicians should capitalize on the notable differences in the way these two devices do their assessment work. Classical test theory has made it clear that using valid tests that have low correlations with each other and high correlations with the criterion will greatly enhance the magnitude of incremental validity. "To complement" means to fill out or make up for what is lacking, and a complementary use of two different tests is what Weiner (1993) is referring to when he points out that contradictions between Rorschach and MMPI results may be generative. The same may be said for the Rorschach and the MCMI-III. Each instrument is unique and provides the examiner with very different "camera angles" that can be very useful in assessment

Case Studies

In this section, two cases are presented to illustrate the advantages and difficulties clinicians may encounter when integrating MCMI-III and Rorschach test results. It may be helpful to make a few comments on the interpretive strategy used in this section. The Rorschach Comprehensive System instructs the clinician to exhaustively review the entire set of clusters in an established sequence, in order to maximize the amount of useful data one may extract from the System. This procedure was followed in the process of the clinical interpretation of the cases presented. However, this process yields a very large number of data. With the addition of the 4 MCMI-III Modifying/ Validity Indices and 24 clinical scales, the potential interpretive combinations multiply exponentially. For these reasons, it is necessary to limit discussion of interpretive possibilities to a few general themes in each case. I am aware that this method oversimplifies the clinical picture and runs the risk of omitting clinically confirming or contradictory data. However, space limitations require parsimony. In the process of data reduction, the admonition to "interpret the person" is followed as closely as possible.

The cases selected for inclusion are neither "neat" nor "clean." In some instances, the data cluster together effortlessly; in others, we face contradictory and challenging discrepancies. It would, however, be a disservice to the reader to report only easy cases. The day-to-day clinical work of the assessment psychologist presents many difficult cases, and these difficulties must be faced, and if possible resolved.

Case 1: Victoria

Victoria is a 24-year-old woman with some college education who lives with one of her boy-friends. She does not have a job, and she is currently not going to school. Her parents are professionals who have well-established careers. She has two siblings; one is doing well, but the other is drifting and unable to establish an affirmative career. Victoria has a history of telling lies and stealing petty things from family members, although this has not happened in recent years. She also has a history of hatching unrealistic career plans, such as migrating to Europe where she hoped to develop a candy business, necessitating her study of foreign languages (neither the move to Europe nor the business ever materialized). She has been successful in attracting the attention of eligible young men, and she usually has one or more suitors at her beck and call at one time. In fact, she was living with her current boyfriend at his college dormitory (which is highly against the rules), and the consequence was that both of them were ejected from this arrangement.

When Victoria was younger, her mother discovered receipts for her motel stays in an area of town known for infestations of prostitution and drugs, but this has not occurred recently. (Parenthetically, she has a long history of involvement in behavior that could place her in harm's way.) Her behavioral history shows serious deficiencies in judgment, but fortunately she has not been harmed in any way, except that she is clearly not actualizing her potential.

As mentioned above, for the sake of brevity and clarity, this review focuses only on variables that appear to bear directly on the case at hand. In a few instances, data from other tests and procedures are included to enhance the clinical picture.

For the reader's information, Victoria's MMPI-2 T-score validity pattern is as follows: L = 47; F = 85; K = 37; Fb = 97; and F(P) = 57. On the basic clinical scales, her scores are as follows: Hs = 69; D = 68; Hy = 68; Pd = 81; Mf = 30; Pa = 74; Pt = 64; Sc = 79; Ma = 76; and Si = 65. In addition, the Pk scale (Post-traumatic Stress) T-score is 75. Victoria's Wechsler Adult Intelligence Scale—Third Edition (WAIS-III) scores are the following: Verbal IQ = 93; Performance IQ = 97; Full Scale IQ = 94; Verbal Comprehension IQ = 96; Perceptual Organization Index = 89; Working Memory Index = 92; and Processing Speed = 99. There is considerable subtest scatter, with Object Assembly and Block Design subscales at 5 each, and Matrix Reasoning and Coding at 13.

Victoria's MCMI-III Profile Report is presented in Figure 7.1. Let us begin with the Modifying Indices, which suggest that Victoria tends to describe herself in fairly negative terms. In view of the degree of her maladaptation, her self-description is honest and realistic. She does not shy away from disclosing her psychopathology. This is a technically and clinically valid profile.

It is suggested that after examining the Modifying Indices, we first examine the Severe Personality Pathology Scales. There is a clinically significant elevation on the Borderline scale, as well as an elevation on the Paranoid scale. The notable elevation on the Borderline scale suggests severe deficiencies in morphological organization. The structure of the personality

MILLON CLINICAL MULTIAXIAL INVENTORY - III
CONFIDENTIAL INFORMATION FOR PROFESSIONAL USE ONLY

Valid Profile

PERSONALITY CODE: 8A ** 2A 3 28 8B * 6B 5 6A + 1 " 4 7 ' ' // - ** C P * //

SYNDROME CODE: -**-* // -**-* //

DEMOGRAPHIC: 000104964/ON/F/23/W/N/12/JO/MA/3004/8/30183/

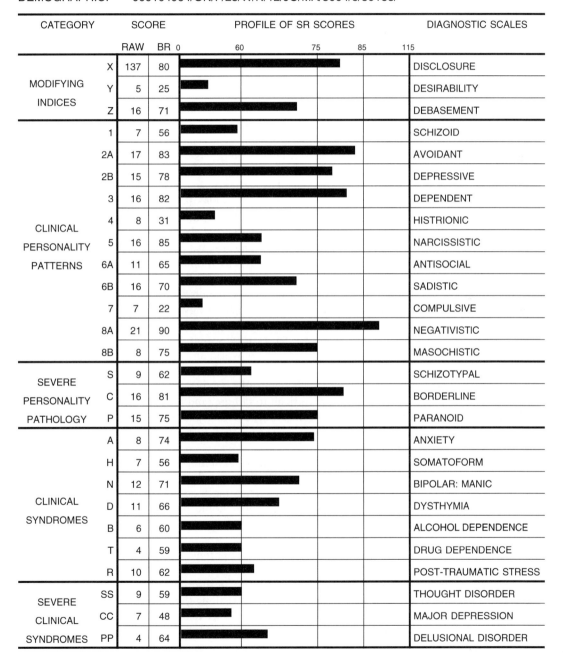

CATEGORY		SCORE		PROFILE OF SR SCORES	DIAGNOSTIC SCALES
		RAW	BR	0 60 75 85 115	
MODIFYING INDICES	X	137	80		DISCLOSURE
	Y	5	25		DESIRABILITY
	Z	16	71		DEBASEMENT
CLINICAL PERSONALITY PATTERNS	1	7	56		SCHIZOID
	2A	17	83		AVOIDANT
	2B	15	78		DEPRESSIVE
	3	16	82		DEPENDENT
	4	8	31		HISTRIONIC
	5	16	85		NARCISSISTIC
	6A	11	65		ANTISOCIAL
	6B	16	70		SADISTIC
	7	7	22		COMPULSIVE
	8A	21	90		NEGATIVISTIC
	8B	8	75		MASOCHISTIC
SEVERE PERSONALITY PATHOLOGY	S	9	62		SCHIZOTYPAL
	C	16	81		BORDERLINE
	P	15	75		PARANOID
CLINICAL SYNDROMES	A	8	74		ANXIETY
	H	7	56		SOMATOFORM
	N	12	71		BIPOLAR: MANIC
	D	11	66		DYSTHYMIA
	B	6	60		ALCOHOL DEPENDENCE
	T	4	59		DRUG DEPENDENCE
	R	10	62		POST-TRAUMATIC STRESS
SEVERE CLINICAL SYNDROMES	SS	9	59		THOUGHT DISORDER
	CC	7	48		MAJOR DEPRESSION
	PP	4	64		DELUSIONAL DISORDER

FIGURE 7.1. MCMI-III Profile Report for Victoria.

organization is likely to lie between the neurotic and psychotic levels of organization, according to Stone's (1980) concepts of psychostructural levels. Victoria is also likely to meet the criteria for the diagnosis of borderline personality disorder. Her internalized representations of significant others may be poorly developed, incomplete, fragmented, and/or stereotyped, and she may have difficulties with interpersonal boundaries. Victoria is likely to have a distorted self-image. Her internalized representations of both self and others are likely to be distorted, pathological, and oversimplified. These difficulties in object representations may lead to considerable difficulties in interpersonal relationships and in general overall adjustment. Her defenses are likely to be primitive, and her capacity to regulate drive and affect will be compromised. The accompanying high elevation on the Paranoid scale suggests the presence of a distrustful, guarded, insular perceptual style. She may be suspicious of the motives of others. Internal representations of others may be fixed, unyielding, and based on unwarranted assumptions, fears, and conjectures.

The notable elevations on these two scales tend to "darken" the interpretation of the Clinical Personality Patterns. The findings are complicated by the elevations on the Avoidant and Dependent scales. This duality represents a major conflict in the interpersonal domain. Dependent persons tend to be needy, and they depend on others to take care of them, to watch out for them, to nurture them, and to be generally emotionally available. On the other hand, persons scoring high on the Avoidant scale tend to be frightened of other people. They do not trust other people. They are constantly testing other people and pushing them away. They exert a great deal of energy in keeping others at bay. This is obviously a major problem for someone like Victoria who is also dependent, because she is likely to put significant others in a double bind. On the one hand, she may send out messages wanting significant others to be helpful; on the other hand, she may push others away, based on her perception that they may be untrustworthy and perhaps out to be hurtful. This tension arch may result in projective identification, in which she may project her own hostile impulses onto others and then enter into a battle with significant others as though the projected hostility may actually be true.

Further muddying the waters is a strong tendency toward a depressive worldview. This does not necessarily translate into an Axis I depressive disorder, but it does suggest the presence of a gloomy, pessimistic, sad attitude toward the world and what the world has to offer. It is not a good sign that Victoria also has a clinically significant elevation on the Negativistic scale. Persons who are elevated on this scale tend to be passive–aggressive, stubborn, resentful, resistant, and discontented. They are difficult to fathom, and likely to be described as vacillating and unpredictable. Rounding out the clinical picture painted by the MCMI-III is the elevation of 75 on the Masochistic scale, suggesting that Victoria may be her own worst enemy.

We now turn to Victoria's Rorschach. The Structural Summary is provided in Figure 7.2. Because there are at least 14 responses and no refused cards, the protocol would appear to be reliable and interpretable. Because the Perceptual Thinking Index (PTI) is greater than three the interpretive search strategy based on key variables should proceed as follows: Ideation, Cognitive Mediation, Information Processing, Capacity for Control and Tolerance for Stress, Affect, Self-Perception, and Interpersonal Perception.

The PTI was derived from revisions of earlier Schizophrenic Indices (SCZI; Exner, 2003). The current index was renamed based on the findings of Hilsenroth, Fowler, and Padawar (1998), who found that the earlier index was effective in discriminating between psychotic disorders and Axis II disorders. These authors suggested calling the index a "Psychosis Index" rather than a Schizophrenic Index. In considering this, Exner renamed it the PTI to identify it as a general marker of psychotic thought.

In examining the Ideation (thinking) cluster, we see evidence of features that are found in persons with schizophrenic spectrum disorders, which include schizophrenia, schizophreniform disorder, schizoaffective disorder, delusional disorder, and schizotypal personality disor-

Structural Summary

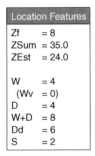

Location Features

Zf	= 8
ZSum	= 35.0
ZEst	= 24.0
W	= 4
(Wv	= 0)
D	= 4
W+D	= 8
Dd	= 6
S	= 2

DQ

		(FQ–)
+	= 8	(3)
o	= 4	(4)
v/+	= 0	(0)
v	= 2	(1)

Form Quality

	FQx	MQual	W+D
+	= 0	0	0
o	= 2	1	2
u	= 4	2	2
-	= 8	3	4
none	= 0	0	0

Determinants

Blends	Single	
M.m.FC'	M	= 4
FM.CF	FM	= 2
M.FM	m	= 1
	FC	= 0
	CF	= 0
	C	= 0
	Cn	= 0
	FC'	= 0
	C'F	= 0
	C'	= 0
	FT	= 0
	TF	= 0
	T	= 0
	FV	= 0
	VF	= 0
	V	= 0
	FY	= 0
	YF	= 0
	Y	= 0
	Fr	= 0
	rF	= 0
	FD	= 0
	F	= 4
	(2)	= 3

Contents

H	= 1
(H)	= 1
Hd	= 3
(Hd)	= 3
Hx	= 5
A	= 6
(A)	= 1
Ad	= 2
(Ad)	= 0
An	= 3
Art	= 0
Ay	= 0
Bl	= 0
Bt	= 0
Cg	= 1
Cl	= 0
Ex	= 0
Fd	= 0
Fi	= 0
Ge	= 0
Hh	= 1
Ls	= 1
Na	= 0
Sc	= 0
Sx	= 0
Xy	= 0
Idio	= 2

S-Constellation

☐	FV + VF + V + FD > 2
☐	Col-Shd Blends > 0
☑	Ego < .31 or > .44
☐	MOR > 3
☑	Zd > ±3.5
☐	cs > EA
☑	CF + C > FC
☑	X + % < .70
☐	S > 3
☑	P < 3 or > 8
☑	Pure H < 2
☑	R < 17
7	Total

Special Scores

		Lvl-1	Lvl-2
DV	=	0 x1	0 x2
INC	=	1 x2	0 x4
DR	=	1 x3	0 x6
FAB	=	1 x4	1 x7
ALOG	=	0 x5	
CON	=	0 x7	

Raw Sum6 =	4
Wgtd Sum6 =	16

AB	= 0	GHR	= 1
AG	= 2	PHR	= 6
COP	= 0	MOR	= 2
CP	= 0	PER	= 0
		PSV	= 0

RATIOS, PERCENTAGES, AND DERIVATIONS

	R = 14		L = 0.40		
EB	= 6 : 1.0	EA	= 7.0	EBPcr	= 6.0
cb	= 6 : 1	cs	= 7	D	= 0
		Adj es	= 6	Adh D	= 0
FM	= 4	SumC'	= 1	SumT	= 0
m	= 2	SumV	= 0	SumY	= 0

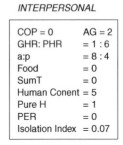

AFFECT

FC: CF+C	= 0 : 1
Pure C	= 0
SumC' : WSumC	= 1 : 1.0
Afr	= 0.40
S	= 2
Blends:R	= 3 : 14
CP	= 0

INTERPERSONAL

COP = 0		AG = 2	
GHR: PHR		= 1 : 6	
a:p		= 8 : 4	
Food		= 0	
SumT		= 0	
Human Conent		= 5	
Pure H		= 1	
PER		= 0	
Isolation Index		= 0.07	

IDEATION

a:p	= 8 : 4	Sum6	= 4
Ma:Mp	= 4 : 2	Lvl-2	= 1
2AB + (Art+Ay)	= 0	Wsum6	= 16
MOR	= 2	M-	= 3
		M none	= 0

MEDIATION

XA%	= 0.43
WDA%	= 0.50
X-%	= 0.57
S-	= 1
P	= 1
X+%	= 0.14
Xu%	= 0.29

PROCESSING

Zf	= 8
W:D:Dd	= 4:4:6
W : M	= 4 : 6
Zd	= +11.0
PSV	= 0
DQ+	= 8
DQv	= 2

SELF-PERCEPTION

3r+(2)/R	= 0.21
Fr+rF	= 0
SumV	= 0
FD	= 0
An+Xy	= 3
MOR	= 2
H:(H)+Hd+(Hd)	= 1 : 4

PTI = 4	☐ DEPI = 3	☐ CDI = 2	☐ S-CON = 7	☐ HVI = No	☐ OBS = No

FIGURE 7.2. Rorschach Structural Summary for Victoria.

der. There is strong evidence of a serious thought disorder; that is, there is evidence of a serious impairment in Victoria's ability to think logically and coherently. She is likely to be much less capable than most people of coming to reasonable conclusions about relationships between events, and of maintaining a connected flow of associations in which ideas follow each other in a comprehensible manner. For this reason, there are likely to be frequent occasions when her adaptation is compromised by instances of arbitrary and circumstantial reasoning, and moments in which her loose and scattered ideation confuses her and may be confusing to others. Her thinking is particularly likely to become strange when she is contemplating the nature of people and their actions.

Another major problem is that Victoria is "pervasively introversive" (EBPer = 6.0). This means that she is overly ideational. She may have an extremely strong preference for dealing with issues primarily through ideational channels at the expense of emotional considerations. The result is excessive cognitive inflexibility. Furthermore, because of her constricted affective style, she may have difficulty dealing comfortably with emotionally arousing situations. Because she has substantial difficulty thinking logically and coherently, her excessive dependency on a cognitive style in dealing with experience is likely to be detrimental to her psychological adjustment.

"Cognitive mediation" can be thought of as one's style of translating information. The Cognitive Mediation cluster tells us something about the way in which people perceive their world, particularly their social world. Healthy adjustment requires that one perceive the world realistically. An inability to view the world in a realistic manner may lead to problems in adjustment. The ego function of reality testing is assessed in this cluster. Victoria's protocol demonstrates severe impairment in her reality testing. She may often misperceive events and form mistaken impressions of people and what their actions may mean. This serious disability is likely to result in a failure to anticipate the consequences of her actions. She may also misconstrue the boundaries of appropriate behavior. Her inaccurate perceptions of people and events are likely to lead her to erroneous conclusions and ill-advised actions. Her faulty judgment is likely to interfere with her attempts to adjust to her world. Victoria's difficulty in separating reality from fantasy may lead to inappropriate behavior, which itself can be a chronic and pervasive source of adjustment difficulties. Most people with this degree of impaired reality testing have difficulty managing basic psychological aspects of everyday living without assistance or supervision.

Victoria seems to have a serious impairment in her social perception. She is likely to form inaccurate impressions of what other people are thinking and feeling and why they act as they do. This tendency to misjudge the attitudes and intentions of others suggests that her empathic capacities are limited, which may increases the chances of inappropriate social behavior. Finally, these distorted impressions of interpersonal situations contribute substantially to impairments in her overall sense of reality.

The Information Processing cluster tells us something about a person's automatic style of taking in information from the environment. It provides a view of how people focus their attention on events in their lives and organize perceptions that enter into their awareness. The main thing we learn in this cluster is that Victoria tends to take in far more information than she needs to function efficiently (Zd = +11.0). She may examine situations more thoroughly than necessary. This "overincorporation" leads her to take in more information than is necessary to address most problems effectively, and leaves her overloaded and confused. She may make things more complicated than they really are. This in turn may lead to difficulties in efficient decision making.

The next cluster to be interpreted is Capacity for Control and Tolerance for Stress. This cluster provides information on the degree to which life's demands result in distress. In interpreting this cluster, it is wise to examine the client's characteristic defenses. A cursory review of the variables in this cluster would indicate that Victoria does not experience much stress.

Although her defenses are primitive, they are effective in protecting her from experiencing stress. She lives in a fantasy world that crowds out impingements from reality, which would indicate that her life is going nowhere. She lives in circumstances that would be very distressing to most people: totally dependent on her boyfriends, no job, no schooling, no money, no insurance, and sometimes even no food. Everyone around her is distressed about her situation, but she remains blissfully unaware of her dire straits. Lack of distress is not always a healthy thing.

The Affect cluster tells us something about how a person processes emotional experiences. Victoria is very disinclined to process emotional stimulation. This tendency is pervasive and is likely to be maladaptive. She will be socially and emotionally withdrawn. It might be said that she has an aversion to emotions. She may avoid social situations because of her aversion to emotionality.

The Self-Perception cluster provides information about how people view themselves. The variables in this cluster seem to suggest that Victoria may purposely avoid self-focus. Her inclination to ignore herself may be due to a low estimate of her personal worth. She may compare herself unfavorably to other people, whom she regards as being more able, attractive, talented, and worthy than she is. Low self-esteem probably translates into a lack of self-confidence. The protocol suggests that Victoria may have a limited capacity to identify comfortably with real people in her life. Instead, she appears inclined to identify with partial objects, imaginary figures, or people who do not regularly participate in her everyday real world. This may contribute to difficulty in establishing a clear and stable sense of personal identity. There may be identity diffusion, and she is likely to have some inaccurate notions about herself. Furthermore, her internal representations of others are likely to be partial (as opposed to whole) and imaginary (as opposed to real). These deficiencies in object representations are likely to contribute to poor decision making, ineffective problem solving, and strained interpersonal relationships.

Finally, the Interpersonal Perception cluster provides information on how the client relates to other people. It provides information on attitudes toward others, degree of interaction with others, and the manner of approaching and managing interpersonal attachments. The information in this cluster provides evidence that Victoria has a limited capacity to form close attachments to other people. Her relationships, including friendship and love relationships, will tend to be distant and detached rather than close and intimate. She notices other people, but she appears subject to feeling uneasy when dealing with them. Interpersonal situations threaten her and make her feel inadequate. She may experience a maladaptive degree of social discomfort. She may expect that social interactions to be characterized more by competition than by cooperation. She may expect interpersonal relationships to be marked by aggressiveness. She sees herself as little and ineffectual, and others as all-powerful, aggressive creatures that she has to struggle against.

Diagnoses

The diagnoses given on the basis of Victoria's Rorschach and MCMI-III (and other clinical data) are as follows:

Axis I: 298.9 Psychotic Disorder Not Otherwise Specified
Axis II: 209.83 Borderline Personality Disorder with Avoidant and Dependent Traits
Axis III: None
Axis IV: Educational and Occupational Problems
Axis V: Current Global Assessment of Functioning (GAF) = 42; GAF for past year = 45

Discussion of Case 1

Although the MCMI-III and Rorschach employ vastly different assessment strategies, both instruments have clearly described the presence of Axis II personality disorder in this case. The MCMI-III does this very directly, beginning with the clinical elevations on the Borderline and Paranoid scales. Indeed, the MCMI-III does what it does best—identify a personality disorder. The profile suggests the presence of severe personality pathology that will be played out in very troubled and conflicted interpersonal relationships. Although the Rorschach was never designed to assess Axis II pathology, it can be very useful in identifying aspects of this kind of difficulty. However, it is especially useful in identifying deficiencies in object representations, a core feature of personality pathology. Variables in the Self-Perception and Interpersonal Perception clusters reveal that Victoria's internalized representations of other people are hazy, distorted, confusing, shallow, and inaccurate. Her H: (H) + Hd + (Hd) ratio of 1:4 clearly suggests that her object representations are severely deficient. The Good Human Representation to Poor Human Representation ratio is 1:6, again providing clear evidence of deficiencies in the capacity to develop rich and accurate object representations. There are no COP responses, and overall the various indices suggest that she sees and experiences others as malevolent threats. Her apperceptive world is not saturated with whole, benevolent internalized representations of significant others. A reading of her M responses is also revealing. Card I response 5: "A sad person, someone who is hurt, someone's heart torn apart, someone going through a hard time." Card III response 6: "Skeleton, looks like these things are happening on the inside and these are things happening on the outside as far as feelings go, because it looks like a skeleton it reminds me of dead emotions, not really a lot going on, reminds me of evil too." Card IV response 7: "Something overbearing, something taking over sides, a powerful force, barrier, standing like a barrier wall force there that will not allow you to go on, crushing your will, weighting you down" (pushes with her hand through the air in pushing motion). Card IX response 13: "Looks like a big force up here and a little force down here and they are going after each other like a battle, a violent struggle for the smaller force to push its way through." And, finally, Card X response 14: "A body looks like a happy person in the middle and the little things outside are the happiness coming out—celebration." In short, the Rorschach has provided ample evidence of serious deficiencies in object representations, in close agreement with the picture provided by the MCMI-III.

The MCMI-III strongly suggests that Victoria will have difficulties in interpersonal relationships. The tension arc between the dependent and avoidant forces speaks of a major approach–avoidance conflict. She needs others to be nurturing and supportive, but she is frightened of others and may actively push them away. Recall that avoidant individuals fall on the active end of the active–passive continuum. Persons high on both the dependent and avoidant dimensions are highly ambivalent. Interestingly, the Rorschach also describes this social ambivalence. Variables in the Self-Perception cluster predict that Victoria may have strained interpersonal relations, whereas variables within the Interpersonal Perception cluster suggest that she has an interest in being around other people. She pays attention to what they say or do, but she appears uneasy when dealing with people, possibly because interpersonal situations threaten her in some way or make her feel inadequate. Clearly, this represents ambivalence.

The Rorschach has done an excellent job of complementing the MCMI-III. It has also provided evidence of personality disorder, but it does a much better job of doing what it does best—the identification of severe Axis I pathology, especially psychosis and deficiencies in the major ego functions of reality testing and thought disorder. Not employing the Rorschach in this case might have resulted in missing the serious thought disorder and faulty reality testing, both signs of a psychotic process imposed on the Axis II pathology. However, used together, the two instruments have given a richer and more complete description of this young woman's clinical picture. This is what Weiner (1993) meant when he wrote that apparent contradictions between the Rorschach and self-report measures are generative and not invalidating.

Case 2: Roxy

Roxy came to the clinic for psychotherapy to help her with various life and marital problems. She was tested as part of a routine intake process. At the time of the intake examination, the patient was a 30-year-old married mother of two children. She was a generally well-dressed and groomed woman of about average height and weight. She appeared to be confident throughout the course of two intake interviews, speaking in a strong voice, maintaining eye contact, and assuming a socially open posture. However, there was a certain affective flatness, in that she shared many troubling symptoms and life experiences (e.g., rape) with a tendency toward joviality or lightness. She seemed motivated to cooperate in her assessment and therapy, but it was often difficult to keep her focused on a particular topic. She could very well be described as a "storyteller" as she related to the examiner (myself).

Roxy's presenting problem was concern about her stressful marriage. She described her marriage as a "can't live with him, can't live without him" relationship. She stated that her husband was very helpful in taking care of the home and the children, yet she couldn't stand being around him. She reported that their marriage was characterized by very poor communication and extremely little sexual activity. It may be of note that prior to their marriage, the couple had had an extensive and passionate sex life. She stated that her husband didn't understand that she would like nonsexual affection. Roxy stated that leaving the marriage was not an option for her in spite of her unhappiness. She felt that because of the children and her financial and emotional limitations, she could not divorce her husband.

The patient felt that the stress of her marriage had exacerbated her long-standing cycle of depressive episodes, for which she had been treated in the past with psychotherapy and medications. It might be helpful to mention that Roxy had a long history of having adverse reactions to psychiatric medications, and she was resistant to a referral to a psychiatrist. She believed that an improvement in the relationship with her husband would help her feel more supported. She reported that she would like to get at the "emotional roots" of her depression.

Roxy's biological parents had divorced when she was very young. Her mother remarried shortly after, and the patient lived with her mother and stepfather until she went to college. She reported that her stepfather made sexually suggestive remarks to her when she was a teenager. In reaction to this, she became suicidal and sought treatment. She reported that the therapist with whom she worked did not see anything wrong with her stepfather's behavior.

Roxy stated that her family had moved from one town to another a number of times when she was very young. She felt picked on and criticized by the other children. Her school problems did not abate as she got older, and she experienced rejection and even violent abuse by her peers. She attempted college, but consumed a great deal of alcohol and ended up dropping out. She did not abuse other substances. She entered the armed services, but was discharged because of extensive interpersonal difficulties. At the time of the intake, she had enrolled again in college and was attempting to earn good grades while raising two small children.

Roxy reported that by the age of 16 she had begun what became a long history of extreme sexual promiscuity. She reported that this was the only way she felt she could gain male acceptance. As she plaintively put it, "It's the only thing I do really well." She said that it was very easy for her to be sexually aggressive. The sexual promiscuity lasted until she married her first husband. This relationship ended in divorce, and she eventually married her current husband, with whom she had been having an affair. By her report she pursued him, and they eventually had the two children prior to their marriage.

Roxy's MCMI-III Profile Report is provided in Figure 7.3. The MCMI-III profile was technically valid. Her Disclosure scale BR score was very high, but in view of her long history of psychopathology, an elevation in this range would not invalidate the profile. It probably represented an honest appraisal of her difficulties. The Debasement scale was also elevated, which indicated that she described herself in a rather negative light. We next move to the Severe Personality Pathology Scales to look for any clinically significant elevations. Her BR score on the Borderline scale was 95, indicating the presence of borderline personality organization (again, according to Stone's [1980] conceptualization of level of psychic structure) as well as the diagnosis of borderline personality disorder. When one or more of the Severe Personality Pathology Scales is significantly elevated, it tends to "darken" the interpretation of the Clinical Personality Patterns. These elevations are considered to provide more evidence of personality disorder than merely personality traits. The BR score was 96 on the Sadistic scale. This indicates that Roxy might be disposed to react in sudden abrupt outbursts of an unexpected and unwarranted nature. She might engage in risky behavior undaunted by danger, and she might be forward and inhibiting to others. This kind of person is often described as strongly opinionated, closed-minded, unbending, energetic, hardheaded, competitive, and malicious. Roxy might be cold-blooded and detached from awareness of the impact of her own actions. Sexual energy might lead to imprudent and unseemly behavior.

The BR score for the Depressive scale was 94. It must be emphasized this scale is not so much a measure of depressive symptomatology as it is an index of a personality that is prone to developing depression. Persons who have elevations on this scale are described as forlorn, somber, heavy-hearted, and discouraged. They feel vulnerable, endangered, and defenseless. Their cognitive style may be described as defeatist and fatalistic. Self-image may be that of an inadequate, unsuccessful person. Such people tend to feel abandoned and unloved. They are harsh in self-judgment, and they may engage in self-destructive acts. Morphologically, they are fragile and impoverished, and their mood is likely to be joyless.

Adding to this gloomy picture were Roxy's high elevations on the Masochistic (BR = 94) and Negativistic (BR = 83) Scales. The Masochistic scale measures a tendency to be self-effacing and to refrain from the pleasures of life. These people may be servile and obsequious, allowing others to take advantage of them. They are overly deferential and diffident. They are self-abasing, and they focus on their worst personal features. They feel worthy of being shamed, humbled, and debased. They focus on past failures and sabotage good fortune. The pain–pleasure polarity is reversed, and they find virtue in suffering. In Roxy's case, the masochism was compounded with passive–aggressiveness. In her self-induced suffering, she might be resentful, resistant, obstinate, and contrary. Interpersonally, she might be unpredictable and cyclic, being contrite on one occasion and hostile on another. Others might find her cynical, doubting, and untrusting, and she might approach positive events with disbelief. Roxy might view the future with pessimism, anger, and trepidation. She might resent the good fortune of others and view herself as misunderstood, luckless, unappreciated, jinxed, and demeaned. The internalized representations of persons like Roxy may be highly conflicted and vacillating. They experience contradictory feelings about significant others and are inclined to degrade the achievements of others. They employ primitive defenses such as projection and displacement, often acting inept or perplexed or behaving in a forgetful manner. There is a clear division in the pattern of their morphological structures, such that coping and defensive maneuvers are often directed toward incompatible goals, leaving major conflicts unresolved; full psychic cohesion is often impossible, by virtue of the fact that fulfillment of one drive or need inevitably nullifies or reverses another. Finally, their mood is likely to be described as irritable, touchy, temperamental, and peevish, followed in turn by sullen and moody withdrawal. They may be petulant and impatient.

MILLON CLINICAL MULTIAXIAL INVENTORY - III
CONFIDENTIAL INFORMATION FOR PROFESSIONAL USE ONLY

Valid Profile

PERSONALITY CODE: 6B 2B 8B ** 8A 2A * 6A 3 1 + − " 5 4 7 ′ ′ // C ** - * //

SYNDROME CODE: N ** - * // - ** - * //

DEMOGRAPHIC: 112965/OP/F/30/W/R/16/MA/MD/3002/09/301/

CATEGORY		SCORE		PROFILE OF SR SCORES					DIAGNOSTIC SCALES
		RAW	BR	0	60	75	85	115	
MODIFYING INDICES	X	169	99						DISCLOSURE
	Y	1	5						DESIRABILITY
	Z	20	77						DEBASEMENT
CLINICAL PERSONALITY PATTERNS	1	14	64						SCHIZOID
	2A	19	80						AVOIDANT
	2B	21	94						DEPRESSIVE
	3	15	67						DEPENDENT
	4	9	23						HISTRIONIC
	5	8	25						NARCISSISTIC
	6A	17	73						ANTISOCIAL
	6B	24	96						SADISTIC
	7	3	0						COMPULSIVE
	8A	22	83						NEGATIVISTIC
	8B	20	94						MASOCHISTIC
SEVERE PERSONALITY PATHOLOGY	S	16	65						SCHIZOTYPAL
	C	22	95						BORDERLINE
	P	10	60						PARANOID
CLINICAL SYNDROMES	A	8	68						ANXIETY
	H	3	16						SOMATOFORM
	N	18	105						BIPOLAR: MANIC
	D	16	73						DYSTHYMIA
	B	7	58						ALCOHOL DEPENDENCE
	T	6	55						DRUG DEPENDENCE
	R	8	54						POST-TRAUMATIC STRESS
SEVERE CLINICAL SYNDROMES	SS	12	58						THOUGHT DISORDER
	CC	11	61						MAJOR DEPRESSION
	PP	3	55						DELUSIONAL DISORDER

FIGURE 7.3. MCMI-III Profile Report for Roxy.

Finally, there was a major elevation (BR = 105) on the Bipolar: Manic scale, which was not incompatible with Roxy's history of mood swings. We now turn to Roxy's Rorschach. The Structural Summary is provided in Figure 7.4.

Because the PTI was greater than 3, the Comprehensive System cluster search proceeds in the following order: Ideation, Cognitive Mediation, Information Processing, Capacity for Control and Tolerance for Stress, Affect, Self-Perception, and Interpersonal Perception.

The Ideation cluster suggests that Roxy's protocol contained many features that are often found in persons with schizophrenic spectrum disorders. Roxy was likely to have serious difficulties in thinking logically and consistently. She might be less likely than most persons to come to reasonable conclusions about how events relate and of maintaining a connected flow of associations in which thoughts follow each other in a meaningful way. Her arbitrary and circumstantial reasoning might negatively affect her attempts to adapt to the demands of her world. She might present with loose and scattered thinking that would confuse her and those around her.

Variables in the Cognitive Mediation cluster suggest that Roxy's reality-testing abilities might be seriously impaired. She might tend to misperceive and misjudge events, and to form erroneous impressions of people and what their actions might denote. Her problems in translating relevant information might result in serious maladaptation, since she might fail to anticipate behavioral consequences. Furthermore, she might not understand the boundaries of appropriate behavior. Due to her faulty perception of people and events, she would be likely to form erroneous conclusions and engage in ill-advised behavior. She might have major difficulties in separating reality from fantasy, which would lead to chronic inappropriate behavior. The severe deficiency in her capacity to test reality would probably lead to major difficulties in managing basic aspects of everyday living, and she might need assistance or supervision in order to make it in society.

The data in the Information Processing cluster clearly suggest that Roxy's style of acquiring information was characterized by "underincorporation." That is, she probably tended to take in too little relevant information that could be useful to her in managing her life. She might examine her experience less thoroughly than most people would believe to be adequate. As a result, she would be likely to arrive at conclusions too quickly, after only a cursory review of relevant information. She might be inclined to scan situations in a superficial manner, which would result in her gleaning too little information from her environment that might be useful to her in forming adaptive life strategies. She might be likely to make decisions quickly, but in an incautious manner. Tasks might be completed rapidly but in an unsatisfactory way.

Children are natural underincorporators. The classic example of the child chasing a ball into the street, heedless of oncoming traffic, serves to describe the possible dangers of this characteristic. As people mature, we hope that they grow out of underincorporation. The Rorschach would suggest that Roxy hadn't.

Accompanying this tendency was a tendency to attend to her experience less precisely than would be optimum. She might be occasionally vague in her processing of information, suggesting that some cognitive immaturity might contribute to adjustment problems.

The elements within the Capacity for Control and Tolerance for Stress cluster provide information about a person's emotional resources, ability to manage stress, and capacity to cope effectively and consistently with life's demands. One of the variables in this cluster that is considered in interpretation is EB. EB is a ratio with the number of human movement responses on the left and the weighted sum C on the right. This is a rough index of a person's coping style. When either side of the ratio is 2 or more points greater than the other side, and the total of both sides is 10 or less, a preferred coping style has been identified. If the sum of both sides is greater than 10, the difference between the numbers on each side must be greater than 2 in order for a preferred style to be marked. If the left side of the EB ratio (human movement) is greater than the right (weighted sum C), an "introversive" style has been identified. If

Structural Summary

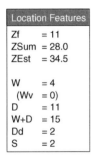

Location Features

Zf	= 11
ZSum	= 28.0
ZEst	= 34.5
W	= 4
(Wv	= 0)
D	= 11
W+D	= 15
Dd	= 2
S	= 2

DQ

		(FQ–)
+	= 7	(3)
o	= 8	(1)
v/+	= 0	(0)
v	= 2	(2)

Form Quality

	FQx	MQual	W+D
+	= 0	0	0
o	= 7	1	6
u	= 4	0	4
-	= 6	1	5
none	= 0	0	0

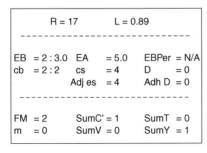

Determinants

Blends	Single	
M.FC'	M	= 1
Fr.FM.CF	FM	= 0
FC.FM	m	= 0
	FC	= 1
	CF	= 1
	C	= 0
	Cn	= 0
	FC'	= 0
	C'F	= 0
	C'	= 0
	FT	= 0
	TF	= 0
	T	= 0
	FV	= 0
	VF	= 0
	V	= 0
	FY	= 1
	YF	= 0
	Y	= 0
	Fr	= 1
	rF	= 0
	FD	= 1
	F	= 8
	(2)	= 5

Contents

H	= 2
(H)	= 2
Hd	= 2
(Hd)	= 0
Hx	= 0
A	= 5
(A)	= 0
Ad	= 2
(Ad)	= 0
An	= 4
Art	= 1
Ay	= 0
Bl	= 1
Bt	= 1
Cg	= 1
Cl	= 0
Ex	= 0
Fd	= 0
Fi	= 0
Ge	= 0
Hh	= 1
Ls	= 0
Na	= 0
Sc	= 0
Sx	= 1
Xy	= 0
Idio	= 0

S-Constellation

☐	FV + VF + V + FD > 2
☐	Col-Shd Blends > 0
☑	Ego < .31 or > .44
☐	MOR > 3
☑	Zd > ±3.5
☐	cs > EA
☐	CF + C > FC
☑	X + % < .70
☐	S > 3
☐	P < 3 or > 8
☐	Pure H < 2
☐	R < 17
3	Total

Special Scores

	Lvl-1	Lvl-2
DV	= 0 x1	0 x2
INC	= 0 x2	2 x4
DR	= 2 x3	3 x6
FAB	= 0 x4	1 x7
ALOG	= 0 x5	
CON	= 0 x7	

Raw Sum6 =		8
Wgtd Sum6 =		39

AB	= 0	GHR	= 2
AG	= 0	PHR	= 4
COP	= 1	MOR	= 0
CP	= 0	PER	= 2
		PSV	= 0

RATIOS, PERCENTAGES, AND DERIVATIONS

R = 17			L = 0.89		
EB = 2 : 3.0	EA	= 5.0	EBPer	= N/A	
cb = 2 : 2	cs	= 4	D	= 0	
	Adj es	= 4	Adh D	= 0	
FM = 2	SumC'	= 1	SumT	= 0	
m = 0	SumV	= 0	SumY	= 1	

AFFECT

FC: CF+C	= 2 : 2
Pure C	= 0
SumC' : WSumC	= 1 : 3.0
Afr	= 0.70
S	= 2
Blends:R	= 3 : 17
CP	= 0

INTERPERSONAL

COP = 0		AG	= 0
GHR: PHR			= 2 : 4
a:p			= 2 : 2
Food			= 0
SumT			= 0
Human Conent			= 6
Pure H			= 2
PER			= 2
Isolation Index			= 0.06

IDEATION

a:p	= 2 : 2	Sum6	= 8	
Ma:Mp	= 2 : 0	Lvl-2	= 6	
2AB + (Art+Ay)	= 1	Wsum6	= 39	
MOR	= 0	M-	= 1	
		M none	= 0	

MEDIATION

XA%	= 0.65
WDA%	= 0.67
X-%	= 0.35
S-	= 1
P	= 4
X+%	= 0.41
Xu%	= 0.24

PROCESSING

Zf	= 11
W:D:Dd	= 4:11:2
W : M	= 4 : 2
Zd	= −6.5
PSV	= 0
DQ+	= 7
DQv	= 2

SELF-PERCEPTION

3r+(2)/R	= 0.65
Fr+rF	= 2
SumV	= 0
FD	= 1
An+Xy	= 4
MOR	= 0
H:(H)+Hd+(Hd)	= 2 : 4

PTI = 4	☐ DEPI = 3	☐ CDI = 2	☐ S-CON = 3	☐ HVI = No	☐ OBS = No

FIGURE 7.4. Rorschach Structural Summary for Roxy.

the right side of the EB ratio is greater than the left, an "extratensive" style has been elevated. If the numbers in the ratio are about equal, it is said that the subject is probably "ambitent." The relevance of this is that it has been found that ambitent persons do not show the consistency of either introversive or extratensive individuals in their decision making or problem solving (Exner, 2003). Instead, they tend to be very inconsistent, and the role their emotions play in coping is inconsistent. Ambitent individuals are inclined to be less efficient in problem solving than either introversive or extratensive persons.

Roxy's EB was 2:3.0, meaning that she was identified as ambitent. That is, she appeared to lack a consistent and well-established coping style. Instead, she would vacillate between affective and ideational modes of coping with the demands of her world. She would be apt to struggle inefficiently and ineffectively without a clear sense of intent. She would probably not adopt a consistent coping strategy of thinking things through versus trial and error. Thus she might be unpredictable even in similar sets of circumstances, and she (and others around her) would have difficulty predicting what she was likely to say, do, and think next.

In considering clients' preferred style of coping with the demands of life, we must also take into consideration their available emotional resources. Psychodynamically oriented workers might use the term "ego strength" here. A variable of relevance to resources is EA, which is the sum of EB. When this number is relatively high, we infer that a client is likely to have sufficient resources to deal with most of life's problems. The norms for nonpatient adults in Exner (2003) indicate a mean EA of 9.43, with a standard deviation of 3.39. The mean for ambitent adults is 7.64, with a standard deviation of 2.53. By contrast, Roxy's EA was 5, which is on the low side. Interpretively, this suggests that she would be likely to have fewer resources available than most people for coping with the ordinary ideational and emotional demands of everyday living.

This would not necessarily be a major problem if the ongoing stressors Roxy faced were minimal. An index of such ongoing stressors is the sum of FM, m, C', V, Y and T. Roxy's sum was only 4, compared to 9.42 for the ambitent adults in the 2003 norm group. On the face of things, Roxy seemed relatively free of stress. However, at this point I must deviate from the classic Comprehensive System crawl through the clusters and reveal some things that have not hitherto been fully revealed. On the basis of the assessment material we have reviewed so far, we should be fairly certain that Roxy exhibited at least borderline personality organization, if not diagnosable borderline personality disorder. We know that such persons tend to use acting out as a defense. Indeed, I have often heard it said that if borderline patients are too happy and stress-free in the therapy sessions, therapists should suspect that they are acting out outside of the sessions! Indeed, Roxy acted out extensively, and her acting out escalated over time. She would come to the session and relate remarkable and dangerous acting out (e.g., dressing in extremely revealing clothes in dangerous areas and going to bars to pick up men to have sex with) and show little to no affect. It could be argued that she managed stress by acting out quickly. This would also explain why her D and Adjusted D scores (which constitute an index of situational and chronic stress) were not elevated.

There is little to comment on within the Affect cluster, except to refer to the points just made about Roxy's extreme acting out and the theorized tension reduction. There was an enormous amount of stress in her life, and this greatly increased later (see "Discussion of Case 2," below): marriage failing, money problems, living in a cheap hotel, children being taken away from her, rejection by her parents, working as a stripper, and getting into fights. But either she acted out the stress, or her cognitive style kept the effects of the stress from expressing itself internally.

Nested in the Self-Perception cluster, the egocentricity index (which includes reflections) was enormously high, indicating a marked tendency for Roxy to overvalue her self-worth. The mean for ambitent adults in the 2003 norms was .40 with a standard deviation of .11.

The average for reflection responses in this same norm group was .10. Only 8% had more than one reflection response. Roxy had two, which is highly clinically significant. This suggests that she was highly narcissistic and that she focused on her own needs without concern about the needs of others. Other narcissistic characteristics would be likely, such as entitlement and a tendency to externalize blame. If she did not receive enough praise, she might become frustrated, negative, and hostile. People with such narcissistic needs often have difficulty establishing and maintaining close and lasting interpersonal relationships. They are more highly involved in themselves than are most people.

Roxy was likely to have a limited capacity to identify comfortably with real people in her life. She appeared to identify with partial representations of others and/or imaginary people. Her internalized representations of others are likely to be split. As a result, she was likely to have difficulty establishing a clear and stable sense of her own personal identity. There might be identity diffusion and some inaccurate notions about herself. Her difficulty in identifying with whole and real human figures might contribute to misguided decision making and strained interpersonal relationships.

Finally, the Interpersonal Perception cluster tells us something about how clients relate to others. Roxy showed evidence of a limited capacity to form close attachments to other people. Her relationships were likely to be distant and detached. Her friendship and love relationships were likely to be at arm's length. She had an interest in people, but she might be uneasy around them, as she probably did not understand them very well. She had limited prospects for becoming socially popular.

Diagnoses

The diagnoses given on the basis of Roxy's Rorschach and MCMI-III (and other clinical data) are as follows:

    Axis Ia: 298.9 Psychotic Disorder Not Otherwise Specified
    Axis Ib: 295.70 Rule Out Schizoaffective Disorder
    Axis II: 209.83 Borderline Personality Disorder with Aggressive, Self-Defeating, Depressive, and Avoidant Traits
    Axis III: Breast Augmentation
    Axis IV: Living and Family Problems
    Axis V: Current GAF = 45; GAF for past year = 48

Discussion of Case 2: Roxy

As in the case of Victoria, the MCMI-III revealed a great deal about Roxy very rapidly. It described a serious personality disorder of a borderline type with several types of accompanying features, including self-defeating, sadistic, and passive–aggressive. It also suggested the presence of a depressive personality style. In addition, the MCMI-III called attention to the possibility of a bipolar disorder. The profile did not indicate the possibility of a psychotic disorder. When I conducted the intake, the only signs of the extent of Roxy's impulse control problems were the sexually explicit drawing in the intake booklet and her history of acting-out behavior. Subsequent to the intake, I had an opportunity to learn about much more extensive acting-out behavior.

As in the first case, the Rorschach also did a good job of identifying dimensions of Axis II problems, but its most important contribution was in identifying the presence of serious deficiencies in reality testing and a thought disorder, as well as several other factors that were cause for concern. The presence of some sort of psychotic process was evident on the Rorschach. The psychometric signs of thought disorder and problems with reality testing were unmistakable and did not seem to emanate from the driven energy of a person in a manic state. Furthermore, Roxy was not in a manic state when I administered the Rorschach. Nor was she depressed. She simply did not deal well with the blots' amorphous ambiguity. Her X–% was .35, Raw Sum 6 was 8, and Weighted Sum 6 was 38. She only had four Populars, and of her two human movement responses, one was minus form. Together, these and other variables led to a PTI of 4, which strongly indicates the presence of a psychotic-like perceptual process.

The importance of identifying the psychotic-like element in this case is demonstrated by the way Roxy's life played out. As time went by, her life began to deteriorate. At the time of the initial assessment, she was attending college classes and hoping to finish her bachelor's degree. However, before too long she got into difficulties with the university by making sexual advances toward her instructors both in the classroom and at a social gathering; as a consequence, her college aspirations were cut short. Her marriage went from bad to worse, and she and her husband separated. To support herself, she began to work as an exotic dancer. She thought that it would enhance her exotic appeal if she got some body piercings, including one in her clitoral area. She reported that "That one hurt." Also during this time she came into a sum of money. She decided to use it to have a breast enlargement, reasoning that her profession was that of a stripper, and such a body modification would increase her earning power. There were ongoing conflicts and altercations in the bars and clubs that she worked and played in. It should be noted that she drank a lot of alcohol but never took drugs of any kind. She developed a fairly notorious relationship with people in the night scene, and she often put herself in dangerous situations. During this time she was referred to another clinician, but I was kept informed of her downward spiral. By this time she was nearly out of money, and she rented a room in a cheap motel night by night, where she lived with her two daughters. That surpassed the threshold for the therapist who was working with her; a call was made to the local child protection agency, and the children were taken from her. She appealed to her parents, who lived in another state, but they made it clear that they wanted nothing to do with her. The last I knew, she had moved back to her home state. Of course, her considerable life difficulties could also be explained on the basis of her severe personality disorder. However, I continue to be struck with the way in which her severe thought disorder and difficulties in reality testing severely limited her capacity to make sense of her world, and thus to adapt to it with some degree of success.

If we focus only on the diagnostic question, the most difficult issue many clinicians face is a differential diagnosis between a bipolar disorder and some psychotic disorder. Roxy was indeed positive on the MCMI-III Bipolar: Manic scale, and much of her irritability, uninviting behavior, and sexual acting out could be explained as manifestations of a bipolar disorder. That may be the most parsimonious diagnostic route to take in such a case. People who suffer from bipolar disorders certainly get into trouble acting out, and they can present with psychotic-like features. However, there may be some problems with this choice of diagnosis. According to *Kaplan and Sadock's Synopsis of Psychiatry* (Sadock & Sadock, 2003), bipolar patients can show psychotic-like features such as perceptual disturbances, thought disorder, and even delirium—but these features are all linked to the mood disorder. For example, delusions are likely to be mood-congruent, as are thought problems (such as self-aggrandizement in the manic phase). Furthermore, in working with this woman for almost 2 years, I never experienced the presence of frank mania and the driven energy that goes with it. I realize that this is not a very scientific impression, but one can usually very quickly feel the presence of mania in the clinical setting.

Concluding Comments

There are many other fascinating and challenging MCMI-III/Rorschach integrative matters to be addressed in these two cases, but space is limited, and these matters will be left for future discourse. Although both instruments have a substantial research base, there is little in the literature about the relationship between the MCMI-III and the Rorschach. Furthermore, there are few models available for guiding the clinician in the principles of integration. Although there are common principles for integration, the clinician begins each case anew, weaving together idiographic and nomothetic principles in an attempt to understand the person being studied.

It would seem that integrating the MCMI-III and the Rorschach is no more or less difficult than integration of other instruments. Indeed, because both instruments measure enduring personality styles, the integration and comparisons are in some ways easier for these two instruments.

Acknowledgment

I would like to thank Stephanie Tilden Dorr for her editorial assistance in preparing this chapter.

References

Archer, R. P., & Krishnamurthy, R. (1993a). Combining the Rorschach and the MMPI in the assessment of adolescents. *Journal of Personality Assessment*, 60(1), 132–140.

Archer, R. P., & Krishnamurthy, R. (1993b). A review of MMPI and Rorschach interrelationships in adult samples. *Journal of Personality Assessment*, 61(2), 277–293.

Bornstein, R. F. (1999). Criterion validity of objective and projective dependency tests: A meta-analytic assessment of behavioral prediction. *Psychological Assessment*, 11, 48–57.

Dorr, D. (1997). Clinical integration of the MCMI-III and the Comprehensive System Rorschach. In T. Millon (Ed.), *The Millon inventories: Clinical and personality assessment* (pp. 75–105). New York: Guilford Press.

Exner, J. E., Jr. (2003). *The Rorschach: A comprehensive system. Vol. 1. Basic foundations* (4th ed.). New York: Wiley.

Ganellen, R. J. (1996a). Comparing the diagnostic efficiency of the MMPI, MCMI-II, and Rorschach: A review. *Journal of Personality Assessment*, 67, 219–243.

Ganellen, R. J. (1996b). *Integrating the Rorschach and the MMPI-2 in personality assessment.* Mahwah, NJ: Erlbaum.

Gronnerod, C. (2003). Temporal stability of the Rorschach method: A meta-analytic review. *Journal of Personality Assessment*, 80, 272–293.

Gronnerod, C. (2004). Rorschach assessment of changes following psychotherapy: A meta-analytic review. *Journal of Personality Assessment*, 83, 256–276.

Hiller, J. B., Rosenthal, R., Bornstein, R. F., Berry, D. T. R., & Brunell-Neuleib, S. (1999). A comparative meta-analysis of Rorschach and MMPI validity. *Psychological Assessment*, 11, 278–296.

Hilsenroth, M. J., Fowler, J. C., & Padawar, J. R. (1998). The Rorschach Schizophrenia Index (SCZI): An examination of reliability, validity, and diagnostic efficiency. *Journal of Personality Assessment*, 70, 514–534.

Jorgensen, K., Andersen, T. J., & Dam, H. (2000). The diagnostic efficiency of the Rorschach Depression Index and the Schizophrenia Index: A review. *Assessment, 7,* 259–280.

Jorgensen, K. Andersen, T. J., & Dam, H. (2001). "The diagnostic efficiency of the Rorschach Depression Index and the Schizophrenia Index: A review": Erratum. *Assessment, 8,* 355.

McClelland, D. C. (1989). Motivational factors in health and disease. *American Psychologist, 44,* 675–683.

Meyer, G. J. (2000). The incremental validity of the Rorschach Prognostic Rating scale over the MMPI Ego Strength Scale and I:Q. *Journal of Personality Assessment, 74,* 356–370.

Meyer, G. J. (2004). The reliability and validity of the Rorschach and TAT compared to other psychological and medical procedures: An analysis of systematically gathered evidence. In M. Hersen (Series Ed.) & M. J. Hilsenroth & D. Segal (Vol. Eds.), *Personality assessment. Vol. 2. Comprehensive handbook of psychological assessment* (pp. 315–342). Hoboken, NJ: Wiley.

Meyer, G. J., & Archer, R. P. (2001). The hard science of Rorschach research: What do we know and where do we go? *Psychological Assessment, 13,* 486–502.

Meyer, G. J., Finn, S. E., Eyde, L. D., Kay, G. G., Moreland, K. L., Dies, R., et al. (2002). Psychological testing and psychological assessment: A review of evidence and issues. *American Psychologist, 56,* 128–165.

Meyer, G. J., & Handler, L. (1997). The ability of the Rorschach to predict subsequent outcome: A meta-analysis of the Rorschach Prognostic Rating Scale. *Journal of Personality Assessment, 69,* 1–38.

Meyer, G. J., & Handler, L. (2000). "The ability of the Rorschach to predict subsequent outcome: A meta-analysis of the Rorschach Prognostic Rating Scale": Correction. *Journal of Personality Assessment, 74,* 504–506.

Meyer, G. J., Mihura, J. L., & Smith, B. L. (2005). The interclinician reliability of Rorschach interpretation in four data sets. *Journal of Personality Assessment, 84,* 296–314.

Millon, T. (with Millon, C., & Davis, R. D.). (1994). *Millon Clinical Multiaxial Inventory–III manual.* Minneapolis, MN: National Computer Systems.

Roberts, B. W., & DelVecchio, W. F. (2000). The rank-order consistency of personality traits from childhood to old age: A quantitative review of longitudinal studies. *Psychological Bulletin, 126,* 3–25.

Rosenthal, R., Hiller, J. B., Bornstein, R. F., Berry, D. T. R., & Brunell-Neuleib, S. (2001). Meta-analytic methods, the Rorschach, and the MMPI. *Psychological Assessment, 13,* 449–451.

Sadock, B. J., & Sadock, V. A. (2003). *Kaplan and Sadock's synopsis of psychiatry* (9th ed.). Philadelphia: Lippincott Williams & Wilkins.

Society for Personality Assessment (SPA). (2005). The status of the Rorschach in clinical and forensic practice: An official statement by the board of trustees of the Society for Personality Assessment. *Journal of Personality Assessment, 85*(2), 219–237.

Stone, M. H. (1980). *The borderline syndromes: Constitution, personality, and adaptation.* New York: McGraw-Hill.

Viglione, D. J., & Hilsenroth, M. J. (2001). The Rorschach: Facts, fiction, and future. *Psychological Assessment, 13,* 452–471.

Weiner, I. B. (1993). Clinical considerations in the conjoint use of the Rorschach and the MMPI. *Journal of Personality Assessment, 60*(1), 148–152.

Weiner, I. B. (2000). Making Rorschach interpretation as good as it can be. *Journal of Personality Assessment, 74,* 164–174.

Wood, J. M., Nezworski, M. T., Lilienfeld, S. O., & Garb, H. N. (2003). *What's wrong with the Rorschach?: Science confronts the controversial inkblot test.* San Francisco: Jossey-Bass.

CHAPTER 8

Studies Relating the MCMI and the MMPI

Michael H. Antoni

For much of the 20th century, distinctions between what are now termed "clinical syndromes" (Axis I) and "personality disorders" (Axis II) were not formally made, although their existence was clearly recognized. Less than three decades ago, the third edition of the *Diagnostic and Statistical Manual of Mental Disorders* (DSM-III; American Psychiatric Association, 1980) made explicit the practice of differentiating long-standing patterns of behavior, mood, thinking processes, and interpersonal style (personality) from more transitory, time-limited, and obvious deviations from characteristic behaviors (clinical syndromes). This approach reflects an evolution in the understanding of psychopathological processes—namely, the acceptance of the idea that the picture a patient presents will depend on his or her characteristic, long-standing perceptual and behavioral tendencies, as well as his or her reactions to the more transitory stressors of everyday life.

As reiterated in DSM-IV-TR (American Psychiatric Association, 2000), comprehensive clinical diagnosis involves a multidimensional assessment featuring at least two major sets of variables. On the one hand, there are "process" variables, including perceptions of self, others, and environmental demands and the responses to these, which occur on the behavioral, interpersonal, and emotional levels. These features, catalogued along Axis II in the DSM scheme, vary in the severity and direction (inward vs. outward) in which they are expressed and tend to perpetuate one another, creating a "loop" that is manifested as a pervasive personality pattern or style. On the other hand, clinical syndromes, indexed in Axis I, encompass more static, newer-onset features that are manifested in overt behaviors and phenomenological reports, and are seen as "outcome" variables in reference to their genesis from the personality loop. From this standpoint, a clinical syndrome (Axis I) may result from several different loops (Axis II), or it may be one of several syndromes' output from the same loop. Knowledge of both the process and outcome variables characterizing a person is necessary (1) for comprehensive diagnostic assessment, because it simultaneously provides broad descriptive information about expected levels of current functioning and sheds light on predicted paths of decompensation after the onset of future stressors; and (2) for determining the person's probable response to specific therapeutic interventions.

Despite the potential for comprehensive case conceptualization, the ability to predict patient responses to future anticipated and unanticipated stressors, and the possibility of optimal treatment triaging that could result from such a test battery, little work has been completed that focuses on the best assessment prescription for achieving these goals at the point of screening and intake. Indeed, *combining* multiple projective assessment instruments (e.g., the Thematic Apperception Test [TAT] and the Rorschach) within a battery is a common practice; however, the ways to *integrate* the information emerging from each into a useful stratagem for addressing the goals just noted have not been laid out.

Similarly, until the mid-1980s, little research had tested the utility of relating two or more "objective" inventories. One reasonable approach to addressing this issue is to examine the ways in which the best available instruments for measuring Axis I and Axis II phenomena covary. The Millon Clinical Multiaxial Inventory (MCMI) was designed to assess personality patterns and disorders (Axis II) specifically as established in the DSM-III. The MCMI is one of the few objective self-report inventories explicitly created to elucidate this realm of psychopathology. The MCMI also assesses levels of personality disorder severity or "organization" (e.g., borderline). The Minnesota Multiphasic Personality Inventory (MMPI) is the best-documented instrument designed to assess the presence of specific clinical syndromes (Axis I). Together, the MMPI and MCMI may provide data on different domains of psychological functioning, both of which are essential to forming a complete clinical picture. Although many of the studies reported in this chapter refer to earlier versions of the MCMI and the MMPI than the present versions (the MCMI-III and MMPI-2), there is good reason to assume that the patterns of covariation found between these two early forms will hold true for later forms of these instruments. The studies reported in this chapter are the only comprehensive investigations based on large patient populations from an extensive national sample; no comparable set of studies exists in the literature.

Emerging Trends in Psychodiagnostics: Another Offspring of the Managed Care Evolution

Despite the fact that the MCMI and MMPI were each designed to focus on a different axis of functioning, it has become commonplace for clinicians to view the MCMI as a "competitor" of the MMPI (Butcher & Owen, 1978; Korchin & Schuldberg, 1981). This sort of "either–or" attitude in clinical assessment is likely to be fueled by current trends in managed health care, designed to cut costs and services remunerated by third-party insurers. The managed care environment that most clinicians in mental health work must operate within has brought about a greater need to justify multiple tests in a psychosocial battery. Weiss (1994) notes some of the ways in which the use of multiple psychological tests are often justified in this climate, including efforts to predict the emergence of psychotic features in major depression and to delineate characterological versus reactive/situational difficulties precipitating current Axis I disorders. He notes that one cost issue at the heart of this strategy—failing to identify characterological dynamic contributions to a currently experienced Axis I condition—could lead to extra days of hospitalization or to repeated hospitalizations (Weiss, 1994). These consequences might be due to a failure to understand the intrapsychic or interpersonal factors precipitating, exacerbating, or maintaining the current presenting problem, as well as those that could increase or decrease a chosen treatment approach's probability of success (Millon, 1988).

In a perfect world, the power brokers in the health insurance industry—those case reviewers who determine the bottom-line services deemed necessary and reimbursable for a given case—would be aware of the cost risks involved in an inadequate clinical assessment, which could be considerably offset with a well-chosen, if somewhat longer, clinical assessment battery. However, in the imperfect and chaotic transition period in which we currently find ourselves, it is not uncommon for the clinician to be required to obtain precertification on a "per-test basis" to receive remuneration for all of the components of a clinical battery (Weiss, 1994). This might constitute a well-controlled, lean, and efficient system if it were not for the fact that the managed care system's decision makers are often not even trained in the use of psychological tests, much less in personality theory and testing.

One specific and growing problem in this climate that is particularly germane to this discussion involves the use of the MMPI and MCMI in clinical practice. Because both tests ostensibly provide information related to personality features and clinical syndromes, they are often deemed interchangeable and redundant by managed care reviewers (Weiss, 1994). Weiss (1994) goes on to note that it may be clinically unwise and financially "inexpedient" for third-party reviewers to discourage clinicians from using both instruments together, because (1) the MMPI is the most widely used objective testing instrument in the world (Greene, 1991) and one that is especially adept at assessing the presence of Axis I symptoms; and (2) the MCMI is the most popular personality (Axis II) instrument of its kind (Choca, Shanley, & Van Denburg, 1992).

Weiss (1994) correctly reasons that the argument of redundancy is substantially weakened by the overwhelming evidence suggesting that the two instruments show little, if any, direct overlap in their measurement of DSM-III-R (American Psychiatric Association, 1987) Axis I diagnoses. Based on studies comparing the MMPI with the MCMI (Patrick, 1988; Smith, Carroll, & Fuller, 1988) and with diagnostic interviews and assorted additional clinical measures (for reviews of this literature, see Wetzler, 1990), it appears that there is considerable divergence in their measurement of a wide variety of commonly diagnosed conditions—including those involving signs and symptoms of anxiety and depression, as well as those involving psychotic features and substance abuse symptoms.

This nonredundancy between the instruments appears to extend to personality disorders as well. Studies examining the comparability of MMPI and MCMI Axis II scales have attempted to determine the zero-order correlation between each of the

MCMI and MMPI personality scales, and have produced mixed results (McCann, 1989; Morey & Levine, 1988; Streiner & Miller, 1988). One study (Morey & Levine, 1988) found correlations ranging from .48 to .78 on 9 out of 11 scales, but negative correlations for the Compulsive and Antisocial scales. McCann (1989) similarly noted Pearson correlations ranging from .41 to .82 on 8 of 11 scales, with the remaining three (Compulsive, Antisocial, and Paranoid) producing negative MMPI–MCMI correlations. Finally, Streiner and Miller (1988) found overall moderate-sized correlations (r's = .29–.66) among scales and noted that 6 of 11 MMPI scales actually showed higher correlations with noncomplementary MCMI scales than with their counterpart scales. Although the small samples (N's = 47–76) and low subject-to-variable ratios extant in these studies may have been responsible in part for the discrepancies observed, it is also arguable that a scale-by-scale correlational analysis of Axis II variables is not the most clinically meaningful way to examine the comparability of these instruments as they are used in clinical diagnostic settings. Because a code type analysis is the method most frequently used by clinicians (Butcher, Dahlstrom, Graham, Tellegen, & Kemmer, 1989; Choca et al., 1992), it seems far more useful to elucidate the code type (e.g., two-point codes) concordance between the MMPI and MCMI to evaluate the degree of overlap that the clinical "consumer" is likely to experience when using the two instruments together in practice. Once this has been done, a reasonable decision can be made about the issue of redundancy and subsequent allocations of remuneration by third-party reviewers. Beyond providing a test of concordance, comparing the patterns of two-point scale elevations between the two instruments may add to the richness of the clinical assessment, if it can be shown that the scale scores/high-point codes from one instrument can be used to create clinically valuable subgroups subsumed under the two-point codes of the other instrument. This would be particularly helpful in the case of two-point codes that have been previously associated with characteristics that appear internally inconsistent, some of which are presented later in this chapter.

One study that tackled the issue of MMPI–MCMI code type concordance was conducted by Weiss (1994). He screened 100 patients admitted to a large general hospital and excluded those with primary diagnoses of organic brain syndromes, psychoses, or alcohol or drug dependence, as well as those with invalid MCMIs (more than one item on Validity scale endorsed) or MMPIs (F scale scores > 100 on the MMPI), resulting in a sample of 72 patients. This sample consisted of predominantly white females with a mean age of 47 years and an average education of 12.8 years. Consistent with previous work (McCann, 1989; Morey & Levine, 1988; Streiner & Miller, 1988), Weiss noted that 9 of 11 scales showed correlations ranging from .27 to .76, with a mean of .44, and that the remaining 2 scales (Compulsive and Antisocial) showed negative or near-zero correlations. He also found, in support of Streiner and Miller (1988), that correlations between counterpart scales (e.g., MMPI Schizoid and MCMI Schizoid) and noncomplementary scales (e.g., MMPI Schizoid and MCMI Avoidant) were not statistically different for 21 of 22 scales.

The two tests also diverged considerably on high-point code frequencies. The most common MCMI single high-point codes were for Dependent (39%) and Passive–Aggressive (18%), while the most frequently observed MMPI high-point codes were for Histrionic (22%), Narcissistic (18%), and Borderline (17%). The two-point code type analysis revealed that the most frequent MCMI two-point types were for Dependent–Passive–Aggressive (11%), Dependent–Avoidant (10%), and Passive–Aggressive–Borderline (8%), while the most frequently encountered MMPI code type patterns included the Histrionic–Narcissistic (25%), Dependent–Avoidant (11%), and Borderline–Histrionic (11%). The code type correspondence analyses for the two tests were particularly revealing: They indicated a total single high-point correspondence of 19.44% and a two-point correspondence of only 9.72%! The scale with the greatest high-point convergence was Dependent (9.72%), and the two-point code with the greatest degree of correspondence was the Dependent–Avoidant code type (5.56%).

As Weiss notes, the lack of correspondence between the MMPI and MCMI in this and prior studies suggests that the scales are not measuring comparable clinical constructs, and that the results emerging from the two instruments are nonredundant (Weiss, 1994). Although this information may be useful in informing third-party reviewers that the two tests can be viewed as nonoverlapping and deserving of separate remuneration, it still leaves open the question of how clinicians might be able to integrate MMPI and MCMI test results to arrive at the most accurate diagnosis and comprehensive understanding of the factors underlying the diagnosis for each patient who completes this test battery. Weiss (1994) concludes that because the MCMI and MMPI are not equivalent measures and appear to measure personality disorders significantly differently, using information obtained from both tests might be a useful way to gather both diagnostic (DSM) and theoretical information for formulating a treatment plan; therefore, the use of the tests concurrently should be reimbursable. Although he alludes to using the instruments in a "complementary fashion" and to synthesizing the tests' output into an "individualized, comprehensive psychological profile," there is no schematic information presented for how to do this. Thus we are back to our original question: *What are the optimal ways to integrate the information from the two most widely used objective instruments to enrich and refine data obtained from either instrument alone (1) to facilitate comprehensive case conceptualizations; (2) to identify factors capable of precipitating, exacerbating, or maintaining current levels of difficulties; and (3) to choose the most efficacious and cost-effective treatments from the resources that are available?* The remainder of this chapter reviews a series of studies conducted over two decades ago, which were designed to provide an analytic strategy for addressing this question.

A Model for Integrating the MCMI and the MMPI

At the time my colleagues and I initiated our research in this area, we were first drawn to examine the ways in which the MMPI and MCMI covaried out of a concern for the fact that MMPI two-point codes often suggest multiple interpretations, some of which contain contradictory "within-code" descriptors. We felt that many tenable hypotheses could be generated for each of the two-point codes presented, which, when taken together, might cloud necessary diagnostic and therapeutic decision-making processes. We reasoned that the addition of MCMI data to the test battery might help to confirm MMPI hypotheses in some cases and to resolve

MMPI descriptive contradictions in others. The model that we formulated for combining information from the MCMI and MMPI was based on the assumption that many of the contradictions in the extant two-point MMPI code descriptions can be sorted out into consistent MCMI-directed subtypes of each MMPI two-point code.

I have chosen here to summarize the large collection of MMPI–MCMI subtypes identified on the basis of our extensive studies conducted in the past two decades (Antoni, Tischer, Levine, Green, & Millon, 1985; Levine, Antoni, Tischer, Green, & Millon, 1985; Levine, Tischer, Antoni, Green, & Millon, 1986; Antoni, Levine, Tischer, Green, & Millon, 1985, 1986, 1987) by viewing them within the framework of a stress–coping model (Antoni, 1993). One of the most valuable benefits of personality diagnoses is that they enable a clinician to predict a patient's course after the onset of new stressors and/or the persistence or exacerbation of extant stressors. While many different personality *styles* present on the surface as similar at regular samplings, it is likely that during periods of acute stress or throughout periods of uncontrollable, unremitting, and severe burden, the pathognomonic signs of different personality *disorders* may be more likely to present themselves. Whereas reactions to acute, short-term stressors may reach extreme levels (manifested as clinical syndromes), the resulting changes in behavior, mood, and psychosocial functioning may be relatively short-lived. More long-term, uncontrollable, and unremitting stressors can be associated with more chronic changes in psychiatric status (e.g., decompensation into a borderline level of psychopathology; Millon, 1981) as well as physical status (e.g., immune system changes; Antoni et al., 1990; McKinnon, Weisse, Reynolds, Bowles, & Baum, 1989). It is plausible that the more precision clinicians are able to develop in characterizing the personality style—by, for instance, combining instruments to identify personality subtypes—the better they might be able to make predictions about a patient's response to future challenges.

A model that we used to guide our empirical investigations is one derived from the personality theory of Millon (1981). This model characterizes reactions to acute stressors along two dimensions: reactive "currency" (or "level") and "direction." In our work, we proposed that one pervasive stressor, loss (or threatened loss) of reinforcement, can lead to responses' taking the form of interpersonal or emotional *currencies* or levels, expressed in an outward or inward *direction*. These dimensions, taken together, make up the individual's coping style—a "program" that sets into motion several strategies that can be employed in demanding situations. When an individual experiences chronic periods of burden, especially to the extent that this burden is perceived as uncontrollable, his or her coping style will ultimately reach a point where it is relatively ineffective in regaining reinforcements and support. According to Millon (1981), the stressed individual's reactions to this loss—expressed in distinct currencies and in a characteristic direction—may spiral him or her into a state of alienation from the self and/or the social environment, possibly followed by decompensation into a more severe level of personality pathology. Millon (1981) has defined these decompensated patterns as "schizotypal," "borderline," and "paranoid." We used this model to interpret the findings of our research with the MCMI–MMPI battery.

To the degree that the MMPI and MCMI can together place individuals along these dimensions, they would offer clinical utility when combined as a battery. Specifically, the resulting information on personality subtypes could be used to generate testable predictions of short-term responses to acute stressors and the more decompensatory sequelae of chronic stressors. I now present a summary of our previous work with this "objective test battery" and suggest how the findings might be useful in making predictions about such stress responses/outcomes. As will be seen, the personality subtypes that result from the integration of these two instruments are also useful in clarifying some of the contradictory descriptions that can result from relying on MMPI two-point codes alone.

Research Strategy

Sampling

Approximately 175 frequent users of both the MMPI and MCMI were approached to participate in the study and to administer the MMPI and MCMI to their patients. We collected data over a 16-month period from 46 of these clinicians in various professional settings at sites located across the United States. In total, 3,283 sets of MMPI and MCMI batteries were returned. Twenty-four of the clinicians responding were in private practice; 15 worked in community mental health centers, shared practices, clinics, or other group settings; and the remaining 7 were in different hospital settings.

The age of the sample was widely distributed, with no systematic bias, and women slightly outnumbered men. Approximately 85% of the subjects were outpatients and 15% were inpatients. DSM-III affective and anxiety disorders were predominant along Axis I, whereas Axis II primary diagnoses included a large number of dependent and borderline personality disorders.

Procedure

Raw score data were reduced to the two highest scores for each instrument, provided that at least two scale scores were above a K-corrected T-score of 70 for the MMPI and a base rate (BR) score of 65 for the first eight or "basic" personality scales of the MCMI. If no MMPI scales were elevated above $T = 70$, then the profile was listed as "flat." It was also noted whether any of the three MCMI severe personality disturbance scales (Schizotypal, Borderline, and Paranoid) were elevated. High-point codes for each subject on the MCMI were tallied, and percentages of the largest and most theoretically relevant code types were computed. Code types were included only when a minimum of 10 cases were used. This cutoff point is somewhat more stringent than those employed in other research designs examining MMPI overlap with measures of psychopathology (Gilberstadt & Duker, 1965; Kelly & King, 1977; Vincent et al., 1983). It was judged that this rule would reduce the possibility of subtypes' emerging spuriously.

From the 3,283 MCMI–MMPI batteries, we anticipated that N's of 200 to 300 would be available for each of the more commonly observed MMPI two-point codes. To date we have published the results of six of the most prevalent MMPI two-point codes. The sample sizes and the relative proportion of the 3,283 cases collected for each of these are displayed in Table 8.1.

TABLE 8.1. Sample Sizes for Each of the Most Prevalent MMPI Two-Point Codes Studied

MMPI code	N	% of overall	Publication
28/82	353	10.8%	Antoni, Tischer, et al. (1985)
24/42	318	9.7%	Antoni, Levine, et al. (1985)
49/94	305	9.3%	Levine, Tischer, et al. (1986)
78/87	272	8.3%	Antoni et al. (1987)
98/89	228	6.9%	Antoni, Levine, et al. (1986)
27/72	228	6.9%	Levine, Antoni, et al. (1985)

Here I summarize the findings from four commonly encountered, though somewhat disparate, two-point code types (28/82, 24/42, 89/98, and 78/87), with an emphasis on stress response predictions that can be made on the basis of MCMI–MMPI covariations. These four MMPI two-point codes are also those that traditionally contain a substantial number of contradictory descriptors, thus providing a demonstration of how such contradictions may be resolved with this "objective test battery" approach. Thus, before describing the results of each set of analyses, I present a sample of the MMPI two-point code description that is widely used when the MMPI is considered alone. Once the discrepancies in this code description are outlined, I present the results of the MCMI–MMPI analysis as related to that MMPI two-point code. For detailed descriptions of the results of each study highlighted here, as well as those done with other MMPI two-point code types, I refer readers to the primary references (Antoni, Levine, et al., 1985, 1986, 1987; Antoni, Tischer, et al., 1985).

MMPI 28/82 (Primary Elevations on Scales 2 and 8 or 8 and 2)

Traditional Description for the MMPI 28/82 Code Type

Individuals with the MMPI 28/82 code type are basically dependent and submissive with difficulties in being assertive. They appear irritable and resentful, fear losing control, deny undesirable impulses, occasionally act-out and express guilt afterwards. Seen by some as stubborn and moody at times, they are considered peaceable and docile to others. These people are judged by some to be in a state of profound inner turmoil over highly conflictual, insoluble problems; others view them as somehow "resigned" to their psychosis. In some cases anxious, agitated depression may be seen while in others soft, reduced speech and retarded stream of thought are noted. Individuals with the 28/82 MMPI code appear most likely to receive a [DSM-II] diagnosis of either manic–depressive psychosis or schizophrenia, schizoaffective type. A significant segment of 28/82 individuals exhibit psychotic upsets, often preceded by hypochondriacal and hysterical episodes. Psychotic symptomatology may include bizarre mentation, delusions, hallucinations, social alienation, sleep disturbance, poor family relationships, and difficulties in impulse control. Unusual thoughts may take a specific form (hallucinations and suicidal ideation) or more diffuse symptomatology (general confusion, disorganization, and disorientation) (Dahlstrom, Welsh, & Dahlstrom, 1972; Graham, 1977). Overall, the 28/82 type appears to suffer from a heterogeneous group of disorders and syndromes characterized by disturbances of thinking, mood, and behavior. (Antoni, Levine, et al., 1985, p. 393)

This collection of descriptors presents several behavioral, interpersonal, and affective facets that at times seem to contradict one another, making clear hypotheses difficult to formulate. These contradictions appear at the behavioral level (denial of undesirable impulses vs. acting-out behaviors), the interpersonal level (withdrawn vs. hysterical), and the emotional level (stubborn and moody vs. peaceable and docile). Whereas some descriptors reflect an outwardly directed response style (hostility and aggression), others portray a more inwardly directed mode (retreat into fantasy via hallucinations). Diagnostic disparities are also prevalent with the 28/82 type, including hysterical and manic syndromes on the one hand, and schizoid and schizophrenic symptoms on the other.

MCMI Subtypes for the MMPI 28/82 Code Type

The results of our first MCMI–MMPI study indicated that the MCMI high-point scales that covary with the MMPI 28/82 code type yield three distinct groups of individuals differing across dimensions. To reiterate some of the aspects of the model proposed previously, the interpersonal style can be detached or ambivalent, while the reaction to loss of reinforcement is manifested in reactive currency (behavioral, interpersonal, or emotional) and direction (inward or outward). Each subtype represents a unique constellation of these dimensions. Persons with the first subtype (elevations on MCMI scales 1 and 2 [12], 21), the "interpersonally acting-in group," anticipate no reinforcement and therefore employ an interpersonal style of detachment or withdrawal. These people tend to react to stress with inwardly directed self-punitive responses on the behavioral and interpersonal levels. Those with the second subtype (elevations on MCMI scales 8, 82, 28), the "emotionally acting-out group," seek reinforcement from external sources; display an ambivalent interpersonal style; and react to loss of support with outwardly directed, unpredictable, and dramatic emotional responses. Those with the third subtype (elevations on MCMI scales 23, 32), the "emotionally acting-in group," seek reinforcements from external sources, move between ambivalent and withdrawn interpersonal styles, and may react to loss of support with inwardly directed negative emotional experiences.

If stress should become excessive in any of these groups, thereby "overwhelming" their interpersonal style, these people may become ineffective in securing reinforcements and support. The reactions to this loss expressed in their distinct currencies and in characteristic direction (inward, outward) could spiral such individuals into a state of alienation followed by decompensation. In the emotionally acting-out group, this alienation is likely to precipitate as self-alienation and identity problems. Our data suggest that decompensation into a borderline pattern appears to follow in this subtype. The interpersonally acting-in group may experience total alienation, with decompensation into a schizotypal pattern when under unremitting stress. Finally, the emotionally acting-in group, possessing traits of both of the other two subtypes, may display borderline and/or schizotypal patterns of decompensation.

To summarize, it appears that the primary sources of ambiguity in the MMPI 28/ 82 code description—the level (emotional vs. interpersonal) and direction (inward vs. outward) on which these individuals react to stress—may be clarified by the use of MMPI–MCMI subtypes, named according to the configuration of these two dimensions.

MMPI 24/42 (Primary Elevations on Scales 2 and 4 or 4 and 2)

Traditional Description of the MMPI 24/42 Code Type

The 24/42 type, often referred to as "psychopaths in trouble," are known for their recurrent acting-out and subsequent periods of guilt and depression. They are noted as impulsive, unable to delay gratification and to have little respect for societal standards. Frustrated by their own limited achievements, resentful of the demands and expectations of others, they often experience a mixture of anger and guilt that manifests itself in agitated depression. Some are overcontrolled, avoid confrontations, and express feelings of inadequacy and self-punitive rumination. Many also engage in asocial or antisocial behaviors, such as stealing, sexual acting-out, and drug or alcohol abuse. Often described as immature and narcissistic, they appear unable to maintain deep relationships. Beneath the carefree and confident facade of many will often reside either worry and dissatisfaction, or an absence of any emotional response. Their failure to achieve life satisfactions results either in self-blame and depression or in a projection of blame and paranoid ideation. In some cases, pre-psychotic behavior and suicide attempts may be seen (Dahlstrom et al., 1972; Graham, 1977). (Antoni, Tischer, et al., 1985, p. 509)

Some of these statements appear contradictory at the behavioral (asocial vs. antisocial) and emotional levels (worry and anger vs. absence of emotional response). Moreover, while some descriptors reflect an outwardly directed response (extrapunitive, projected blame), others indicate a more inwardly directed response (self-blame, depression).

MCMI Subtypes of the MMPI 24/42 Code Type

Analysis of the MCMI–MMPI battery for subjects classified with the MMPI 24/42 code type produced three subtypes, with at least one of these appearing to break into two variants. For this reason, I discuss our findings for this code type in somewhat more detail, emphasizing the predicted stress responses within each subtype.

Interpersonally Acting-Out Group

One of these subtypes is the "interpersonally acting-out group"; the tendency is to react to stress on the behavioral and interpersonal levels through impulsive, outwardly directed, and projected responses. For these patients, it is possible that MMPI scale 4 elevations approximate their personality core, and scale 2 elevations reflect a clinical outcome that is more likely to occur when they are unable to acquire the reinforcements they need. Individuals falling within this subtype (those with elevations on MCMI scales 6, 65, 67, 5) are related in their arrogance, aggressiveness, and self-centeredness. When criticized, they may become explosive and display overtly antisocial behaviors such as brutality, alcoholism, drug addiction, and other forms of acting out.

ACUTE STRESS RESPONSE

Persons with the first variant of this subtype (MCMI scale 6, primary elevation) may be prone to display behavior and affect driven by fear and a mistrust of others, taking the form of hostile acting out, angry rejection of social norms, and an undercurrent of inadequacy and self-dissatisfaction. This desire to provoke fear and intimidate others may come either from a need to compensate for a sense of inner weakness or from a wish to vindicate past injustices (Millon, 1969, 1981).

Individuals who fit more into the second variant of this subtype (primary elevations on MCMI scale 5) are more likely to be guided by their high self-esteem, leading to arrogance and a disregard for social constraints. They may come across as charming and exhibitionistic, yet manipulative. These people are rarely likely to experience self-doubt, though psychosocial stressors may trigger acting-out behaviors (addictions, sexual excesses) as a means of restoring equilibrium.

CHRONIC STRESS SEQUELAE

Should the individuals with the high scale 6 variant of this subtype meet with repeated failure in their attempts to secure support and reinforcement, paranoid-like behaviors may become evident. In support of this notion, we found that over half of the interpersonally acting-out group (primary elevations on MCMI scale 6) also showed high elevations on the MCMI Paranoid scale—a scale measuring symptoms such as ideas of reference, vigilant mistrust, and grandiose self-image. It is noteworthy, however, that those people characterized by the other variant (primary elevations on MCMI scale 5) showed no elevations on the three, more severe syndrome scales.

Interpersonally Acting-In Group

ACUTE STRESS RESPONSE

A second subtype of the MMPI 24/42 code type composes a more unitary group, which we have referred to as an "interpersonally acting-in group" to emphasize their tendency to react to stressors on the behavioral and interpersonal levels through withdrawal, self-deprecation, and self-punitive responses. Individuals in this subtype (those with elevations on MCMI scales 1 or 138) may be self-belittling and possess a weak and ineffectual self-image. The intrapunitive nature of this subtype seems to be at the other end of the pole from the extrapunitive and blaming nature of the acting-out group. According to Millon (1981), this subtype may include individuals who have neither internal nor external sources of reinforcement, and therefore turn neither inward nor outward to acquire psychic pleasure or support. Their high endorsement of MMPI scale 2 items may be accounted for by the deflated self-esteem and daily experience of a pansocial isolation that are predicted by Millon's theory. Importantly, isolation for this group is likely to reflect an indifference to social interaction rather than an active disdain or rejection of others, the latter being more characteristic of the interpersonally acting-out group.

CHRONIC STRESS SEQUELAE

Should individuals with this MMPI 24/42 subtype continue to experience both self- and social alienation, they may display behavioral eccentricities, ideas of reference, cognitive slippage, magical thinking, and depersonalization anxieties—symptoms in line with a schizotypal personality pattern. Not surprisingly, we found that a large proportion of patients in the interpersonally acting-in group showed distinct and frequent elevations on the Schizotypal scale of the MCMI.

Emotionally Acting-Out Group

ACUTE STRESS RESPONSE

The two subtypes discussed thus far, both representing variations of the MMPI 24/42 type, differ in both the "direction" of their expressive functioning (acting out vs. acting in) and in their likely course of decompensation. Those with a third MMPI 24/42 subtype, referred to as the "emotionally acting-out group," are best characterized by their tendencies to exhibit demodulated, labile, and outwardly expressed affect to gain attention and support. These people's coping patterns may toggle between the traits of MMPI scales 2 and 4. In their case, the contradictory nature of the traditional MMPI 24/42 code type descriptors portray, to some extent, the intrinsically contradictory nature of ambivalent interpersonal styles (Millon, 1969, 1981). Individuals included in this subtype (those with elevations on MCMI scales 34/43, 83, 84) may vacillate between irritable, depressive moods and manic-like euphoric or hostile episodes. The unifying element in the emotional expressions is the dramatic nature. According to Millon (1981), these displays may be motivated by a desire to regain a "lost" source of reinforcement or support. Accordingly, these individuals can be characterized by both extreme dependence and self-alienation; they display a resentful ambivalence, possibly generated by conflict between dependence needs and a desire to be autonomous.

CHRONIC STRESS SEQUELAE

We hypothesized that when individuals with this subtype fail to gain and sustain attention and support, a mixed and conflicting set of emotions such as rage, guilt, and love may emerge. During these periods, these persons may be plagued by cognitive confusions over goals and identity, as well as desultory energy levels and sleep irregularities. Supportive of this notion is the fact that a significant proportion of those in the emotionally acting-out group showed marked elevations on the MCMI Borderline scale—a scale that reflects difficulties in identity confusion and physiological phenomena such as sleep patterns.

Based on the results of the MCMI–MMPI analysis just summarized, it appears that the MMPI 24/42 code represents in the interpersonally acting-out group an acting-out type in which scale 4 relates to the personality, whereas scale 2 reflects a more transient clinical outcome occurring when these individuals are unable to acquire reinforcements. High scale 2 scores in the interpersonally acting-in group seem to reflect the personality style, whereas scale 4 elevations represent the clinical outcome of withdrawal via asocial behaviors and interpersonal indifference. The contradictory descriptors of the MMPI 24/42 code appear to accurately reflect the essential ambivalent nature of the third, or emotionally acting-out group, whose coping style vacillates between the aspects of the MMPI scales 2 and 4.

MMPI 89/98 (Primary Elevations on Scales 8 and 9 or 9 and 8)

Traditional Description of the MMPI 89/98 Code Type

Individuals with the 89/98 code type have been described as being self-centered and infantile in their expectations of others, demanding a great deal of attention, and responding with resentment and hostility when demands are not met. Fearing emotional involvement they avoid close relationships and tend to be socially withdrawn and isolated. Characterized as hyperactive, emotionally labile and unrealistic in self-appraisal, these individuals may im-press others as grandiose, boastful and fickle. Their feelings of inadequacy and low self-esteem tend to limit the extent to which they involve themselves in competitive and achievement-oriented activities. However, these individuals usually emphasize achievement as a means of gaining status and recognition. Their affect is characterized by some as inappropriate, unmodulated, irritable and hostile, yet they may also tend to be ruminative, overideational and withdrawn, fearing any type of outward communication with others. Highly suspicious and distrustful of others, these individuals may display unusual and unconventional thought processes including delusions of a religious nature, feelings of grandiosity, hallucinations, poor concentration and negativism. These individuals may receive a diagnosis of either schizophrenia, stressing an interpersonal element, or manic depression, manic type, stressing the emotional features. Drug abuse is a common accompanying symptom (Dahlstrom et al., 1972; Graham, 1977). (Antoni et al., 1986, pp. 66–67)

As we have noted previously (Antoni et al., 1986), the phrases making up the description of this MMPI code type, taken as a whole, seem to contradict one another at the behavioral level (avoidance of achievement-oriented activities vs. emphasis on achievement as a means of gaining status and recognition), the interpersonal level (socially withdrawn and inadequate vs. grandiose and boastful), and the emotional level (ruminative and fearful of emotional involvement vs. overt hostility and emotional lability). Diagnostic disparities also appear possible in the 89/98 MMPI type, including schizophrenia on the one hand, and bipolar syndromes on the other. This range of variability seems to suggest a strong likelihood of the presence of subtypes within this code type.

MCMI Subtypes of the MMPI 89/98 Code Type

Our work integrating the MCMI and MMPI results for these individuals identified three subtypes that begin to explain the roots of these discrepancies. Because the chronic stress sequelae of the first two groups are likely to be similar, I first list the acute stress responses of each before moving on to describing the predicted responses to more chronic burdens.

Interpersonally Acting-Out Group

ACUTE STRESS RESPONSES

The largest subtype, consisting of individuals with elevations on MCMI scale 6 (Antisocial), (including 65/56, 61, 6, and 67), was referred to as the "interpersonally acting-out group" to describe these persons' tendency to respond to stressors with impulsive, outwardly directed, and projected responses. We hypothesized that acute stressors taking the form of criticism and assaults on their self-image may result in explosive antisocial behaviors such as substance abuse and frank brutality. The behaviors of persons of this subtype may be "driven" by a fear and mistrust of others, resulting in hostile acting out, rejection of social norms, and an avoidance of close relationships stemming from a need to compensate for an inner sense of weakness or from a wish to vindicate past injustices (Millon, 1969, 1981).

Interpersonally Grandiose Group

ACUTE STRESS RESPONSES

Individuals with the second subtype (with primary elevations on MCMI scale 5, including codes other than 56) are primarily motivated by high self-esteem, feelings of grandiosity, disregard for social constraints, and interpersonal arrogance. These individuals, though charming and exhibitionistic during periods of low stress, may be prone to periods of acting out (e.g., substance abuse, sexual excesses) when they experience mounting stressors.

CHRONIC STRESS SEQUELAE

Should persons of either of the two MMPI 89/98 subtypes just discussed encounter periods of unremitting stress during which they are unable to secure support and reinforcement, they may evince paranoid-like changes (e.g., magnifying the incidental remarks of others). We did indeed observe that a large proportion of individuals in both subtypes showed clear elevations on the MCMI Paranoid scale, indicating that they were experiencing such symptoms as ideas of reference, vigilant mistrust, and grandiose self-image.

Emotionally Acting-Out Group

The third MMPI 89/98 subtype is made up of individuals with primary elevations on MCMI scale 8 (Passive–Aggressive) and scale 3 (Dependent), including codes 85, 86, 35, 34/43, and 83. These individuals were referred to as the "emotionally acting-out group" to describe their tendency to react to stressors with demodulated, labile, unpredictable, and intense affective responses.

ACUTE STRESS RESPONSES

Because these individuals actively seek reinforcers from external sources, they are susceptible to periods of extreme dependence and self-alienation, and may be particularly hard hit when encountering interpersonal losses due to deaths and relocation. These individuals are also untrusting, fearful of domination, and suspiciously alert to efforts to undermine their veiled movements toward closeness and intimacy. As such, their coping style for dealing with interpersonal stressors is marked by ambivalence.

CHRONIC STRESS SEQUELAE

When these individuals' attempts at securing social support and attention fail, perhaps due to self-inflicted damage to their social network or unavoidable losses, conflicting emotions of guilt, rage, and love may emerge. We hypothesized that such periods may be characterized by cognitive confusions over identity, extreme suspiciousness, and unpredictable succession of moods. In support of this notion, we observed that a substantial proportion of those people in the emotionally acting-out group showed elevations on both the MCMI Borderline and Paranoid scales.

MMPI 78/87 (Primary Elevations on Scales 7 and 8 or 8 and 7)

Traditional Description of the MMPI 78/87 Code Type

Individuals with the 78/87 code type are often described as experiencing a good deal of psychic turmoil. Usually introspective and obsessional, they spend much of their time being worried, tense, and depressed. Often indecisive, these individuals usually show poor judgment when they do act and may appear to others as jumpy and socially inept. In interpersonal situations, the 78/87 type comes across as shy and hard to get to know at times, yet sentimental, sensitive, and softhearted on other occasions. These individuals characteristically maintain a rigid hold on affect, yet may be prone to displays of immaturity and emotionality. These people tend to deal with their psychic and social discomfort by withdrawal into a rich fantasy experience, often of a sexual nature (Dahlstrom et al., 1972; Graham, 1977). (Antoni, Levine, et al., 1987, p. 377)

What is immediately apparent in the description of the MMPI 78/87 code type is that DSM-III diagnoses can range from the neurotic to psychotic level, with primary emphasis placed on Axis I in some cases and on Axis II in others. In terms of Axis II diagnoses, these range from passive–dependent and schizoid to schizotypal and borderline. Several inconsistencies and ambiguities occur across interpersonal, behavioral, and emotional spheres of functioning as well. Within the interpersonal sphere, as noted above, people with this code type are characterized as introverted and hard to get to know on the one hand, yet sentimental, sensitive, and softhearted on the other (Dahlstrom et al., 1972). We have portrayed these descriptors as presenting a simultaneous "moving away from" and "moving toward" others (Antoni et al., 1987). In the behavioral domain, those with the 78/87 code type have been described with terms that emphasize both compulsivity and impulsivity (Dahlstrom et al., 1972; Graham, 1977). Finally, on the emotional level of functioning, those with the 78/87 code type have been characterized by some as rigid, affectively restrained, and introspective, yet by others as immature and emotional (Dahlstrom et al., 1972). The DSM-III diagnoses often associated with this code type also vary in the degree to which they emphasize behavioral (compulsive behaviors), interpersonal (schizoid, passive–dependent), and affective (depression) features. Some have utilized the relative elevations of scales 7 and 8 for differentiating neurotic from psychotic or schizoid disorders (Graham, 1977).

MCMI Subtypes of the MMPI 78/87 Code Type

Based upon the study examining the MMPI 78/87 code type (Antoni et al., 1987), we found three MCMI subtypes: an "interpersonally acting-in group," an "emotionally acting-out group," and an "emotionally acting-in group."

Interpersonally Acting-In Group

ACUTE STRESS RESPONSES

One subtype of the MMPI 78/87, made up of individuals with elevations on MCMI scales 1 (Schizoid) and 2 (Avoidant), including codes 12 and 21, was termed the *interpersonally acting-in group* to describe these persons' predicted tendency to react to stressors on the interpersonal level with indecision, withdrawal, pervasive anxiety, and obsessional thoughts. Millon (1969, 1981) theorizes that the withdrawal and acting-in quality of this group results from an inability to experience pleasure. This subtype can be seen interpersonally as a group of individuals who are often socially and self-alienated, and who experience a chronic state of psychic turmoil. Because these people are unsuccessful in reducing this chronic turmoil through interpersonal channels, they may engage in repetitive and ritualistic behaviors. Individuals who fit this MMPI 78/87 subtype may be those who are the most likely to receive a diagnosis of obsessive–compulsive disorder.

CHRONIC STRESS SEQUELAE

Because individuals with this MMPI 78/87 subtype are isolated from social feedback, they may under periods of persistent and severe stress decompensate into a pattern of behavioral eccentricities, ideas of reference, depersonalization anxieties, cognitive slippage, and magical thinking—a schizotypal pattern. Relatedly, we observed that a large proportion of people fitting into this subtype also showed elevations on the MCMI Schizotypal scale.

Emotionally Acting-Out Group

ACUTE STRESS RESPONSES

Other features making up traditional descriptions of the MMPI 78/87 code type focus on a more agitated clinical picture featuring outwardly expressed affect. These features mirror a second subtype, which we termed the emotionally acting-out group to describe the tendency to react to stressors with labile emotional responses that alternate between angry defiance and sullen moodiness. As opposed to people falling into the formerly described MMPI 78/87 subtype, these individuals actively seek reinforcement from others and are characterized by extreme dependence, self-alienation, and interpersonal ambivalence. We hypothesized that their ambivalence over relationships could be manifested as hostility and demonstrative emotional displays, perhaps to repel the significant others that they desperately need. As such, this subtype fits the MMPI 78/87 descriptors that pertain to an immature expression of affect.

CHRONIC STRESS SEQUELAE

We reasoned that when under periods of chronic, uncontrollable demands, individuals with this subtype may become frustrated in their attempts to secure support and attention from others, especially to the extent that they have rebuffed members of their social network in the past. During such periods, they may experience conflicting emotions related to others (e.g., guilt, love, rage), identity confusion, and physiological changes such as sleep irregularities. These predictions are supported by our observations that individuals in the emotionally acting-out group obtain elevations on the MCMI Borderline scale, which taps many of these symptoms.

Emotionally Acting-In Group

ACUTE STRESS RESPONSE

A final subtype with the MMPI 78/87 code includes individuals with primary elevations on MCMI scales 2 (Avoidant) and 3 (Dependent), whom we have designated as the emotionally acting-in group. They are likely to respond to stress with inwardly directed anger and frustration, which Millon (1981) has hypothesized to result from an intense conflict between opposing sources of reinforcement (other, self, none) and alternating approaches to securing that support (active, passive). It could be further speculated that out of a fear of rejection by others, they may actually withdraw from their only sources of reinforcement, resulting in loneliness and mixed feelings of anxiety, sadness, anger, and guilt.

CHRONIC STRESS SEQUELAE

If reinforcers are unavailable for extended periods, these individuals may become emotionally drained and may translate anger at others into self-degradation and feelings of worthlessness. Because of this relentless, downwardly spiraling conflict, they may decompensate into either a schizotypal pattern, a borderline pattern, or some mixture of both, including such symptoms as acute emotional turmoil, irrational thinking, and extended periods of despondency. In support of these predictions, we noted that a large proportion of individuals with this subtype also obtained elevations on both the MCMI Borderline and Schizotypal scales.

Conclusions

We believe that conceptualizing the various MMPI two-point codes as distinct MCMI-indexed subtypes will facilitate making predictions concerning the coping responses that these individuals will employ in periods of acute stress and the route of decompensation that they will take, should stressors persist and coping resources become insufficient. A pattern that runs consistently through the results of the studies reviewed here is that individuals with a given MMPI two-point code type can display marked heterogeneity across many spheres of functioning (Antoni, Levine, et al., 1985; Antoni, Tischer, et al., 1985). The variability described for these groups may be found across behavioral, interpersonal, and affective realms and is manifested in specific "styles" of reinforcement acquisition and decompensation. This variance describes the configurations of assorted clinical features, some describing a core issue and others representing more or less "spinoffs" of this central feature. Here we have demonstrated a format that gives a focus to the clinical picture by specifying particular spheres of psychosocial functioning and impairment (behavioral, cognitive, interpersonal, emotional), thereby establishing subtypes with distinct clusters of clinical symptoms. The goal of our work was to lay the groundwork for empirical tests of diagnostic categories assessed by an "objective" test battery made up of the most widely used and researched instruments available for addressing personality-related phenomena. This descriptive stage in this process was the aim of our previous studies. The next step (the empirical stage) necessarily involves external criteria against which these categories can be compared (e.g., clinical observations).

On a practical level, it remains uncertain, according to the set of descriptions provided for MMPI two-point code types, which axis should be considered primary and which secondary in arriving at a diagnosis. It is equally unclear which Axis II disorder is most likely to "coexist" with an accompanying Axis I syndrome. One consistent bias in our work has been to assign primacy to Axis II; hence all of the subgroups identified and described had a primary label along this axis. However, this formulation allowed for the explanation of clinical syndromes that would be very likely to be present in each subtype and, in so doing, united the most likely Axis I–Axis II combinations. The elucidation of these combinations is essential for accurate and comprehensive diagnosis, and may help predict probable clinical course and treatment prognosis. As such, the discriminations that become available with this test battery may be useful in cases in which a clinician needs to determine the salience and centrality of behavioral, interpersonal, and affective issues and observations to plan the most efficacious and cost-effective therapeutic interventions. With an understanding of the central clinical features and a clear picture of the primacy of syndrome and disorder in a given case, the clinician may be better prepared to decide on a treatment approach based on the efficacy of one intervention modality over another. Also, having available a better understanding of the spheres of functioning (e.g., interpersonal vs. emotional) that their patients tend to be most comfortable operating within may help clinicians with general rapport and communication issues, allowing them to work more efficiently with patients in familiar ways. Ultimately, wider use of this integrated test battery approach, supported by a more assessment-literate managed care system, will greatly facilitate the most comprehensive case conceptualizations. Clinicians should then be far better able to identify factors precipitating, exacerbating, or maintaining current levels of difficulties, as well as the treatments that are the most efficacious and cost-effective routes to patient management, remediation, and recovery.

References

American Psychiatric Association. (1980). *Diagnostic and statistical manual of mental disorders* (3rd ed.). Washington, DC: Author.

American Psychiatric Association. (1987). *Diagnostic and statistical manual of mental disorders* (3rd ed., rev.). Washington, DC: Author.

American Psychiatric Association. (2000). *Diagnostic and statistical manual of mental disorders* (4th ed., text rev.). Washington, DC: Author.

Antoni, M. H. (1993). The combined use of the MCMI and MMPI. In R. Craig (Ed.), *The Millon Clinical Multiaxial Inventory: A clinical research information synthesis* (pp. 279–302). Hillsdale, NJ: Erlbaum.

Antoni, M. H., Levine, J., Tischer, P., Green, C., & Millon, T. (1985). Refining MMPI code interpretations by reference to MCMI scale data: Part I: MMPI code 28/82. *Journal of Personality Assessment, 49*(4), 392–398.

Antoni, M. H., Levine, J., Tischer, P., Green, C., & Millon, T. (1986). Refining personality assessments by combining MCMI high point profiles and MMPI codes: Part IV. MMPI code 89/98. *Journal of Personality Assessment, 50*(1), 65–72.

Antoni, M. H., Levine, J., Tischer, P., Green, C., & Millon, T. (1987). Refining personality assessments by combining MCMI high point profiles and MMPI codes: Part V. MMPI code 78/87. *Journal of Personality Assessment, 51*(3), 375–387.

Antoni, M. H., Schneiderman, N., Fletcher, M. A., Goldstein, D., Ironson, G., & LaPerriere, A. (1990). Psychoneuroimmunology and HIV-1. *Journal of Consulting and Clinical Psychology, 58*(1), 38–49.

Antoni, M. H., Tischer, P., Levine, J., Green, C., & Millon, T. (1985). Refining personality assessments by combining MCMI high point profiles and MMPI codes: Part III. MMPI code 24/42. *Journal of Personality Assessment, 49*(5), 508–515.

Butcher, J. N., Dahlstrom, W., Graham, J., Tellegen, A., & Kemmer, B. (1989). *MMPI-2: Manual for administration and scoring*. Minneapolis: University of Minnesota Press.

Butcher, J. N., & Owen, P. L. (1978). Objective personality inventories: Recent research and some contemporary issues. In B. B. Wolman (Ed.), *Clinical diagnosis of mental disorders: A handbook*. New York: Plenum Press.

Choca, J. P., Shanley, L., & Van Denburg, E. (1992). *Interpretative guide to the Millon Clinical Multiaxial Inventory*. Washington, DC: American Psychological Association.

Dahlstrom, W. G., Welsh, G. S., & Dahlstrom, L. E. (1972). *An MMPI handbook: Vol. 1. Clinical interpretation*. Minneapolis: University of Minnesota Press.

Gilberstadt, H., & Duker, J. (1965). *A handbook for clinical and actuarial MMPI interpretation*. Philadelphia: Saunders.

Graham, J. R. (1977). *The MMPI: A practical guide*. New York: Oxford University Press.

Greene, R. L. (1991). *The MMPI-2/MMPI: An interpretive manual*. Boston: Allyn & Bacon.

Kelly, C., & King, G. D. (1977). MMPI behavioral correlates of spike 5 and two-point code types with scale 5 as one elevation. *Journal of Clinical Psychology, 33*, 180–185.

Korchin, S. J., & Schuldberg, D. (1981). The future of clinical assessment. *American Psychologist, 36*, 1147–1148.

Levine, J., Antoni, M. H., Tischer, P., Green, C., & Millon, T. (1985). Refining MMPI code interpretations by reference to MCMI scale data: Part II. MMPI code 27/72. *Journal of Personality Assessment, 49*(5), 501–507.

Levine, J., Tischer, P., Antoni, M. H., Green, C., & Millon, T. (1986). Refining personality assessments by combining MCMI high point profiles and MMPI codes: Part VI. MMPI code 49/94. *Journal of Personality Assessment, 51*, 388–401.

McCann, J. T. (1989). MMPI personality disorder scales and the MCMI: Concurrent validity. *Journal of Clinical Psychology, 45*(3), 365–369.

McKinnon, W., Weisse, C., Reynolds, C., Bowles, C., & Baum, A. (1989). Chronic stress, leukocyte subpopulations, and humoral responses to latent viruses. *Health Psychology, 8*(4), 389–402.

Millon, T. (1969). *Modern psychopathology: A biosocial approach to maladaptive learning and functioning*. Philadelphia: Saunders.

Millon, T. (1981). *Disorders of personality: DSM-III, Axis II*. New York: Wiley-Interscience.

Millon, T. (1988). Personologic psychotherapy: Ten commandments for a post-eclectic approach to integrative treatment. *Psychotherapy, 25*, 209–219.

Morey, L. C., & Levine, D. (1988). Multitrait–multimethod examination of the MMPI and MCMI. *Journal of Psychopathology and Behavioral Assessment, 19*(4), 333–343.

Patrick, J. (1988). Concordance of the MCMI and MMPI in the diagnosis of three DSM-III Axis I disorders. *Journal of Clinical Psychology, 44*(2), 186–190.

Piersma, H. L. (1987). The MCMI as a measure of DSM-III Axis II diagnoses: An empirical comparison. *Journal of Clinical Psychology, 43*(5), 478–483.

Smith, D., Carroll, J., & Fuller, G. (1988). The relationship between the MCMI and MMPI in a private outpatient mental health clinic population. *Journal of Clinical Psychology, 44*(2), 165–174.

Streiner, D. L., & Miller, H. R. (1988). Validity of MMPI scales for DSM-III personality disorders: What are they measuring? *Journal of Personality Disorders, 2*(3), 238–242.

Vincent, K. R., Castillo, I., Hauser, R. I., Stuart, H. J., Zapata, J. A., Cohn, C. K., et al. (1983). MMPI code type and DSM-III diagnoses. *Journal of Clinical Psychology, 39*(6), 829–842.

Weiss, E. (1994). Managed care and the psychometric validity of the MMPI and MCMI personality disorder scales. *Psychotherapy in Private Practice, 13*(3), 81–97.

Wetzler, S. (1990). The MCMI: A review. *Journal of Personality Assessment, 55*(3–4), 445–464.

CHAPTER 9

Using the Millon Inventories in Forensic Psychology

Frank J. Dyer

The Role of the Forensic Expert and the MCMI-III

Ever since the concept of the therapeutic alliance was first discussed among psychoanalytic practitioners in the early part of the 20th century, clinicians have viewed themselves as being advocates for their patients. That is to say, the process of producing positive therapeutic change in a therapy patient or counseling client is universally recognized as being intrinsically bound up with the development of a relationship in which the patient has trust and confidence in the therapist and views the therapist as being on his or her side (periods of negative transference excepted, of course). Clinicians—whether engaged in psychiatric hospital work, therapy in a clinic, or other types of therapeutic consultations—generally perceive what they do as helping their patients to grow, healing the patients' psychic pain, or enhancing the patients' capacity to adapt to interpersonal reality. Clinicians tend to see themselves in this role even when their interventions may impose frustration on a patient or inflict an unavoidable blow or two to the patient's ego in the process of therapeutic work.

It is therefore something of a culture shock when psychologists who are used to doing clinical work step into the forensic arena and find that their alliance with their clients, if such exists, is actually a hindrance rather than a help. This is due to the extremely specialized division of labor in the court system and the rigidly circumscribed roles in which the main parties in courtroom proceedings are cast. In the typical situation where a psychologist becomes involved as an expert in the legal system, there are only two figures in the courtroom, among the primary participants in the litigation, who are expected to be absolutely neutral and unbiased in everything that they say and do. The first of these figures is the judge, who is expected to make impartial rulings on admissibility of evidence, to rule on attorneys' objections to certain aspects of testimony on the part of witnesses, to give a fair charge to the jury that does not favor either side, and to perform similar functions with a strict adherence to due process of law. From the very earliest days of their legal training, judges have been inculcated with the concept that any deviation from an unbiased stance will provide grounds for an appeal, which may result in the judge's decision being overturned on the grounds of a prejudicial ruling favoring one side or the other. This mindset of strict neutrality, then, comes relatively automatically to judges.

Attorneys, on the other hand, are the adversaries in this particular drama. They are charged by law to provide zealous representation to their clients, and as such are required to assert interpretations of points of law, facts, evidence, and even expert opinions, skewed in a direction that is favorable to the interests of their clients. Neutral is perhaps the last thing that they want to be perceived as being. The sanction for deviating from that role is a charge of ineffective assistance of counsel or incompetent representation. It is not all that uncommon for attorneys to be sued for failing to take some action in the representation of their clients' legal interests. Their responsibility for advocacy is extremely well defined and trumps everything else, even attorneys' own personal beliefs about the validity of the arguments that they so vigorously pursue.

Enter the clinical psychologist, with a mindset focused on providing therapeutic assistance to the client. It is surprising that many psychologists coming into the domain of forensic psychology from the ranks of clinicians have so little idea of what is expected of them on the witness stand. In many cases, no one seems to have told them that the only other party in the proceedings besides the judge who is expected to be entirely neutral and unbiased is, in fact, the expert witness. Even many attorneys, who should know better, reinforce the inappropriate generalization of the clinician's helpful attitude of advocacy to include the role of expert witness. An attorney will often comment that the attorney and the clinician make a good team in assisting certain types of clients, much as the clinician teams up with a psychiatrist, clinical social worker, and other specialists in assisting the hospitalized patient with a comprehensive treatment plan.

In fact, the expert witness has one and only one function in court, that being to provide information for the trier of fact. This information must be of the type that assists the trier of fact in resolving the legal question at issue in a just manner. The expert witness, strictly in terms of role definition, is not there to assist the client of the attorney who has put the expert forward; nor is the expert there to undermine the interests of the client of the attorney's adversary. The expert is expected to perform a neutral and unbiased assessment that addresses the specific referral questions; to collect data, including those favorable and unfavorable to the interests of the client that the attorney represents; to formulate conclusions in a logical manner that adequately addresses the referral questions; and to state those conclusions fully, including any findings that may be at odds with the overall conclusions of the expert. The standard that experts are expected to adhere to is one of writing the same basic report, regardless of which side engages the expert.

Over the course of the past few decades, it has become more and more widely accepted that experts are not merely testifying on the basis of their own individual training and experience, but are representing the discipline in which they received their training. As scientific disciplines such as psychology mature and develop a greater knowledge base in a particular area, experts are expected to familiarize themselves with the relevant research findings and assessment techniques, and to structure their procedures and their testimony accordingly. In this vein, experts' claims to credibility on the witness stand are based on the principle that their testimony rests on a foundation outside their own subjective judgment. That is, experts are not going to be believed by judges and juries simply on the basis of their having completed extensive training in their field and having had a certain number of years of experience. One can guarantee with just about 100% certainty that if an expert comes to court and testifies based only on his or her experience and training, then the other side will put forward a similarly qualified expert who will testify on the basis of that expert's experience and training, but will reach an entirely opposite conclusion in line with the interests of the client represented by the attorney who engaged the expert.

The basis on which psychological experts testify in regard to their evaluations is enhanced in this regard by the use of assessment instruments and techniques that supplement the clinical interview. Such assessment techniques as projective drawings, Rorschach protocols, and the like have the advantage of providing something of an objective basis for arriving at conclusions in regard to psychological issues. This can sometimes be rather dramatic, as in the case of a bizarre drawing by a floridly psychotic individual that speaks volumes without any additional clinical interpretation. On the other hand, there are disadvantages as well. The very structure of projective techniques makes it exceedingly difficult to evaluate them in terms of traditional psychometric characteristics such as internal consistency, stability, and validity. Even though they may yield valid results that are relevant to the legal issue before the court, the subjective element in interpreting them and the absence of solid psychometric data supporting them make them vulnerable to attack under the right type of cross-examination.

The most promising assessment techniques to provide a solid basis for psychological expert testimony regarding diagnosed mental disorders have clearly been self-report clinical personality inventories. In contrast to, say, the Rorschach, in which pathological characteristics of individuals are inferred from their responses to unstructured inkblots, the conclusions of self-report clinical inventories rest on the statements that test subjects endorse about themselves. The true–false (or in some cases Likert) format of this type of inventory lends itself to psychometric analysis yielding evidence of the internal consistency of the instrument's scales, stability of the results over time, and validity against external criteria.

In spite of the decided psychometric advantages of self-report clinical personality inventories, there is still a major pitfall associated with the use of many of these instruments in forensic work. It is fairly commonly accepted that just about every forensic psychological evaluation should include a *Diagnostic and Statistical Manual of Mental Disorders*, fourth edition, text revision (DSM-IV-TR; American Psychiatric Association, 2000) diagnosis, or a statement that the subject does not qualify for any such diagnosis. The nexus between the findings of psychometric measures and the formulation of a particular diagnosis for the client is not always clear. Scales for some commonly used psychometric measures are derived through lexical analysis, or in some cases reflect archaic diagnostic labels such as "psychaesthenia." Thus, while the results of psychometric testing may indicate that the individual scores high on characteristics such as aggressiveness, mistrust of others, or neuroticism, there is little in these findings to provide a direct basis for assigning a specific DSM-IV-TR diagnosis. Even in the case of an instrument that yields a score high in "depression," there may be little in the record to help the clinician differentiate among DSM-IV diagnoses such as Dysthymia, Major Depressive Episode, Adjustment Disorder with Depressed Mood, or simply a pessimistic and helpless outlook on life that is more characteristic of a personality disorder than an Axis I condition.

It is here is that the Millon Clinical Multiaxial Inventory–III (MCMI-III) provides a solid, reliable, well-documented psychometric footing for the formulation of a DSM-IV-TR diagnosis. The very structure of the MCMI-III is closely aligned to the diagnostic categories of the DSM-IV and DSM-IV-TR. This is no accident; Theodore Millon served on the committees that developed the personality disorders sections for both the DSM-III and DSM-IV. In fact, the diagnostic criteria for these sections of the manuals reflect Millon's theoretical concepts to a great extent. Thus, instead of the more usual trait scales found in many clinical instruments, the MCMI-III comprises scales that assess the actual diagnostic constructs contained in the DSM-IV(-TR). The validity evidence for the MCMI-III (discussed in greater detail below) indicates that when the instrument diagnoses someone as having a particular condition, then it is likely that the person is actually diagnosable as having that condition—whether it is traits or features of a personality disorder, the full-blown personality disorder itself, an Axis I clinical syndrome, or designation of that Axis I clinical syndrome as a prominent feature in the overall diagnostic picture. A detailed discussion of the advantages of classification efficiency statistics over the more traditional Pearson product–moment correlation coefficient for presentation of validity evidence in court is found in McCann and Dyer (1996).

This brings up an additional advantage of the MCMI-III over other commonly used clinical self-report personality inventories in forensic work. With many of the other inventories, the evaluator has to play something of a guessing game in regard to the question of what level of score elevation should trigger a particular diagnostic statement. It has been increasingly evident in the field of psychopathology research that the use of a single cutoff score, such as a T-score of 65, is a rather arbitrary procedure that ignores the differential frequencies of particular disorders in the population. In other words, a cutoff score that does not take into account baseline frequency of the disorder in the population is subject to error on the basis of this arbitrary cutoff score procedure alone. Millon (2006) points out that an inflexible cut score will overdiagnose conditions with a very low frequency in the population and underdiagnose conditions with a relatively high frequency in the population. Deviation from the prescribed uniform cutoff score involves something of a guessing game for the evaluator in deciding what alternative score should trigger the diagnosis.

The MCMI-III offers a solution for the forensic witness that removes the subjective element from this aspect of the diagnostic process as well. The formulation of scale scores on this instrument in terms of the base rate rather than the traditional T-score measuring the distance of the individual's raw score on a particular scale from the mean of raw scores of the standardization sample, confers quite an advantage. The proper interpretation of a BR score of 75, for example, is that it indicates the

point on the *raw score* scale at which evaluating or treating clinicians begin to diagnose clients as having particular personality traits, features, or disorders, or begin to
diagnose clients as having particular Axis I clinical syndromes. A BR score of 85 indicates the *raw score* point at which clinicians begin to diagnose their patients as having a full-blown Axis II personality disorder, or the point at which an Axis I clinical
syndrome occupies a prominent place in the overall diagnostic picture. Thus, when
cross-examined as to decision-making processes, experts who rely on the MCMI-III
or other Millon inventories can adduce psychometric evidence for the objectivity of
their use of the appropriate cutoff score, rather than having to search for justification
for their use of a particular *T*-score level. In this respect, the MCMI-III bears more of
a resemblance to a criterion-referenced test than to a normed test, because raw scores
are directly tied to an external criterion of clinical diagnosis.

Finally, the role of the forensic expert as a neutral and objective evaluator testifying on the basis of the accumulated knowledge of a scientific discipline, rather than
individual experience, training, and authority, is further supported by the fact that
the MCMI-III was not developed in a theoretical vacuum. In virtually every single
training publication and workshop on the use of the Millon inventories since the
inception of this series of tests, it has been stressed that they are grounded in a fully
elaborated theory of psychopathology. In addition, the introductory workshops on
the inventories stress that practitioners need to familiarize themselves with Millon's
basic concepts of the polarities of human experience, existential aims, and replication
strategies, as well as the functional and structural domains of personality. Millon's
theory includes the functional domains of expressive behaviors, interpersonal conduct, cognitive style, and intrapsychic regulatory mechanisms. The theory also
includes the structural domains of self-image and object representations, morphological organization, and (at the biophysical level) mood/temperament. As will be discussed in the section on individual cases below, the analysis of each of these domains
in light of specific personality disorders that may be diagnosed from the MCMI-III
sheds light on numerous specific characteristics of the type that are frequently issues
in various forensic psychological contexts. Thus the inferences that the expert draws
from test results receive the support of an objective theory—one that incorporates
well-accepted concepts from the behavioral, dynamic, and neurological streams of
psychological research. Furthermore, there are often clear and reasonably well-
supported linkages between a subject's diagnosed personality disorder(s) and specific
behavioral tendencies, cognitive processes, aspects of personality organization, and
social competencies, based on Millon's clinical theory. These linkages frequently
prove useful in answering even the most narrowly focused referral questions that one
encounters in forensic work.

Case Studies

Mental State at Time of Offense

In criminal law, certain crimes as such as the offense of murder are defined by two
elements. The first is the criminal act itself, or *actus reus*, which is solely behavioral.
The second element is the criminal mental state, or *mens rea*, which refers to an attitude of mind associated with the severity of the offense. For example, in many juris-

dictions the offense of murder requires a knowing and purposeful mental state. In other words, in order to be convicted of that particular offense, the defendant must be shown to have had an awareness that his or her behavior toward the victim had a high probability of causing that individual's death. This constitutes the "knowing" aspect of the requisite mental state. Furthermore, it must be shown that the individual had a specific criminal intent to cause the death of the victim. This is the "purposeful" element of the mental state required for the offense of murder.

The U.S. judicial system treats those with certain classes of mental problems differently from typical defendants in regard to punishment for certain severe criminal offenses. For example, the judicial system recognizes that someone who is in an acute psychotic episode and is completely divorced from reality is incapable, by virtue of that pathological mental condition, of formulating the requisite mental state for a serious offense such as murder. There are other mental disorders that, while falling short of a complete psychotic break with reality, nevertheless reduce the criminal culpability of the defendant to a level below the offense of murder, because these disorders are also deemed to render the individual incapable of formulating the requisite mental state.

The most highly publicized mental health defense is the insanity defense. There are a number of definitions of legal insanity. The most conservative of these, the *M'Naghten* standard, requires that defendants, by virtue of mental disease or defect, suffer a degree of impairment such that they are unaware of the nature or quality of the acts that they are committing, and also unaware of the wrongfulness of the acts. Other definitions of legal insanity discuss "irresistible impulse" and other factors (Parry & Drogin, 2000).

Very few defendants qualify for the insanity defense, and it is successful in only a small fraction of cases. Much more common is the situation in which an individual accused of murder pleads "diminished capacity." In other words, the defendant claims that by virtue of some mental disorder he or she had a diminished capacity at the time of the offense to formulate the requisite mental state. It is argued that either (1) the defendant's judgment was so clouded that he or she did not fully grasp that the actions were highly likely to result in the death of the victim, or (2) the defendant was rendered incapable of formulating a specific criminal intent to cause the victim's death. A New Jersey Supreme Court case, *State v. Galloway* (1993), provides guidance as to the types of disorders that qualify for diminished capacity. In this case, the defendant, Galloway, physically assaulted his girlfriend's child, causing the infant's death. The New Jersey Supreme Court ruled that the defendant's borderline personality disorder should be considered as a mental disorder as defined in the law, and therefore should qualify as a pathological condition that rendered the defendant incapable of formulating the requisite mental state for the crime of murder.

One such case in which the presence of traits of a personality disorder was cited to support the legal defense of diminished capacity to commit the offense of murder was that of Herman. Herman was a normally intelligent but socially unsophisticated 22-year-old man who had relocated to a northern industrialized state from his native Midwest, where he was brought up in a rural environment. Landing in a midsize town almost at random, Herman secured employment as a day laborer, and had started to form superficial friendships with others on his work crews shortly before the time of the offense for which he was indicted. Herman had gone out drinking at various bars with a couple of these friends, and eventually found himself alone in an unfamiliar part of town in the early hours of the morning after he and his friends became separated. Herman was already mildly intoxicated and was feeling a bit disoriented; therefore, he accepted the offer of a ride from an individual who happened to be driving by.

According to Herman's statement to the police, the man who picked him up, George, drove to a location where there were some individuals on the street selling drugs, and bought cocaine. He then drove Herman back to his apartment, which was in a section of town that Herman was completely unfamiliar with. After they used cocaine together, George proceeded to fellate Herman. Although Herman had not had any previous homosexual experiences, he allowed George to perform the act on him and found it pleasurable. After they used cocaine a second time, George disrobed and asked Herman to penetrate him anally. Again Herman complied, and found the experience pleasurable. A short time later, George announced that he was going to penetrate Herman anally, and began to approach him. Herman related to the police that he "blanked out" at that point, and only recalled grabbing George around the throat. He related that George struggled and then became limp. Actually, there had been a noisy scuffle as George resisted being strangled. Herman placed George on the bed and covered him up. He was about to leave the apartment when he encountered the police, summoned by a neighbor who had heard what sounded like a fight going on.

The police determined that the George was still breathing, and called the emergency medical technicians, who transported him to a hospital. Herman actually thanked the police for coming, and stated that he and George had gotten into a fight earlier in the evening. The police arrested Herman for aggravated assault; the charge was upgraded to murder when George expired at the hospital later that evening.

The task before the forensic expert was to make sense out of the events of that evening, in which an unsophisticated individual with no criminal record whatsoever wound up causing the death of a man who had been a stranger to him only a few hours previously. Furthermore, the death was caused in a manner that was suggestive of raw, primitive rage—namely, strangulation. The central psycholegal question was that of mental state at the time of the offense. Was there any pathological condition in Herman's background that would have negated his ability to formulate the requisite knowing and purposeful mental state for the offense of murder in such circumstances? In this regard, it was noted that Herman had not had any previous history of mental health treatment, or even a referral to any type of mental health facility. The collateral sources interviewed by his attorneys all described Herman as a well-adjusted individual who had never shown any propensity toward violence.

Herman's MCMI-III record (see Figure 9.1) showed the classic defensive pattern of an elevation on Desirability and relatively low scores on Disclosure and Debasement. This was actually a helpful finding for the defendant, as the demand characteristics of the situation were such that it might have seemed advantageous to Herman to exaggerate pathology in order to appear too impaired to be guilty of murder. There was an elevation on Anxiety, which may have been completely explainable on the basis of Herman's incarceration on a serious criminal charge; no other Axis I scales were elevated. There was an elevation on the Schizoid scale and an elevation on the Dependent scale in the Clinical Personality Patterns section of the test record. No elevations appeared in the Severe Personality Pathology section of the record, which includes the Schizotypal, Paranoid, and Borderline scales.

The examiner reconstructed the homicide in the following manner. Herman came from a rural culture dominated by fundamentalist Christian beliefs that regarded homosexuality as an abomination. It appeared that any prior homosexual proclivities that Herman might have had were subjected to rigid repression. On the evening of the offense, being disinhibited by the effects of the alcohol and cocaine that he consumed, Herman did allow himself to engage in homosexual acts that he was able to rationalize as providing a substitute for a woman. Specifically, he was able to allow the victim to fellate him and to penetrate the victim anally by

MILLON CLINICAL MULTIAXIAL INVENTORY - III
CONFIDENTIAL INFORMATION FOR PROFESSIONAL USE ONLY

Valid Profile

ID NUMBER: 1109

PERSONALITY CODE: - ** 3 1 * 5 8B 2B + 2A 7 4 6A 6B " 8A ' ' // - ** - * //

SYNDROME CODE: - ** A * // -**-* //

DEMOGRAPHIC: 1109

CATEGORY		SCORE		PROFILE OF SR SCORES				DIAGNOSTIC SCALES
		RAW	BR 0	60	75	85	115	
MODIFYING INDICES	X	94	60					DISCLOSURE
	Y	17	80					DESIRABILITY
	Z	5	49					DEBASEMENT
CLINICAL PERSONALITY PATTERNS	1	11	77					SCHIZOID
	2A	5	59					AVOIDANT
	2B	4	63					DEPRESSIVE
	3	11	80					DEPENDENT
	4	17	52					HISTRIONIC
	5	17	71					NARCISSISTIC
	6A	6	45					ANTISOCIAL
	6B	5	43					SADISTIC
	7	17	53					COMPULSIVE
	8A	3	22					NEGATIVISTIC
	8B	4	67					MASOCHISTIC
SEVERE PERSONALITY PATHOLOGY	S	7	66					SCHIZOTYPAL
	C	2	19					BORDERLINE
	P	8	64					PARANOID
CLINICAL SYNDROMES	A	6	80					ANXIETY
	H	1	30					SOMATOFORM
	N	6	62					BIPOLAR: MANIC
	D	0	0					DYSTHYMIA
	B	4	60					ALCOHOL DEPENDENCE
	T	3	45					DRUG DEPENDENCE
	R	2	30					POST-TRAUMATIC STRESS
SEVERE CLINICAL SYNDROMES	SS	2	30					THOUGHT DISORDER
	CC	4	61					MAJOR DEPRESSION
	PP	3	63					DELUSIONAL DISORDER

FIGURE 9.1. MCMI-III Profile Report for Herman.

regarding these acts as amounting to his turning George into a woman and satisfying himself that way in the absence of an available female.

It was at the point when George announced that he was now going to penetrate Herman anally and began to approach him that Herman was evidently affected by extremely powerful, emotionally loaded material of which he had not had much conscious awareness. George was considerably older than Herman and not in very good physical condition, in contrast to Herman, who was rather athletic and muscular. Thus the victim did not present any physical threat. It was the examiner's view that the dynamic that aroused such primitive physical aggression in Herman was the result of internal psychic turmoil, rather than a realistically self-protective reaction to any external threat. Herman simultaneously experienced a revulsion at the victim's attempts to make him into the woman by approaching him for that sexual act, and at the same time the passive component of his homosexuality seemed to have been mobilized. It was felt that the pressure of this rigidly repressed passive homosexual component was what precipitated the aggressive physical assault on George.

In terms of mental state at the time of the offense, the MCMI-III record provides a good deal of useful information. The elevation on the Schizoid scale provides insight into the subject's cognitive processes. With reference to the characteristics of the cognitive domain associated with schizoid personality disorder in Millon's theoretical system, we find that the cognitive processes of an individual with this disorder can be characterized as vague and obscure. This type of thinking, combined with the disinhibition associated with cocaine and alcohol abuse that evening, impaired Herman to such an extent that he was unable to formulate a rational approach to the dilemma that confronted him. Rather than an intentional, well-thought-out assault on the victim that had the express purpose of causing his death, Herman's behavior was more reflective of a lashing out in response to homosexual panic. It was a blind, aggressive physical discharge fueled by the arousal of rigidly repressed passive homosexual impulses.

One could well ask, given this explanation, why Herman, who appeared to have some physical advantage over the victim, did not simply adopt a more assertive strategy to resolve the situation. Indeed, Herman could have spoken sharply to George (warning him not to approach any further and stating flatly that he was not interested in that type of homosexual activity), or could even have reacted physically in a manner short of strangling the victim if verbal warnings proved insufficient. The elevation on the Dependent scale in Herman's MCMI-III record provides insight here as well. In terms of the expressive behaviors domain, Herman's capacity for autonomy was deficient. By virtue of this disorder, he would not be expected to be able to muster a degree of responsible self-assertiveness to resolve this type of emotionally loaded situation. Again, it is stressed that this behavior was highly unusual for Herman, who had never before been involved in any type of physical altercation that required the intervention of law enforcement. It seemed that the instant situation offered the "perfect storm" of disinhibition due to substance abuse, mildly eccentric thinking processes impairing capacity for rationality, and mobilization of extremely powerful and threatening repressed sexual impulses in an individual with a deficient capacity to stand his ground convincingly.

The examiner's reconstruction of Herman's mental state at the time at the time of the offense and the associated dynamics was greatly facilitated by the information that Herman's MCMI-III record yielded, in spite of his defensive response set. In terms of the three types of expert knowledge cited in the Federal Rules of Evidence (scientific, technical, and other specialized knowledge), this type of application of the MCMI-III involves both scientific and other specialized knowledge. In this respect, it does not differ from most psychological testimony, which relies on a social science basis; however, it also requires clinical judgment and reasoning in the application of scientific findings to a rather restricted set of circumstances that are much too narrow and fact-specific to be addressed through any type of empirical research.

Risk Assessment in Child Protective Services Consultation

One of the most stressful activities for forensic evaluators is that of risk assessment. It is particularly so in the field of child protective services work, where a wrong decision to return a child to a dysfunctional birth parent may have fatal consequences. Although the use of structured risk assessment instruments is now routine in many jurisdictions, child protective services and family courts often rely on psychologists to provide opinions about risk to a child in situations where a parent has filed a motion for a return of custody.

The case of Crystal presented something of an unusual set of circumstances with respect to pressure to return a child currently in placement. Crystal's father was a prominent matrimonial attorney with a reputation for providing extremely zealous representation for his clients. When Crystal's daughter, Tracy—his granddaughter—was removed from Crystal's custody, he very actively involved himself in the case. The first family court judge assigned to the matter had to recuse herself because Crystal's father frequently appeared before her in matrimonial manners.

Crystal, now 25 years old, had been a special education student because of emotional and behavioral problems. Although her local school district had decided to provide services to her in a special class housed in the town high school, her father filed suit and forced the district to fund Crystal's special education at a private school 45 minutes out of town. Crystal apparently profited a great deal from this school's educational program, as she was reasonably well adjusted at the time of her high school graduation; she went on to live independently, with some parental assistance, while working at a local retail establishment. The severe temper problems that had resulted in her classification for special education, and had included physical assaults on some of her classmates in school, had disappeared entirely.

Crystal's life adjustment took a downward turn when she became romantically involved with an individual who both used and sold drugs. Shortly after she gave birth to Tracy, who was fathered by that individual, Crystal ended her relationship with him. From that point onward, she expended a great deal of time, effort, and energy in attempting to collect child support payments from Tracy's birth father, whom she repeatedly had jailed for nonsupport.

The state child protective services became involved with Crystal because of an incident in which, while visiting a new boyfriend, Crystal left 5-year-old Tracy with the boyfriend's housemates, who were supposed to watch her. The police found Tracy wandering the streets at 3:00 in the morning looking for her mother. When the child protective services worker made contact with Crystal, Crystal minimized the incident—stressing that Tracy had been found only a few doors away from the boyfriend's house, and repeating that she had left the child with her boyfriend's housemates, who were supposed to have been caring for her. Crystal also stated that this was not the first time Tracy had wandered out of the house, and added that the child would do this frequently. She seemed to be attempting to convey to the child protective services worker that the present incident was nothing unusual that warranted concern, because the child's wandering away was merely a routine occurrence. She also seemed to be conveying that the incident had not placed Tracy in any danger because she was found only a few doors away, and that it was not Crystal's fault anyway because she had left the child with unspecified individuals who were supposed (by Crystal) to take care of her. Tracy was placed with the maternal grandparents, who then pressured the agency to return the child to Crystal.

During the clinical interview that formed part of the examination in which she was administered the MCMI-III, Crystal related that she had become extremely angry with the child protective services worker, who had accused her of lying. Crystal stated that on another occasion, she came close to actually slapping the caseworker when she was told that she (Crystal) did not really have to be present at a court hearing that she had gone out of her way to attend. Crystal also reported a history of having been arrested for assaulting a police officer, although she minimized the significance of that incident and insisted that the assault charge had been dismissed. Crystal also related that she had been in therapy after the incident with the police officer, but that she had left treatment after a "very nasty dispute" with her therapist. When questioned further about the nature of the therapy, Crystal admitted that she had become suicidal in her late teens, and that her parents had sent her for treatment because they were concerned about the possibility of self-harming behavior. Crystal denied any problematic consumption of alcohol or any use of illicit drugs. There were no allegations regarding drug or alcohol abuse anywhere in the case history. The examiner regarded Crystal's statement about having come close to striking the child protective services worker as having considerable significance, in light of the demand characteristics of the evaluation, in which subjects usually attempt to put their "best foot forward" and impress the examiner as being fit candidates for custody of the child in placement.

Crystal's MCMI-III record contained an elevation on the Desirability scale and suppressions of the Disclosure and Debasement scales, suggesting that at least in the area of psychometric testing Crystal did attempt some positive impression management. The Clinical Personality Patterns section of the record, however, was notable for elevations on Schizoid, Narcissistic, and Antisocial. No Axis I conditions were indicated in the record.

It was the examiner's impression that the MCMI-III results were consistent with Crystal's behavioral presentation during the interview. She impressed the examiner as a volatile young woman with extremely little insight into the impact of her behavior upon others. She was entirely preoccupied with her own social and romantic needs, to the exclusion of an investment of any depth in the needs of her child. Crystal's statement that Tracy had wandered away from the house on quite a few occasions—coupled with her minimizing the incident by stating that the child was found only a few doors away from the house, and her projection of blame and responsibility for the child's disappearance onto the unspecified housemates of her boyfriend—provided further evidence of her narcissistic self-involvement and lack of commitment to the child's safety and welfare.

Other aspects of this young woman's personality organization complicating the clinical picture included an inner emotional blunting and detachment (as reflected in the elevation on the Schizoid scale), as well as a tendency to be irresponsible, exploitive, and contemptuous of rules and laws (as reflected in the elevation on the Antisocial scale). Consistent with the case history and interview impressions of Crystal, it was the examiner's opinion that the MCMI-III results indicated problems in adaptive ego functioning. That is, Crystal lacked certain fundamental competencies that assist most people in meeting the challenges of daily living. These include a fundamental awareness of the needs of other people (and perhaps even the basic reality of other people), an ability to follow rules and to obey the law, and the capacity to connect in a meaningful way with other people and to experience modulated emotions. Evidently Crystal, by virtue of her inner emotional blunting, did not have much of a reaction to anything unless she felt thwarted, criticized, or threatened in some manner, in which case the only type of emotional responsiveness of which she was capable was an explosive one.

The examiner commented that this was a young woman who would have a rather difficult time in simply managing her own affairs without getting into trouble or becoming embroiled in very severe interpersonal conflicts. She was clearly very poorly equipped to provide the kind of consistent structure, nurturance, physical protection, vigilant supervision, and stimulation that a young child would require. The report outlined a program of therapy that represented the optimal plan for attempting to rehabilitate Crystal so that she might achieve adequate parenting capacity, although the accompanying prognosis was listed as guarded. The report concluded with a strong recommendation that Tracy remain in placement with the grandparents until such time as Crystal might demonstrate substantive and lasting progress in overcoming her emotional and behavioral problems.

Crystal's MCMI-III record is a striking example of the failure of the subject's attempts at impression management. Even though Crystal displayed the typical positive impression management configuration on the Modifying Indices, she nevertheless registered elevations on certain scales indicating a great deal of severe psychopathology. This phenomenon was attributable to Crystal's lack of insight into the impact of her statements on others, as well as the ego-syntonic nature of her problems, which were not experienced as distressing symptoms, but merely as a natural part of the self.

Risk Assessment in Evaluations for Professional Boards

The work of forensic psychologists is not confined to the courtroom, but also extends to quasi-judicial entities such as professional boards. Typically, professional boards have all three functions of government—executive, legislative, and judicial—incorporated into their sphere of responsibility. They perform the executive function of enforcing regulations of practice. They are also frequently responsible for revising and adapting existing regulations, which they then vote to adopt, thus exercising a legislative function. Finally, they are empowered to sit as judicial bodies to hear cases of licensees whose competence to practice has been called into question, and to resolve complaints by consumers of professional services.

Forensic psychologists are frequently engaged by professional boards to evaluate licensees and candidates for licensure about whom there are questions regarding mental health and fitness to practice. They also sometimes testify before such boards sitting as judicial bodies, or before an administrative law judge in cases where the matters cannot be resolved by consent orders between the licensees and the boards.

The case of Kirby illustrates how MCMI-III findings can be useful in addressing questions of risk to the public if a dysfunctional professional is allowed to continue in practice. Typically, the referral question posed by a board's counsel is not an either–or proposition, but involves a request for recommendations regarding any restrictions of the individual's license or scope of practice that the examiner may feel are warranted.

Kirby was a 39-year-old registered pharmacist who had been arrested for child endangerment as a result of his 8-year-old daughter's disclosure to her therapist that he had sexually fondled her when she was 4 and 5 years old during weekend visits. (Kirby was a divorced, noncustodial father.) Kirby's response to his daughter's disclosure of the sexual abuse and his arrest was to volunteer a full statement of the events leading up to the repeated incidents of molestation, and to enter voluntarily into individual psychotherapy with a practitioner specializing in the treatment of sex offenders. In addition, Kirby voluntarily sought out a self-help support group for individuals who had committed acts of child sexual abuse, and met with that group on a weekly basis.

Kirby's ex-wife was actually supportive of his efforts to reform himself, and she did not insist that he bear the full weight of the legal punishments to which he was exposed. She spoke positively about him to the prosecutor, and stressed the fact that no molestation of the child had occurred from age 5 years until the daughter disclosed the previous abuse at age 8 years. The ex-wife's support, coupled with Kirby's admission of the offense and his voluntarily seeking appropriate treatment, enabled him to secure a plea bargain under which he would not be incarcerated or sent for any type of inpatient sex offender treatment, but would become a registered sex offender on the lowest tier of risk under the state's registry law, which only required yearly reporting to a local police station to submit his current address. The concern of the licensing board's members was whether they were dealing with a compulsive and repetitive offender who would become sexually aroused by children entering his place of business. The board wanted an opinion as to whether Kirby was likely to engage in "grooming" behavior toward the children themselves, or gain the trust of adults who accompanied them and then manipulate the situation so that he could be alone with children in a private area of the establishment and molest them.

Kirby presented at the time of his evaluation as an anxious, passive, inadequate individual who appeared to have a rather impoverished inner mental life. He described the sexual molestation of his daughter between the ages of 4 and 5 in terms suggesting that he was lonely and depressed as a result of the divorce, and that he had turned to his preschool child as a source of physical contact comfort to gratify infantile emotional needs. He also described a scene that had followed the last incident in which he fondled the child: He had apologized to her, telling her that it was wrong for daddies to touch their children in that way, and expressing concern that it would affect her in the future. It was of interest that although the 5-year-old victim did not really comprehend at the time what her father was trying to communicate to her, she remembered that conversation very well, and this formed a part of her disclosure to her therapist.

Another noteworthy theme that emerged in Kirby's clinical interview was his extreme enmeshment with his family of origin. His parents had been heavily involved with all aspects of his academic and social life when he was a student, even into the college years. There were also a number of family members working in his pharmacy business and associated side businesses, with whom he had contact on a daily basis. Finally, his ex-wife's family was also in the pharmacy business, and Kirby's parents had seen a great deal of the ex-wife's parents socially since Kirby was a child, with the children visiting back and forth as well.

Kirby's MCMI-III record was quite sparse, reflecting the inner barrenness of his emotional life that had been apparent during the clinical interview. In contrast to the "right-pointing arrow" pattern on the Modifying Indices (scale X depressed, scale Y elevated, scale Z depressed), often seen in forensic evaluations where the demand characteristics call for positive impression management, Kirby's scores on these scales were uniformly depressed. There were no elevations on any of the Clinical Syndrome or Severe Personality Pathology Scales. The only elevation seen on the Clinical Personality Patterns portion of the record was on the Schizoid scale.

The MCMI-III results served as an adjunct to other data sources in formulating opinions about the risk concerns cited by the Board of Pharmacy. In this particular case, the behavioral predictors were given the most weight, consistent with current thinking in regard to risk assessment in sexual offenders (Quinsey, Harris, Rice, & Cormier, 1998). Among the sex offender population, Kirby was extremely unusual in that he did not exhibit any denial whatsoever when confronted with his daughter's disclosure of the abuse. Another unusual factor in this case was that he immediately entered therapy on a voluntary basis, prior to any such recommendation by his attorney. His apology to the victim, while representing a curious reversal of parent–child roles (with the parent seeking forgiveness from the child for misbehavior), did indicate that Kirby was aware of the potential effects of the sexual abuse on his daughter. Furthermore, he evidently possessed sufficient ego resources to cease the behavior on his own. Other significant behavioral predictors associated with the case included abuse restricted to a single victim (there was nothing to suggest that Kirby had ever been interested sexually in any other child, let alone acted on it), absence of grooming behavior, and opportunistic nature of the offense (actor alone with victim during court-ordered weekend visits). Finally, the incestuous dimension appears to have held particular significance for Kirby, who came from a pathologically enmeshed family and who did not even venture very far outside the family for a spouse. The parent–child role reversal also appeared to have been an important part of the offense. Thus the behavioral picture of this offender was not one of a predator who sought out young children to molest, but rather that of a father inappropriately seeking nurturance and sexualized comforting from his preschool daughter when he was alone with the child.

The MCMI-III provides ancillary information to round out the assessment. Kirby's elevation on the Schizoid scale was consistent with the behavioral impression of him as having an impoverished emotional life. According to Millon's theory, in schizoid personality disorder, the morphological organization domain is characterized by an inner barrenness and a feeble drive to fulfill needs. The interpersonal conduct domain is characterized by a lack of engagement with others and a general lack of social competence. This picture contrasts sharply with the kind of socially adept, engaging predator who cons parents into trusting him with a young child, only to betray that trust by molesting dozens of victims in the service of a powerful compulsion to achieve erotic gratification with a physically immature sexual object (see, e.g., Salter, 1997). In regard to the specific referral question posed by the Board of Pharmacy, it was recommended that Kirby be permitted to continue in practice as a registered pharmacist without any restrictions on his scope of practice or any supervision requirement, but with the condition that he continue in his current self-help group and in his current individual psychotherapy, with mandatory quarterly reporting by the therapist regarding progress in treatment and any risk factors that might become apparent. The convergence of behavioral predictors and the MCMI-III findings in this case reinforced the validity of the bottom-line opinion about the possibility of risk to the public.

Cross-Examination Traps and Counters in Forensic Use of the MCMI-III

The MCMI-III, more than any other instrument (with the possible exception of the Minnesota Multiphasic Personality Inventory), has been the subject of criticism as to its use in court-related psychological evaluations. Much of the criticism appearing in the technical and professional literature is a product of flawed logic and misinformation. Nevertheless, in the courtroom, where the only information in that the trier of fact receives is through testimony or items admitted into evidence, it is important for psychological experts to be aware of some of the current controversies surrounding the forensic use of the test and to have ready answers when challenged on these issues by opposing counsel.

One widely disseminated piece of misinformation about the MCMI-III, which has actually assumed something of a mythic status by now, is the curiously anthropomorphic assertion that the test "assumes that you have a disorder and then goes about determining which disorder you have." Although this argument is grist for the rumor mill of Internet sites discussing forensic psychology, it also appears in some of the professional literature as well (Brodie, 2003; Butcher & Miller, 1999; Hess, 1998). This criticism of the MCMI-III is based on the fact that the test was standardized on a clinical sample rather than on a community sample.

The argument for the MCMI-III's "assumption" that all test subjects have a disorder is this: Standardization of the test on a clinical sample automatically means that examinees are being compared inappropriately to clinically disturbed individuals, where in fact the appropriate comparison group should be psychologically "normal" subjects. The conclusion of this argument is that the use of a clinical standardization group results in a tendency to overpathologize nondisturbed subjects (i.e., to classify as pathological those individuals who are actually free of pathology, simply because they are being compared to the wrong group).

When confronted with this argument on cross-examination, the expert witness only needs to make two points. In the first place, anybody with even a rudimentary knowledge of psychometrics will instantly realize that normative comparison of a nondisturbed person with a pathological group will simply make that person appear *more* "normal" than he or she actually is. In other words, if one is comparing a test subject to a pathological group and the test subject scores at the mean for the pathological group, and if one assumes that the test validly measures the construct, then this means that the individual is as pathological as the comparison group. If the test subject is actually nonpathological, then instead of having an average score (as would be the case if a community sample had been used as the standardization group), the nondisturbed individual will have an extremely *low* score against a pathological standardization sample.

The second response to this argument is that it treats the scores of the MCMI-III and other Millon inventories as though they were *T*-scores. That is to say, it treats the scores as if they represent comparisons of the individual's test scores with the means of test scores for the standardization sample. As described earlier, the Millon inventories do not use *T*-scores, but BR scores. The BR score format results in an instrument that is much closer in its concept to a criterion-referenced test than to a norm-referenced test. BR scores tie the individual's raw scores directly to the criterion diagnoses by the treating or examining clinicians who formulated diagnoses for each member of the standardization group. Thus, for each personality disorder, a BR score of 75 represents the raw score point at which clinicians begin to diagnose their clients as having traits or features of the target disorder, while a BR score of 85 represents the raw score point at which clinicians begin to diagnose their clients as having the full-blown disorder. For individuals who in fact do not display the pathology measured by a particular scale of the MCMI-III, it is extremely unlikely that they will respond in the keyed direction on scale items to amass enough raw score points to match the scores of standardization clients who are diagnosed with the target disorder or its traits and features.

This last proposition receives ample support in a study of child custody litigants conducted by McCann et al. (2001). The overpathologizing argument is one that appears very frequently in these types of cases, where the lawyer for each spouse tends to portray his or her client as a saint and to demonize the partner. Thus an expert witness who, on the basis of MCMI-III results, arrives at some clinical diagnosis for a child custody litigant is fair game for the overpathologizing argument. McCann et al. (2001) found that the mean elevation on MCMI-III scales for child custody litigants was extraordinarily low, with the exception of three scales: Histrionic, Narcissistic, and Compulsive. All three of these scales are well known as being affected at least in part by considerations of social desirability. Thus individuals who display the typical defensive response set of child custody litigants are likely to have elevations on some or all of those three scales purely as artifacts of their defensiveness. Clearly, there is no overpathologizing of "normal" individuals associated with the use of a clinical sample.

One further point: The MCMI-III does not contain any overall psychopathology scale; it measures individual Axis I and Axis II disorders. Thus, for each of the Clinical Syndrome, Clinical Personality Pattern, and Severe Personality Pathology Scales, subjects in the standardization group who did not in fact have the particular disorder could be considered "normal" with respect to that disorder. For example, someone who actually presented with obsessive–compulsive disorder would have been highly likely to register an elevation on the MCMI-III Compulsive scale, but would almost certainly not have done so on the Antisocial scale. Similarly, a standardization subject who presented with antisocial personality disorder would almost certainly not have shown an elevation on the Dependent scale. Most standardization subjects scored high on only a few of the instrument's scales, and were free of pathology with respect to the great majority of scales. When taken scale by scale, the MCMI-III effectively distinguishes "pathological" from "normal" subjects, as evidenced by the test's impressive operating characteristics.

One occasionally hears the sophisticated counterargument that individuals who present with any type of psychological disorder cannot truly be considered "normal" for standardization purposes, even with a scale-by-scale approach. To this argument, the expert using the MCMI-III might respond that even in a randomly selected community sample, "normality" is scarcely guaranteed. Fully one out of every five adults has some diagnosable DSM-IV-TR disorder; therefore, we might say that even the vaunted nonclinical community sample is fully 20% pathological.

Psychologist expert witnesses may be confronted on the stand with an article by Rogers, Salekin, and Sewell (1999) asserting that the MCMI-III should not be admitted as evidence under federal standards because of a purported lack of criterion-related validity. This issue has received extensive treatment in the forensic psychological literature (Dyer & McCann, 2000; Retzlaff, 2000). Briefly, the Rogers et al. (1999) piece criticized the test's empirical validity on the basis of results of the preliminary study using the item analysis sample that appeared in the first edition of the test manual; it ignored an updated validity study of the MCMI-III by Davis, Wenger, and Guzman (1997) demonstrating classification efficiency statistics as good as or better than those developed for the MCMI-II. The Davis et al. (1997) study employed a structured rating instrument as the clinical criterion, yielding a substantial enhancement of criterion reliability over the previous study's criterion of unaided clinical judgment. It therefore behooves experts who testify about MCMI-III results to acquaint themselves with the literature on the test's empirical validity, including the critiques and responses to those critiques. If unanswered by citations of literature supportive of the forensic use of the test, the Rogers et al. (1999) article, with its categorical rejection of all but the most limited forensic applications, can prove fatal to the credibility or even the admissibility of MCMI-III findings.

Grossman Facet Scales in Forensic Cases

The first major addition to the MCMI-III in terms of new report content is a series of subscales known as the Grossman Facet Scales. Introduced in 2006, these scales and their development are described in detail in the third edition of the test manual (Millon, 2006; see also Grossman, Chapter 6, this volume). Briefly, the Grossman Facet Scales are factorially derived subscales of the primary personality scales on the MCMI-III. They are intended to enable clinicians to engage in a finer-grained analysis of an individual's personality than is possible from a review of the BR scores on the Clinical Personality Patterns and Severe Personality Pathology Scales alone. The Facet Scales also represent a psychometrically more sophisticated method of analyzing the personality scales than the more usual method of simply eyeballing the individual scale items.

The Grossman Facet Scales are not automatically generated by the Q Local software for the MCMI-III. Users who wish this additional output are required to check a box on the screen immediately preceding the print screen. Checking the box results in an additional section of the report that lists the Facet Scale scores for the three personality scales with the highest scores. This is followed by a complete printout of the Facet Scale scores for each of the Clinical Personality Patterns and Severe Personality Pathology Scales.

The Facet Scale scores are derived from raw score frequency distributions for each of the target scales. Even though they are labeled as BR scores, they cannot be properly given this label, because they are not externally linked to any type of diagnostic frequency in the way that the main scales of the MCMI-III are connected. They are also framed in a different metric from the personality scale BR scores, in that the Facet Scale scores range between 0 and 99 rather than 0 and 115. This is because the Facet Scales have far fewer items than do the personality scales. At this writing, there have not been any empirical studies of the validity of the Facet Scales. There is also no listing in the MCMI-III manual of the correlations among the various Facet Scales. Thus, even though the content differs among the scales, and even though the individual scales represent the different constructs of Millon's evolutionary personality theory, depending on which constructs are felt to be salient for the specific personality disorder, there is no empirical evidence that the Facet Scales within each personality disorder are actually measuring characteristics that are fundamentally different from one another. On the positive side, the coefficient alpha values are impressively high, considering the limited number of items in these subscales.

Notwithstanding the unresolved question as to whether the Facet Scales are actually measuring weakly correlated constructs that are fundamentally different from one another or merely differ in terms of theoretical concept only and lack empirical separation, they do appear useful in formulating a nuanced understanding of test takers' behavioral and emotional response tendencies. From this perspective, they are potentially of great value in terms of clinical work, and can also inform opinions and recommendations in forensic cases.

There are two potential problems in using the Grossman Facet Scales as a direct basis for forensic testimony. The first problem is the absence of any sort of criterion-related validity. Although the advantages of this type of fine-grained analysis are clear to clinicians who are familiar with the underlying theoretical basis, as elaborated in many publications by Millon and various collaborators, the current climate in regard to expert testimony stresses empirical research as the basis for conclusions offered to a reasonable degree of professional certainty. Once the empirical data on the Facet Scales have become available, however, such findings could very effectively bolster the type of linkage among an individual's test responses, diagnosed disorder, and specific behavioral or structural characteristics elaborated in Millonian theory (as discussed above).

A second problem, which empirical research may not be able to address satisfactorily, resides in the tendency of scales that are so highly specific and so numerous to yield superficially or apparently contradictory results. For example, in a recent examination that I performed with the Facet Scales, the test subject registered an elevation on the Immature Representations subscale (Dependent) and an elevation on the Uncertain Self-Image subscale (Borderline). These two fairly consistent findings are jarringly at odds with the same subject's elevation on the Reliable Self-Image subscale (Compulsive). Based purely on the semantics of these subscales' titles, a skilled cross-examining attorney could portray the entire system of the Facet Scales as a jumble of self-contradictions, thus vitiating the impact of the witness's overall testimony about the MCMI-III personality findings. Although a thorough clinical analysis of the subject's personality organization may disclose dynamics that would resolve the apparent inconsistency in this record, forensic witnesses do not have the luxury of such analysis. Every trial or hearing is a learning situation in which a large set of complex facts is presented, with contradictory "spin" by each side, and finders of fact have only a limited time available to process all this information. Unfortunately, the apparent contradictions and inconsistencies tend to have the greatest staying power in the minds of judges and jurors, with the recollection of these potentially eclipsing the recollection of all the valid information offered by the witness.

Bearing in mind these two obstacles to effective forensic use of the Grossman Facet Scales, I suggest that practitioners review them as ancillary information, but that they not rely on them in formulating their conclusions in forensic cases.

Content Validity

Although it is generally considered as less important than criterion-related validity evidence for the usefulness of a psychometric measure, content validity occupies a special status in regard to the evaluation of scales such as the MCMI-III that are used extensively in forensic work. So frequently is the DSM-IV (American Psychiatric Association, 1994) cited in legal decisions that this document and its subsequent text revision, the DSM-IV-TR (American Psychiatric Association, 2000), have become the forensic standards for psychological diagnosis (McCann & Dyer, 1996). The MCMI-III was developed to reflect the specific diagnostic criteria of the DSM-IV, which required the replacement of half the content of its predecessor, the MCMI-II. Elsewhere (Dyer, 1997), I have noted that the MCMI-III is unique among self-report clinical personality inventories in its close links with the content of the DSM-IV.

Rogers et al. (1999) criticize the content validity of the MCMI-III, citing an absence of any controlled interrater studies of the similarity of personality disorder scale items to the corresponding DSM-IV(-TR) criteria. It is therefore not unlikely that at some point forensic experts who use the MCMI-III will be forced to respond to a cross-examination attack on the instrument's content validity based on this criticism. The question might be phrased thus: "Isn't it true, Doctor, that there is no statistical evidence for the content validity of the MCMI-III?" Elsewhere (Dyer, 2005), I have pointed out that the test manual contains a scale-by-scale comparison of relevant test items and DSM-IV(-TR) diagnostic criteria. The similarities are so striking that the content validity of the test against the DSM-IV(-TR) is entirely self-evident. Experts facing this sort of attack should be able to deflect it readily by pointing out these extremely close parallels. If one does this while equipped with a copy of the test manual to illustrate specifics, the effect will be enhanced.

In conclusion, the extensive validity support for the MCMI-III in the form of content validity evidence coupled with empirical research against criteria of clinical diagnosis—in conjunction with the clear connections between diagnosed disorders and specific cognitive, behavioral, and structural characteristics of the test subject provided by Millon's theory of personality—make this a uniquely useful instrument in forensic work.

References

American Psychiatric Association. (1994). *Diagnostic and statistical manual of mental disorders* (4th ed., text rev.). Washington, DC: Author.

American Psychiatric Association. (2000). *Diagnostic and statistical manual of mental disorders* (4th ed., text rev.). Washington, DC: Author.

Brodie, L. A. (2003). *Child custody: Issues and techniques—part I*. Retrieved from *www.e-edCredits.com/PsychCredits/article.asp?TestID=5*

Butcher, J. N., & Miller, K. B. (1999). Personality assessment in personal injury litigation. In A. K. Hess & I. B. Weiner (Eds.), *The handbook of forensic psychology* (2nd ed., pp. 104–126). New York: Wiley.

Davis, R., Wenger, A., & Guzman, A. (1997). Validation of the MCMI-III. In T. Millon (Ed.), *The Millon Inventories: Clinical and personality assessment* (pp. 327–359). New York: Guilford Press.

Dyer, F. J. (1997). Application of the Millon inventories in forensic psychology. In T. Millon (Ed.), *The Millon inventories: Clinical and personality assessment* (pp. 124–139). New York: Guilford Press.

Dyer, F. J. (2005). Forensic application of the MCMI-III in light of current controversies. In R. Craig (Ed.), *New directions in interpreting the Millon Clinical Multiaxial Inventory–III* (pp. 201–226). New York: Wiley.

Dyer, F. J., & McCann, J. T. (2000). The Millon inventories, research critical of their forensic application, and *Daubert* criteria. *Law and Human Behavior, 24,* 487–497.

Hess, A. K. (1998). Review of the Millon Clinical Multiaxial Inventory–III. In *Mental measurements yearbook*. Lincoln: University of Nebraska Press.

McCann, J. T., Campana, V., Flens, J., Campagna, V., Collman, P., Lazzaro, T., et al. (2001). The MCMI-III in child custody evaluations: A normative study. *Journal of Forensic Psychology Practice, 1,* 27–44.

McCann, J. T., & Dyer, F. J. (1996). *Forensic assessment with the Millon inventories*. New York: Guilford Press.

Millon, T. (with Millon, C., Davis, R. D., & Grossman, S. D.). (2006). *Millon Clinical Multiaxial Inventory–III (MCMI-III) manual* (3rd ed.). Minneapolis, MN: Pearson Assessments.

Parry, J., & Drogin, E. Y. (2000). *Criminal law handbook on psychiatric and psychological evidence and testimony*. Washington, DC: American Bar Association.

Quinsey, V. L., Harris, G. T., Rice, M. E., & Cormier, C. A. (1998). *Violent offenders: Appraising and managing risk*. Washington, DC: American Psychological Association.

Retzlaff, P. D. (2000). Comment on the validity of the MCMI-III. *Law and Human Behavior, 24,* 499–500.

Rogers, R., Salekin, R. T., & Sewell, K. W. (1999). Validation of the Millon Clinical Multiaxial Inventory for Axis II disorders: Does it meet the *Daubert* standard? *Law and Human Behavior, 23,* 425–443.

Salter, A. C. (1997). *Listening to sex offenders: Truth, lies and sex offenders*. Thousand Oaks, CA: Sage.

State v. Galloway, 133 N.J. 631, 628 A.2d 735 (1993).

CHAPTER 10

Using the MCMI in Correctional Settings

John W. Stoner

Personality and Corrections

At the most fundamental level, personality disorders represent the patterns of poor decisions made by individuals in their efforts to cope with the demands of life. The personality theory developed by Theodore Millon and his associates provides an excellent model of the chronic ways in which individuals can make poor decisions, and a theoretical structure for understanding why those particular patterns were developed. The criminal justice system in general, and the correctionals system in particular, represent the social response to individuals who make these unacceptably poor decisions in our culture. The very nature of the correctional industry is the management and (when successful) the alteration of these patterns of poor decision making.

Although the mental health programs associated with corrections have traditionally focused on the classical forms of mental illness, usually categorized on Axis I in the several *Diagnostic and Statistical Manuals of Mental Disorders* (DSMs) of the American Psychiatric Association, the reality is that only about 15% of the offenders entering state correctional systems have a major Axis I mental illness, while it is estimated that 75% have identifiable personality disorders. Even more crucial to the efforts of corrections, it is usually the personality disorders that produce the behaviors of interest to criminal justice, rather than the Axis I clinical syndromes.

In providing screening for mental health issues for corrections, it is therefore at least as important to identify the primary personality disorders in offenders as it is to identify the Axis I mental illnesses. This does not diminish the importance of identification, management, and treatment of those with Axis I syndromes within corrections. Rather, it provides a balance in understanding the critical role played by personality disorders. The personality disorder patterns are tied not only to the crimes for which offenders are incarcerated, but also to the problems they experience while incarcerated. Much of this chapter will look at the problems experienced by these individuals while incarcerated.

Offender and Officer Personalities

Although most efforts at dealing with the impact of personality on corrections focus on the personalities of the offenders as the primary issue, it is obvious for even the casual observer that the staff personalities also play a major role in the quality of interaction that occurs in a correctional setting. Even more important, it is the interaction between offender and officer personalities that guides many of the most troublesome management issues in corrections. Although administrators can write policies that fill volumes about humane conditions and treatment of offenders, it can only work when the line staff is able to accept the structure in which those values are created. It is easy, when putting characters on a page, to talk about human rights and dignity. It is quite something else to remember those values when feces and urine are running down the front of your uniform and you are being verbally abused by an offender.

Prison Personalities: A Three-Part Structure

In preparation for the extension of an officer training program to include material on personality, it was decided that any attempt to reflect the many personality types and characteristics would interest a few officers and glaze the eyes of many. Instead of the many forms and levels of personality functioning, these constructs were converted to a simpler three-part structure centered around components of primary concern to correctional officers. Specifically, the focus of this design was on the most typical types of responses that might be expected by an officer in interaction with an offender. The personality designations for the offender and the officer were converted into this three-part structure to permit easier review of interactions and problems.

Since interpersonally aggressive behavior is a particular problem for correctional settings, a number of the basic personality patterns were subsumed into the "aggressive" patterns. These included the sadistic, antisocial, negativistic, and narcissistic patterns. A second major group of personalities consists of those who are generally socially withdrawn and who will often lose the ability to function effectively when under conditions of moderate to strong stress. This group was identified as the "reserved" patterns and included the schizoid, avoidant, and depressive personality disorders. The third group was classified as the "compliant" patterns; these included the dependent, compulsive, masochistic (self-defeating), and histrionic personality disorders. (Note that the three "severe" personality disorders in Millon's theory of personality—the schizotypal, borderline, and paranoid personality disorders—were not included in this three-part structure. The reason for this is that these disorders

TABLE 10.1. Offender–Staff Personality Interactions

Staff personality patterns	Inmate personality patterns		
	Aggressive	Compliant	Reserved
Aggressive	1. Angry; challenge; aggression 2. Aggressive 3. Firm	1. Neutral 2. Dominate 3. Simple	1. Irritated 2. Dominate 3. Nurturant
Compliant	1. Guarded 2. Delay 3. Firm	1. Neutral 2. Simple 3. Simple	1. Nurturant 2. Nurturant 3. Nurturant
Reserved	1. Fearful; anxiety; stress; uncertainty 2. Withdrawal 3. Firm	1. Relieved 2. Nurturant 3. Simple	1. Anxious 2. Nurturant 3. Nurturant

Note. Key to numbers: 1. Typical emotions felt during encounter. 2. "Native" reaction or impulse. 3. Professional reaction.

represent not just chronic ways of making bad decisions, but more serious disabilities that require more sophisticated schemes for treatment and management. Because of their importance in correctional settings, however, they are discussed in a separate section later in this chapter.)

On the basis of this three-part classification structure, it has been possible to outline a number of areas in which the "natural" interactions of staff and offenders are likely to create problems. In addition, it has been possible to develop three alternative management patterns for staff members to utilize in adapting their behavior to the behavior of the offenders with whom they work. For convenience, these three patterns have been identified as the "simple," "nurturant,", and "firm" management styles. This has resulted in the interaction matrix shown in Table 10.1.

A basic assumption of this approach is that staff members will often have the greatest difficulty dealing with offenders whose personality patterns most closely resemble those of the staffers. If, for example, a staff member with a "forceful" (active, independent) personality is attempting to manage an offender with an "antisocial" (active, independent) personality, each will have as a personal goal the establishment of social dominance over the other. No one is likely to resist such efforts at dominance as much as another active, independent personality attempting to do the same thing. Another example can be found in an interaction between a "narcissistic" (passive, independent) offender and a "confident" (passive, independent) officer. The person least likely to recognize and acknowledge the fundamental wonderfulness of a narcissistic offender is an officer who has somewhat similar needs and drives.

The Colorado Study of the MCMI-III in Correctional Settings

In 1995, the Colorado Department of Corrections (CDOC), Theodore Millon, and National Computer Systems (the publisher of the Millon Clinical Multiaxial

Inventory–III [MCMI-III] at that time began a cooperative effort to assess the applicability of the test to screening a general correctional population. The initial results of that study were published in the June 2002 issue of the *International Journal of Offender Therapy and Comparative Criminology*. This paper (Retzlaff, Stoner, & Kleinsasser, 2002) presented the relationship of the screening scores obtained at the time of intake with subsequent correctional needs and behavior. This same data set is utilized here to describe in more detail the frequencies of various personality patterns and the relationship of those personalities to various correctional issues.

This data set was constructed by examining 10,804 consecutive admissions to the CDOC. As a part of the intake process, the MCMI-III was administered to these offenders. From this initial sample, 9,468 of the MCMI-III tests administered produced results that were "valid" profiles by the more stringent standards utilized in this study. These results were entered into the computer data system used by the CDOC. Relevant information obtained as a routine part of the correctional system's operations were then obtained on these 9,468 offenders and used to assess the utility of the MCMI-III as an intake screening instrument.

The most significant feature of the information obtained in this study is well demonstrated in Figure 10.1. The offenders sentenced to the CDOC (and this is probably true of all other correctional systems) had a wide range of personality patterns and were not limited to just antisocial personality disorder, the most popularly diagnosed pattern in this setting. They were not even limited to the "big three" of antisocial, histrionic, and narcissistic personality disorders. Certainly those diagnoses were well represented in this sample, but to limit the management and program design to just these patterns would result in less effective management for over half of

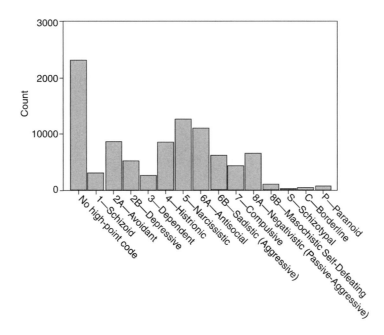

FIGURE 10.1. Frequency of highest-point personality code for each of the 14 MCMI-III personality scales in the Colorado sample.

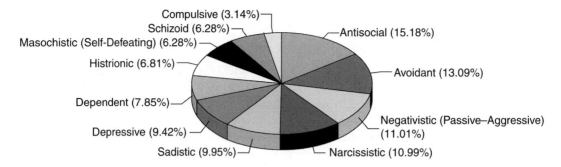

Compulsive (3.14%)
Schizoid (6.28%)
Masochistic (Self-Defeating) (6.28%)
Histrionic (6.81%)
Dependent (7.85%)
Depressive (9.42%)
Sadistic (9.95%)
Antisocial (15.18%)
Avoidant (13.09%)
Negativistic (Passive–Aggressive) (11.01%)
Narcissistic (10.99%)

FIGURE 10.2. Distribution of high-point codes for offenders with elevations on at least one MCMI-III personality scale.

all offenders. Figure 10.2 represents the distribution of MCMI-III high-point codes for offenders with elevated personality pattern scales. It clearly shows the significant impact of the "rest" of the personality patterns on the correctional system. In particular, note the number of offenders with avoidant, depressive, dependent, and schizoid personality patterns, which are characterized by fear and withdrawal from others. Traditional correctional practice usually leaves these offenders as the "prey" for the more predatory offenders. The remainder of this chapter examines the characteristic manifestations of the major personality disorders in a correctional setting.

Aggressive Personality Patterns

The personality types that have been grouped into the "aggressive" patterns include the three basic patterns with markedly "self-centered" components, antisocial, sadistic, and narcissistic. It also includes the negativistic pattern, which often responds aggressively to its ambivalence. These personality patterns are marked by an egocentrism that is one of their most powerful characteristics. Individuals with each will have little empathy for the impact of their behavior on others. Persons exhibiting two of these patterns, the antisocial and the sadistic, have adopted an active strategy for achieving their own needs. The fundamental difference between these two categories lies in the pleasure–pain dimension. The antisocial pattern is actively driven by a need to attain pleasure and is defective in pain avoidance learning. The sadistic pattern, on the other hand, is primarily motivated by pain avoidance. Although sadistic individuals do seem to acquire a perverse pleasure in inflicting pain on others, the underlying motivation seems to be in their own pain avoidance by inflicting overwhelming pain on others before it can be done to them. The third pattern found in this group is the narcissistic personality disorder, which involves a more passive strategy for meeting needs. This pattern focuses on an unrealistic sense of self-worth and specialness, and the assumption that all desires should have already been met. It is not proper or necessary for such individuals to pursue needs actively, since it is only through the interference or ignorance of others that such needs have been denied to begin with. The final pattern is the negativistic (passive–aggressive) personality, marked by an underlying resentment and burning anger toward others that often becomes aggressive when the opportunity presents itself.

Antisocial Personality Disorder

Antisocial personality disorder is certainly the most written about and discussed of the personality disorders. It has been described in literature for centuries. The modern formulations are usually attributed to Cleckley's book *The Mask of Sanity,* first published in 1941 and revised several times (see, e.g., Cleckley, 1976). Cleckley was the first to use the term "psychopathic personality," and "psychopathy" has become the term preferred by Hare (1993) and his associates.

The current label of "antisocial personality disorder" was created by the committee of the American Psychiatric Association in developing the modern DSMs. The process of moving from the more restrictive construct of psychopathy to the broader one of antisocial personality disorder has been well described by Millon and Everly (1985) and others.

Manifestations in a Correctional Population

In spite of the popular impression that most inmates in prison have antisocial personality disorder, there were only 2,759, or 29.14% of the 9,468 inmates in the Colorado sample, who had elevations above 75 on the Antisocial scale of the MCMI-III. Of these, only 1,151 had the Antisocial scale as their high-point scale. Although this is a large group of inmates, it also suggests that we must program our prisons for the management of many other personality types as well.

Of the 1,151 profiles where the Antisocial scale of the MCMI-III was the high-point scale, 35 (3.04%) were elevated on only the Antisocial scale (see Table 10.2). Such offenders will typically display the prototypal antisocial traits. In a correctional setting, the constant struggle for dominance over others will be one of the most noteworthy of these traits. These offenders will consistently challenge officers over issues of authority. They will also constantly challenge each other in vying for social position. Perhaps the most consistently observed behavior for these offenders is their high level of verbal banter. Although much of this will have an "edge" to it related to social dominance issues, it will often be overtly aggressive in nature. These same offenders will contribute regularly to the apparent chaos and disruption of facility operation. Most often, this will take the form of agitating other offenders just for the excitement it produces. "Door warriors," who challenge and threaten other offenders or officers through the doors of their cells, are common in this group. Millon (1999) describes such individuals as exhibiting the "covetous" subtype of antisocial personality: "[They will] feel intentionally denied and deprived; rapacious, begrudging, discontentedly yearning, envious, seek[ing] retribution, and avariciously greedy; pleasure more in taking than in having" (p. 479). They will tend to focus their energies on aggrandizement and will often resemble narcissistic individuals in this quality. The major differentiation between them is the amount of energy expended in forcing the world to recognize their wonderfulness or power. Whereas a truly narcissistic person has a presumption of worth and expectation that all others will recognize it, a

TABLE 10.2. Comorbid Personality Patterns for Antisocial High-Point Profiles

Anti only (6A)	6A + Schiz	6A + Avoid	6A + Depres	6A + Depend	6A + Histr	6A + Narcis	6A + Sadis	6A + Comp	6A + Neg
35	90	91	84	59	123	194	280	8	94
3.04%	7.82%	7.91%	7.30%	5.13%	10.69%	16.85%	24.33%	0.70%	8.17%

Note. Abbreviations in this and similar tables: Anti, Antisocial; Schiz, Schizoid; Avoid, Avoidant; Depres, Depressive; Depend, Dependent; Histr, Histrionic; Narcis, Narcissistic; Sadis, Sadistic; Comp, Compulsive; Neg, Negativistic (Passive–Aggressive).

covetous antisocial individual actively and aggressively pursues such acknowledgment. The other major difference will be in the emphasis on the material trappings of power and status rather than just acknowledgment.

As can be seen in Table 10.2, the most common comorbid pattern in the Colorado sample for profiles with the Antisocial scale as the high-point code was a secondary elevation on the Sadistic scale, which was found in 280 (24.33%) of the Antisocial high-point profiles. In Millon's (1999) subtypes, this pattern, in combination with an elevation on the paranoia scale of the MCMI-III, produces the "malevolent" antisocial subtype. Such persons will be seen as "belligerent, mordant, rancorous, vicious, malignant, brutal, resentful; anticipates betrayal and punishment; desires revenge; truculent, callous, fearless; guiltless" (Millon, 1999, p. 483). These individuals perceive constant attempts on the part of others to victimize them, and their coping style emphasizes preemptive "retaliation." This antisocial subtype is the one most often portrayed in movies and literature as a generally "nasty" individual. Whereas the prototypal antisocial personality will tend to focus on the status-enhancing components of a social interaction, the malevolent subtype will emphasize retribution and revenge.

The second most common of the comorbid patterns of profiles with the Antisocial scale as the high-point scale was a secondary elevation on the Narcissistic scale. This pattern was found in 194 (16.85%) of the Antisocial high-point codes. This pattern was identified by Millon as the "reputation-defending" subtype of antisocial personality. These individuals "need to be thought of as unflawed, unbreakable, invincible, indomitable, formidable, inviolable, intransigent when status is questioned, overreactive to slights" (Millon, 1999, p. 481). Such offenders will closely resemble those with the prototypal or *covetous* antisocial personality. They will be focused on the acknowledgment of their uniqueness, worth, or status, rather than on the material trappings that accompany such status. They will be more active than narcissistic individuals in their pursuit of this status, but similarly reactive to challenges or threats to this sense of worth.

The third common comorbid pattern with an Antisocial high-point scale was a virtual tie between a secondary elevation on the Schizoid scale and one on the Avoidant scale. This pattern has also been recognized by Millon, who labeled it the "nomadic" subtype of antisocial personality. With secondary elevations on either the Schizoid or the Avoidant scale, individuals tend to feel "jinxed, ill-fated, doomed, and cast aside; peripheral drifters; gypsylike roamers, vagrants, dropouts and misfits;

itinerant vagabonds, tramps, wanderers; impulsively not benign" (Millon, 1999, p. 481). They usually have a sense of victimization or rejection common to many antisocial persons, but rather than actively act out against those who impose such a deprivation, individuals with this subtype actively escape from the situation and wander on the periphery of society, taking opportunistic advantages as they occur. These offenders are more likely to be characterized by sudden, impulsive, aggressive reactions to a gradual buildup of pressures, and the noticeable event will be quite out of proportion to whatever event finally triggered the reaction. In spite of their tendency to avoid most challenge and threat, however, they are capable of strong outbursts of violent behavior.

Patterns of Institutional Offenses

In the total sample of 10,804 inmates, 9,468 of the MCMI-III profiles were "valid" profiles by the more stringent standards utilized in this study. Among these, we had complete and useable data on all of the indexed disciplinary infractions for 4,474 of the subjects/inmates. Of this subsample, 1,452 (32.45%) had an elevation of 75 or more on the Antisocial scale of the MCMI-III.

True to form, this group of inmates was overrepresented in almost all categories of disciplinary infractions. Inmates with an elevation on the Antisocial scale of the MCMI-III were likely to offend in only one or two categories. As can be seen in Table 10.3, however, only 0.18% of such offenders obtained no disciplinary infractions. In that same table, we can see that offenders with an elevation on the Antisocial scale were significantly more likely than those without such an elevation to have disciplin-

TABLE 10.3. Code of Penal Discipline (COPD) Violations for Antisocial Profiles

Type of violation	No. of violations	% with this profile who did this	Chi-square signif.
Disobey	666	45.90%	0.009
Wontwork	237	16.30%	0.002
Verbabuse	230	15.80%	0.049
Drugs	229	15.80%	0.806
Fight	210	14.50%	0.049
Tattoo	170	11.70%	0.001
Assault	160	11.00%	0
Threats	155	10.70%	0.049
Escape	103	7.10%	0.671
Sxmiscon	51	3.50%	0.516

Note. Abbreviations for types of violations in this and similar tables: Disobey, disobeying a direct order; Wontwork, refusal to work; Verbabuse, verbal abuse; Drugs, drug offenses; Fight, fighting; Tattoo, tattooing; Assault, assault; Threats, threats; Escape, attempts to escape; Sxmiscon, sexual misconduct.

ary infractions for assault, disobeying a lawful order, fighting, refusal to work, tattooing, threats, and verbal abuse. Of particular significance is the incidence of write-
ups for disobeying a lawful order: The offenders with elevations on the Antisocial
scale made up just under half (45.90%) of all offenders receiving this charge. This
suggests that especially in their verbal behavior, the antisocial offenders will be more
likely than others to challenge orders and instructions given by staff. It would appear
that the most common pattern of conflict with these offenders devolves into a childlike "You can't make me; yes, I can" form of interaction.

Management Recommendations

Even though the antisocial offenders are not in a numerical majority in a correctional
system, they will be among the most conspicuous. This will come largely from their
continuing conflicts with authority and efforts to establish themselves as dominant.
Their continuing conflict with authority will frequently lead to confrontation with
staff members who define their job as one of personally making inmates behave as
demanded and to punish them if they should fail to respond as directed. To "win"
such encounters, offenders must only be willing to endure the imposed consequences.
They will have demonstrated, at least to themselves and often to their peers, that the
staff was incapable of making them perform as demanded.

A much more effective management strategy is generally available, but it
involves systemic as well as individual changes in common correctional officer
behavior. The foundation of this strategy is the recognition that it is the responsibility
of the system, not any individual officer, to manage offender behavior. At least emotionally, an officer should not care whether an offender responds or not. Whatever
the offender does, the officer has a proper and predefined response. The condition
that one tries to achieve is "What if you gave a war and no one showed up?"

For example, if Officer John Smith comes to the door to distribute mail and the
offender, Jim Jackson, refuses to come to the door, Officer Smith can just move on.
He doesn't have to argue, threaten, or bully—just move on. In the face of this form of
response, the only issue confronting Jackson is whether he wants his mail. There is
no status or power to be derived from the encounter. It is likely, at least initially, that
the offender will attempt to escalate the encounter into more familiar patterns. Jackson might demand that Officer Smith return to the door and give him his mail, now
that he is ready for it. Ignoring this challenge will probably lead to further escalation
and to increased threat and verbal abuse. If Officer Smith continues to respond in a
professional manner and refuses to play "door warrior" with Jackson, such encounters will diminish. This is not to say that an officer should make no response to
improper offender behavior. If, in the scenario above, Jackson violates facility rules
regarding verbal behavior, Officer Smith will write up the offense, even though he
does not engage Jackson in verbal battle. Under this circumstance, the offender faces
the consequence of his behavior without the social or "moral" victory to make it
worthwhile.

In general, correctional systems must recognize that they cannot "punish"
behavioral infractions by offenders of this type in a manner that will significantly
control or reduce the rate of such infractions. Indeed, the stereotypical strategy of
personal confrontation with these offenders only sets the stage for encounters that

the offenders will almost always "win." A particularly significant feature of the modern high-security prison is the ability to control the consequences imposed as a response to an inmate's behavior. It is important to maintain a powerful connection between the behavior of inmates and the consequence of such behavior. One of the difficulties with most less secure facilities is that much of an inmate's behavior is unobserved and it is possible for the system to react to only a small portion of the inappropriate behaviors that occur. The typical problem behaviors in prisons, such as selling drugs, gambling, extortion, assault, and so on, go unpunished much more often than they are discovered and punished. For inmates, it is the same kind of "risk of being caught" that they ignored on the streets. For predatory inmates, it "works" most of the time, and when caught, they serve the consequence as the "cost of doing business."

All limitations and restrictions in privileges must be made entirely contingent upon the behavior of inmates. They should never face a consequence other than the incarceration itself because of the crime(s) they committed. Rather, all limits and specific restrictions imposed upon the inmates in this setting should be a direct and predictable result of their own behavior. This consequence should occur as immediately as possible after the offending behavior, and should be as predictable as possible. Under equal conditions, the consequences should also be equal and never reflect the momentary irritation, social views, or outside lives of the staff members.

Although it is necessary to impose consequences on behavior—and, indeed, this is the most important feature of a good prison program—it cannot be assumed that most aversive consequences are likely to lead to positive changes in behavior. Instead, the deprivation imposed as a consequence to a behavior creates a starting point from which the individual can again "earn" privileges through appropriate behavior. It is not the *deprivation* that leads to the improvement in behavior, but the *earning* of privilege.

Sadistic Personality Disorder

Sadistic personality disorder is not one of the personality disorders formally identified in DSM-IV-TR. Although it was present in the early DSMs, it was deleted from DSM-IV for a variety of reasons. According to Millon (1999), who was present for much of this discussion, this decision reflected a series of social and political reasons rather than a logical response to the professional literature. This disorder is included here for several reasons. Perhaps the most important is that the sadistic personality fills a logically derived niche in Millon's personality theory and can be logically inferred on the basis of the underlying variables. It is also included because it is more likely to be present in a correctional population than in any other segment of society.

Manifestations in a Correctional Population

In the Colorado sample, there were 653 profiles that had a high-point elevation on the Sadistic scale of the MCMI-III. Of these, only 2 (0.31%) had only the Sadistic scale elevated (see Table 10.4). The remainder of the profiles with a high-point code on the Sadistic scale had a secondary elevation on one of the other scales. The most common comorbid pattern was a secondary elevation on the Antisocial scale. This

TABLE 10.4. Comorbid Personality Patterns for Sadistic High-Point Codes

Sadis only (6B)	6B + Schiz	6B + Avoid	6B + Depres	6B + Depend	6B + Histr	6B + Narcis	6B + Anti	6B + Comp	6B + Neg	6B + Masoc
2	32	60	26	15	14	92	238	5	157	12
0.31%	4.90%	9.19%	3.98%	2.30%	2.16%	14.09%	36.45%	0.77%	24.04%	1.84%

Note. Masoc, Masochistic (Self-Defeating). For other abbreviations, see Table 10.2.

combination was found in 36.45% of the profiles with a Sadistic high-point scale. This profile is close to the prototypal sadistic personality. The strong need for social dominance is coupled with the perverse enjoyment of inflicting pain on others.

These offenders will be notable for their opportunistic infliction of pain in a gratuitous manner on any convenient victim. They are the offenders most likely to encourage self-destructive behavior in fellow offenders and to be generally viewed as "troublemakers" in the cellhouse. They are likely to harass peers who are about to be released to see if they can make them misbehave in ways that will void their parole before release, or to encourage suicidal offenders to "do it."

The second most common comorbid pattern was a secondary elevation on the Negativistic (Passive–Aggressive) scale. This pairing was found in 24.04% of the offenders with a high-point code on the Sadistic scale. This combination was identified by Millon (1999) as the "tyrannical" subtype of sadistic personality; he characterized such individuals as "menacing and brutalizing others, forcing them to cower and submit; verbally cutting and scathing, accusatory and destructive; intentionally surly, abusive, inhumane, unmerciful" (Millon, 1999, p. 511). To the already distressing and frightening pattern of the sadistic personality, this subtype adds the resentfulness and ambivalence of the negativistic personality. These individuals will couple the uncertainty and resentment about their relationships with others with the angry desire to inflict pain on others to control social environments. The result is the most aggressively hurtful and unpredictable of all personality types. Because offenders with this personality combination will lack a stable internal reference for their relationship with others, they will generally have acquired the reputation of being "snakes" who can bite almost at random, even when it serves no purpose.

The third most common comorbid pattern in the group with a Sadistic high-point code was a secondary elevation on the Narcissistic scale. This group of personalities was also identified by Millon (1999) as the "reputation-defending" subtype of disorder (see the earlier description of this subtype).

Patterns of Institutional Offenses

There were 1,003 inmates in the subsample of 4,474 for whom disciplinary infraction data were available who had an elevated score on the Sadistic scale of the MCMI-III. This represents 22.42% of that subsample. Compared to the inmates without an elevation on this scale, those with sadistic traits were significantly more likely to be disciplined for assault, disobeying a lawful order, fighting, refusal to work, tattooing, threats, and verbal abuse. They were significantly less likely to be charged with attempting to escape. These data are found in Table 10.5.

TABLE 10.5. COPD Violations for Sadistic P

Type of violation	No. of violations	% with this profile who did this	Chi-square signif.
Disobey	463	46.20%	0.026
Verbabuse	171	17.00%	0.006
Wontwork	165	16.50%	0.012
Drugs	160	16.00%	0.711
Fight	150	15.00%	0.04
Threats	125	12.50%	0
Tattoo	121	12.10%	0.003
Assault	114	11.40%	0.001
Escape	55	5.50%	0.05
Sxmiscon	40	4.00%	0.142

Note. See Table 10.3 for abbreviations.

Consistent with the description of this disorder, inmates with elevated scores on the Sadistic scale were generally "bad actors." The issue of social dominance is highlighted by the frequency of disciplinary infractions that involved disobeying a lawful order. This group accounted for just under half of all individuals who obtained this infraction. This is important, because it is an infraction that is a response to an assertion of authority by staff. It is also informative to compare this table with Table 10.3, which presents the offense rates for the offenders with an elevation on the Antisocial scale. Both of these disorders represent active self-centered personality patterns, and both generate high levels of disciplinary problems.

Management Recommendations

The best management strategies for offenders with sadistic personality disorder are essentially the same as those for offenders with antisocial personality disorder. Sadistic offenders are also socially aggressive and seek to dominate those around them. The particular problem posed by these offenders as compared to those with the prototypal antisocial personality is that the former are more likely to elicit strong emotional responses in officers. Whereas the antisocial offenders will trigger competitive impulses in officers with "forceful" (independent/active) personalities, these impulses will typically remain at emotionally manageable levels. Sadistic offenders, on the other hand, are likely to identify vulnerabilities in officers (and other offenders) and exploit them, producing strong fearful or painful emotional responses.

Narcissistic Personality Disorder

Narcissistic personality disorder is another of the "big three" disorders found in a correctional setting. These individuals have an exaggerated sense of self-worth and a profound assumption that the rest of the world can and does have the same interest in themselves as they do. Their coping strategy in life appears focused on maintaining a high level of social feedback from others that they can use to confirm these beliefs.

In addition to their unrealistic sense of uniqueness and worth, these individuals have a tremendous need to be admired by others. Although they have no qualms about manipulating others for their own advantage, they differ from antisocial individuals in that they more often take passive advantage of what is presented to them, rather than actively creating that advantage. Because they view themselves as unique and special, they expect treatment in kind. That is, they expect to be granted special privileges and considerations that are justified by their "specialness."

Unfortunately for individuals with narcissistic personality disorder, there is a relative deficiency in their access to such feedback in a correctional environment. Most of their peers have their own personality disorders, which interfere with their willingness to feed the social needs of the narcissist offenders. Even worse, the system itself is controlled, at least in part, by staff members who believe that it is important for the narcissistic inmates to accept responsibility for their behaviors, which would be incompatible with their elevated sense of self-worth.

It is important to note that several recent research studies have identified individuals with narcissistic personality disorder as those most likely to exhibit extremely violent behavior in prison and hospital settings. Bushman and Baumeister (2002) suggest that the most dangerous people are "those who have a strong desire to regard themselves as superior beings" (p. 228). According to Twenge and Campbell (2003), the kids who become violent after rejection are those who are strongly narcissistic. Another study out of Canada found similar effects when examining domestic violence:

> Although one might expect antisocial personality to be the most common disorder across all groups, the finding that narcissism and borderline personalities are overrepresented, especially among the family-violent group, is noteworthy. One of the diagnostic criteria of borderline personality is having "physical fights," and narcissism is characterized by reacting to criticism with rage, shame and humiliation. Clearly, either reaction would increase the probability of inclusion in a violence group. (Dutton & Hart, 1996)

Manifestations in a Correctional Population

In the Colorado sample, there were 1,556 profiles with a high-point code on the Narcissism scale of the MCMI-III. Of these profiles, 175 had only an elevation on the Narcissism scale and no comorbid pattern (see Table 10.6). Such offenders will generally exhibit prototypal narcissistic traits, with a profoundly elevated sense of self-worth and entitlement. Within the correctional environment, the available sources of support for this self-concept are limited and require exaggerated efforts to maintain, as noted above. Many of these offenders will use outside family, associates, or attorneys as the primary sources of support for this image of self-worth. Others will establish complementary relationships with offenders who have other personality disorders, such as dependent personality disorder. Overall, however, the correctional system is a very stressful environment for "purely" narcissistic inmates. The most common response of staff members to such an inmate is a profound urge to "find a hatpin and burst his [or her] overinflated ego" within minutes of first meeting. These offenders' sense of entitlement not only runs counter to the basic management philosophy of most institutions, but outrages the overworked staff, whom they expect to

TABLE 10.6. Comorbid Personality Patterns for Narcissistic High-Point Profiles

Narcis only	(5) 5 + Schiz	5 + Avoid	5 + Depres	5 + Depend	5 + Histr	5 + Anti	5 + Sadis	5 + Comp	5 + Neg	5 + Masoc
175	133	61	56	27	220	287	138	341	83	35
11.25%	8.55%	3.92%	3.60%	1.74%	14.14%	18.44%	8.87%	21.92%	5.33%	2.25%

Note. See Tables 10.2 and 10.4 for abbreviations.

meet whatever need is most current. In addition, their sense of entitlement serves as a "red flag" to other predatory and socially dominant offenders, who often take it as a challenge to overcome.

Narcissistic offenders have a relatively high risk of episodes of dysthymia or even major depression. These episodes are almost always the result of a traumatic confrontation or other experience that challenges the assumption of self-worth. The episodes are typically brief, however, because the depressive experience is inherently contradictory to the underlying sense of self-worth.

Among the offenders with a Narcissistic high-point scale and a comorbid scale, the most frequent pattern was a secondary elevation on the Compulsive scale; this was seen in 21.92% of the Narcissistic high-point profiles. This comorbid pattern combines the elevated sense of self-worth with a strategy of rigid expectation that all others must follow the formal rule structures. This reliance on rules permits these offenders to justify their strong expectations about how others should respond. This reliance on rules also provides such individuals with ample demonstration that it was not their fault whenever something goes wrong, and makes it easy to assign blame to others for their failings.

Patterns of Institutional Offenses

Of the 4,474 offenders for whom we had complete and useable data on all of the indexed disciplinary infractions, 1,062 (23.74%) had an elevation of 75 or more on the Narcissistic scale of the MCMI-III. Data for these inmates are presented in Table 10.7. Inmates with an elevation on this scale were significantly more likely to obtain disciplinary infractions for assault, disobeying a lawful order, threats, and verbal abuse than were inmates without such an elevation. These results are consistent with the patterns of disciplinary infractions found in the other self-centered personality profiles. Although the narcissistic offenders were less likely than those with the other patterns to have exceptionally high numbers of infractions in many categories, it is important to note that the categories in which they were disciplined are among the most dangerous for a correctional setting.

Management Recommendations

Narcissistic offenders present particularly difficult management problems in correctional settings. Most of these problems stem from the strong reaction of most line staff, who almost immediately want to "burst their bubble." The arrogant sense of entitlement is particularly irritating in a correctional setting, where staff members are

TABLE 10.7. COPD Violations for Narcissistic Profiles

Type of violation	No. of violations	% with this profile who did this	Chi-square signif.
Disobey	490	46.10%	0.022
Verbabuse	181	17.00%	0.004
Drugs	173	16.30%	0.464
Fight	155	14.60%	0.083
Wontwork	144	13.60%	0.625
Assault	127	12.00%	0
Threats	120	11.30%	0.017
Tattoo	111	10.50%	0.301
Escape	61	5.70%	0.099
Sxmiscon	41	3.90%	0.21

Note. See Table 10.3 for abbreviations.

usually aware of the behavior that resulted in the incarceration. There is frequently a desire on the part of the staff to help these offenders understand the "thinking errors" that are reflected in this excessive sense of entitlement. Unfortunately, such efforts produce exactly the kinds of experiences that are most likely to threaten the core self-concept structures of the narcissistic inmates, and often result in a surprising burst of aggressive behavior quite out of proportion to the situation as it would be most often seen.

It is with the management of narcissistic offenders that the correctional staff will have its greatest test of professionalism. To the extent that an officer can focus on the behavior required of such an offender at the moment and slide past the entitlement that marks most of the offender's verbal behavior, there should be relatively little problem. Strategies such as those described by Thompson and Jenkins (1993) are optimal for this task. Confrontation, on the other hand, is likely to result in a burst of aggressive behavior as described above.

Negativistic (Passive–Aggressive) Personality Disorder

Negativistic or passive–aggressive personality disorder is not one of the personality disorders formally identified in DSM-IV-TR. It was present in the early DSMs, but it was deleted from the main text of DSM-IV for various reasons and is now found in the appendix titled "Criteria Sets and Axes Provided for Further Study." Rather than emphasizing the underlying personality characteristics, DSM-IV and now DSM-IV-TR have focused on the overt behavior manifested in this disorder, and thus have missed its cardinal qualities. This personality disorder is characterized by an underlying negativity and pessimism that permeates almost all aspects of an individual's life. These individuals feel cheated and deprived of their proper benefits from this life, and resent others who have such good fortune. They continually struggle with the authority of others and find passive strategies to subvert demands made on them.

Their behavior is dominated by such excuses as "I forgot," "I can't find it," and "You never told me to do that."

The term "passive–aggressive" for this personality disorder was first introduced in a U.S. War Department technical bulletin in 1945. The term was coined by wartime psychiatrists who found themselves dealing with reluctant and uncooperative soldiers who followed orders with chronic, veiled hostility and smoldering resentment. Their style was a mixture of passive resistance and grumbling compliance (Stone, 1993, p. 361). Such individuals frequently act out their resentments against others in indirect ways that leave them with "plausible deniability" for both the actions and the underlying feelings.

Millon and Davis (1996) have presented a much more comprehensive description of negativistic/passive–aggressive personality disorder than that found in the DSMs. They suggest that underlying the behavior characterizing this personality pattern are profound confusion and ambivalence about self and others—similar to that seen in the compulsive personality, but with very different coping strategies. These are individuals who have failed to develop a clear sense of self and their relationship to others. As a result, these individuals are constantly angry at the world for its unpredictable nature and their inability to adequately control what happens to them. Like children, they vacillate between anger over their dependency on others and their desire for autonomy. This pattern—naturally found in early adolescence in most individuals, but retained by those with negativistic/passive–aggressive personality disorder—leads to the frequent observation of "childish" emotionality. These persons have adopted a very active style of coping with the challenges presented by other people, but they focus that effort on resistance to the wishes or desires of others.

Manifestations in a Correctional Population

There were 742 profiles in the Colorado sample with a high-point code on the Negativistic (Passive–Aggressive) scale of the MCMI-III. Of these, only 6 (0.81%) had an elevation only on the Negativistic scale (see Table 10.8). On the others, the Negativistic elevation was comorbid with an elevation on another of the personality scales. This means that fewer than 1% of the offenders with negativistic traits would display the prototypal pattern described above.

The most frequently occurring comorbidity pattern was a secondary elevation on the Avoidant scale. A very similar pattern is described in more detail later in the section on avoidant personality disorder—that is, a primary elevation on the Avoidant scale and a secondary elevation on the Negativistic scale. This combination has been identified by Millon (1999) as the "conflicted" subtype of avoidant personality.

Almost as common was the second comorbid pattern, which coupled a Negativistic primary elevation with an Antisocial secondary elevation. This profile produces angry, retaliatory behavior very similar to that seen in the third most common comorbid pattern. There were 114 (15.36%) of the profiles with this third pattern— that is, the high-point elevation on the Negativistic scale and a secondary elevation on the Sadistic scale. This pattern produces a type of behavior that has been discussed earlier in the section on sadistic personality disorder; as noted there, this combination was identified by Millon (1999) as the "tyrannical" subtype of sadistic personality.

TABLE 10.8. Comorbid Personality Patterns for Negativistic High-Point Profiles

Neg only (8A)	8A + Schiz	8A + Avoid	8A + Depres	8A + Depend	8A + Histr	8A + Narcis	8A + Anti	8A + Sadis	8A + Comp	8A + Masoc
6	48	169	69	48	13	65	168	114	7	35
0.81%	6.47%	22.78%	9.30%	6.47%	1.76%	8.76%	22.64%	15.36%	0.94%	4.72%

Note. See Tables 10.2 and 10.4 for abbreviations.

Patterns of Institutional Offenses

Of the 4,474 offenders for whom we had complete and useable data on all of the indexed disciplinary infractions, 1,097 (24.52%) had an elevation of 75 or more on the Negativistic (Passive–Aggressive) scale of the MCMI-III. Data for these inmates are given in Table 10.9. Inmates with an elevation on this scale were significantly more likely to obtain disciplinary infractions for assault, disobeying a lawful order, refusal to work, tattooing, and threats. This pattern of offenses is consistent with the expected behavior in negativistic personality disorder.

Management Recommendations

The offenders with various "blends" of the negativistic personality pattern are among the most difficult to manage in a correctional setting. Their anger augments or intensifies the anger qualities of other personality disorders, and the strategy of searching for "plausible deniability" for their behavior stretches the quasi-legal structure of a correctional setting to its limits in having to respond to their common challenge of "Oh, yeah? Prove it!" Their erratic hostility and their pursuit of "justifiable

TABLE 10.9. COPD Violations for Negativistic Profiles

Type of violation	No. of violations	% with this profile who did this	Chi-square signif.
Disobey	512	46.70%	0.006
Wontwork	187	17.00%	0.001
Verbabuse	187	17.00%	0.492
Drugs	151	13.80%	0.057
Fight	145	13.20%	0.832
Tattoo	132	12.00%	0.002
Assault	125	11.40%	0
Threats	124	11.30%	0.015
Escape	66	6.00%	0.202
Sxmiscon	44	4.00%	0.109

Note. See Table 10.3 for abbreviations.

vengeance" make them difficult for fellow inmates as well as staff to manage. This is clearly reflected in the fact that they were significantly overrepresented in half of the disciplinary infractions examined in this study.

Reserved Personality Patterns

The "reserved" personality patterns in a correctional setting include the schizoid, avoidant, and depressive personality disorders. In spite of the common misconception of prisons as the domain of the brutal, "knuckle-dragging," aggressive portion of our population, the "reserved" forms of personality disorders are strongly represented in this setting. Although they are often easy to overlook, these offenders play an important, if unfortunate, role in prison life: They frequently serve as the "prey" for the more predatory offenders. They also find themselves in disciplinary trouble because of their efforts to withdraw and isolate themselves in an environment that does not permit such individual choices. In addition, this group of offenders is overrepresented in many crimes that are despised by most other offenders, such as sexual assault against children (Kleinsasser, Stoner, & Retzlaff, 2000).

Avoidant Personality Disorder

Individuals with avoidant personality disorder try to make life choices on the basis of which option is least likely to produce an immediate experience of stress. They tend to avoid social situations largely because stress is most often experienced in the company of other people. Unlike schizoid persons, avoidant individuals would generally like to be more social, and refrain from such contact to avoid the associated pain. It is frequently this same avoidance quality that results in criminal behavior for such individuals, who would otherwise greatly prefer not to face the stress of court and incarceration. By making short-term stress avoidance choices, such as not preparing tax returns or reconciling checkbooks, avoidant individuals will place themselves in circumstances that ultimately produce even greater stress. Or, rather than confront a gang recruiter, they will just try to blend in and not reject or refuse the demand/offer to join.

Manifestations in a Correctional Population

There were 1,181 profiles in the Colorado sample with a high-point code on the Avoidant scale of the MCMI-III. Of these, 258 (21.85%) had an elevation only on the Avoidant scale. For the others, avoidant personality disorder was comorbid with at least one of all the other personality disorders. These results can be seen in Table 10.10.

The most common comorbidity was a secondary elevation on the Depressive scale, which occurred in 14.56% of offenders with the Avoidant scale as the high-point code. This comorbid pattern has been identified by Millon (1999) as the "self-deserting" subtype of avoidant personality. These avoidant characters will often suppress or repress awareness of uncomfortable experiences or perceptions, particularly perceptions of self. Gaps in social memory should be common, and a higher risk of

TABLE 10.10. Comorbid Personality Patterns for Avoidant High-Point Profiles

Avoid only (2A)	2A + Schiz	2A + Depres	2A + Depend	2A + Histr	2A + Narcis	2A + Anti	2A + Sadis	2A + Comp	2A + Neg	2A + Masoc
258	138	172	148	2	48	114	31	44	137	89
21.85%	11.69%	14.56%	12.53%	0.17%	4.06%	9.65%	2.62%	3.73%	11.60%	7.54%

Note. See Tables 10.2 and 10.4 for abbreviations.

self-harm is expected. In fact, 31.97% of the inmates with this type of profile were also scored as having significant risk for self-harm in the intake assessment on this sample.

The second most common comorbidity was a secondary elevation on the Schizoid scale, which occurred on 11.69% of all profiles where the Avoidant scale was the high-point scale. Persons with this combination will reflect the social withdrawal common to both problems. These offenders will be less reactive than those with the prototypal avoidant personality, and more fearful than those with the prototypal schizoid personality.

Almost as frequent a comorbidity with a high-point elevation on the Avoidant scale was a secondary elevation on the Negativistic scale. As noted earlier, this combination has been identified by Millon (1999) as the "conflicted" subtype of avoidant personality. It manifests the anxiety and social withdrawal of the avoidant personality, with the interpersonal ambivalence of the negativistic (passive–aggressive) personality. These individuals fear both independence and dependence, and cannot find a comfortable "middle ground" in interpersonal relationships. They want to be detached from others, but fear independence. They will feel chronic guilt and low self-esteem, while continually berating others for the problems they experience.

The least common secondary elevation when the Avoidant scale was the high-point scale was on the Histrionic scale. As might be expected, there is almost no overlap between the sociable and outgoing histrionic personality and the socially isolated and withdrawn avoidant personality.

Patterns of Institutional Offenses

In the subsample of 4,474 valid and useable records, 1,129 (25.23%) had elevations of 75 or more on the Avoidant scale of the MCMI-III. Data for these inmates are provided in Table 10.11. Inmates with an elevation on this scale obtained significantly more disciplinary infractions for assault, fighting, and refusal to work. They were significantly less likely to be charged with a drug infraction.

The relationship between assault and fighting on the one hand, and the social withdrawal of avoidant individuals on the other, may initially appear contradictory. However, it is essential to understand the social context for these behaviors. In a prison environment, there is little institutional tolerance for people who just "want to do their own thing," and considerable pressure to engage in the activities and programs designed by the institution for the majority of offenders. This institution has a high need to know where each offender is and what he or she is doing at any moment

TABLE 10.11. COPD Violations for Avoidant Profiles

Type of violation	No. of violations	% with this profile who did this	Chi-square signif.
Disobey	482	42.70%	0.753
Wontwork	185	16.40%	0.008
Fight	177	15.70%	0.002
Verbabuse	169	15.00%	0.492
Drugs	146	12.90%	0.005
Assault	117	10.40%	0.021
Tattoo	116	10.30%	0.398
Threats	115	10.20%	0.316
Escape	68	6.00%	0.197
Sxmiscon	39	3.50%	0.676

Note. See Table 10.3 for abbreviations.

in time. Given these institutional realities, the pressure on avoidant offenders to behave in ways other than what they find most desirable is obvious.

In addition, a prison environment has far more predatory individuals than most of us have ever experienced. Even when the avoidant offenders are able to minimize conflict with the institution, the pressures applied by the more predatory offenders are likely to lead to intolerable conflict, which will in turn lead to episodes of fighting or assault as a method of leaving a situation that has become intolerable.

Management Recommendations

On the surface, it would seem that offenders with avoidant personality disorder would be ideal inmates to manage, because their dominant drive is to avoid all forms of stress and conflict. Unfortunately, as noted above, prison provides little opportunity for the avoidance strategies that were at least marginally successful in the free world. The programs and structure of prison life permit these offenders few chances to remain quietly in their cells, avoiding the demands of daily life. In addition, efforts at avoidance mark the offenders as easy prey for the more aggressive offenders.

The most successful management strategies for offenders with avoidant personalities require that the choices to behave in the manner desired by the prison create less stress than alternative choices will. Officers will need to be aware of the motivating conditions for these offenders and to respond in a more supportive and helpful manner. "In-your-face," "drill instructor" styles of commanding behavior will be clearly counterproductive with this group of offenders.

Depressive Personality Disorder

Depressive personality disorder is another of the personality disorders that is not covered in the main DSM-IV-TR text and is included in the appendix "Criteria Sets and

Axes Provided for Further Study." The DSM-IV-TR (American Psychiatric Association, 2000) notes that "it remains controversial whether the distinction between
depressive personality disorder and Dysthymic Disorder is useful" (p. 788). As with
several other personality patterns in this chapter, it is included because it identifies
the common behavior of a sufficiently large number of correctional inmates that it
becomes a useful designation in at least that setting.

Individuals with depressive personality disorder have a powerful sense of personal inadequacy and impaired self-esteem. Although often misunderstood and
misdiagnosed as dysthymia or some other Axis I mood disorder, depressive personality disorder is truly an Axis II disorder because it derives from a distorted perception
of the world and deviant efforts to cope with that distorted perception. The
depressive-like behavior does not stem from a disturbance of mood, alteration of
brain chemistry, or other major elements of the an Axis I mood disorder. Indeed, one
of the features we often see is the failure of traditional therapies and medications to
ameliorate the symptoms. The "depression" of depressive personality disorder is a
picture of the world as a dismal place of little hope and frequent failure.

Manifestations in a Correctional Population

There were 768 profiles in the Colorado sample with the Depressive scale of the
MCMI-III as the high-point code. Of these, only 41 (5.31%) had the Depressive scale
as the only significant elevation (see Table 10.12). The remainder demonstrated a
"blending" with other personality disorders.

By far the most common comorbid elevation on protocols that had the Depressive scale the high-point scale was on the Avoidant scale, which is theoretically
closely allied. The primary difference between these two disorders is that avoidant
individuals actively seek to avoid or escape from painful circumstances, whereas
depressive individuals seem to have given up and are just passively waiting for these
circumstances to go away. In this respect, the depressive personality includes many of
the characteristics described years ago by Seligman and others as "learned helplessness" (Seligman, Maier, & Geer, 1968). This comorbid pattern has been described by
Millon (1999, p. 355) as the "restive" subtype of depressive personality. This is the
more active and agitated form of expression of the depressive pattern, and will be
associated with increased risk of self-harm.

The second most common comorbid pattern for Depressive high-point profiles
was a secondary elevation on the Antisocial scale. This pattern was found in 14.06%
of the profiles with a Depressive high-point code. It is likely that this particular pat-

TABLE 10.12. Comorbid Personality Patterns for Depressive High-Point Profiles

Depres only	(2B) 2B + Schiz	2B + Avoid	2B + Depend	2B + Histr	2B + Narcis	2B + Anti	2B + Sadis	2B + Comp	2B + Neg	2B + Masoc
41	85	150	68	14	45	108	31	33	100	93
5.34%	11.07%	19.53%	8.85%	1.82%	5.86%	14.06%	4.04%	4.30%	13.02%	12.11%

Note. See Tables 10.2 and 10.4 for abbreviations.

tern will be unusual in any population other than an incarcerated one, where the base rate for antisocial behavior is so high. This blend will emphasize the angry, blaming aspects of antisocial personality with the generally hopeless and negativistic features of depressive personality.

The other common comorbid pattern is a secondary elevation on Negativistic (Passive–Aggressive) scale. This pattern occurred in 13.02% of the Depressive high-point profiles. This pattern has been identified by Millon (1999, p. 355) as the "ill-humored" subtype of depressive personality. Offenders with this profile will emphasize the ill-tempered, cantankerous, pessimistic components of the depressive pattern.

The least common comorbidity was a secondary elevation on the Histrionic scale, which occurred in only 1.82% of the profiles with the Depressive scale as the high-point scale. The histrionic personality's sociability and outgoing nature are unlikely to blend easily with or be commonly found with the cardinal features of the depressive personality.

Patterns of Institutional Offenses

Of the subsample of 4,474 useable profiles in this study, 871 (19.47%) had an elevation of 75 or more on the Depressive scale of the MCMI-III. Table 10.13 gives data for those inmates. Compared to offenders without an elevation on the Depressive scale, these offenders were significantly more likely to obtain disciplinary infractions for refusal to work and verbal abuse.

Management Recommendations

Like offenders with the other reserved personality patterns, personalities, offenders with depressive personality disorder are not generally going to present serious management problems. When they do require greater system resources, these will gener-

TABLE 10.13. COPD Violations for Depressive Profiles

Type of violation	No. of violations	% with this profile who did this	Chi-square signif.
Disobey	482	42.70%	0.753
Wontwork	185	16.40%	0.008
Fight	177	15.70%	0.002
Verbabuse	169	15.00%	0.492
Drugs	146	12.90%	0.005
Assault	117	10.40%	0.021
Tattoo	116	10.30%	0.398
Threats	115	10.20%	0.316
Escape	68	6.00%	0.197
Sxmiscon	39	3.50%	0.676

Note. See Table 10.3 for abbreviations.

ally need to come from clinical services. Compared to offenders without such an elevation, offenders with an elevated score on the Depressive scale of the MCMI-III were significantly more likely to be assessed as having higher mental health needs and were significantly more likely to be given a psychiatric diagnosis.

Schizoid Personality Disorder

Schizoid personality disorder is marked by individuals' emotional disconnection from the social world around them. Although such individuals are usually socially isolated and withdrawn, the key feature is their emotional isolation from others. These individuals are not always physically isolated from others like hermits, but will not be emotionally connected even when surrounded by coworkers.

The second defining quality of these individuals is a general lack of pleasurable experience. Rather than being morose or unhappy, these individuals tend to live life on a flat emotional plane marked by small emotional variations of either a positive or negative nature. This also means that they are not particularly motivated by the typical experiences of "pleasure" that motivate most of us. They can "coast" through long periods of little change in stimulation without the distress over a sense of boredom that most other offenders would experience in a similar situation. Lack of sexual drive is commonly found with this personality disorder and associated with this lack of pleasure experience.

A correctional interpretive description of this high-point code on the MCMI-III might include the following ideas. (Following the Colorado study, this statement was suggested as an addition to reports of the screening evaluations where the Schizoid scale was the high-point scale. The content of the statement was ultimately seen as correct, but too lengthy, and a shorter statement was developed for inclusion in reports.)

> This inmate is a "loner" who lacks the capacity to enjoy life and tends to lead a seclusive life focused on "things" rather than people. He [sic] is unaware of the subtle variations in social relationships and gets into social difficulties by misreading the needs or intent of others. He will usually spend most of his time involved with the mastery or manipulation of things. Often, if sufficiently bright, he will be involved in technical activities such as computers. Alternative interests might be in fixing or modifying automobiles, hunting, or manual skills. He will have few friends and will not maintain intimate bonds well.

Manifestations in a Correctional Population

Of the Colorado sample, 11.62% obtained an elevated base rate score of 75 or above on the Schizoid scale of the MCMI-III. Of the 1,100 offenders with such an elevation, many had elevations on other scales as well. Table 10.14 shows the number of profiles in which the Schizoid scale was the highest scale, and identifies the next highest scale when at least one more scale was also above 75. The pattern of two-point codes shown is generally consistent with the subtype patterns of schizoid personality described by Millon (1999).

Clearly, the majority of offenders with their highest elevation on the MCMI-III Schizoid scale had no other personality disorder elevation (69.87%). This would suggest that schizoid personality disorder as reflected by that scale is a coherent personality pattern and will most often be seen in a prototypal form. Profiles with a second elevation were distributed across all the other personality disorders. The most common second-point elevation was on the Antisocial scale (9.27%). This apparently contradictory combination of traits is most likely to manifest itself as a "porcupine personality"—that is, as an individual who tries to remain withdrawn when possible, and bristles aggressively when that withdrawal is threatened. It is most likely that the predominant characteristics for this combination will be those of the schizoid personality, and that the aggressiveness of the antisocial personality will be apparent only when threatened. Such individuals are unlikely to have the outgoing, social dominance drive characteristic of the antisocial personality.

The second most common comorbid pattern was a secondary elevation on the Avoidant scale, which was present in 8.45% of the profiles with Schizoid as the highest scale elevation. This is the comorbid pattern that would be expected to be the most common, since both patterns involve social withdrawal and highly controlled emotional expression. Offenders with this personality pattern can be expected to display higher levels of anxiety than would be expected in those with the prototypal schizoid personality, and are therefore more likely to exhibit an actively aggressive pattern of offenses when "cornered." This profile was identified by Millon (1999) as the "remote" subtype of schizoid personality.

The third most common comorbid pattern of profiles with the Schizoid scale as the high-point scale was a secondary elevation on the Depressive scale. Such offenders are still most likely to be predominantly schizoid in nature and presentation, but will include an increased display of depressive behaviors as a part of their overall pattern. These offenders are more likely to show the self-deprecation and sense of failure of the depressive personality, but with significantly diminished affect. This combination of traits was characterized by Millon (1999) as the "languid" subtype of schizoid personality.

Although it is apparent that several other personality disorders (e.g., antisocial) have a more visible relationship to crime, a prison population will include a fair sampling of all the major personality disorders, as noted throughout this chapter. In a prison setting, the schizoid personality is in many ways the ideal personality. These will be offenders who are interested in doing their own time, can manage the boredom of institutional life much better than many, and will tend to avoid the "mix" of the general population.

The major problems for these inmates seem to come from two primary sources. First, prison is a relatively structured environment in which isolated and autonomous behavior is usually not rewarded and sometimes punished. The typical correctional

TABLE 10.14. Comorbid Personality Pattern for Schizoid High-Point Profiles

Schiz only (1)	1 + Avoid	1 + Depres	1 + Depend	1 + Histr	1 + Narcis	1 + Anti	1 + Sadis	1 + Comp	1 + Neg	1 + Masoc
1092	93	69	12	4	54	102	28	62	26	21
69.87%	8.45%	6.27%	1.09%	0.36%	4.91%	9.27%	2.55%	5.64%	2.36%	1.91%

Note. See Tables 10.2 and 10.4 for abbreviations.

officer (and, for that matter, the typical correctional program) will have difficulty differentiating the verbal expressions of the schizoid inmate who is just seeking isolation from the often similar statements of the more aggressive inmate who is being defiant and rebellious as part of asserting personal dominance. This problem can be minimized in programs where the correctional officers have the opportunity for observations of the inmates' behavior over a long period of time to gain a historical perspective on their typical behavior. It also requires advanced training for these officers on the differences among various offender personalities and the implications of these differences. These discriminations will become increasingly important as the custody/security levels of facilities and programs increase. As the personal choice options decrease with increased security, the need for the programs and staff members to make these discriminations increases. Management programs and strategies that are appropriate and necessary for the classical antisocial offender can often time be inappropriate or even counterproductive for the schizoid offender.

The other major problem for schizoid inmates is the difficulty they will have avoiding the attentions of the more predatory inmates concentrated in the same environment. It is likely that many of the disciplinary problems elicited by schizoid offenders are the results of their efforts at avoiding unwanted attention either from other inmates or from staff.

Patterns of Institutional Offenses

Of the 4,474 offenders for whom we had complete and useable data on all of the indexed disciplinary infractions, 557 (12.45%) had an elevation of 75 or more on the Schizoid scale of the MCMI-III. Table 10.15 provides data for these offenders.

This typically quiet group of inmates had significantly more institutional drug offenses than did those inmates with a Schizoid scale score of 74 or below. They were significantly less likely to be involved in charges of refusal to work or assault. The most common infraction for all inmates was disobeying a lawful order, and this infraction was most common for the schizoid offenders as well, but at a lower rate than for nonschizoid offenders. Another disciplinary finding of particular importance for this group was the low incidence of sexual misconduct, which is again consistent with the prototypal behavior pattern. It is particularly likely that the higher rates of drug offenses were efforts at self-medication to isolate these offenders emotionally from the social mix surrounding them. The lower rates of refusal to work and assault might reflect the efforts of schizoid inmates to avoid the social conflict such behavior would entail.

Management Recommendations

When they can be correctly identified, inmates with schizoid personality disorder can be best managed by examining the particular prison environment in which they are found and trying to balance the institutional needs for proper inmate management and programming with the greatest opportunities for withdrawal from threatening, intimate, or demanding social encounters. In general population environments,

TABLE 10.15. COPD Violations for Schizoid Profiles

Type of violation	No. of violations	Expected no.	% with this profile who did this
Sxmiscon	24	18.2	4.30%
Escape	30	38.2	5.40%
Tattoo	52	53.7	9.30%
Threats	66	52.5	11.80%
Assault	68	48.4	12.20%*
Drugs	72	86.8	12.90%*
Verbabuse	81	79.9	14.50%
Fight	84	72.6	15.10%
Wontwork	103	78.1	18.50%*
Disobey	238	240	42.70%

Note. See Table 10.3 for abbreviations.
*Significant at .05 level.

among the most useful sources for identifying such settings would be the job board, case management, or other parts of the system that regularly deal with job and educational assignments.

Compliant Personality Patterns

The third group of basic personality patterns relevant for a correctional setting consists of those in which offenders will usually be cooperative with requests and instructions. This group includes the compulsive, masochistic, and histrionic dependent, personality patterns. Offenders with these patterns will typically work to comply with requests and expectations. In the "us versus them" milieu of corrections, however, this compliance is likely to be perceived by offenders as "sucking up" to officers, and by officers as "manipulation."

Compulsive Personality Disorder

The cardinal feature of individuals with compulsive personality disorder (labeled "obsessive–compulsive personality disorder" in DSM-IV-TR) is the need to maintain control of their relationship to the world by maintaining careful organization of themselves and the world around them. The underlying emotional dynamic for this personality disorder is similar to that of the negativistic (passive–aggressive) personality, but the coping strategy is very different. Millon (1999) notes that, like negativistic persons, compulsive individuals are "torn between their leanings toward submissive dependence on the one hand and defiant autonomy on the other" (p. 524). Millon further notes that by

clinging grimly to rules of society and insisting on regularity and uniformity in relationships and life events, these individuals help restrain and protect themselves against their
own aggressive impulses and independent strivings. Although this behavioral and cognitive rigidity may effectively shield the individual from intrapsychic conflict as well as
social criticism, it may also preclude growth and change, cause alienation from inner feelings, and interfere with the formation of intimate and warm relationships. (p. 524)

In other words, compulsive individuals will struggle to maintain the facade of
socially desirable feelings and behavior without the underlying substance to support
such a facade. "If I can't be/feel normal, I can at least look normal" is their theme.

In a correctional population, these offenders will be most noteworthy for their
insistence on having the institution follow its own rules. In this regard, they can often
be misidentified as antisocial manipulators, who can also periodically try to use institutional rules for personal advantage. The difference will be in the regularity and
intensity of the need for such institutional consistency. Compulsive offenders will
usually be identified as "paper hangers" and will tend to file many grievances in
which they ask that the institution and staff comply with their own rules. They will
often incur disciplinary infractions secondary to such requests, although these will
usually be verbal in nature, such as verbal abuse or threats. They will often be identified by housing staff as troublemakers, even though there are significant differences
between their typical offenses and those of more aggressive offenders.

For institutional management, it should be recognized that an elevation on the
Compulsive scale of the MCMI-III is one of the strongest positive prognostic measures for successful completion of programs. The same traits that are so frustrating to
staff members when applied to the staff will also make it easier for these offenders to
comply with the rules and expectations of programs. Compulsive offenders will generally perform well above their native ability level in the highly structured programs
typically available in a correctional setting.

Manifestations in a Correctional Population

There were 1,016 profiles in the Colorado sample with a high-point code on the
Compulsive scale of the MCMI-III. Of these, a little fewer than half (40.75%) had
only an elevation on the Compulsive scale (see Table 10.16). Such offenders will
exhibit the prototypal compulsive personality traits as described above. As a group,
they will be the best prognostic risks for any program for which their security level
permits access.

The most frequent comorbid pattern was a secondary elevation on the Histrionic
scale, which occurred in 20.57% of the profiles with Compulsive as the high-point
scale. Although the orderly, rule-following features of the compulsive component of
this profile will be readily apparent, the dominant focus of such individuals will come
from the histrionic need to meet the needs of others in order to obtain personal
rewards. This profile will most closely approximate the one described by Millon
(1999) as the "appeasing" subtype of histrionic personality. These individuals will be
constantly scanning the environment for more powerful and/or authoritative people,
and will try to anticipate their needs and appease them in order to obtain their own
rewards. While much of their behavior will resemble that of dependent individuals in

TABLE 10.16. Comorbid Personality Patterns for Compulsive High-Point Profiles

Comp only (7)	7 + Schiz	7 + Avoid	7 + Depres	7 + Depend	7 + Histr	7 + Narcis	7 + Anti	7 + Sadis	7 + Neg	7 + Masoc
414	102	16	25	35	209	184	24	3	1	3
40.75%	10.04%	1.57%	2.46%	3.44%	20.57%	18.11%	2.36%	0.30%	0.10%	0.30%

Note. See Tables 10.2 and 10.4 for abbreviations.

attachment to others, this is a much more active personality form that seeks to go "overboard" to please powerful people as a strategy for gaining benefits later. Unfortunately for offenders with this personality style, the numbers of generous personalities who will reward such strivings are very limited in a correctional population, and their efforts will often go unrecognized by either staff or other offenders. Such an individual is at high risk for being identified, fairly or unfairly, as a "snitch" and being subjected to the consequences of such a label.

The second most common comorbid pattern in the correctional sample was a secondary elevation on the Narcissistic scale of the MCMI-III. This pattern was identified by Millon (1999) as the "bureaucratic" subtype of compulsive personality. These offenders will combine a self-centered sense of worth with a strong reliance on a formal rule structure to support their officious behavior. Although it is easier to see this coping strategy on the other side of the bars, offenders with this personality will tend to move into similar functions within whatever group they are affiliated. Within gangs and security-threatening groups, they will tend to gravitate into roles such as group historian and codifier. The meticulously created and formalized by-laws that are sometimes associated with even the most aggressively violent of these groups testify to the ability of some of these individuals to adapt to such incongruous settings.

The third most frequent comorbid pattern was a secondary elevation on the Schizoid scale of the MCMI-III. This pattern has been previously identified by Millon (1999) as the "parsimonious" subtype of compulsive personality. It is described as follows: "miserly, niggardly, tight-fisted ungiving, hoarding, unsharing; protects self against loss; fears intrusions into vacant inner world; dreads exposure of personal improprieties and contrary impulses" (p. 543). Particularly in the usually Spartan world of corrections, these individuals will tend to hoard what little they have and to protect it from the official intrusions of staff (property shakedowns) and the unofficial intrusions of other offenders. These individuals will exhibit the lack of emotional experience characteristic of the schizoid personality, while relying on a compulsive pattern of hoarding to protect their sense of security and well-being.

Patterns of Institutional Offenses

As might be expected from the descriptions above, offenders with high-point codes on the Compulsive scale were less likely than those without elevations on this scale to violate many different disciplinary infraction codes. While 26% of this group had no disciplinary infraction at all, another 40.5% had only one category of infraction, and 22.9% had infractions in only two categories.

TABLE 10.17. COPD Violations for Compulsive Profiles

Type of violation	No. of violations	% with this profile who did this	Chi-square signif.
Sxmiscon	12	8.2%	0.124
Escape	21	6.8%	0.181
Drugs	45	6.5%	0.113
Threats	24	5.7%	0.644
Verbabuse	33	5.1%	1.000
Disobey	94	4.9%	0.454
Fight	22	3.8%	0.109
Wontwork	24	3.8%	0.119
Tattoo	13	3.0%	0.030
Assault	10	2.6%	0.006

Note. See Table 10.3 for abbreviations.

Of the 4,474 subjects/inmates, for whom we had complete and useable data on all of the indexed disciplinary infractions, 232 (5.19%) had an elevation of 75 or more on the Compulsive scale of the MCMI-III. Table 10.17 gives the infraction data for these offenders. Inmates with an elevation on this scale were not more likely than others to receive disciplinary infractions in any category of offense. They were, however, significantly less likely to receive write-ups for assault and tattooing.

Management Recommendations

Management of compulsive offenders is, to a great degree, a problem of education and management of the correctional staff. Offenders with this personality pattern are more likely than those with any other personality pattern to be successful in assigned programs and cooperative with work and program assignments. They will be substantially irritating to line staff members, however, largely because of their insistence that the facility and staff follow their own rules. In this arena, they will be legalistic and demanding. They will have typically memorized the rulebook outlining the expectations of the facility and will use this to challenge the staff whenever possible. They are also most likely to make use of the officially prescribed procedures for handling complaints and grievances.

Dependent Personality Disorder

Like several of the preceding personality disorders, dependent personality disorder is characterized by a sense of personal inadequacy and impaired self-esteem. Dependent individuals attempt to cope with these perceptions of themselves in relationship to the world by finding a person they perceive to be more competent and powerful. They attempt to develop a relationship with the more powerful person in which they can be protected and nurtured. They then relinquish responsibility for choices and decisions to the powerful person, and try to adapt their lives to whatever is needed by that person. Their primary needs in life appear to be expressions of acceptance and affection. They are more likely than individuals with most other personality disorders to experience stress, anxiety, and depression, since they are sensitive to all evidence of rejection and are helpless to change things on their own. They view themselves as weak, fragile, and utterly reliant on others. They avoid social conflict at all costs and will placate others to avoid such conflict.

Manifestations in a Correctional Population

There were 340 MCMI-III profiles in the Colorado study with the high-point elevation on the dependent scale. Of these, 19 (5.59%) were elevated only on the dependent scale (see Table 10.18). The remainder were "blended" with other personality traits.

The Dependent scale was remarkable in this study for its wide range of comorbidity patterns. The most common of the comorbid scales was the Depressive scale, which was found in 21.47% of the profiles with Dependent as the high-point scale. Offenders with this pattern can be expected to display a passive strategy for coping with the world, in which they are powerless to control the events that happen to them. The dependent component of this profile will lead such an individual to seek out the nurturance or protection of a more powerful individual, while the depressive component will emphasize the ultimate futility and hopelessness of any effort.

The Dependent high-point profile was combined with the Avoidant scale in 16.18% of the cases. This combination has been previously identified by Millon (1999, p. 385) as the "disquieted" subtype of dependent personality. The strategy of passively accommodating a more powerful individual will be blended with the increased anxiety and desire to withdraw of the avoidant personality and produce a chronic state of anxiety, dread, and fear of abandonment. This latter quality is also found in the borderline personality (to be discussed later), but the dependent–avoidant personality will not have the perceptual and affective swings that mark the borderline pattern.

In this sample, the third most common comorbid pattern with a Dependent high-point profile was a secondary elevation on the Antisocial scale, which occurred in 12.35% of the cases. As with several previous high-point scales, the addition of the Antisocial scale to the Dependent scale will increase the likelihood that the more powerful individual on whom an offender with this comorbid pattern is dependent is a more predatory antisocial inmate and will have encouraged or demanded various antisocial behaviors as the price of the continuing dependency. This pattern will also

TABLE 10.18. Comorbid Personality Patterns for Dependent High-Point Profiles

Depend only (3)	3+ Schiz	3+ Avoid	3+ Depres	3+ Histr	3+ Narcis	3+ Anti	3+ Sadis	3+ Comp	3+ Neg	3+ Masoc
19	32	55	73	18	11	42	11	13	29	37
5.59%	9.41%	16.18%	21.47%	5.29%	3.24%	12.35%	3.24%	3.82%	8.53%	10.88%

Note. See Tables 10.2 and 10.4 for abbreviations.

demonstrate greater resentment and anger than the prototypal dependent personality, although it will often be focused on the self or a third party, rather than the powerful individual on whom the person is dependent.

There were no personality scales that had remarkably low comorbidity with the Dependent scale. The two least frequent comorbid patterns were with the Narcissistic scale and the Sadistic scale. The low-frequency relationship with the Sadistic scale is likely to have been an artifact of the low base rate for elevations on that scale overall. The low frequency of comorbid patterns with the Narcissistic PD scale would be expected from the almost direct contradiction between the excessive sense of self-worth in the narcissistic personality and the low self-esteem in the dependent personality.

Patterns of Institutional Offenses

Of the 4,474 subjects/inmates, for whom we had complete and useable data on all of the indexed disciplinary infractions, 656 (14.66%) had an elevation of 75 or more on the Dependent scale of the MCMI-III. Table 10.19 presents data for these offenders. Inmates with this scale elevated were significantly more likely than those without such an elevation to be charged with disciplinary infractions involving refusal to work and tattooing. The increased rate of conviction for tattooing is certainly consistent with their primary personality pattern. This activity can be easily viewed as "branding" themselves to affiliate with a particular group or individual, and proclaiming that identity as a way of acceptance.

Management of Recommendations

Dependent offenders usually do not present particular management problems and can typically be expected to comply with simple requests. They are most likely to become problematic when they agree to violate behavior codes at the instigation of the more powerful person to whom they have attached themselves. Individuals with this pattern can be easily encouraged to join "group" dissension activities, particularly when such activities have a built-in level of anonymity. Verbal harassment of staff members, beating on cell doors to create disruptions, and similar activities are good examples of this kind of conduct. Such offenders can also be influenced into carrying contraband to protect the individual to whom that contraband belongs.

When such individuals attempt to become dependent on facility staff members, such as officers or mental health staffers, they are often identified as "snitches" by their peers and further ostracized. Although this pattern is commonly recognized by staffers and occasionally encouraged, it is a particularly destructive strategy for such offenders and usually leads to frequent bouts of Axis I syndromes, such as dysthymia or depression. Table 10.20 shows the number of MCMI-III profiles with elevated scores on the Dependent scale and the frequency with which these offenders scored high on the Axis I Clinical Syndrome Scales. As can be seen, offenders with elevations on the Dependent scale were significantly more likely than those without such elevations to be overrepresented on all of the Axis I scales. As a result, these same offenders were significantly more likely to be assessed as having high mental health needs, and significantly more likely to be given psychiatric diagnoses while incarcerated.

TABLE 10.19. COPD Violations for Dependent Profiles

Type of violation	No. of violations	% with this profile who did this	Chi-square signif.
Disobey	280	42.70%	0.818
Wontwork	109	16.60%	0.038
Drugs	93	14.20%	0.284
Verbabuse	90	13.70%	0.618
Fight	89	13.60%	0.659
Tattoo	82	12.50%	0.007
Assault	65	9.90%	0.232
Threats	50	7.60%	0.086
Escape	48	7.30%	0.618
Sxmiscon	26	4.00%	0.275

Note. See Table 10.3 for abbreviations.

Masochistic (Self-Defeating) Personality Disorder

Self-defeating or masochistic personality disorder is not formally identified in DSM-IV-TR, and there is controversy over the existence of this personality. Millon (1999) notes that the attempts to minimize controversy by renaming the disorder as "self-defeating" did little to change the problems associated with this syndrome, because all personality disorders are "self-defeating." His formulation of this disorder (Millon, 1999) emphasizes the passive coping strategy inherent in almost all historical descriptions of this personality. The critical feature, however, is a mixing or confusion of the usual pleasure-seeking drive with the pain avoidance. As a result, these individuals appear to create personal and social discomfort in their lives. Although it is often reported that they seem to feel comfortable only with guilt and shame, they

TABLE 10.20. Axis 1 Disorders for Dependent PD

Syndrome	Observed d	Expected	Chi-square signif.
Anxiety	1130	530.0	0.000
Somatoform	60	15.2	0.000
Bipolar: Manic	104	44.2	0.000
Dysthymia	688	208.8	0.000
Alc. Depend.	609	380.4	0.000
Drug Depend.	371	255.5	0.000
PTSD	280	84.9	0.000
Thought Dis.	84	20.1	0.000
Maj. Depres.	154	39.4	0.000
Delusional Dis.	59	25.5	0.000

are also believed to use their self-deprecation as a social strategy to gain support from others. This personality pattern seems to range from the culturally normal level of self-sacrificing behavior encouraged by many parts of our culture to people who display their failure and ruin at every turn.

This personality disorder shares many traits with depressive personality disorder, in that both masochistic and depressive individuals see themselves as relatively powerless, incapable, and unable to cope with the world. The person with depressive personality disorder, however, displays a passive resignation to his or her fate, while people with masochistic personality disorder seem to proclaim their problems almost proudly. It is also important to note that masochistic individuals seem to revel in a "victim" role, and will also resent and feel further victimized by others who exaggerate that role. They will resent those who add to the list or who judge their failures as exceeding the levels they personally acknowledge. In this way, they perpetuate the image of themselves as failures, but justify finding fault with others as well.

Manifestations in a Correctional Population

There were only 221 protocols in the Colorado study with a high-point code on the Masochistic scale of the MCMI-III. Of these, 16 (7.24%) had only the elevation on that one scale and were likely to exhibit the prototypal traits described above. The remainder exhibited a comorbid mix of traits with other personality disorders (see Table 10.21).

The most common comorbid pattern was with the Antisocial scale and occurred in 22.17% of the protocols where Masochistic was the high-point scale. Individuals with this pattern are likely to present with a resentful sense of victimization similar to, but much more passive than, what might be expected in negativistic personality disorder.

The second most common comorbid pattern was with the Depressive scale. This combination was the one most expected of those with masochistic personality disorder, and it tends to reflect the pessimism and sense of failure common to both disorders. The manipulative use of this presentation, however, will be somewhat different from the prototypal depressive personality.

The third most common comorbid pattern was a secondary elevation on the Schizoid scale. Individuals with this pattern are more likely to exhibit the withdrawal of the schizoid personality, coupled with the sense of failure of the masochistic personality.

TABLE 10.21. Comorbid Personality Patterns for Masochistic High-Point Profiles

Masoc only	8B + Schiz	8B + Avoid	8B + Depres	8B + Depend	8B + Histr	8B + Narcis	8B + Anti	8BA + Sadis	8B + Comp	8B + Neg
16	27	23	37	13	9	16	49	6	15	10
7.24%	12.22%	10.41%	16.74%	5.887%	4.07%	7.24%	22.17%	2.71%	6.79%	4.52%

Note. See Tables 10.2 and 10.4 for abbreviations.

Patterns of Institutional Offenses

In the Colorado sample, 516 (11.53%) had an elevation of 75 or more on the Masochistic scale of the MCMI-III. Inmates with an elevated score on this scale were significantly more likely to obtain disciplinary infractions for escape, refusal to work, and sexual misconduct than were inmates without an elevation on this scale. Escape is usually the charge for individuals who "walk away" from a facility, rather than those who aggressively "break out of jail," as in the movies; however, the offense carries similar high penalties. This increased risk is certainly consistent with the masochistic personality's characteristic pattern of choices that lead to punitive long-term consequences.

The significant relationship with sexual misconduct is also consistent with this personality disorder. This is particularly notable because, of the 31 offenders with an elevation on the Masochistic scale who were written up for sexual misconduct, 21 were males and 10 were females. However, the difference between high and low scorers on this scale was significant only for the males.

Management Recommendations

In the usually aggressive and active world of corrections, inmates with masochistic personality disorder face problems because of their tendency to elicit inappropriate behavior from others. In the "free" world, this strategy may have some adaptive value by eliciting sympathy from others, or at least by not stimulating competitive reactions. In a prison setting, however, such offenders are likely to be used by more predatory inmates as sources of distraction or excitement. These offenders are unlikely to actively resist any program or order; their style is clearly more acquiescent. Nevertheless, they will also elicit resentment from officers and abuse from other offenders.

Histrionic Personality Disorder

Histrionic personality disorder is one of the "big three" disorders common in correctional environments, along with narcissistic and antisocial personality disorders. The essential feature of persons with this disorder is the creation of a coping strategy for life that focuses on having their needs met by others. They do this by reacting to those others in such a manner that the others choose to give them what they want. This strategy requires histrionic individuals to be particularly adept at understanding the feelings and needs of others, and able to create the proper social responses to make themselves desirable to and trusted by the other persons. This disorder is "seductive" in almost all senses of the word; these individuals have exceptional skills at insinuating themselves into the lives of those around them in a way that makes it "reasonable" for those other people to respond in a supportive and nurturant way.

In general, these individuals exhibit high levels of energy, which at times can become hypomanic in intensity. They are powerfully oriented toward others and define themselves and the world in general in terms of the social relationships they experience. This strong other-directedness is accompanied by a lack of insight into themselves or their own feelings. They will tend to have difficulty concentrating and will prefer the awareness of social dynamics to any logical or structured approach to problem solving.

Although histrionic individuals are aware of the emotions and other motivational factors in others, they tend to be unaware of most of their own drives and to lack empathy for others. They have intense needs for attention and adulation from others, and will go to great lengths to be the center of attention. This individuals will almost always be viewed as charming and pleasant, at least on initial meeting. Their flair for the dramatic will often present as emotional lability and will often be seen as "overreactive." Their high need for excitement will often place them in the company of more antisocial personalities who more actively pursue that excitement.

Manifestations in a Correctional Population

There were 985 profiles in the Colorado sample with a high-point code on the Histrionic scale of the MCMI-III. Of these, 141 or 14.31% had only the elevation on the Histrionic scale (see Table 10.22). The remainder demonstrated comorbid relations with significant elevations on at least one other scale.

The most common comorbid pattern for profiles with a Histrionic high-point code was with the Narcissistic scale. This is the pattern identified by Millon (1999) as the "vivacious" subtype of histrionic personality. These energetic and outgoing individuals will evidence high apparent self-esteem and will be distressed by any event that might challenge this self-esteem. They will often be seen as overly cheerful and exhibit primitive denial patterns when confronted with unpleasant experiences. They will be "flighty" and undependable in social relationships, and will frequently generate brief, intense relationships that fall apart as the individuals move on to new needs and associates.

The second most common of the comorbid patterns was with the Compulsive scale. This pattern occurred in 21.62% of the profiles with a Histrionic high-point code. Such offenders will tend to emphasize structured expectations for others, in addition to the socially manipulative qualities of the histrionic personality. Although predominantly histrionic in nature, these offenders will show high expectations for others to perform as expected, and will have intense emotional reactions to the failure of others to act out their assigned script. They will also tend to be more rigid and unable to adapt to variations in the responses of others.

The Colorado offender sample also had a strong representation of the comorbid Antisocial pattern, which made up 18.88% of the Histrionic high-point profiles. This

TABLE 10.22. Comorbid Personality Patterns for Histrionic High-Point Profiles

Histr only	4 + Schiz	4 + Avoid	4 + Depres	4 + Depend	4 + Narcis	4 + Anti	4 + Sadis	4 + Comp	4 + Neg	4 + Masoc
141	4	1	27	23	346	186	20	213	10	14
14.31%	0.41%	0.10%	2.74%	2.34%	35.13%	18.88%	2.03%	21.62%	1.02%	1.42%

Note. See Tables 10.2 and 10.4 for abbreviations.

profile has been identified by Millon (1999) as the "disingenuous" subtype of histrionic personality. This particular subtype will display somewhat less of the seductive quality of the prototypal histrionic personality, and more of the cunning, manipulative, and scheming qualities.

As was noted for some of the earlier personality profiles, the Histrionic high-point profiles included relatively few comorbidities with the Avoidant, Depressive, Dependent, and Schizoid scales. This was particularly true of the Schizoid and Avoidant scales, which were elevated less than 1% of the time in Histrionic high-point profiles.

Patterns of Institutional Offenses

Of this subsample, 600 (13.41%) had an elevation of 75 or more on the Histrionic scale of the MCMI-III. Data for these offenders are presented in Table 10.23. Inmates with an elevation on this scale were not significantly more likely than inmates without such an elevation to be charged with any of the indexed disciplinary infractions.

Severe Personality Disorders

Whereas the basic personality disorders are seen as extensions of normal personality processes that have become self-defeating and self-perpetuating, the severe personality disorders represent even more disorganized and maladaptive social strategies. Severity of personality disorders is not an element of the DSM-IV-TR schema and is derived from the theorizing of Millon and others. In particular, the model of severe structural disorganization of personality presented by Millon and Everly (1985) has considerable applicability to correctional psychology and is utilized here.

TABLE 10.23. COPD Violations for Histrionic Profiles

Type of violation	No. of violations	% with this profile who did this	Chi-square signif.
Disobey	245	40.80%	0.23
Drugs	109	18.20%	0.06
Wontwork	96	16.00%	0.132
Verbabuse	89	14.80%	0.716
Fight	65	10.80%	0.086
Tattoo	56	9.30%	0.789
Escape	49	8.20%	0.174
Threats	45	7.50%	0.082
Assault	42	7.00%	0.113
Sxmiscon	21	3.50%	0.726

Note. See Table 10.3 for abbreviations.

Each of the three severe patterns to be considered here represents the extreme end of a behavioral continuum that flows from the normal manifestations of personality traits through the basic personality disorders and into these most deteriorated patterns. Each of the patterns discussed here sits on the logical border between the poor life management strategies of the basic personality disorders, and distortions so severe as to fall into the psychotic realm of Axis I disorders. Indeed, one of the most troublesome aspects of these patterns for clinicians is the difficulty of determining when the "strangeness" of the severe personality disorders gives way to fundamentally psychotic disorganization.

Schizotypal Personality Disorder

Schizotypal personality disorder is a severe personality disorder that in many ways appears to be a subclinical expression of schizophrenia. The major observable characteristic of individuals with this disorder is the general sense of "oddness" that permeates their lives. In most major spheres of life, these individuals are "not quite bad enough for a diagnosis," but their thought and behavior are clearly outside the commonly expected range. The dominant feature of schizotypal personality disorder is a profound quality of social and self-alienation. In this sense, this disorder shares some features with avoidant and schizoid personality disorders and is thought to represent a more structurally defective or deteriorated version of these other disorders. Schizotypal individuals will certainly have an impaired social life and unusual quality of thinking, which can also be seen in persons with these less severe disorders. There seems to be a powerful self-perpetuating quality to schizotypal personality disorder: These individuals' profound social isolation results in increasing reliance on their own internal perceptions and beliefs, which do not have the chance to be measured against external norms and therefore become increasingly skewed from conventional beliefs without the self-correcting advantage of normal social relationships. These persons will manifest eccentric or idiosyncratic beliefs that are not shared by their general subculture and that frequently have a strong "magical" quality to them. They will usually appear to be "out of step" with those around them, and their behavior is just far enough away from social expectations to make others feel uncomfortable.

Manifestations in a Correctional Population

In the Colorado sample, 312 or 3.30% obtained a high-point code on the Schizotypal scale of the MCMI-III. This would suggest that schizotypal individuals are more frequently found in a correctional system than in the population at large. Of these offenders, all had elevations on other MCMI-III scales as well. Over half of these offenders had at least five of the basic personality disorder scales elevated, and 93.3% had three or more scales elevated. It is clear from these data that when the Schizotypal scale is elevated, many other problems exist as well. This does not mean that such individuals will have diagnoses in these other areas as well. Rather, it shows that the problems associated with the basic personality disorders are frequently manifested in schizotypal individuals, and that the severe schizotypal diagnosis will supersede most of the alternative diagnoses.

Patterns of Institutional Offenses

There were 312 (3.3%) offenders who had an elevation of 75 or more on the Schizotypal scale of the MCMI-III. This small, but distressed and distressing, group of offenders showed no remarkable propensity to commit or avoid most disciplinary offenses. The exceptions to this were in the two cases of threats from the females with an elevated Schizotypal scale and the greater rate of verbal abuse charges in the males with an elevation on this scale. Because of the very small number of cases, it is not clear that these findings would be replicated in subsequent studies.

Management Recommendations

Individuals with an elevation on the Schizotypal scale at the time of intake represent a high risk for needing clinical services throughout their period of incarceration. These individuals are significantly more likely to have clinical histories at the time of intake, which results in their being identified as having higher psychiatric needs. They are also significantly more likely to be given psychiatric diagnoses during their incarceration. Their "oddball" social behavior is unlikely to be tolerated as well by other inmates as it is in life outside prison, and they are also more likely to attract the predatory interest of other inmates.

Like inmates with several of the less severe disorders, these offenders will do best in circumstances in which demands for social behavior are relatively low, and their ability to avoid others with whom they have a risk of conflict is high. Typically, prison is not structured to produce such an environment. As a result, offenders with this profile are at increased risk of acting out in clinically significant ways, to attempt to cope with the demands of prison life in a general population setting. There is a high risk that many of these offenders will be identified as "malingering" because of these efforts. With this group, a more careful assessment is likely to reveal the more profound underlying personality disorder, and steps can be taken to intervene before the individuals decompensate into a psychiatric crisis.

Borderline Personality Disorder

The construct of "borderline personality disorder" suffers from a naming problem that has yet to be resolved. Originally conceived as a pathology falling "on the borderline" between psychosis and neurosis, the disorder to date has failed to acquire a name that adequately reflects the diverse symptom presentations included under the clinical definition. It is not yet even clear that this represents a single coherent symptom pattern that can be expected to respond in a consistent way to etiological development or treatment.

Regardless of the as yet unintegrated research literature on this disorder, several characteristic features dominate the symptom pattern. Of these, perhaps the most profound are the powerful dependence and fear of rejection that permeate the social relations of those with borderline personalities. They attempt to form tenacious attachments to the few individuals in their lives, and then follow an extreme pattern of elation and distress as these emotionally vital relationships are periodically confirmed and disconfirmed. This confirmation is often through "testing" to make sure that the other persons will be there the borderline individuals are being unlovable. This gives rise to the common characterization of borderline behavior as "I hate you, don't leave me."

Another characteristic of borderline personality disorder is a propensity for perceptual extremes. Particularly in their social relationships, these individuals tend to see the world as wonderful when their attachments are confirmed and to see the world as dismal when they believe they have been abandoned. Their moods during these times appear congruent with their social perceptions: They are elated when they feel safely attached, and in profound despair when they see themselves as abandoned. Because both states are overgeneralizations of momentary experience, they can exhibit the third cardinal feature of borderline personality disorder, which is rapid mood swings. It is common for persons who expressed delight that their lives were better than ever just a short while ago to present as in total despair when seen again.

Although the general characteristics of borderline personality disorder described above are more than sufficient to create misery for these individuals and for those around them, the most significant problem associated with this disorder is the very high rate of self-harming behavior. In the Colorado sample, offenders with an elevated score on the Borderline scale of the MCMI-III were significantly more likely to be rated as having self-injury risk at the time of intake than were offenders without an elevation on that scale. Since this rating is based almost entirely on history of self-harming behavior or expressions of current suicidal thoughts, it provides powerful evidence of the chronic nature of these issues over time. It is estimated that the rate of completed suicides in individuals with borderline personality disorder is about 8–10% (Association d'Aide aux Personnes avec un "État Limité" [AAPEL], 2003).

These offenders are often known as "cutters" within prison settings and are generally viewed by clinicians as among the most difficult of all people to treat. Most individuals with borderline personality disorder do not commit suicide, but the risk is higher than for any other personality disorder. This risk can never be ignored and must be included in the treatment plan. The more frequent issue, however, is the prevalence of "parasuicidal" behavior. Parasuicidal behavior involves an action usually associated with suicide, but exhibited at a level that is likely to be nonlethal. An example of parasuicidal behavior would betaking a fingernail or other sharp object and digging or cutting at the skin until it bleeds. Another example would be fabricating a noose, placing it around one's neck, and then waiting to be discovered by others who can intervene.

Sometimes the parasuicidal behavior in an offender with borderline personality disorder is driven entirely by internal needs and is not intended to elicit any particular response from others. Often the pain associated with cutting oneself is the goal in itself. The pain can be understood as inflicting punishment on oneself for bad behavior, as creating an external distraction from the emotional pain being experienced, or sometimes as just establishing or confirming one's continued existence. At other times, the behavior is designed to influence the responses or perceptions of others. Forcing an important person to rescue one from self-destruction, for example, can be a profound confirmation of the continuing existence of a needed relationship.

Manifestations in a Correctional Population

There were 614 profiles in the Colorado study with a high-point code on the border-line scale of the MCMI-III. Of these, there was only 1 profile that had no other eleva-tions. The remainder had additional elevations on many of the other MCMI-III scales. Three-quarters of all profiles with an elevation on the Borderline scale also had an elevation on the Negativistic scale. About two-thirds also had elevations on the Avoidant, Depressive, and Antisocial scales.

Patterns of Institutional Offenses

There were 354 (7.91%) profiles in the Colorado sample that had an elevation of 75 or more on the Borderline scale of the MCMI-III. These offenders were significantly more likely than offenders without such an elevation to be charged with disobeying a lawful order, refusal to work, tattooing, and sexual misconduct. The tattooing and sexual misconduct offenses can easily be seen as congruent with the offenders' efforts to form and retain some significant relationship. The other two categories of viola-tions are high-base-rate offenses in general. It is not apparent how they fit into the pathological coping patterns of borderline personality disorder, but they are likely to result from a number of dynamics, including the depressive withdrawal and despair during a period of perceived rejection.

Management Recommendations

Effective management of this complex and difficult group of offenders requires care-ful coordination between a correctional facility's clinical services and other opera-tions. It is not reasonable to attempt to suppress the self-injurious behavior itself through increasingly severe restraint and punitive sanctions. The common misunder-standing that "They are just doing it for attention" is usually incorrect and mislead-ing. Treating this self-harming activity merely as a disruptive behavior that is entirely volitional in nature and motivated by simple social attention as a goal will seldom remove the risk of further self-harm.

A carefully crafted multidisciplinary management plan needs to be developed that includes the major operations staff, such as line officers and case managers, along with the mental health staff. This program must include carefully structured contingencies that provide regular access to a stable relationship with a staff person, very clear and consistent contingencies on self-harming or disruptive behaviors, and short-term consequences for those behaviors that permit a rapid return to the main plan. It is reasonable, for example, to establish a contingency that a therapist will not directly respond to an offender while the offender is in seclusion or observation for a recent self-injurious behavior, and that the observational interactions will be made by a different clinical staff member. This same consequence becomes inappropriate when the time in seclusion exceeds more than a few days. Extended consequences may fit the punitive scheme for the disciplinary process, but will not effectively alter this form of behavior.

The essence of an effective plan will center on an offender's being able to main-tain a close relationship with an important individual during periods in which behav-ior is appropriate, and the short-term loss of such a relationship when the offender misbehaves. The treatment program recommended by such authors as Linehan (1993) includes a therapeutic balance (dialectic) between acceptance and understanding of the borderline individual on the one hand, and maintaining a requirement for change on the other. Such programs require a much greater commitment of clinical time than is typically provided to offenders with most other disorders. It becomes cost-effective only when we consider the immense response required of a system when an offender plays the self-harm "trump card." When an offender threatens or actually commits self-harm, there is a clear legal responsibility on the part of all correctional facilities to respond with effective intervention strategies. Almost all systems now have "suicide protocols" that must be put into effect when an offender poses a credible threat or engaged in actual self-injury. This response almost always requires immediate action from correctional staff, as well as notification of responsible mental health staff, who must determine the level of additional action required. Frequently this episode will also require some special housing, transportation to a more suitable facility, and/or intervention by medical services.

Paranoid Personality Disorder

Paranoid personality disorder is marked by a distrust of others and the belief that the world is a malignant place that poses constant risks. Tied to this perception is these individuals' most basic fear that they will lose their ability to determine or control their lives. In response to these perceptions, such individuals limit their relations with others and often take preemptive steps to protect themselves from the evil they expect from others. Their expectation of a hostile world often leads them to misinterpret the intent and motives of others. This personality disorder is characterized by a rigidity that makes it difficult for individuals to alter mistaken beliefs even in the face of overwhelming contrary evidence. They tend to have a disagreeable social nature that leaves them isolated and perpetuates the sense of conflict. They refuse to adapt to the world as commonly perceived, and instead reconstruct their internal representation of the world to remain consistent with their expectations. Millon (1999) suggests that paranoid personality disorder may develop from the collapse of any of several basic personality disorders. In particular, there is a tendency for the narcissistic, avoidant, compulsive, sadistic, or negativistic personality pattern to devolve into a paranoid pattern after enough stress and failure.

It should be noted that paranoid thinking is a common outcome of many human disorders in which the world becomes less predictable or understandable. It is often found, for example, in individuals who have an insidious loss of hearing. As these people struggle with trying to interpolate meaning from increasingly sparse bits of data, it is easy to believe that other people are becoming untruthful or deceitful.

Manifestations in a Correctional Population

Of the 634 offenders with a high-point code or more on the Paranoid scale of the MCMI-III, only 3 had no elevations on any of the basic personality disorder scales. Of this same group, 231 had an elevation on at least one of the other severe personality disorder scales, 548 had elevations on at least one of the basic Axis I clinical scales, and 195 had an elevation on one of the severe clinical scales. All of this is consistent with common clinical beliefs that this disorder is severe and represents the presence of a wide range of other pathological qualities.

Patterns of Institutional Offenses

In the Colorado sample, there were 343 (7.67%) offenders who had an elevation of 75 or more on the Paranoid scale of the MCMI-III. This severe personality disorder was not differentially associated with any of the indexed disciplinary infractions except for assault: Offenders with an elevation on the Paranoid scale were significantly more likely to be charged with this disciplinary infraction than those who did not have an elevation on this scale.

Management Recommendations

Given the severe and pervasive nature of paranoid personality disorder, offenders with this disorder are likely to be seen as particularly difficult inmates by correctional officers. Even if these offenders do not overtly misbehave, their pervasive belief that staff members will be bad, evil, and malicious is likely to offend even the most patient staffers. Their "porcupine" personality is likely to feed into a social cycle of less adequate responses from staff members, which will in turn serve to strengthen the paranoid beliefs and produce more defective social encounters.

Even though staff members are likely to believe that paranoid offenders would "test the patience of a saint," it is essential for staffers to understand the self-perpetuating quality of the social interactions involving such offenders and the importance of limited, objective, and professional behavior. These are offenders for whom the best response is a matter-of-fact presentation of all information and requests. The skills taught in the book *Verbal Judo* (Thompson & Jenkins, 1993) are particularly important for this population. Staff members must get done what needs to be done and remove themselves from encounters with these inmates without accepting the many offers for conflict. For offenders with paranoid personality disorder—like those with the antisocial, sadistic, narcissistic, and compulsive patterns from which the paranoid pattern derives—verbal engagement by staff members provides an important opportunity to escalate personal and social dominance issues into a win–lose conflict. If an offender gives a war and staff members do not choose to come, the facility wins. The other critical features for this group of offenders are identification and careful monitoring by clinical services. Even though they are more likely than not to believe that mental health services are part of a government conspiracy or other sinister plot, it is important for at least collateral information on the offenders' adjustment to be obtained on a regular basis. This permits earlier intervention, should these individuals begin to exhibit more serious decompensation.

Gender and Personality

Gender Differences in Manifestations in a Clinical Population

In the Colorado study, there were MCMI-III profiles on 9,468 offenders. Of these, 8,574 profiles were obtained from male offenders and 894 (9.44%) from female offenders. These figures are consistent with other measures of gender proportions in Colorado and other state correctional systems. A chi-square analysis of the data shows that there were significant gender differences on all MCMI-III personality scales except the Dependent scale (see Table 10.24).

Proportionally, females obtained elevated scores on the Schizoid scale significantly more often than did males. The traits described in the section on schizoid personality disorder will be found more often in female facilities than in male facilities. These women will usually be socially isolated and withdrawn, and will particularly show emotional isolation from others.

Female offenders obtained elevations on the Avoidant scale significantly less often than did males. The pattern of making life choices on the basis of the option that is least likely to produce an immediate experience of stress will occur less frequently in female facilities than in male facilities. There will be fewer females who will tend to avoid social situations largely because stress is most often experienced in the company of other people.

Females were also less likely than males to show significant elevations on the Depressive scale. There will be fewer women with this pattern of personal inadequacy and impaired self-esteem. This particular result is counterintuitive, because there is a common observation in female facilities of high frequencies of low self-esteem. It suggests that there are other dynamics involved in this process, such as perhaps an ego-dystonic component to these perceptions of inadequacy, because they derive from a distorted perceptions of the world and deviant efforts to cope with those distorted perceptions.

TABLE 10.24. Frequency of Elevations above 75 on the MCMI-III by Gender

Scale	Male	Female	Scale	Male	Female
Schizoid			Antisocial		
Count	952	148	Count	2,461	298
Expected	996.1	103.9	Expected	2,498.5	260.5
Avoidant			Sadistic		
Count	2,248	92	Count	1,496	295
Expected	2,119.0	221.0	Expected	1,621.9	169.1
Depressive			Compulsive		
Count	1,595	124	Count	403	162
Expected	1,556.7	162.3	Expected	511.7	63.3
Dependent			Negativistic		
Count	1,276	125	Count	1,871	137
Expected	1,268.7	132.3	Expected	1,818.4	189.6
Histrionic			Masochistic		
Count	888	361	Count	882	204
Expected	113.1	117.9	Expected	983.5	102.5
Narcissistic					
Count	1,715	248			
Expected	1,777.6	185.4			

There were no significant gender differences noted in the occurrence of elevations on the Dependent scale, as noted above.

Consistent with stereotypes and other literature, female offenders were significantly more likely to have elevations on the Histrionic scale. This suggests that, at least for females who get sentenced to prison, the essential histrionic coping strategy is more often effective and adopted than for males. As noted in the earlier section on this disorder, this coping strategy focuses on getting personal needs met by reacting to others in such a manner that the others choose to respond in a supportive and nurturant way. The fact that this quality is more often defined as acceptably "feminine" in our culture undoubtedly contributes to the frequency of this disorder in female offenders. These women are powerfully oriented toward others and define themselves and their world in terms of the social relationships they experience. This quality is almost always noted as characteristic of the social "mix" in female facilities. These women will also exhibit the lack of insight, difficulty concentrating, avoidance of any logical or structured approach to problem solving, and lack of empathy described in the earlier discussion.

Women were also significantly more likely to have elevated scores on the Narcissistic scale of the MCMI-III. These women will have an exaggerated sense of self-worth, a profound assumption that the rest of the world can and does have the same interest in them as they do, and other characteristics described in the section on narcissistic personality disorder.

Another surprising result of the Colorado study was that female offenders obtained elevated scores on the patterns of personality most associated with aggressive behavior. In particular, the Antisocial scale was elevated significantly more often than in males. This should not be interpreted as suggesting that women in general are more likely to have this disorder. Rather, it suggests that the women who have this disorder are the ones who are more likely to commit serious enough offenses to result in incarceration, in spite of gender bias against female incarceration. These women will be most powerfully characterized by their need for social dominance. They will seek to dominate those people with whom, and situations in which, they interact, and will tend to pursue such a goal even when it is likely to be self-destructive or contrary to their best interests. They have little flexibility in adopting a cooperative or subservient role except as a temporary expedient in their long-term quest for ascendancy. These women will also be marked by significant difficulty in learning from adverse experience, and will not respond well to control and management strategies based on punitive consequences for behavior. Finally, like antisocial men, antisocial women will show a much-increased need for external stimulation and excitement in their lives. They will regularly be seen as parties to the chaos and uproar of life in the general prison population.

Female offenders were also proportionately more likely than males to have elevations on the Sadistic scale. The essence of this inherently aggressive and usually violent personality is the pattern of actively inflicting pain on others. Particularly among female offenders, this infrequent pattern is likely to be reflected in the use of verbal skills to inflict emotional pain on those around them, rather than relying only on physical abuse. These women will utilize the infliction of pain as the primary method of social control and will employ it in most social environments. The infliction of pain on others will become a goal in itself and can be maintained far beyond what would be required to obtain an external goal.

On the more positive side, there were also significantly more females than males who had elevations on the Compulsive scale. As noted in the section on compulsive personality disorder, these women will be "torn between their leanings toward submissive dependence on the one hand and defiant autonomy on the other" (Millon, 1999, p. 524). These women will display an exceptional need to impose structure and regularity on all aspects of their lives, and will exhibit the other characteristics described in the earlier section.

Proportionally, females obtained elevated scores on the Negativistic scale significantly less often than did males.

Finally, proportionally, females obtained elevated scores on the Masochistic scale significantly more often than did males.

The relationships of gender and several personality variables are shown in Figure 10.3. In this graph, we see the average values for the Antisocial, Sadistic, Histrionic, and Narcissistic scales of the MCMI-III. The mean values obtained by the females in this sample were clearly higher than those obtained by males on all but the Antisocial scale.

Gender Differences in Patterns of Institutional Offenses

In the Colorado study, females had significantly fewer disciplinary charges than males for tattooing, making threats, verbal abuse, fights, and disobeying a lawful order (see Figure 10.4). Most of these behaviors reflect aggressive social behaviors that are more closely associated with male roles in our culture.

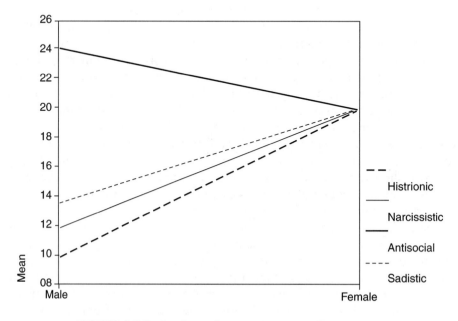

FIGURE 10.3. Gender and aggressive personality patterns.

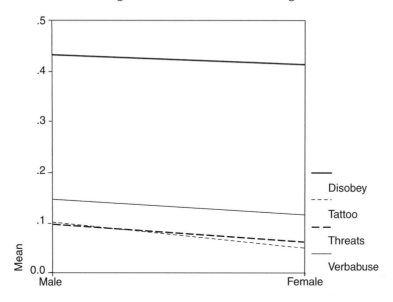

FIGURE 10.4. Less frequent disciplinary charges among women. (See Table 10.3 for abbreviations.)

On the other hand, the female offenders had signiicantly more charges than the males for attempted escapes, refusal to work, sexual misconduct, abuse of drugs, and assault (see Figure 10.5). With the exception of the charges of assault, most of these charges may be incurred through somewhat more passive resistance to the rules of a facility. We tend to think of escape, for example, in terms of the exciting scenes from action movies, but in the real world of corrections, that almost never happens. What does happen is that an offender will walk away from a minimum-security center or fail to appear for appointments while on parole.

Conclusions

In many ways, the correctional system serves as a laboratory for the study and management of personality disorders. This system is confronted with the multiple challenges of a society dealing with individuals who violate the standards and rules we impose upon ourselves. It is challenged with the management of individuals who have not conformed their behavior to social rules and expectations. Corrections officers are also challenged to make their management strategies in their care of these incarcerated individuals conform to the values that the rest of society holds to be important in the management of other human beings. This effort is further challenged by the value society places on these efforts, as defined by the various legislative bodies that provide the funds for these efforts.

It is in this context that we can begin to understand the importance of our growing knowledge of personality patterns and disorders. Our slowly growing understanding of the similarities and differences between offenders and the rest of society

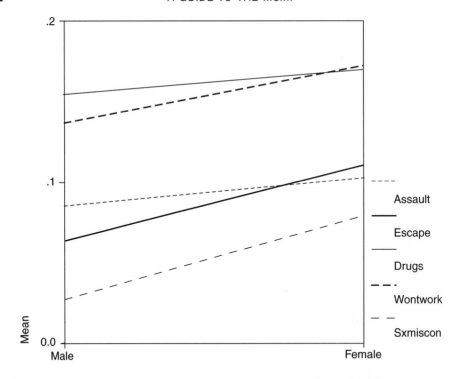

FIGURE 10.5. More frequent disciplinary charges among women. (See Table 10.3 for abbreviations.)

is helping us focus our efforts at more humane and effective management of offenders while in prison, and will ultimately help us develop strategies that will permit more effective reintegration of these individuals into free society. It is only when we begin to understand the differences in offenders' perceptions and motivations that we can begin to design management systems that will compensate for these differences and minimize the social distress that they produce. As a group, these individuals present significant differences from unincarcerated society in their perception of social rules and the need to conform to them. Even more important, this "group" is much less homogeneous than was previously thought. The old correctional philosophies assumed that one basic highly structured environment was the proper way to manage "the group" of offenders. We now see that there are many different types of individuals in a correctional environment, and that the management strategies most appropriate for one type will often be detrimental to others. Utilizing the correctional "laboratory" to define these differences more clearly is crucial to the ultimate mission of the criminal justice system.

References

American Psychiatric Association. (2000). *Diagnostic and statistical manual of mental disorders* (4th ed., text rev.). Washington, DC: Author.

Association d'Aide aux Personnes avec un "État Limité" (AAPEL). (2003). *The borderline personality disorder and suicide*. Retrieved from *www.aapel.org/bdp/BlsuicideUS.html*

Bushman, B., & Baumeister, D. (2002). Threatened egotism, narcissism, self-esteem, and direct and misplaced aggression: Does self-love or self-hate lead to violence? *Journal of Personality and Social Psychology, 75*(1).

Cleckley, H. (1976). *The mask of sanity* (5th ed.). St. Louis, MO: Mosby.

Dutton, D., & Hart, S. (1996). Risk markers for family violence in a federally incarcerated population. *Forum of Correctional Research, 5*(2). Retrieved from *www.csc-scc.gc.ca/text/pblct/forum/e052/e052i_e.shtml*

Hare, R. D. (1993). *Without conscience: The disturbing world of the psychopaths among us.* New York: Simon & Schuster (Pocket Books).

Kleinsasser, D., Stoner, J., & Retzlaff, P. (2000, November). *Differential treatment and monitoring of sex offenders.* Paper presented at the 19th Annual Conference of the Association for the Treatment of Sexual Abusers, San Diego, CA.

Linehan, M. M. (1993). *Cognitive-behavioral treatment of borderline personality disorder.* New York: Guilford Press.

Millon, T., & Davis, R. (1996). *Disorders of personality: DSM-IV and beyond.* New York: Wiley.

Millon, T., & Everly, G., Jr. (1985). *Personality and its disorders: A biosocial learning approach.* New York: Wiley.

Millon, T. (with Grossman, S., Meagher, S., Millon, C., & Everly, G.). (1999). *Personality-guided therapy.* New York: Wiley.

Retzlaff, P., Stoner, J., & Kleinsasser, D. (2002). The use of the MCMI-III in the screening and triage of offenders. *International Journal of Offender Therapy and Comparative Criminology.*

Seligman, M. E. P., Maier, S. F., & Geer, J. (1968). The alleviation of learned helplessness in dogs. *Journal of Abnormal Psychology, 73,* 256–262.

Stone, M. H. (1993). *Abnormalities of personality, within and beyond the realm of treatment.* New York: Norton.

Thompson, G. J., & Jenkins, J. B. (1993). *Verbal judo: The gentle art of persuasion.*

Twenge, J., & Campbell, W. K. (2003). "Isn't it fun to get the respect that we're going to deserve?": Narcissism, social rejection, and aggression. *Personality and Social Psychology Bulletin, 29,* 261–272.

CHAPTER 11

Using the MCMI-III in Neuropsychological Evaluations

Sally L. Kolitz Russell
Elbert W. Russell

Objective measures of affective conditions—that is, the personality and emotional status of an individual—make an indispensable contribution to any neuropsychological examination. The Millon Clinical Multiaxial Inventory–III (MCMI-III) provides such a contribution with its relationship to the *Diagnostic and Statistical Manual of Mental Disorders*, fourth edition (DSM-IV), and its text revision, DSM-IV-TR. It also provides the best measure of personality characteristics, as well as examination of types of psychopathology. Although such objective measures of personality are neither designed nor intended to be methods of assessing neurological conditions, they are necessary to identify or rule out a number of affective conditions that may interfere with an accurate neuropsychological evaluation. They are also necessary to assess emotional reactions to the psychological trauma of brain damage.

The Purposes of the Neuropsychological Evaluation

Neuropsychological assessment examines the functioning of the whole brain. The affective and personality components are as much a part of brain functioning as is cognition. Nevertheless, as usually constituted, a neuropsychological examination is primarily composed of cognitive measures. Brain damage tends to impair cognitive abilities in a more direct and obvious manner than it does affective functions. Nevertheless, affect and personality are related to brain pathology both directly and indirectly. Consequently, affective components must be assessed.

Related to this somewhat theoretical reason for utilizing affective tests in a neuropsychological examination, there are practical issues that require the use of such tests. A neuropsychological assessment is usually conducted for the purpose of determining the status of an individual's brain functioning with reference to various neuropathological conditions. Prior to the advent of computerized tomography (CT) and magnetic resonance imaging (MRI), ascertaining diagnosis and localization were the major reasons for a neuropsychological examination. There are certain conditions that still require such information—for instance, mild to moderate head trauma and dementia of the Alzheimer's type.

At present, however, neuropsychological assessment makes its major contribution by providing information concerning a patient's brain functioning in regard to many psychological conditions. Such information is essential for rehabilitation, vocational/educational planning, disability ratings, forensic compensation in personal injury cases, and differential diagnosis between neurological and psychiatric conditions. Indeed, such contributions require affective assessment even more than earlier neuropsychological examinations.

Therefore, for all of these reasons, any neuropsychological assessment is incomplete without a thorough affective evaluation. No matter how accurate the measures of cognition may be in the neuropsychological evaluation, if any substantial impairment is primarily the result of an emotional problem, the cognitive evaluation is useless. No neuropsychological evaluation is valid without an accurate measure of emotional and personality functioning, including effort testing. Yet it is disturbing how often a neuropsychological report does not include objective affective tests.

The Affective Examination

In order to evaluate the affective aspects of a neuropsychological condition, the examiner must understand the relationships between neuropsychological test results and measures of affective conditions. The MCMI-III is a battery of scales that provides objective information concerning affective conditions, both personality and psychopathology.

Problems with Alternatives to Objective Affective Testing

Although objective tests provide public, verifiable information concerning the affective aspects of neuropsychological disorders, there are many neuropsychologists who discount objective testing. While Lezak, Howieson, and Loring (2004) state that evaluating the affective status of a neuropsychological patient is important (p. 738), they are highly critical of objective affective tests. In the place of objective tests, Lezak et al. (2004) advocate the use of either an interview involving clinical judgment or a self-report questionnaire to assess the emotional condition of a neuropsychological patient.

Clinical Judgment

Clinical judgment involves the use of informal inferences to make assessments. The inferences may be drawn from an interview, from test scores, or simply from observation of the patient's behavior. On the basis of personal training and experience, the neuropsychologist decides that the person has a particular affective condition.

The primary problems with clinical judgment are its reliability and validity. The whole area of clinical judgment has been examined by Garb (1998), who found that such judgment, particularly outside the field of neuropsychology, was generally quite inaccurate. However, the more formalized and structured was the information on which the judgment was based, the more accurate it was. Use of the criteria supplied by the DSM-III increased reliability (Garb, 1998, pp. 41–44) and validity (pp. 82–83). In general, presumed expertise, including that indicated by diplomate status (p. 244), and experience beyond graduate-level training are not related to diagnostic accuracy (pp. 14–17, 55–57). A more extensive discussion of clinical judgment is beyond the scope of this chapter, but may be found in Garb's (1998) book.

Self-Report Scales

As another alternative to the use of an objective inventory, Lezak et al. (2004) support the use of self-report scales. However, these authors deem even self-report questionnaire general scores useless, as this statement indicates: "As summary scores obscure the pattern of responses to individual scales, they do not constitute data on which the reasonableness of a response pattern should be judged" (p. 754). They apparently do not realize that scales are summaries of items.

Self-reports may be quite inaccurate, particularly in forensic patients. Reitan and Wolfson (1997) have thoroughly reviewed this situation, particularly in regard to head trauma. It was found that subjects without formal medical training knew the general symptoms related to various kinds of organic conditions. In addition, such self-report questionnaires are quite transparent. Consequently, if a person answering such a questionnaire has anything to gain from certain answers to questions, the accuracy of the instrument may be severely compromised; again, this is a particular possibility in forensic cases. As Reitan and Wolfson (1997) have put it, "personal complaints scarcely serve as a valid or reliable basis for assessing after effects of mild head injury" (p. 11).

Utility of Objective Tests

Objective tests are created through a standardization process that formalizes the scores and the specific interpretation. As such, they can be directly validated.

Formal Assessment Methods

The advantage of formal methods is that they permit the objective psychometric procedures of science to be applied directly to the test items and test measures. Thus, in contrast to clinical judgment and other forms of subjective evaluation, formal methods derive interpretive information directly from test scores or the mathematical and/or logical analysis of combinations and comparisons of test scores. Formal methods provide numerical scores that have well-defined meanings.

In contrast to self-report questionnaires, objective tests are composed of items that are much less transparent. In addition, there are validity scales designed to measure the veracity of the patient's answers. Such tests provide objective relatively nontransparent validated measures of various pathological affective conditions. They bring to affective measurement the objectivity and accuracy that formal tests have brought to neuropsychological assessment.

Criticism of Objective Inventories

Although Lezak et al. (2004) direct their critique of objective tests to the Minnesota Multiphasic Personality Inventory (MMPI), their judgment applies to all objective affective inventories. Their chief objection is summarized as follows:

> These scales have all been evaluated for their effectiveness in discriminating between various brain injured and psychiatric patient groups. None reached a level of accuracy that would permit clinical judgments. With the increasingly common use of imaging combined with appropriate neuropsychological evaluations, neurodiagnostic applications of the MMPI have become irrelevant. (p. 750)

It is not clear what imaging has to do with the validity of the MMPI or any other affective inventory. However, the accuracy of the MMPI-2 in regard to neuropsychological diagnosis was thoroughly examined by Gass (2006, pp. 301–325), and it was found to be quite accurate when utilized correctly.

The primary difficulty with Lezak et al's. (2004) criticism is that apparently they are stating that objective affective tests do not diagnose the existence and types of brain damage with much accuracy. This demonstrates how little they understand the ways in which affective inventories are utilized in neuropsychological assessment. The authors apparently conceive of affective tests only in terms of their ability to diagnose brain damage. This type of evaluation was never the intention of these inventories. Neither the MMPI-2 or the MCMI-III is designed to be a measure of brain damage, although they may be utilized (as will be discussed) to separate certain affective conditions from the effects of brain damage.

Nowhere is this more evident than in regard to schizophrenia. The most recent version of the Lezak reference manual (Lezak et al., 2004, pp. 748–750), in contrast to the previous one (Lezak, 1995, pp. 784–785), completely avoids discussing the accuracy of the MMPI in discriminating schizophrenia from brain damage. In fact, the MMPI rate of correct separation of schizophrenia from brain damage varies from 75% to 80% (Russell & Russell, 1997, pp. 155–156), which is equivalent to the accuracy of neuropsychological batteries in assessing the existence of brain damage (Russell, 1995). As such, Lezak et al.'s (2004) statement in regard to research studies that "None reached a level of accuracy that would permit clinical judgments" (p. 750) is just plain wrong.

Relationship between Neuropsychological and Affective Measures

In order to provide an understanding of the contribution that objective affective inventories can make to a neuropsychological examination, their psychometric relationship to neuropsychological tests must be delineated. The questions are whether there are effects of brain damage on affective tests and whether emotional reactions impair performance on brain damage tests. Over the years, there has been a great deal of speculation on this subject. Reitan and Wolfson (1997) examined this speculative discussion in the literature quite thoroughly. They demonstrated that much of the speculation was incorrect.

As in much of psychology, this maxim holds: One does not know whether a function or condition exists until there is a test for it. The test may be as rudimentary as the criteria in the DSM-IV-TR (American Psychiatric Association, 2000), but the measures must be objective and public. When actual objective tests have been utilized to examine the interaction between affective tests and neuropsychological cognitive tests, the situation has become clear.

Early Research Studies of Objective Inventories

In this area of psychological assessment, research studies have been able to validly determine the relationships between objective affective tests (particularly the MMPI) and brain damage tests. Although these results have only been partially duplicated for the MMPI-2 and the MCMI-III, the more recent forms of these inventories are sufficiently similar to the early forms that the previous results undoubtedly apply.

Reitan began to study the relationship between affective tests and brain damage tests as early as 1955. Major attempts to study this relationship of psychological measures to neurological conditions were conducted in a series of studies by Dikemen and Reitan, using the MMPI and the Halstead–Reitan Battery (HRB). Wiens and Matarazzo (1974, 1976, 1977) also examined this relationship in nondisabled subjects. No significant correlation was found in any of these studies between personality tests and any of the subtests of the HRB.

More recently, Reitan and Wolfson (1997) thoroughly reviewed the relationship between neuropsychological tests and affective measures. They concluded that most emotional conditions have relatively little effect on neuropsychological tests, and that brain damage has very little direct effect on affective tests. There is, however, an expected emotional reaction to having brain damage, particularly head trauma, which is reflected in scores on affective and personality tests. This pattern also occurs in people under stress who do not have brain damage.

MCMI Studies

In regard to the MCMI in its various forms, apparently only a few studies that are related to brain damage have been conducted. However, some results have been fairly consistent. Primarily, no significant effects of brain damage per se have been found with any version of the MCMI.

In a study of the MCMI-II, Alyman (1999) found no significant differences on the MCMI-II among groups with the moderate, mild, and no head trauma. No groups had mean scores in the pathological range. Another study of psychiatric patients with a simultaneous brain damage diagnosis (Brazil, 1995) obtained only low and not significant correlations between varying types of brain damage and scores on all scales of the MCMI-II. Millikan (2002) did find that head injury claimants demonstrated some psychopathology on the MCMI-II, but that the pathology was not related to the amount of impairment produced by head injury. Consequently, the psychopathology appeared to be an emotional reaction to being injured and to litigation. In a final study (Ruttan & Heinrichs, 2003), scores on the MCMI-II related to depression were largely independent of cognitive performance on a selected group of neurocognitive tests for patients with mild traumatic head injury.

In regard to the MCMI-III, an exhaustive review of the literature found only one study, a dissertation (Oden, 2000), that was concerned with neuropsychological testing. A group of battered women were divided into those with and without head injury. As would be expected, the women in both groups suffered from anxiety, depression, and posttraumatic stress disorder (PTSD). However, since there was no significant difference in the amount of measured neuropsychological impairment between these groups, the MCMI-III scores could not be due to the consequences of head injury.

In short, no relationship has been found between neuropsychological measures of brain damage and any form of the MCMI. The emotional effects of trauma were often evident, but these were not related to physical brain damage.

An Unpublished Study of Brain Damage and the MCMI-II

Since no study of the relationship between the MCMI, in any version, and brain damage other than brain trauma, has been published, such a study by one of us (Elbert W. Russell) is briefly presented here. Data on the MCMI-II and the MMPI were gathered at the Department of Veterans Affair Medical Center in Miami as part of the study used to norm the Halstead–Russell Neuropsychological Evaluation System—Revised (HRNES-R) battery (Russell & Starkey, 1993, 2001). These data were used to examine the statistical relationship of brain damage to these two personality tests.[1]

Although the results of this study do not directly apply to the MCMI-III, the MCMI-II and MCMI-III are structurally quite similar (Millon, 1997, pp. 62–64). Consequently, the findings of this study should apply generally to the MCMI-III. The same is true of the MMPI in relationship to the MMPI-2.

Data on nondisabled control subjects had been collected, but only brain-damaged subjects were examined in this study. Of these, 406 subjects, with a mean age of 47.3 and a mean education level of 12.4 years, were administered the MMPI. The MCMI-II was added to the battery later, so that the MCMI-II was given to 75 subjects, with a mean age of 51.6 and a mean education of 12.7 years. There were 20 patients with left-hemisphere damage, 19 with right-hemisphere damage, and 36 with diffuse damage.

Three studies were completed for both the MMPI and MCMI-II. The profiles of the scale means were obtained. The scales were correlated (Pearson r) with a general index of brain damage, the HRNES-R Average Impairment Score (AIS), and a factor analysis was performed for each inventory.

For the factor analyses, a matrix was created for each inventory; this matrix included all of the subtests in the inventory, the Category Test, Trails B, Tactual Performance Tests total time, Sensory-Perceptual Examination total score, the AIS, and the three IQ scores from the Wechsler Adult Intelligence Scale—Revised (WAIS-R). These two matrices were subjected to a principal-components factor analysis using an orthogonal varimax rotation. In order to examine the affect of an increasing variance, two, three, and four factors were obtained.

The most obvious and important result in regard to both the MCMI-II and the MMPI was that there was almost no statistical relationship between these two affective inventories and the brain damage test scores. When three rotated factors (63% of the variance) were derived from the MCMI-II analysis, two of the factors were composed of MCMI-II tests, and one was composed of the neuropsychological tests (WAIS-R and HRB tests). Four factors (70% of the variance) had to be obtained before any factor contained both affective and cognitive brain damage test loadings. The MMPI required four factors (62% of the variance) before any factor contained both types of tests.

In regard to the correlations between the AIS (again, a measure of the severity of brain damage impairment), and each MCMI-II test, none was significant. The correlations clustered around zero, with the highest two correlations being .39 for Drug Addiction and .35 for Bipolar: Manic. The correlations for the MMPI scales were also not significant. All were below .16.

The profiles of the MCMI-II scale means presented a somewhat different picture. The elevated base rate (BR) means were as follows: Anxiety, 78; Dysthymia, 72; and the Depressive personality scale, 70. The rest of the scales were below 70. The first two of the elevated scales represented Axis I acute conditions, whereas the Depressive personality score indicates that this emotional reaction probably has a more enduring emotional effect on personality. These elevated scales would be expected to be affected for any type of emotionally disturbing situation. The brain damage situation did not elevate the somatic scale to any extent, since it was 67. The usual pattern of elevations (Gass, 2006; Russell, 1977) on the MMPI was found, in which Hs (69), D (72), Hy (67), and Sc (70) were elevated. This corresponds to the pattern demonstrated by the MCMI-II.

These results concerning the MCMI-II have in general supported the previous findings for the MMPI. The pattern of elevations is consistent with an Axis I neurotic reaction that occurs in any form of stress or emotional trauma. Cognitive functioning tends to be preserved under the pressure of the testing situation, even in fairly seriously depressed or anxious individuals. Again, since both inventories are fairly strongly related to their more recent versions, one would expect the same findings if the MCMI-III and the MMPI-2 were utilized.

Summary

The lack of any correlation of brain damage measures with affective measures means that in general, scale elevations on the MCMI-II and presumably the MCMI-III are not due to the direct effects of brain damage. They generally represent Axis I acute emotional reactions to a traumatic event. The clinical examiner can therefore feel comfortable in interpreting the MCMI-III elevations as being due to emotional disturbances and not to the effects of brain damage. Such elevations represent either preexisting emotional or personality conditions, or expected emotional reactions to having brain damage. Consequently, the MCMI-III research that has been conducted on personality disorders and affective conditions applies to brain-damaged persons in much the same way that they apply to non-brain-damaged persons. The only caveat is that with severe brain damage, there may be a personality change in the form of an organic disturbance.

Utility of the MCMI-III

As the most advanced form of the MCMI, the MCMI-III provides a valuable addition to a neuropsychological battery. It was designed to be equivalent to the DSM-IV categories. Consequently, the items on the MCMI-III provide descriptions of personality styles congruent with the DSM-IV-TR diagnostic guide. In addition, the PTSD scale is a welcome advance, as a large segment of the neuropsychological population seen by clinicians comes from subjects with head trauma.

Although a personality test cannot be used to assess cognitive functioning, differentiating between long-existing personality styles and current or transient emotional dysfunction is essential, particularly in the forensic arena. The MCMI-III provides this information, which of course, has to be evaluated in the light of background information and a clinician's judgment. Although there has been almost no research directly relating the MCMI-III to organic conditions, there has been considerable research into personality pathology and personality disorders. In the area of head trauma, there has been some research using either the MCMI-II or MCMI-III (Alyman, 1999; Millikan, 2002; Oden, 2000; Ruttan & Heinrichs, 2003). Since the accuracy of the MCMI-III in assessing the existence of schizoid and schizophrenic symptoms has been greatly improved over that of previous versions (Davis, Wenger, & Guzman, 1997), it will be much more discriminating in regard to schizophrenic conditions.

The severity of psychopathology is quite important to assess, since the results of a neuropsychological examination can be influenced when an individual is seriously emotionally compromised. Particularly in the area of a thought disorder such as schizophrenia, the neurobiological health of the brain may be affected. Although it is rare, an organic personality disorder may occur as a result of head trauma or neurological disease; for this diagnostic entity, an objective psychological test is a necessity.

One of the major advantages of the MCMI-III over other objective tests of psychopathology is that it specifically examines personality characteristics. No other test provides personality information as completely and accurately as this objective inventory.

It is perhaps the "user-friendliness" of the inventory that is one of the strongest points of the MCMI-III. A test that accurately assesses personality with the least number of questions necessary for accurate diagnosis is preferable, due to the length of a thorough neuropsychological examination. In a neuropsychological evaluation, "if the set of tests in a battery is to be an adequate representation of the brain, then coverage is an essential concern" (Russell, 2000). It is standard practice that a complete neuropsychological evaluation may require 6 or more hours of testing, exclusive of the clinical interview and psychological testing.

Although the MMPI is often administered as part of a battery, its length may make it difficult to include in a neuropsychological evaluation. The reliability and validity of MMPI short forms are compromised, and their use is not considered advisable (Pope, Butcher, & Seelen, 1993, p. 24). The advantage of the shorter length of the MCMI-III cannot be underestimated. In our experience of administering neuropsychological evaluations, almost no patients have balked when given the MCMI, but there have been more than several instances where a patient has reacted to administration of the MMPI with a disgruntled attitude. Since the attitude of the examinee can affect the outcome of the test results, this is no small matter.

In general, the MCMI-II has been found to have good concurrent validity (Craig & Olson, 1992) as well as temporal stability (Overholser, 1990). The results of the latter study showed that similar symptom patterns were displayed over time. This finding held true whether these patterns were part of personality traits or patterns of responding when patients were symptomatic.

An audiotaped version of the MCMI-III is particularly useful for patients with either some types of organic damage or a low reading level. Visual impairments or difficulties with attention and concentration are fairly common in this population; this shorter audiotaped version of a personality test is more feasible in such cases.

The Spanish version of the MCMI-III brings with it added cultural fairness and is a welcome addition to a neuropsychologist's armamentarium, because relatively few tests are offered in Spanish. The audiotaped Spanish version is usually administered to these patients, as it is difficult to assess the reading level of a Spanish-speaking individual unless the examiner him- or herself is a fluent Spanish speaker.

The MCMI-III in Neuropsychological Assessment: Special Conditions

As discussed earlier, the independence of measures of brain damage and those of affective states means that in general the neuropsychologist can interpret the MCMI-III for brain-damaged subjects in the same manner as for those without damage. Nevertheless, there are a number of rather specific exceptions to this general understanding. A neuropsychologist must be able to recognize these special conditions in order to avoid rather gross misinterpretations of neuropsychological data. These special conditions are examined in the remainder of this chapter.

The remainder of this chapter is based on clinical experience and actual case studies in the use of the MCMI-II and MCMI-III. Topics concerned with strictly clinical as well as forensic issues are covered. We have employed the MCMI-II and MCMI-III in our practice for about 20 years as part of our neuropsychological evaluation process. We are familiar with how it aids the neuropsychological assessment and consider it a necessary part of any thorough neuropsychological evaluation.

There are several major types of affective conditions that interact with neuropsychological assessment conditions. These may be separated into (1) organically based affective conditions; (2) schizophrenia; (3) emotional reactions to head trauma, especially PTSD; (4) emotional conditions with somatic symptoms; and (5) intentional deception.

Organically Based Affective Conditions

The Effects of Brain Damage on MCMI-II and MCMI-III Results

The only study that directly examined the relationship between aspects of the MCMI-II and types of brain damage was completed by Chitwood (1989) as part of a doctoral dissertation. When subjects with irritative lesions were removed, some mild lateralized differences were found. These differences indicated more characteristics of the avoidant personality in patients with left-hemisphere damage. In patients with right-hemisphere damage, more histrionic features were found. Chitwood (1989) pointed out that the MCMI-II differentiated lateralized effects better than the MMPI.

Postconcussive Syndrome

The DSM-IV(-TR) criteria generally do an inadequate job of helping neuropsychologists find diagnostic labels for brain damage, especially if the damage is not severe. The use of an affective instrument describing both personality and Axis I disorders is essential in making the transition between the psychological evaluation and the diagnosis. In this regard, the MCMI-III has been indispensable in our neuropsychological evaluations.

The postconcussion syndrome consists of many of the following symptoms: headaches, concentration deficits, memory problems, irritability, increased anxiety, emotional lability, loss of self-worth, and depression. A fair number of people with mild head traumas report all or some of these symptoms. The more subtle effects of mild head injury (duration of loss of consciousness less than 15 minutes) are sometimes difficult to detect with standard neuropsychological tests. Closed head injury commonly affects the frontal lobes, temporal lobes, and midbrain. These areas, containing the brain structures traditionally referred to as the "limbic system," are concerned with emotional reactions. Emotional sequelae are thus sometimes demonstrated in the postconcussion syndrome even when cognitive deficits are not seen. The medical profession and the public at large are often insensitive to the needs and problems of patients with mild head injuries, even though they represent the greatest percentage of head-injured patients.

A 49-year-old man was in a motor vehicle accident in which he sustained significant injuries to his pancreas and diaphragm, requiring surgery. Although he did suffer a closed head injury, there was no loss of consciousness even though he was somewhat obtunded at the scene of the accident. A validated neuropsychological evaluation (HRNES-R) was performed almost 4 years after the accident, and this did not demonstrate any permanent cognitive impairment.

The MCMI-III described a moody and somewhat volatile individual who was endorsing a multitude of physical symptoms. He was hypervigilant and severely fatigued. The MCMI-III protocol was consistent with an adjustment disorder with depressed mood. Psychological and pharmacological treatment was recommended for this patient. Once his case had been settled for psychological and not brain injury damages, some of his stress was alleviated. He was able to be treated for the appropriate condition and was relieved to learn that he did not have brain damage. Interestingly, after having been "disabled" for all 4 years, he returned to his former work as an electrician.

Organic Mood Disorder

Although the usual need is to differentiate functional from organic conditions, both can coexist when there is an organic mood disorder. Moderate to severe head trauma can produce this condition. The degree of brain injury is best assessed on the basis of length of loss of consciousness, the rating of the Glasgow Coma Scale, and the presence and duration of retrograde or anterograde amnesia. As part of an organic mood disorder, brain damage itself can produce depression. Recommendations for treatment are extremely important in the case of an organic mood disorder, and the amount of compensation will be increased in forensic cases if such a condition is diagnosed.

Recently we saw a case of a 43-year-old man who had been working on a construction site when over 50 pounds of steel beams fell from the ceiling, trapping him underneath. He sustained not only multiple physical injuries but brain damage. Organic damage was found to be diffuse, with significant frontal lobe dysfunction. This type of frontal brain damage typically results in intense mood swings, lack of impulse control, and aggressive behavior. The MCMI-III demonstrated a pattern of high scores on the Thought Disorder (SS) and Delusional Disorder (PP) scales. Since there had been no premorbid history of personality problems, the severe brain damage was consistent with a person who showed bizarre thought patterns, regressive behavior, patchy hallucinatory experiences, and delusions of a persecutory nature. Thus the diagnosis of an organic mood disorder was made, and inpatient psychiatric treatment was recommended.

Since this was a forensic case, the defense had attempted to discredit the findings concerning neurological impairment, as well as psychological findings. The use of the MCMI-III strongly supported our contentions of an organic mood disorder. An objective psychological test is mandatory in a court case, since it provides objective evidence to support a contention. The MCMI-III is gaining in such recognition in the forensic arena. In fact, in this particular case the actual graph was replicated in the form of an exhibit, so that the neuropsychologist could explain its significance to the jury.

Dementia versus Depression

Perhaps the most frequent nonforensic reason for a neuropsychological assessment referral is to differentiate dementia from depression. This referral question can only be answered by administering a thorough neuropsychological and psychological evaluation.

As an example of this type of assessment problem, a 63-year-old woman was referred by her neurologist because she had been complaining of memory problems for about a year. She was a nurse in an intensive care unit, and the changes in the health care system were making the intensity of her job extremely difficult, particularly for an older woman. In addition, her husband had been diagnosed with esophageal cancer, and she had been under even more stress with his medical treatments.

The results of the neuropsychological testing were benign, and there was no evidence of early dementia. By contrast, her MCMI-III was consistent with the clinical diagnosis of major depression, severe, without psychotic features. Additionally, she reported extreme fatigue and feeling, apathetic and discouraged. Her usual upbeat mood had been replaced by what she called "my gray cloud." The MMPI-2 further supported this diagnosis with elevations on D (Depression) and Hy (Hysteria).

In our feedback session, she was relieved to know that her cognitive functioning was well within the average range for her age and educational level. Although she had always thought of herself as a "strong" person who needed no professional help, she did enter psychotherapy, and the reduction of her extreme depression improved her mentation.

A differential diagnostic case with a different conclusion was that of a 67-year-old man who had been referred by his neurologist for neuropsychological testing because he reported memory and word-finding problems. Complicating the diagnosis of possible dementia was the fact that his wife of 46 years had died 1 year previously. In the clinical interview, this gentleman appeared rather stoic and guarded with his feelings. He described his memory problems in an understated manner and only displayed minimal word-finding problems. Although he described the death of his wife as a significant loss to him, he did not evidence much emotionality.

The neuropsychological test results demonstrated a clear left parietal problem. That is, the patient was found to have significant anomia (word-finding problems), as well as memory deficits for verbal material, both rote (in the form of word lists) and semantic (stories). Right-hemisphere tests such as spatial relations tasks were intact.

The MCMI-III showed BR scores that were all below 75. The profile was constricted and described a man who endorsed no psychosocial or environmental problems. The audiotaped version had been administered to him because of his left-hemisphere problems and hence difficulties with reading. He had scored within the average range on the Comprehension subtest of the WAIS-R and had understood all the directions given to him during the testing. It was decided that this man's test results were unfortunately consistent with a dementia of the Alzheimer's type, which was more prominent in his left-hemisphere functioning.

It is a characteristic of patients with Alzheimer's dementia that they often do not suffer from much depression. Emotional problems and stress are more characteristic of the families of these patients. In this case, the MCMI-III had been extremely helpful in showing the typical picture of such a patient's rather flat emotional status, and the neuropsychological testing had served to corroborate a cognitive pattern found in patients with dementia.

Substance Abuse

There is a high correlation between traumatic brain injury and substance abuse, occurring either before or after the injury. The neuropsychologist must evaluate not only the person's brain functioning, but also the proclivity for substance abuse in accordance with personality style.

In this case, a 57-year-old man had suffered subdural hematomas in a motor vehicle accident occurring 6 months previous to testing him for a legal case. He had graduated from high school, but had dropped out of college because of poor grades. A review of his academic records revealed someone who had always been a poor student, with nonexistent motivation. Interestingly, his father had been a physician. This litigant had always wandered from unskilled job to unskilled job, never finding any type of work that suited him. Although his brain injury had been rather severe, his IQ level indicated superior intelligence. IQ testing is often less sensitive in detecting brain injury than neuropsychological tests are. As such, some of the neuropsychological tests known to be more sensitive to brain injuries demonstrated moderate brain damage. This man was able to be administered the MCMI-III, and interestingly, the profile did indicate a substance abuse pattern. He had presented a negative alcohol history when questioned. However, when questioned further (after the MCMI-III had been scored), he finally admitted to a prolonged history of alcohol abuse beginning in his teens. Not only did this change the interpretation of his cognitive test results; because now alcoholic encephalopathy in addition to his brain injury had to be considered, it also resulted in a recommendation for alcohol abuse treatment, as this gentleman was continuing to drink heavily.

Often individuals such as this patient have an easier time admitting to their problems on a psychological questionnaire than in a face-to-face interview situation.

Adult Attention-Deficit/Hyperactivity Disorder and Learning Disabilities

Many congenital organic problems, such as attention-deficit/hyperactivity disorder (ADHD) and learning disabilities (LD), are often accompanied by emotional problems that must be fully assessed. Much research has concentrated on the increased incidence of emotional problems in children who are diagnosed with ADHD or LD. These children are often labeled with multiple diagnoses (Biederman, Gillis, Toner, & Goldberg, 1991).

The increased interest in adult ADHD has resulted in a need for accurate assessment of this disorder in this population and an increase in referrals reflecting this entity. It is important to be able to distinguish ADHD from an affective condition and to assess personality style accurately. The MCMI-III can help to accomplish this. In many instances, a parent recognizes his or her own ADHD after having had a child diagnosed with this disorder. Although the heritability factor is prominent, a systematic diagnosis must be made of the adult, as in the case of the child. One of the important facets of this evaluation is to rule out a primary emotional problem as the cause of the adult's distractibility and/or hyperactivity. Information from the MCMI has been essential in many cases in which we diagnosed ADHD, as well as in cases in which this diagnosis was ruled out.

A 42-year-old gentleman was referred by his physician because of problems with attention. The patient was a college-educated business executive who had considerable difficulty following through on projects, organizing his work, and focusing on conversations both at work and at home. He described himself as always feeling bored and needing to participate in risk-taking behaviors in order to make life interesting. His latest escapade had resulted in his losing a considerable amount of money from his wife's inheritance.

His neuropsychological test results indicated memory, executive, psychomotor, and attentional deficits. However, all of these functions may be sensitive to psychological problems as well as ADHD. The MCMI-III portrayed a man who viewed his emotional adjustment as adequate, but who endorsed a mild depression concerned with an inability to concentrate, difficulty with organization, and frequent periods of restlessness. He presented himself as being in a stable and loving marriage, with strong ties to family and close friends. Since there were no apparent significant problems, the diagnosis of ADHD was made. He was placed on Ritalin, which has helped him considerably. Therefore, the combination of the abnormal neuropsychological markers with the relatively normal MCMI-III protocol proved essential in this determination.

Adults who have difficulty with learning, despite the fact that their intellectual capacity is determined to be normal, are considered to have LD. ADHD and LD often coexist. This disability may relate to verbal or nonverbal (spatial-perceptual) abilities. Dyslexia is the most common of the learning problems.

Research has now begun to focus on the so-called "right-hemisphere" types of LD as well. In fact, where problems in the verbal area have often created frustration and a feeling of low self-worth, the emotional problems connected with nonverbal LD can be even greater. There may be a lack of social awareness and difficulty with understanding nonverbal communication as a result of a nonverbal LD. Thus an objective psychological test is an important part of an evaluation for LD as well as for ADHD.

Schizophrenia

Schizophrenia has been an especially vexing disorder for neuropsychology, since the pattern of neuropsychological test results for a schizophrenic or schizophreniform patient often resembles a brain damage pattern. In the late 1960s, it was discovered that schizophrenia will impair performance on neuropsychological tests (Watson, Thomas, Anderson, & Felling, 1968). As such, neuropsychological tests in themselves cannot distinguish schizophrenia from brain damage. This finding has been quite consistent throughout subsequent studies of schizophrenia (Goldstein, 1986).

Differentiation of Schizophrenia and Brain Damage

One way in which neuropsychologists have tried to solve this problem is to consider schizophrenia to be an organic condition. If schizophrenia is a "brain condition," one would expect deficits in neuropsychological test results.

However, though considering schizophrenia to be an organic condition may resolve this problem theoretically, it does not solve the practical problem of distinguishing schizophrenia from "other forms" of brain damage. In all respects of diagnosis and treatment, schizophrenia is a separate entity. In hospital settings and in forensic situations especially, it is quite important to distinguish impairment on a neuropsychological battery due to schizophrenia from impairment due to standard forms of brain damage.

The contribution of objective affective tests to this differential diagnosis is often crucial. Although such measures cannot diagnoses brain damage, the MMPI and probably the MCMI-III can separate schizophrenia from organic conditions at a very acceptable rate (Golden, Sweet, & Osman, 1979; Russell, 1975; Watson, 1977). For the MMPI, the rate of correct separation of schizophrenia from brain damage falls between 75% and 80%. This level of accuracy is equivalent to that of neuropsychological batteries in assessing the existence of brain damage (Russell, 1995).

These studies have not been duplicated with the MMPI-2 or the MCMI-III. However, the accuracy of the MCMI-III in assessing the existence of schizoid and schizophrenic conditions is now quite acceptable (Davis et al., 1997). This will probably make it as discriminating in regard to the separation of schizophrenic conditions from brain damage as the MMPI-2. Nevertheless, this should be validated.

Triangulation

The procedure for making a differential diagnosis when a brain condition is involved was delineated by Watson (1977). Although it was designed for the differential diagnosis of schizophrenia versus brain damage, the same method applies to the differential diagnosis of many other Axis I disorders versus brain damage.

The method utilized by Watson (1977) involves comparing two tests and may be called "triangulation." The concept is analogous to the technique of this nature that is employed in surveying. Using trigonometric data concerning spatial relationship lines drawn between two points enables one to locate a third point. For instance, in the U.S. Forest Service, fire towers are used to determine the location of a fire through triangulation. The locations of, and distance between, the two towers are known. If a line is drawn on a map to the fire from each of the two towers, the angle of intersection precisely locates the fire.

By analogy, triangulation as used in psychological measurement enables one to obtain information from two tests that is not obtainable from either test alone. As used in regard to the assessment of schizophrenia, the method is to administer both a neuropsychological battery and an objective test of psychopathology. Comparison of scores from these will produce accurate differentiation among nondisabled individuals, persons with schizophrenia, and persons with organic brain damage. If the neuropsychology battery indicates impairment and the psychopathology tests are relatively benign, then a patient probably has an organic condition. If the neuropsychological battery indicates impairment and the psychopathology tests indicate schizophrenia, then the diagnosis is probably schizophrenia. If neither set of tests suggests impairment, then the patient is probably nondisabled.

In support of this concept, a preliminary study by Brown (1987) was designed to use an algorithm based on the preceding method. With the MMPI, when the most accurate cutting points were used, the algorithm's overall separation of "normal," organic, and psychiatric (largely schizophrenic) cases was 73%. The chance probability for making this separation among three categories is only 33.3%. In terms of the three separate categories, 69% of the organic subject, 94% of the schizophrenic subjects, and 89% of the "normal" subjects were correctly identified.

Triangulation is a form of pattern analysis. It is a formalization of the psychological assessment method for making certain diagnostic differentiations that is commonly utilized in clinical judgment. In contrast to clinical judgment, this formal procedure provides an exact measure of the accuracy of the differentiation. Consequently, it has been validated for the MMPI, and could be for the MCMI-III as well.

Finally, a neuropsychological assessment may provide additional information concerning schizophrenia. Since neuropsychological tests are affected by schizophrenia, and they measure the amount of cognitive impairment, they may reflect the severity of schizophrenia. Certainly, they provide a measure of how much cognitive impairment the schizophrenia is producing.

This important differentiation of a preexisting schizophrenic spectrum condition from traumatic brain injury can be exemplified by an assessment in a forensic case. This case, in fact, was settled in favor of the defense, based on the use of the MCMI-III.

A 28-year-old male who worked as a laborer on a construction site fell off the back of a truck as he was being transported to the site. He broke his left arm, but there was no report in the medical records or in the patient's own self-report of his having hit his head. However, the plaintiff sued for brain damage on the basis of a whiplash-type injury, which supposedly caused an axonal shearing resulting in brain damage.

The plaintiff performed in the brain-damaged range on tests of memory, executive functioning, and language functions. His Verbal IQ on the WAIS-R was 75. His answers to some of the questions on the Comprehension subtest were found to be somewhat bizarre. For example, he said that "people needed a license to get married because they might need to put the other person in jail." His reading ability as determined by an achievement test was at the 10th-grade level, so he was able to be administered the MCMI-III. His personality code was noted as Schizoid, Avoidant, and Dependent, with the Schizotypal scale extremely elevated.

The premorbid history was consistent with this man's MCMI-III results: He had never married; had not formed close relationships with anyone, including his own family, and had an inconsistent work history, with more periods of being unemployed than employed. He presented in the clinical interview as devoid of affect, never making eye contact, displaying ideas of grandeur, and being tangential in his responses. The conclusions of the neuropsychological evaluation were not consistent with the pattern of test results found in head trauma and were more consistent with schizoaffective disorder. In addition, the possibility of secondary gain could not be ruled out. Needless to say, this condition would have existed before the alleged mild head trauma occurred. Depositions taken from various employers and acquaintances who had known the plaintiff before the accident had confirmed that this person was previously considered to have had rather severe personality problems. The case was dropped after the depositions.

Emotional Reactions to Head Trauma

Emotional reactions to head trauma are to be expected. As demonstrated in the previous research reviews and the research presented in this chapter, an Axis I type of acute "neurotic" reaction usually accompanies brain damage. This emotional reaction generally occurs in the same manner as do such reactions that are not related to brain damage. A detailed examination of such acute reactions is beyond the scope of this chapter. However one form of reaction that is specific to traumatic injury situations is important to discuss. This is PTSD.

Posttraumatic Stress Disorder

In forensic cases, PTSD is among the most common alleged sequelae of accidents. Assessing people who have undergone an emotional trauma requires knowledge of PTSD in order not to confuse these symptoms with brain injury. DSM-IV-TR lists 17 symptoms or behaviors as criteria for PTSD, with specified numbers that have to be present in certain categories in order to make this diagnosis.

There has been considerable controversy over whether someone who has amnesia for an event because of organic memory problems can suffer from PTSD, since memory is important in this psychological condition. However, it is beyond the scope of this chapter to pursue this controversy.

As an illustration, a man exiting a movie theater was accosted in the parking lot by thugs who beat him brutally. Fortunately, they were frightened off by some people who had parked in the same area, and his life was saved. The lawsuit against the movie theater was our reason for being retained on the case to assess this man for both cognitive damage and emotional status.

While fortunately no brain impairment was found, his cognitive complaints resembled those of a brain-damaged individual. The MCMI-III showed not only a significant elevation on the PTSD scale (above BR = 85), but also elevations on the Anxiety and Dysthymia scales. Psychological testing was thus vital in enabling the separation of the cognitive from the emotional components as accurately as possible. The diagnosis of PTSD was important not only for determining appropriate treatment recommendations, but also for damage assessment.

Further research may tell us whether there is a representative pattern of neuropsychological test results in these patients. For the present, the neuropsychologist should be aware that a patient with PTSD may resemble a brain-damaged patient, especially in a self-report. Cognitive and emotional variables are all too closely intertwined.

One study supports this interrelationship. Dysfunctional cognitions were found in a group of 31 Vietnam veterans with PTSD (Muran & Motta, 1993). This group was compared with a group of patients with other anxiety disorders or depressive disorders, and a nonclinical group of college students. One of the measures the subjects completed was the MCMI-II. There was supporting evidence for the uniqueness of thought processing in the group with PTSD.

Thus, as a form of triangulation, the administration of neuropsychological measures, along with the psychological measures, is essential for a definitive diagnosis. Scale R (the PTSD scale) on the MCMI-III is a welcome addition to this inventory.

Emotional Conditions with Somatic Symptoms

Although the emotional reactions just discussed are related to head trauma, they are expected symptoms produced by a stressful situation. However, different sets of symptoms are related to the reactions of persons with certain preexisting types of conditions, in which a particular event is utilized as a basis for exhibiting physical symptoms. These symptoms often mimic true organically produced symptoms, such as the inability to use an arm or leg or the loss of memory. This type of somatic reaction is due to either a somatoform disorder (hypochondriasis, somatization disorder, conversion disorder, etc.) or to some other type of condition that may involve somatic symptoms (some personality patterns, some dissociative states). These symptoms are unconsciously utilized by an individual because they provide a form of secondary gain, such as attention from a distant cold family member or the prospect of financial gain from a legal suit.

The distinction between these types of disorders and malingering is often more difficult to make than the distinction between real brain damage and malingering. However, this differential assessment is important, since the person with a psychiatric condition involving somatic symptoms genuinely believes that his or her symptoms are produced by physical brain damage. Consequently, this person's treatment both in regard to medical treatment and to a legal situation must be quite different. It is obvious that the MCMI-III may be of great importance in helping to make this differentiation.

Somatoform disorders such as hypochondriasis are quite common in the brain injury field, and an accurate differentiation between such a diagnosis and other diagnoses is essential. The MCMI-III is most helpful in this area.

An illustration of such a somatoform disorder was the case of a 52-year-old man who worked in the computer field and had been a victim of a mugging. He complained of memory loss, agitation, fatigue, headaches, neck pain, hip pain, knee pain, shoulder pain, numbness of hands and feet, inability to sleep, and indigestion. He was sent for a neuropsychological assessment by his attorney to rule out a cognitive disorder and to assess damages for his claim. The incident had occurred a full 2 years previously. Cognitive functions were found to be well intact, but his psychological testing revealed somatoform disorder with prominent hypochondriacal features. His doctors had cleared him medically 6 months after his incident, but he had continued to suffer from all of the above-stated ailments. He was convinced that he was physically ill as well as brain-damaged. The Somatoform scale on the MCMI-III was significantly elevated (BR = 83). The MMPI-2 was consistent with this finding, since the Hy (Hysteria) scale was dramatically elevated. We sometimes administer the MMPI-2 in conjunction with the MCMI-III when we want to make as strong a case as possible for litigation purposes. Psychological counseling and an evaluation for medication were recommended to this gentleman. He followed up on both suggestions, and his attorney related that he had become more functional in his work and in his interpersonal relationships even before his court case was heard.

Although there is no iron-clad rule or definitive test to distinguish a histrionic personality pattern or conversion disorder from malingering, neuropsychological testing along with reliable and valid objective psychological tests can usually rule out brain damage. Premorbid history as well as experienced clinical judgment must also be utilized in the determination. The neuropsychologist needs to assess whether or not the neuropsychological test results are consistent with a neurological condition; in other words, do the results make neuropsychological or neurological sense? In order to answer this question, the clinician needs to have not only a knowledge of neuroanatomy, but also an understanding of the neurological entities and the various patterns each condition typically produces in neuropsychological protocols. Objective personality tests, especially the MCMI-III, are often helpful in making this separation. One study (Webb, 1999) has demonstrated that the MCMI-III can be an aid in making this distinction.

In a relatively typical case, a 52-year-old woman was evaluated for brain damage 2 years after an accident. She had been in an elevator that had malfunctioned, causing it to jolt rather strongly when it arrived at the first floor. There had been no physical indications that this woman had hit her head (no loss of consciousness, no cuts or bruises on the head). However, 2 years later she was still experiencing severe headaches and backaches, an inability to concentrate, and a decreased libido. Her performance on the battery of neuropsychological tests was all in the average to above-average range as normed for her age and educational level. Although she was only a high school graduate, her IQ testing placed her in the superior range on the WAIS-R. Based on her high cognitive test performance, there was obviously no indication for malingering.

Administration of the MCMI-II resulted in elevations on the Histrionic, Dependent, and Narcissistic personality scales. It was surprising and significant that in the history session, she spoke about a situation earlier in her life in which she was hospitalized for 5 days in a psychiatric unit because she had "lost my voice after my divorce." Her medical records revealed that she had been hospitalized at least four additional times for various physical problems, for which no organic cause was ever found. One of us had to appear in court to describe to the jury the characteristics of a histrionic personality style. Utilizing the results from the MCMI, the jury was better able to understand the personality dynamics involved, and, in fact, the plaintiff was not awarded any compensation. It was obvious that her personality dynamics had been long-standing.

Two of our more fascinating patients were referred by neurologists for evaluation. One had pseudoseizure activity; the other patient had episodic cluster headaches, which resulted in dissociative states.

In the first case, a 21-year-old woman had been experiencing seizure-like activity for 2 years. These "seizures" manifested themselves in the form of sleepwalking, in which she would be aware of her surroundings but was in a dreamlike state, unable to speak. She would clench her jaw and hands during these episodes, shake, and have difficulty breathing. Her parents had witnessed these "seizures," which would awaken them during the night. They would occur on an average of once a week.

An MRI was noted to be negative. Adding to the mystery, however, the electroencephalogram (EEG) showed nonspecific signs that could either point in the direction of a neurological problem or be interpreted as a normal variation.

This young woman presented herself at the first testing session as guarded with depressed affect. She responded to questions during the clinical interview in a highly defensive and constrained manner. Projective testing was administered, and the Rorschach, which was quite defensive, produced a paucity of responses for someone of her age and intellectual level (which was average). She responded to many of the cards by stating, "I have no idea," or "I have no imagination."

Neuropsychological testing was negative, in that there was no temporal lobe pattern of the type that may be found in seizure patients, nor were there any signs of focal or diffuse impairment. Her neurologist had placed her on an antiseizure medication as both a precautionary and a diagnostic measure, but the medication had not reduced her "seizure" activity.

Both the MMPI-2 and the MCMI-III were administered. Consistent with the information found in the technical manual (Millon, 1997) describing the test pattern related to hysteria, the scales on the MCMI-III that were elevated were Somatoform and Major Depression. The Hysteria scale (Hy) on the MMPI-2 was elevated to a T-score of 90. It was concluded that this young woman was suffering from conversion disorder, and it was recommended that she seek psychiatric treatment.

In the second case, a 54-year-old divorced woman had been experiencing migrainous headaches along with dissociation for several months. Following the headaches, she would regress to a childlike state and call to her mother, who had been dead for 10 years. Her adult children had witnessed this phenomenon and had described her behavior, as the patient herself had no memories of the episodes. Her neurologist had hospitalized her and administered several EEGs. While undergoing one of the EEG tests, she began dissociating, but the EEG had been unremarkable.

Neuropsychological testing results did not indicate any cognitive deficits. In fact, her performance was well above the average range for all brain functions. Her WAIS-R Full Scale IQ was 127.

The MCMI-II revealed high scores on the Histrionic personality scale, as well as on the Axis I Anxiety and Somatoform scales. The pattern of results indicated a woman who needed extreme attention as well as approval from others. However, due to her problems with self-assertion it was difficult for her to obtain approval, and she most often went with her needs unmet. Desirability on the Modifying Indices was elevated (BR = 85). In addition, she was shown to lack insight and to avoid introspection. Hostile urges were denied, and as a result, her constrained feelings tended to produce psychosomatic problems.

Consistent with the MCMI-II result was this woman's previous medical history. She had suffered from severe bouts of gastrointestinal problems, as well as extreme periods of fatigue. No physical causes had been documented for her problems, despite consistent medical attention.

Psychotherapy and psychopharmacological medications were suggested under the MCMI-II's prognostic and therapeutic implications. Consistent with the narrative, this woman did consider therapy as a threat to her self-image, and withdrew from counseling after her second session. Interestingly and perhaps predictably, she was unhappy with the neuropsychological test results and refused to believe that she did not have a neurological problem. Upon follow-up with her neurologist, it was learned that her cluster headaches with the accompanying dissociative states had disappeared. However, several months later it was learned that she was now being evaluated medically for heart palpitations of unknown etiology.

Intentional Deception

A final category of affective conditions not due to an organic condition involves intentional deception. In these conditions, the symptoms of an organic condition are knowingly exhibited in order to obtain some gain. Whereas malingering is a well-known attempt to profit from a mishap, the purpose of another form of deception, factitious disorder, is not to obtain an obvious monetary or some other tangible gain.

Factitious Disorder

Factitious disorder may look like malingering, since the person is aware that he or she is pretending to have a condition. Nevertheless, it is a separate entity. In the absence of external incentives such as monetary gain or a determination of disability, a person who pretends to be suffering from physical or emotional problems can be said to have factitious disorder. Again, this category is different from malingering, in which there is an intentional purpose to feign symptoms for economic or some other tangible gain. It is very difficult to diagnose this disorder, as it is easily confused with malingering or disorders involving somatic symptoms.

The following case of a woman with factitious disorder was one that we misdiagnosed. We knew that this was not a case of brain damage and diagnosed the person as having a somatoform disorder and PTSD. In this case, the MCMI-II had been consistent with schizophrenia as well as with paranoid personality disorder. However, schizophrenia was ruled out on the basis of this woman's history, as she had been married, had children, and had been steadily employed. Clinical judgment of her behavior in the interview also ruled out this diagnosis. The diagnosis of paranoid personality disorder was also found not to fit the woman's history, as she was a black person from the deep South who had little education and strong fundamentalist religious beliefs, coupled with an understandable distrust of people based on her life experience of discrimination.

This 55-year-old woman had been preparing to go to work in the housekeeping department of the hospital where she had been employed as a janitor for 15 years. She was sitting by a window in her house eating her lunch when a hammer crashed through the window, hitting her on the forehead. A workman had been repairing a neighbor's roof and had thrown the hammer to a coworker in jest.

The results of the neuropsychological tests showed mild to moderate deficits across many brain functions. It was felt that the emotional sequelae brought on by her accident were interfering in her cognitive processing. In addition, her low level of premorbid academic and intellectual functioning was an important factor compromising her performance. Since there had been a question in our minds about possible monetary gain factors, there was the possibility of malingering.

As it turned out, unbeknownst to us, her legal case had been settled months before the evaluation. She was referred to a psychologist for supportive and behavior modification counseling following the testing. The therapy uncovered the fact that this woman had always been responsible for taking care of family members since she was 8 years old, when she had to take care of three younger siblings. This caretaker pattern had been predominant from then on, culminating with her nursing both of her parents the past few years until their deaths. She admitted to the psychologist that she had wanted to be cared for herself by her live-in boy-friend, whom she had helped through a crisis with drug addiction. Her goal had been achieved, as she was now dependent on him both physically and financially.

We decided to include this example of factitious disorder as a caution concerning any objective psychological test. Clinical judgment and detailed history are extremely important. The MCMI-II could not have assessed the situational parameters sur-rounding this individual's life.

Malingering

Perhaps there is no greater challenge in the forensic area than in detecting a true case of malingering. This is always a possibility in a forensic case. Multiple factors can be operating other than a patient's purposeful intent to deceive. One of the most cogent articles in this area was written by Weissman (1990). This article speaks to the fact that we often underestimate the influence of litigation on a person's psychological and physical condition. The stress upon the individual who has been ordered to be examined by multiple expert witness physicians and psychologists takes its toll. The plaintiff may feel angered at the process and believe that he or she is not trusted, and the defense expert witnesses thus can appear as professionals to be deceived and out-witted. Weissman (1990) makes the important point that often the plaintiff is not sent to defense expert witnesses for several years from the date of the accident and thus has had an extended period of time to experience the stressors that often exacer-bate preexisting personality styles, such as those found in individuals with histrionic, narcissistic, or antisocial traits.

To complicate the situation, malingering and conversion disorder are often con-fused. It is also important to keep in mind that conversion disorder and malingering are not mutually exclusive; people with conversion disorder can also malinger. The behaviors of individuals with a diagnosis of conversion disorder or malingering are also similar in nature, as they both may attempt to be declared disabled, and both may be reporting atypical symptomatology. Both of these conditions can be sub-sumed under the category of a functional disorder. The MCMI-III may also help dis-tinguish malingering from a dissociative disorder (Webb, 1999).

It is generally easier to determine that the patient does not have significant brain damage than to separate malingering from a disorder involving somatic symptoms. Especially in forensic cases, the determination of the existence of brain damage takes priority. There are several effects on neuropsychological tests that may help separate functional problems from organic damage. In a functional case, psychological factors can have the effect of overwhelming a person over time, so that the person may appear to be regressing. In neuropsychological assessment, serial testings on such an individual often show a pattern of decreasing performance on cognitive tasks over time. This type of pattern is not one produced by brain damage.

The neuropsychological test profile itself provides information that helps the cli-nician detect malingering. Variable and inconsistent test results that do not make neurological nor neuropsychological sense are a major clue. Even a neurologically sophisticated person may find it difficult to fake successfully on an entire test battery. For example, a test profile is suspect when the memory tests are performed so poorly that a person who has dementia could do better, but tests that are highly sensitive to brain damage, such as the Tactual Performance Test, are within normal limits.

In his book on malingering, Rogers (1988) wrote: "Nearly all psychological measures are susceptible to dissimulation. The notable exception is defensiveness on intellectual and neuropsychological testing, since patients cannot perform better than their organic impairment will allow" (p. 295). Clearly, someone cannot perform better than his or her own best effort, but it is important to realize that a person can perform poorly for reasons other than brain damage.

There are also tests in neuropsychology specifically designed to help detect malingering. In these tests, missing more items than would be expected by chance alone provides important information. The objective personality tests, especially the validity scales, are often of great help in separating the functional from the organic case.

Along the same line of reasoning, a study was conducted to determine whether there was a relationship between the validity scales on the MMPI-2 and the personality scales on the MCMI-II (Grillo, Brown, Hilsabeck, Price, & Lees-Haley, 1994). The authors concluded that there was indeed a relationship between these two sets of scales. Whether the effect on the MCMI-II personality scales indicated a malingering type of person was not completely clear, since there was also the possibility that the elevations on the personality scales themselves may have been exaggerated.

A personality inventory itself must have the ability to discriminate among different testing styles. In one study of the MCMI-II, eight different test-taking styles were analyzed in order to determine whether clinically relevant separation of the profiles could be found (Retzlaff, Sheehan, & Fiel, 1991). Good statistical and clinically relevant separation of the profiles was found for "normal," "fake good," "fake bad," and randomly generated profiles. However, the percentage of profiles identified by validity scales was not as good. In a related study, the effectiveness of three validity scales from the MCMI-II was analyzed (Bagby, Gillis, Toner, & Goldberg, 1991). The overall rate of classification was found to be quite high. At this point, no studies attempting to utilize the MCMI-III in distinguishing malingering from real brain damage appear to have been completed.

The clearest example of malingering in our case histories was a woman who had fallen down a few stairs with no evidence of head injury. Of course, she was suing for brain damage—and there were huge sums of money involved, as she was suing a hospital. This 49-year-old woman was well educated and had held a professional position in the educational field prior to her "brain damage." In the testing environment, she presented as bright and articulate, and no problems were noted with either her expressive or receptive language abilities. However, upon formal testing, it was apparent she was malingering. She was unable to recite the alphabet, could not count from 1 to 10, and performed all neuropsychological testing worse than a person who had been severely brain-damaged and in a coma for months would have.

Noteworthy was the fact that although this woman was first administered the MCMI-III in the publisher's audiotaped version, she asked for the written version. Since she had failed the reading test, the use of the audiotaped version had seemed prudent. However, she completed the written version in 20 minutes, and the Desirability scale score was below BR = 30. She obviously did not want to appear to have psychological problems, but rather concentrated on pretending to have cognitive problems. She failed all the tests of motivation and effort administered to her. It was most revealing that she could even understand the MCMI-III, since she had pretended to have lost all reading abilities!

Rehabilitation

Neuropsychology and rehabilitation are closely allied as parts of an interdisciplinary entity. Rehabilitation experts depend on a neuropsychological assessment to provide them with the information necessary to perform their work. A person's emotional functioning and personality style influence the course of remediation for brain injury. Thus an objective personality inventory is essential for the complete assessment of a patient. The MCMI is making its contribution in this area.

The utility of the MCMI-III is illustrated by a study (Campbell, 2006) that used the inventory, along with neuropsychological tests (including tests of cognition and memory), to predict the functional outcome of mild traumatic brain injury. As expected, those who did more poorly on certain neuropsychological tests and the WAIS-R also did more poorly at the follow-up 3 to 12 months after the original assessment. However, subjects who scored higher on the MCMI-III Major Depression and PTSD scales also reported less favorable outcomes in terms of their reintegration into the community at follow-up.

Thus it is necessary to assess patients psychologically in the acute stage of neurological problems, as well in the chronic stage. In rehabilitation planning, knowledge of positive personality and character traits is as important as knowledge of types of psychopathology. Just as neuropsychological measures are important in determining the success of a rehabilitation program, so are psychological measures vital in order to provide for the most optimal functioning of the brain-injured patient, as well as to ensure compliance with treatment.

Suggestions for Future Research

As we have mentioned at the beginning of this chapter, there has been very little research on the MCMI-III in relation to neuropsychological variables. This is unfortunate, as the complex and vital interrelationship between emotional and cognitive functioning is only beginning to be understood.

The study by Swirsky-Sacchetti et al. (1993) demonstrates how the MCMI can be used in neuropsychological investigations. This study used the MCMI as one of the major measures used in diagnosing borderline personality. The study investigated the question of whether borderline personality disorder might be a subtle organic condition, or at least might have an organic component. It was found that defects impairing performance on neuropsychological tests were found in patients assessed as having borderline personality disorder.

The area of differential diagnosis is one in which the MCMI-III may make a significant contribution. As we have noted earlier, the scales related to schizophrenia and other forms of psychosis have been greatly improved (Davis et al., 1997, pp. 327–359). Therefore, the psychosis scales as well as the personality scales on the

MCMI-III may now be able to separate certain types of schizophrenia from brain damage better than any other test. The case histories in this chapter demonstrate that both patients with Alzheimer's dementia and malingering patients may have particular patterns on the MCMI-III. Considering the gravity of their disease, patients with Alzheimer's disease appear to have a remarkably bland pattern on the MCMI-III; they show little of the expected depression or other emotional disturbances. This could reinforce the typical pattern found for the HRB (Russell & Polakoff, 1993).

The finding of a schizophrenic-like pattern in a person who has no historical or interview characteristics typical of schizophrenia, in our experience, is a strong indication of malingering. If this could be verified in a research study, the MCMI-III would greatly enhance the ability to detect malingerers in neuropsychology cases.

Substance abuse and its influence on brain functioning have produced considerable and controversial research. The relationship between psychopathology and neuropsychological deficits also needs to be explored further. An important research study for the MCMI-III would be to verify the finding with earlier forms of the MCMI that emotional conditions such as depression, anxiety, and personality styles do not influence neuropsychological performance,.

An area in neuropsychology that is continually expanding is the influence of toxins on neuropsychological processes, and their interaction with emotional factors is obvious. Biochemical explanations for both neuropsychological deficits and psychological deficits may fruitfully be further explored (Coffman, 1998).

Currently, the relationships between emotions and health are being explored in the exciting field of psychoimmunology. In the same manner, we must continue to explore how psychological functioning relates to mental functioning. The MCMI-III is a valuable personality instrument to use in conducting this research because of its reliance on personality theory.

Syndromes involving frontal and temporal lobe damage have been researched from both the neurological and psychological vantage points. However, we are discovering that these syndromes cannot be considered as single entities, and that there appears to be a wide spectrum of emotional and cognitive changes occurring with such damage, either bilaterally or with only one affected hemisphere (Chitwood, 1989). The MCMI-III would be useful in conducting such studies. The whole area of lateralized brain damage and depression needs additional research, in order to understand more thoroughly the specialized hemispheric functions as well as the functions shared by both hemispheres. The differences in the psychological problems incurred because of damage to a particular hemisphere are still not fully understood.

Return-to-work studies related to neuropsychological assessment will constitute another important research area. The return to work is a major indicator of successful rehabilitation in brain-injured patients. In the area of closed head injury, there are indications that patients with more optimal psychological functioning perform better cognitively and rehabilitate more quickly (Campbell, 2006). Discovering markers for which individuals are at the highest risk for a lifetime of disability is crucial for the whole field of rehabilitation and for society's productivity. Personality variables as assessed by the MCMI-III can increase the likelihood of achieving a predictive model.

Thus in clinical cases, forensic cases, and issues of treatment and rehabilitation, the MCMI-III is making a considerable impact. Continued research with this personality instrument may open even more vistas for the field of neuropsychology.

Note

1. Complete data and detailed analysis for this study can be obtained from the author, Elbert W. Russell.

References

Alyman, C. A. (1999). The relationship of personality disorders and persistent post-convulsive syndrome in mild head injury. *Dissertation Abstracts International, 59*(12), 6482B.

American Psychiatric Association. (2000). *Diagnostic and statistical manual of mental disorders* (4th ed., text rev.). Washington, DC: Author.

Bagby, M. R., Gillis, J. R., Toner, B. B., & Goldberg, J. (1991). Detecting fake-good and fake-bad responding on the Millon Clinical Multiaxial Inventory–II. *Psychological Assessment: A Journal of Consulting and Clinical Psychology, 3*, 496–498.

Biederman, J., Gillis, J. R., Toner, B. B., & Goldberg, S. (1991). Comorbidity of attention deficit hyperactivity disorder with conduct, depressive, anxiety and other disorders. *American Journal of Psychiatry, 148*, 564–567.

Brazil, P. J. (1995). Use of the neuropsychological spectrum as a frame of reference in psychometric assessment of a dual diagnosis population. *Dissertation Abstracts International, 55*(10), 4319B.

Brown, J. (1987). *A screening key to differentiate normals from organics and patients with functional disorders.* Unpublished doctoral dissertation, Nova University.

Campbell, C. A. (2006). Predictors of functional outcome in mild traumatic brain injury: Findings from an archival study at John Muir Medical Center/Trauma Services. *Dissertation Abstracts International, 66*(8-B), 44–75.

Chitwood, R. P. (1989). *Objective assessment of personality characteristics related to cerebral lesions and cognitive deficits in persons with unilateral brain damage.* Unpublished doctoral dissertation, Florida State University.

Coffman, S. G. (1998). MCMI-III categories predict physiological responses. *Dissertation Abstracts International, 58*(11).

Craig, R. J., & Olson, R. E. (1992). Relationship between MCMI-II scales and normal personality traits. *Psychological Reports, 71*, 699–705.

Davis, R. D., Wenger, A., & Guzman, A. (1997). Validation of the MCMI-III. In T. Millon (Ed.), *The Millon inventories: Clinical and personality assessment* (pp. 327–359). New York: Guilford Press.

Garb, H. N. (1998). *Studying the clinician: Judgement research and psychological assessment.* Washington, DC: American Psychological Association.

Gass, C. S. (2006). Use of the MMPI-2 in neuropsychological evaluations. In J. N. Butcher (Ed.), *MMPI-2: A practitioner's guide* (pp. 301–326). Washington, DC: American Psychological Association.

Golden, C. J., Sweet, J. J., & Osman, D. C. (1979). The diagnosis of brain-damage by the MMPI: A comprehensive evaluation. *Journal of Personality Assessment, 43*, 138–142.

Goldstein, G. (1986). The neuropsychology of schizophrenia. In I. Grant & K. M. Adams (Eds.), *Neuropsychological assessment of neuropsychiatric disorders* (pp. 147–171). New York: Oxford University Press.

Grillo, J., Brown, R. S., Hilsabeck, R., Price, J. R., & Lees-Haley, P. R. (1994). Raising doubts about claims of malingering implications of relationships between MCMI-II and MMPI-2 performances. *Journal of Clinical Psychology, 50*, 651–655.

Lezak, M. D. (1995). *Neuropsychological assessment* (3rd ed.). New York: Oxford University Press.

Lezak, M. D., Howieson, D. B., & Loring, D. W. (2004). *Neuropsychological assessment* (4th ed.). New York: Oxford University Press.

Millikan, C. P. (2002). Empirically derived psychopathology subgroups in traumatic brain injury. *Dissertation Abstracts International*, 62(10), 4795B.

Millon, T. (with Millon, C., & Davis, R. D.). (1997). *Millon Clinical Multiaxial Inventory–III manual* (2nd ed.). Minneapolis, MN: National Computer Systems.

Muran, E. M., & Motta, R. W. (1993). Cognitive distortions and irrational beliefs in post-traumatic stress, anxiety, and depressive disorders. *Journal of Clinical Psychology*, 49, 166–176.

Oden, T. M. (2000). Insult denied: Traumatic brain injury and battered African-American women. *Dissertation Abstracts International*, 61(4-B), 1864.

Overholser, J. C. (1990). Retest reliability of the Millon Clinical Multiaxial Inventory. *Journal of Personality Assessment*, 55, 202–208.

Pope, K. S., Butcher, J. N., & Seelen, J. (1993). *The MMPI, MMPI-2, and MMPI-A in court*. Washington, DC: American Psychological Association.

Reitan, R. M. (1955). Affective disturbances in brain-damaged patients: Measurements with the Minnesota Multiphasic Personality Inventory. *Archives of Neurology and Psychiatry*, 73, 530–532.

Reitan, R. M., & Wolfson, D. (1997). Emotional disturbances and their interaction with neuropsychological deficits. *Neuropsychological Review*, 7, 3–19.

Retzlaff, P., Sheehan, E., & Fiel, A. (1991). MCMI-II report style and bias: Profile and validity scales analyses. *Journal of Personality Assessment*, 56, 466–477.

Rogers, R. (1988). *Clinical assessment of malingering and deception*. New York: Guilford Press.

Russell, E. W. (1975). Validation of a brain-damage versus schizophrenia MMPI key. *Journal of Clinical Psychology*, 31, 659–661.

Russell, E. W. (1977). MMPI profiles of brain-damaged and schizophrenic subjects. *Journal of Clinical Psychology*, 33, 190–193.

Russell, E. W. (1995). The accuracy of automated and clinical detection of brain damage and lateralization in neuropsychology. *Neuropsychology Review*, 5, 1–68.

Russell, E. W. (2000). The cognitive-metric, fixed battery approach to neuropsychological assessment. In R. D. Vanderploeg (Ed.), *Clinician's guide to neuropsychological assessment* (2nd ed., pp. 449–481). Hillsdale, NJ: Erlbaum.

Russell, E. W., & Polakoff, D. (1993). Neuropsychological test patterns in men for Alzheimer's and multi-infarct dementia. *Archives of Clinical Neuropsychology*, 8, 327–343.

Russell, S. L. K., & Russell, E. W. (1997). Using the MCMI in neuropsychological evaluations. In T. Millon (Ed.), *The Millon inventories: Clinical and personality assessment* (pp. 154–172). New York: Guilford Press.

Ruttan, L. A., & Heinrichs, R. W. (2003). Depression and neurocognitive functioning in mild traumatic brain injury patients referred for assessment. *Journal of Clinical and Experimental Neuropsychology*, 25(3), 407–419.

Swirsky-Sacchetti, T., Gorton, G., Samuel, S., Sobel, R., Genetta-Wadley, A., & Burleigh, B. (1993). Neuropsychological function in borderline personality disorder. *Journal of Clinical Psychology*, 49, 385–396.

Watson, C. G. (1977, March 10–12). Brain damage tests in psychiatric settings. *The INS Bulletin*.

Watson, C. G., Thomas R. W., Anderson, D., & Felling, J. (1968). Differentiation of schizophrenics from organics at two chronicity levels by use of Reitan–Halstead organic test battery. *Journal of Consulting and Clinical Psychology*, 32, 679–684.

Webb, L. M. (1999). Clinical assessment of malingering utilizing the Minnesota Multiphasic Personality Inventory–II, Millon Clinical Multiaxial Inventory–III, and Dissociative Experiences Scale. *Dissertation Abstracts International*, 59(12).

Weissman, H. N. (1990). Distortions and deceptions in self-presentation: Effects of protracted litigation in personal injury cases. *Behavioral Sciences and the Law*, 8, 67–74.

Wiens, A. N., & Matarazzo, J. D. (1977). WAIS and MMPI correlates of the Halstead–Reitan Neuropsychology Battery in normal male subjects. *Journal of Nervous and Mental Disease*, 164, 112–121.

CHAPTER 12

MCMI Applications
in Alcohol and Drug Dependence

Robert C. McMahon
Stephanie E. Diamond

Millon Clinical Multiaxial Inventory (MCMI)[1] studies of those with addictive disorders have revealed personality dimensions (McMahon, 2001; McMahon, Malow, & Jennings, 2000) and psychopathology subtypes (Fals-Stewart, 1992; McMahon, Malow, & Penedo, 1998; Messina, Farabee, & Rawson, 2003; Messina, Wish, Hoffman, & Nemes, 2002; Ball, Nich, Rounsaville, Eagan, & Carroll, 2004) associated with the nature and severity of substance abuse problems and with treatment response. Examination of co-occurring psychiatric disorders and dimensions of psychopathology among well-defined groups of these individuals holds promise for better understanding important clinical status characteristics and for developing more carefully tailored interventions.

MCMI dimensional and subtyping analyses have been useful in predicting important aspects of clinical status and treatment response. We will begin with a brief review of studies that have helped define MCMI cluster subtype relationships to important dimensions of clinical status. Ball et al. (2004) points out that most studies designed to classify substance-abusing patients in patient × treatment matching efforts have focused on "antisocial," "neurotic/affective," and "high-psychiatric-severity" subgroups. MCMI classification studies identify these three broad groupings and help clarify their clinical significance. Next, we focus on MCMI studies involving prediction of treatment retention. It has been demonstrated that treatment retention is among the strongest predictors of posttreatment abstinence (i.e., Messina et al., 2002). Until recently, most MCMI treatment outcome studies have involved evaluation of treatment retention (Ball et al., 2004; McMahon, Kelley, &

Kouzekanani, 1993; Stark & Campbell, 1988; Haller, Miles, & Dawson, 2002; Haller & Miles, 2004). However, of late, several studies have targeted a broader range of treatment outcomes—including relapse, quality of employment functioning, HIV risk, and psychiatric symptom status (i.e., Fals-Stewart, 1992; McMahon & Tyson, 1990; McMahon, 2001; Messina et al., 2002). Furthermore, an important recent study has tested hypotheses involving matching MCMI-III subtypes with substance abuse treatment conditions in a manner coordinated with Millon's theory of personality and psychopathology (Ball et al., 2004).

Clinical research studies involving the MCMI have been very helpful in articulating group relations among personality–psychopathology, clinical status, and treatment response among those presenting with substance dependence. However, clinicians are ultimately required to understand and plan effective treatments for individuals. We present a case that illustrates the usefulness of carefully examining the coincidence of personality disorder, clinical symptom status, and substance use in individual clinical conceptualization and treatment planning.

Clinical Status and MCMI Subgroup Membership

In the majority of classification studies of alcohol- and drug-dependent individuals, an MCMI-defined "antisocial" cluster subgroup has emerged; its members might be described as dominating, manipulative, and interpersonally exploitive. Substance use by members of this cluster type may be associated with a self-indulgent and stimulation-seeking lifestyle. Among alcohol-dependent samples, members of this cluster type have been found to deny the importance of substance abuse in their lives (Donat, Walters, & Hume, 1991), but to reveal relatively serious alcohol problems (Corbisiero & Reznikoff, 1991) and high alcohol consumption rates (Matano, Locke, & Schwartz, 1994). These individuals have been considered poor candidates for psychotherapy, because their fierce sense of independence clashes with externally imposed expectations for attitude and behavior change. However, more recent research raises questions about this conclusion (Messina et al., 2002; Ball et al., 2004).

A second MCMI cluster type identified with considerable consistency consists of individuals with substance abuse and evidence of rather severe personality pathology. Craig and Olson (1990) have described this type as characterized by pessimistic attitudes, unstable moods, and erratic behavior. Paranoid features involving feelings of being misunderstood, unappreciated, and exploited may be associated with edgy irritability and interpersonal acting out. Among cluster studies involving drug-abusing samples, the "high-psychopathology" type has been found to have higher prevalence of posttraumatic stress disorder, more suicide attempts, and more frequent drug and psychiatric treatments, compared to other types (Craig, Bivens, & Olson, 1997). This group has also been associated with more frequent substance use, more severe psychiatric problems, and poorer attitudes related to HIV risk reduction than those found in antisocial and subclinical cluster groups, as well as less sexual self-efficacy, less frequent condom use, and more HIV anxiety than antisocial cluster group members (McMahon et al., 1998). In addition, members of a severely disturbed subtype identified among opioid-dependent inpatients have demonstrated more depression, substance-related problems, and family conflicts than those found in low-psycho-pathology patients (Ball et al., 2004).

A third MCMI cluster type involves those who abuse substances and also experience self-depreciatory attitudes, excessive social dependence or avoidance, anticipation of failure in interpersonal relations, and high levels of depression and anxiety. This subtype is often characterized as "neurotic" or as revealing "affective disturbance." Within this cluster type, substance use may be associated with attempts to cope with chronic or recurrent anxiety and depression. Among alcohol-dependent samples, the neurotic type has been found to be more likely than others to drink alone, and to have more difficulty tolerating interpersonal anxiety, frustration, and discouragement than the narcissistic–antisocial type (Donat et al., 1991). Members of this subtype are also characterized by more serious life disruption and more distress associated with alcohol use than other cluster types (Corbisiero & Reznikoff, 1991). Furthermore, in a drug-abusing sample, members of an MCMI affective type have reported more years of opiate use, more distress due to substance-related issues, higher levels of depression, and more medical and psychological problems on a structured clinical interview, compared to a type without affective disturbance (Ball et al., 2004).

Treatment Retention

Retention in substance dependence treatment is often found to be an important determinant of drug use outcomes (Messina et al., 2002). A number of investigators have used the MCMI in efforts to predict treatment dropout. McMahon, Kelley, and Kouzekanani (1993) argued that a patient's personality style could be a useful predictor of dropout from residential therapeutic community drug abuse treatment. Patients with prominent detached (schizoid or avoidant) personality features were judged likely to have few interpersonal coping skills, to receive little reinforcement from social participation, and to find pressures for group involvement in typical residential treatment as aversive. Those with independent (narcissistic and antisocial) personalities, tending to be self-oriented, manipulative, and exploitive in social interactions, were expected to resist the pressure for attitude and behavior change inherent in therapeutic-community-oriented treatment. In contrast, those with significant passive/dependent characteristics, disposed to seek guidance and approval from caretakers, were expected to find the structured and supportive therapeutic community appealing.

Discriminant analysis was used to differentiate between treatment dropouts and completers, based upon scores on MCMI-II personality scales from an intake assessment among men receiving treatment for cocaine dependence. Dropouts were differentiated from completers by a discriminant function defined, in part, by elevated scores on MCMI-II personality scales that tap a ruggedly independent orientation with dominating, exploitive, and manipulative features. MCMI-II scales measuring opposing characteristics, such as a strong need for social approval and a compliant, respectful, and conscientious interpersonal pattern, also contributed to the function. Those with this pattern demonstrated a greater likelihood of treatment completion.

Fals-Stewart (1992) used hierarchical agglomerative cluster analysis of intake MCMI personality scales to identify homogeneous subgroups among drug-abusing individuals in therapeutic community residential treatment. He then compared these cluster subgroups for length of stay in treatment and for proportions that remained abstinent during a follow-up period. Consistent with predictions, clusters defined by elevations on the MCMI Antisocial scale and on the Schizoid and Avoidant scales had substantially shorter stays in treatment and significantly smaller proportions abstinent during the follow-up interval than clusters characterized by peaks on the MCMI Narcissistic, Dependent, and Histrionic scales. Members of the Antisocial cluster were most likely to be removed from treatment for rule infractions, whereas those in the Schizoid/Avoidant cluster were most likely to leave against staff advice. Members of these two clusters not only relapsed in greater percentages, but also did so faster than those in other clusters. Fals-Stewart (1992) concludes that those with personality features associated with membership in these clusters are not as appropriate for traditional therapeutic-community-oriented treatment as are those in the other clusters.

Furthermore, Craig and Olson (1988) found that dropouts from treatment for drug dependence had lower needs for affiliation and nurturance and higher needs for autonomy and aggression than did treatment completers. However, although Stark and Campbell (1988) found that treatment completers showed more evidence of interpersonal dependence on the MCMI, no differences between dropouts and completers were found on MCMI scales measuring independent personality features. Interestingly, Craig (1984) found that histrionic features predicted treatment completion, whereas passive/dependent features were associated with dropout. Craig (1984) suggests that results may vary, depending upon mode of treatment (therapeutic community, methadone maintenance, detoxification), duration of treatment, and the type of substance abuse for which treatment is sought.

Haller et al. (2002) examined differences in treatment retention among MCMI-II cluster subtypes of drug-dependent women in day treatment at the Center for Perinatal Addiction (CPA), a treatment and research program sponsored by the National Institute on Drug Abuse. Most participants were young (mean age 29 years), single (62%), African American (77%) women who were on probation, were on parole, or had a court date pending. The most frequently reported drug of abuse was crack cocaine.

The sample was cluster-analyzed, and a three-cluster solution was identified as optimal. Cluster 1 was characterized as subclinical; cluster 2 was described as severely disturbed, with many elevations on personality and symptom scales; and cluster 3 was described as revealing moderate psychopathology, with fewer Axis I elevations but prominent externalizing (antisocial) personality disorder features. In relationship to treatment retention, there was rapid attrition for those in cluster 2 (severely disturbed). Interestingly, those with moderate psychopathology (cluster 3) had the lowest attrition rate. The fact that cluster 1 (subclinical) had a higher attrition rate than cluster 3 may reflect less perceived need for treatment among the relatively healthy members of the first cluster.

A more recent study by Haller and Miles (2004) examined the treatment completion rates among clusters of drug-dependent women in residential treatment at the CPA Residential Project (CPA-RP). As in the Haller et al. (2002) study, most participants were single, pregnant African American women involved with the criminal justice system for whom crack cocaine was the most frequently reported drug of abuse. Three cluster subgroups based on level of psychopathology (mild, moderate, and severe psychopathology) were identified, based on the patients' MCMI-III records. The authors found that the groups' treatment completion rates varied by cluster, with the mild-psychopathology group having the highest completion rate (66%), followed by the moderate group (45%), and finally the severe-psychopathology group (29%).

Messina et al. (2002) found no relationship between the presence–absence of MCMI-II-identified antisocial personality and treatment dropout among a group of predominantly African American male participants receiving therapeutic community treatment for cocaine and heroin addiction. Finally, Ball et al., (2004) found no relationship between membership in three separate MCMI-III-based psychopathology subgroups (antisocial/narcissistic, affective/neurotic, and high psychiatric severity) and dropout among a group of opioid-dependent participants in a study involving a variety of outpatient treatment options. However, the significance of this finding may be difficult to interpret, because nearly half of the individuals approached about participation in the study apparently left treatment prior to classification.

Pretreatment versus Posttreatment MCMI Comparisons

A number of investigators have used repeated administrations of the MCMI to gauge improvement in clinical status among substance-dependent individuals over the course of treatment and follow-up. McMahon and Richards (1996) examined changes in MCMI-II base rate (BR) scores between intake and discharge administrations in a group of cocaine-dependent men in residential treatment. They found mean scale elevations (BR > 74) on the MCMI-II Antisocial, Aggressive/Sadistic, Narcissistic, Passive–Aggressive, Borderline, Drug Dependence, and Alcohol Dependence scales at treatment intake. Although there were some mean changes between intake and discharge, few involved a change from clinically elevated levels to subclinical levels. Furthermore, examination of intake–discharge stability coefficients suggests the relative consistency of these scale-linked characteristics over time.

In a study by de Groot, Franken, van der Meer, and Hendriks (2003), patients who met diagnostic criteria for opiate or cocaine abuse or dependence in residential treatment in the Netherlands were assessed over time in effort to examine the extent of change in scores on MCMI-II personality scales during treatment. Subjects completed the MCMI-II at 3-month intervals, and only those who had completed the instrument at least four times were selected for study. Subjects were included in the study if they completed 9 months of treatment and had valid MCMI profiles. Most had polydrug dependence. Repeated measures analyses demonstrated significant decreases in Schizoid, Avoidant, Dependent, Schizotypal, Passive–Aggressive, and Borderline scores. There was no evidence of increases in personality scale scores during treatment.

Schinka et al. (1999) were interested in change over time on the Beck Depression Inventory (BDI), Hamilton Anxiety Scale (HAM-A), and MCMI-II scores of cocaine-dependent women in therapeutic community treatment. Intake assessment revealed elevated scores on the BDI and HAM-A, as well as on the Avoidant, Dependent,

Antisocial, Passive–Aggressive, Self-Defeating, and Borderline scales of the MCMI-II. Follow-up results revealed that BDI and HAM-A scores decreased, and that scores on the Avoidant, Dependent, Self-Defeating, and Borderline MCMI-II scales changed from the clinical to the subclinical range. No change was found for the Antisocial and Passive–Aggressive scales of the MCMI-II.

Caslyn, Wells, Fleming, and Saxon (2000) were interested in examining whether changes in MCMI scores of opiate-dependent individuals were related to methadone maintenance treatment retention and recent drug use. Assessments using the MCMI, Addiction Severity Index, and AIDS Initial Assessment Questionnaire were administered within the first month of treatment and at 18 months. Results indicated that scores on many MCMI scales decreased significantly. No changes were evident on the Histrionic, Narcissistic, Antisocial, Schizotypal, Paranoid, and Psychotic Thinking scales. Scores on the Compulsive scale increased significantly. As anticipated, almost all Axis I scores decreased, and there was less change on Axis II scores.

Caslyn et al. (2000) also divided their sample into subgroups with heavy and light drug use. To make this distinction, participants were asked to report their use of opiates, cocaine and benzodiazepines in the 6 months prior to the 18-month follow-up. "Heavy use" was defined as self-reported weekly use or more of any of the above-mentioned substances; "light use" was defined as self-reported use of any of the substances less than four times per month. The researchers found that MCMI scores changed over time in a manner linked with the extent of drug use in the 6 months prior to follow-up. The scores of those who reported light drug use decreased more than the scores of those reporting heavy use. Significant decreases were found in the percentage of cases with clinically elevated scores on the Anxiety, Dysthymia, Alcohol Abuse, Avoidant, Passive–Aggressive, and Borderline scales for the participants who reported light drug use. No similar decreases were evident in the heavy-use group.

HIV Risk Behavior Outcomes

There has been increasing interest in personality disorders and other psychiatric conditions among substance-dependent individuals that might elevate risk for HIV infection and influence response to HIV prevention intervention. Antisocial personality disorder (ASPD) has received particular attention. ASPD has been conceptualized as including impulsive behaviors and reckless disregard for personal safety and that of others—characteristics that might increase risk for HIV infection. Gill, Nomilal, and Crowley (1992) found that those diagnosed with ASPD were more likely to report needle-sharing, a greater number of needle sharing partners, recent injection drug use, earlier first sexual contacts, a greater number of sexual partners, and involvement in prostitution than were those without ASPD. Compton, Cottler, Spitznagel, Ben-Abdallah, and Gallagher (1998) found ASPD was linked with having multiple sexual partners, being intoxicated during sex, paying for sex, giving drugs for sex, and receiving drugs for sex. This trend for higher rates of HIV risk behaviors applied both at baseline and after HIV risk reduction intervention at 18-month follow-up. However, those with ASPD demonstrated similar rates of risk reduction after completion of HIV transmission risk reduction intervention.

In contrast, however, Abbott, Weller, and Walker (1994) found no association between ASPD diagnosis made with the Structured Clinical Interview for DSM-IV Axis II Disorders (SCID-II) and HIV risk scores on the Risk Assessment Battery). Tourian et al. (1997) suggested that the diagnosis of ASPD may insufficiently capture features that contribute to risky behavior and is complicated by including antisocial behaviors that may be associated with drug use. They found that sex-related risky behavior was predicted more consistently by measures of personality traits associated with antisociality than by a diagnosis of ASPD.

Although Axis II disorders other than ASPD have been given less emphasis, a number of personality disorders involve deficits in judgment, planning, and interpersonal problem solving connected to transient, exploitive, and coercive sexual contacts (Kelly, Murphy, Bahr, & Brasfield, 1992). Indeed, there is evidence that psychiatric patients with Axis II disorders are at higher risk for HIV exposure than those with Axis I syndromes only (Kalichman, Carey, & Carey, 1996), and borderline personality disorder has been linked with impulsive high-risk sexual behaviors (Kelly et al., 1992; Chen, Brown, Lo, & Linehan, 2007). McMahon et al. (1998) found that a group with polysubstance abuse and with high levels of personality pathology (identified via cluster analysis of MCMI-II records) revealed relatively little confidence in their ability to enact safer sexual practices, little commitment to condom use, and higher anxiety associated with risk of contracting HIV, compared to those without evidence of such pathology.

McMahon et al. (2000) studied linkages between maladaptive personality characteristics measured by the MCMI-II (Millon, 1981; Millon & Davis, 1996) and HIV risk behaviors among those with polysubstance abuse. Factor-analytic studies of the MCMI-II have identified avoidant, dependent, and antisocial personality dimensions that predict such clinically meaningful outcomes among substance-abusing samples as treatment dropout and drug use relapse (McMahon, Kelley, & Kouzekanani, 1993; McMahon, 2001). Associations between these personality dimensions and high-risk sexual practices among those receiving treatment for substance abuse were hypothesized.

McMahon et al. (2000) hypothesized that substance-abusing individuals with avoidant personalities would have limited involvement in sexually intimate relationships, due to their hypersensitivity to social rejection, frequently anxious and depressed mood, and limited interpersonal coping skills. These qualities were also expected to limit successful enactment of safer sexual practices (including condom use) in sexual encounters that did occur. Furthermore, avoidant individuals were predicted to experience little benefit from HIV risk reduction intervention that requires sharing personal information about risky sexual behaviors and practicing sexual negotiation skills in group counseling. Elevated sexual risk behavior among substance-abusing individuals with dependent personalities was hypothesized to be related to overreliance on others for direction and support, especially on those with whom there is sexual intimacy. Risk reduction interventions designed to encourage assertive negotiation of safer practices were hypothesized to be of limited value for these persons. Finally, individuals with antisocial personalities are characterized as rejecting conventional norms and social values, and as being behaviorally hedonistic and erotically impulsive (Millon & Davis, 1996). These qualities were expected to dispose antisocial individuals to promiscuous and coercive sexual encounters and sensation-seeking behaviors inconsistent with safer sexual practices. Interventions targeting HIV risk reduction behaviors (including consistent condom use) were expected to have limited effect among those with this orientation.

Participants in the McMahon et al. (2000) study were male veterans who met *Diagnostic and Statistical Manual of Mental Disorders*, third edition, revised (DSM-III-R) criteria for substance dependence, and who participated in a 6-week Department of Veterans Affairs-based therapeutic community drug dependence treatment program that included an HIV prevention intervention. The HIV prevention component (Corrigan, Thompson, Malow, & Sorensen, 1992) involved four 2-hour group sessions aimed at encouraging HIV risk reduction by increasing perceived susceptibility to HIV infection, encouraging beliefs and attitudes that would promote risk reduction, and fostering development of communication and behavioral skills associated with safer sexual practices and methods of syringe use.

Sequential multiple-regression analysis was used to determine whether personality dimensions and then perceived stress and social support improved prediction of 12-month follow-up percentage of unprotected sex among treatment completers after the researchers controlled for important covariates, including pretreatment percentage of unprotected sex and both pretreatment and 12-month follow-up substance abuse levels. Results of this study revealed that those with dependent personalities were more likely to engage in unprotected sex at follow-up, perhaps because of their excessive reliance upon others for direction and because of their limited ability to negotiate consistent condom use assertively. Those with significant avoidant personality features revealed lower risk levels associated with limited sexual involvement during follow-up. However, no association was found between level of this personality style and level of risk behavior among those who reported sexual activity. Perhaps avoidant characteristics are more likely to inhibit development of sexual relationships than to compromise enactment of safer sexual practice among those who do engage in sexual intimacies. The authors also found a significant bivariate relationship between antisocial personality and unprotected sex prior to intake, but not during follow-up. The failure to find stronger and more consistent associations may be related to the very high scores on the MCMI-II Antisocial personality scale earned by the majority in this sample: Nearly three-fourths of the group scored in the clinically elevated range (BR > 74) on this scale. Perhaps there was insufficient variability on this dimension to allow for an adequate test of this hypothesis.

Employment Functioning Outcomes

Whereas most studies predicting drug treatment outcome focus (appropriately) on relapse, another important aspect of recovery involves adequacy of employment functioning. In addition to being an important outcome in its own right, several studies have identified links between posttreatment employment functioning and maintenance of drug abstinence (e.g., Gregoire & Snively, 2001; Hser, Hoffman, Grella, & Anglin, 2001; Siegal, Li, & Rapp, 2002). Unfortunately, relatively little is known about factors that influence employment outcomes among those treated for alcohol and other drug abuse, or about the relevance to employment outcomes of stress and personality factors found important in substance use relapse prediction (cf.

Compton, Cottler, Jacobs, Ben-Abdallah, & Spitznagel, 2003; McMahon, 2001; Fals-Stewart, 1992; Ball et al., 2004). In an investigation involving 304 male cocaine-dependent participants in residential treatment, McMahon and Enders (2005) hypothesized that stress and avoidant, dependent, antisocial, and delusional/paranoid personality factors would predict severity of employment problems at treatment completion (intercept) and change in level of employment problem severity over three follow-up intervals, reflected in the shape factor derived from latent growth curve analysis. This investigation included a lagged time-varying covariate to capture the influence of relapse status (0 = no relapse, 1 = relapsed or lost to follow-up) on employment problem severity scores at 6 and 9 months following discharge and controlled for a number of potentially important factors, including age, education, employment problem severity at treatment intake, length of current treatment, and number of prior treatments. Not surprisingly, those with delusional/paranoid personality characteristics showed relatively limited recovery of employment functioning. More intensive and long-term psychiatric treatment and vocational rehabilitative services may be required for improvement in employment functioning among those with such characteristics.

MCMI Studies Involving Depression Subtypes

Several studies by McMahon and colleagues have investigated the link between personality and depression in alcoholism (McMahon & Davidson, 1985b; McMahon & Tyson, 1990; McMahon, Schram, & Davidson, 1993). Alcoholic individuals entering treatment frequently present with clinical depression. It is commonly believed that the depressive symptoms exhibited are results of ethanol ingestion and withdrawal (Schuckit, 1983). Typically, once detoxification is complete, depressive symptoms abate within several weeks. However, for a significant number of those with alcohol dependence, depressive symptoms persist after treatment completion. As evidenced by the work of McMahon and colleagues, this more enduring depression may be linked to underlying personality disorder (McMahon & Davidson, 1985a; McMahon & Tyson, 1990). McMahon and Tyson (1990) argued that personality styles at treatment intake may help to distinguish between alcoholic individuals who would be likely to experience an early remission of depressive symptoms and those who would be more likely to experience enduring depressive symptoms. According to Millon (1981), enduring depressive syndromes may result from rigidly dysfunctional ways of perceiving and relating to self and others.

For instance, alcoholic individuals with avoidant personalities were hypothesized to be vulnerable to enduring depression because of their alienated and devalued self-images and hypersensitivity to social rejection. Similarly, for those with passive–aggressive personalities, enduring depression was predicted to be associated both with discontented self-images and with unstable, conflict-laden, and fault-finding interpersonal behaviors that result in low rates of positive reinforcement and high rates of punishment.

In contrast, those with narcissistic, histrionic, and compulsive personalities were assumed to have characteristics associated with less vulnerability to enduring clinical depression. Millon (1981) suggests that enduring depression is not consistent with narcissistic individuals' highly developed sense of self-assurance and self-worth. Failures to live up to inflated self-estimations are typically rationalized and externalized and infrequently lead to enduring depression. Those with histrionic personalities may experience transient depressions associated with predictable disruptions in social attachments. Such depressive reactions often reflect dramatic but superficial emotionality, and should dissipate rather quickly as supportive social relationships are reestablished. Finally, those with compulsive personalities may be vulnerable to depression when they have failed to live up to self-imposed performance standards, or when they receive negative evaluations from those upon whom they depend for guidance and approval. However, their depressions are considered likely to be transient, because they have been punished for signs of vulnerability and inadequacy and are likely to respond to structured and supportive residential treatment.

McMahon and Tyson (1990) found that in their sample of alcoholic women, approximately two-thirds suffered from significant clinical depression at treatment intake. Clinical depression was then subcategorized as enduring or transient. Slightly more than half of those suffering from depression met criteria for the enduring subtype. Associations between depression subgroup membership and MCMI personality measures at both intake and discharge were examined via discriminant analysis. Strong and moderate positive associations at intake and discharge, respectively, were found between scores on the Passive–Aggressive and Avoidant scales and membership in the enduring-depression group. Moderate positive associations were found at both intake and discharge between scores on the Compulsive scale and membership in the transient-depression group. A moderate association was also found between scores on the Narcissistic scale and transient depression at discharge.

Results from the McMahon and Tyson (1990) study of alcohol-dependent women are generally consistent with the results of an earlier study of alcohol-dependent men (McMahon & Davidson, 1985b) in demonstrating that personality features are useful in distinguishing between transient and enduring depression. Yet some differences were identified in the factors that distinguished depression subgroup membership. Whereas the passive–aggressive personality style was most strongly linked with enduring depression in the study of alcoholic women, the MCMI scales associated with clinical features including irrational, confused, and disorganized thinking and behavior and an avoidant personality pattern were more strongly predictive of enduring depression in the study of alcoholic men. However, the authors noted similarities between cognitive and interpersonal features of the passive–aggressive and avoidant personalities, and those emphasized in influential cognitive and interpersonal models of depression (Beck, 1967; Klerman & Weissman, 1986).

Another study (McMahon, Schram, & Davidson, 1993) examined relationships among three MCMI-II-defined personality subgroups and depression among predominantly male alcoholic participants in residential treatment. The first MCMI subgroup (detached/ambivalent) had peak mean scale elevations on the Schizoid or Avoidant scales, with secondary elevations on the Passive–Aggressive scale. The second MCMI group was defined by elevations on the Dependent scale. The third group (independent) was characterized by elevations on the Narcissistic and/or Antisocial scales.

It was hypothesized that the avoidant/passive–aggressive (detached/ambivalent) group would be more likely than the other two groups to report high levels of depression, due to their limited interpersonal coping skills, tendencies toward disturbing cognitions, and withdrawal from potentially supportive relationships. Cognitive and interpersonal models of depression suggest that these characteristics may contribute directly to depression (Beck, 1967; Klerman & Weissman, 1986). Results indicated that the detached/ambivalent group did indeed report significantly greater depression than found in the dependent and independent groups.

Additional hypotheses were that vulnerability to negative life events and/or responsiveness to the effects of social support would vary by personality group. As predicted, the detached/ambivalent group reported significantly more depression under high-stress than low-stress circumstances. Furthermore, as hypothesized, there was no evidence that this group profited from either direct or stress-buffering effects of social support. Consistent with expectations, the dependent group also reported significantly more depression under high-stress than low-stress conditions. However, anticipated directly beneficial and stress-buffering social support effects were not found in this group. Finally, as hypothesized, significant relationships were not found between stress or support levels and depression in the independent group. However, an unexpected stress × support interaction was found. This interaction highlights the possibility that when stress is low, independent types in treatment for substance abuse may experience social support as unwanted pressure for attitude and behavior change, which may be linked with depression. The authors note that these results must be interpreted with caution. Although subjects reported about stressors that occurred during the year prior to their treatment admission, it is possible that the depression preceded the reported life stressors. Furthermore, the fact that current depression may have led to overreporting of stressful life events must be considered.

Substance Use Relapse

In the past decade or so, a number of researchers have drawn upon Millon's theory of personality and psychopathology and have used various versions of the MCMI in predicting substance use outcomes after treatment for alcohol, cocaine, and opiate dependence (Fals-Stewart, 1992; McMahon, Kelley, & Kouzekanani, 1993; McMahon, Schram, & Davidson, 1993; Messina et al., 2001; 2003; Ball et al., 2004). These studies have involved MCMI cluster-analytic, profile-sorting, and scale-level factor-analytic methods.

McMahon (2001) conducted a study designed to examine stress, social support, and personality as predictors of both cocaine relapse and drug abuse severity in cocaine-dependent males during the 12 months after residential treatment. It was hypothesized that relapse and severity of drug abuse would be associated with (1) higher levels of detached, dependent, and antisocial personality traits; (2) more negative life events, less perceived social support, and smaller support network size; and (3) effects of negative life events and social support among those with dependent personalities, and effects of negative life events among those with detached personality styles.

Vulnerability to relapse in those with detached personalities was hypothesized to be linked to their preoccupation with disturbing cognitions that interfere with social communication and lead to dysphoric mood, their inability to tolerate close relationships or benefit from social support, and their limited capacity to cope effectively with life stressors. Vulnerability to relapse among those with dependent personalities was considered connected to their excessive reliance upon others, as well as their limited initiative, autonomy, and capacity for assuming adult responsibility, including coping with inevitable stressors during attempts at drug abuse recovery (Millon, 1981; Millon & Davis, 1996). Those high on the antisocial factor were viewed as strongly independent, because of either a deeply rooted confidence in themselves, a pervasive mistrust of others, or both (Millon, 1981; Millon & Davis, 1996). Characterized as interpersonally manipulative and exploitive, they were judged likely to be unconcerned with the needs and expectations of others, and relatively resistant both to the effects of negative life events and to supportive social influences. They were expected to resist demands for admission of personal failings and elimination of substance use. Those with strong antisocial features were considered unlikely to make a serious commitment to treatment or recovery in the posttreatment period, and likely to resume a sensation-seeking (rather than a stress-coping) pattern of substance abuse.

The McMahon (2001) sample included 304 cocaine-dependent males recruited from three residential therapeutic communities for the treatment of drug dependence. Intake evaluation was conducted within 2 weeks after treatment admission but after completion of detoxification. Follow-up evaluations were conducted prior to treatment discharge and at 3, 6, 9, and 12 months posttreatment. Nearly half of the subjects were African American, about one-third were European American, and most of the rest were Hispanic. The mean age was 29.3 years, the average education level was 12.2 years ($SD = 2.2$), and few (<14%) were currently married and living with a spouse prior to treatment entry.

MCMI-II factors tapping antisocial and dependent personality characteristics did not predict drug outcomes. However, higher levels of detached personality traits predicted both cocaine relapse and drug abuse severity prospectively in main-effects analyses. Less favorable drug outcomes in those with this orientation may have been associated with their difficulty in participating fully in therapeutic community treatments that emphasized social participation and confrontation of attitudes and behaviors relevant to drug use. Also, lack of attention during treatment to long-standing personality problems may have limited participants' prospects for enduring maintenance of abstinence. More personality-sensitive residential or aftercare treatments may be necessary for cocaine-dependent individuals with detached personality characteristics (Beck, Freeman, & Associates, 1990). Those with prominent avoidant personality features may have considerable reluctance to discuss stressful interpersonal events that serve as drug use triggers. Indeed, many group-confrontation-oriented residential drug treatment approaches may overwhelm their most basic defense, which is detachment. It has been recommended that those with prominent detached personality characteristics be approached gradually and supportively. Initially, an emphasis on positive attributes and on social skills training designed to enhance confidence and self-esteem is recommended (Millon, 1981; Millon & Davis, 1996; Beck et al., 1990). Results of this study are consistent with previously identified associations between negative affective states and relapse among those treated for alcohol, tobacco, and opiate addictions (Wills, 1990; Brownell, Marlatt, Lichtenstein, & Wilson, 1986; Ball et al., 2004), because the detached factor predicting cocaine relapse and outcome abuse severity had moderate or higher loadings on the Anxiety and Major Depression scales.

It is unclear what contributed to the failure to establish associations between dependent and antisocial personality characteristics and relapse. Only a few participants earned significant elevations on the MCMI Dependent scale, and fewer showed such elevations in the absence of similar or more pronounced elevations on one or several other scales (e.g., Antisocial). Dependent characteristics were probably not particularly salient in the personalities of most participants. In contrast, most (> 80%) scored in the clinically elevated range on the Antisocial scale. In this investigation, there were perhaps too few participants without antisocial characteristics to allow for an adequate test of the relationship between antisociality and relapse. However, current findings are consistent with a series of studies (Carroll et al., 1994; Cacciola, Alterman, & Rutherford, 1995; Messina et al., 2002, 2003) suggesting that opioid- and cocaine-dependent patients with antisocial personalities do not experience less favorable treatment outcomes. We note that Ball et al. (2004) did find less favorable treatment outcomes among MCMI-III-defined antisocial/narcissistic opioid-dependent treatment participants (see reviews of Messina et al., 2001, 2003, and Ball et al., 2004, in this chapter).

Hypotheses relating to the stress vulnerability of those with detached and dependent personalities, and the support responsiveness of those with dependent personalities, were not confirmed. However, important direct effects of stress and social support were found. Wills (1990) suggested the possibility that negative life events and limitations in social support predict relapse because of their link with underlying psychopathology. In this investigation, both stress and social support prospectively predicted outcome drug abuse severity, and they both prospectively predicted relapse after three separate dimensions of psychopathology were controlled. These findings reveal the importance of considering both personality and social context factors in understanding the process of recovery from drug dependence.

Messina et al. (2002) examined the relationship between MCMI-II-identified ASPD and response to two therapeutic community treatment programs that were part of the District of Columbia Treatment Initiative. The standard treatment involved 10 months of inpatient care and 2 months of outpatient care. The comparison condition involved a briefer program consisting of 6 months of inpatient care and 6 months of outpatient care. Participants (72% male, 98% black) were administered the MCMI-II, and those with valid records (88%; n = 275) and BR scores greater than or equal to 75 on the MCMI-II Antisocial scale were classified as having ASPD. One hundred and thirty-six participants had been randomly assigned to standard inpatient treatment, and 139 to abbreviated inpatient treatment. More than 90% had arrest histories, with a mean of 8.6 adult arrests prior to treatment. The primary drug of abuse was crack cocaine; however, nearly half had problems with both cocaine and heroin. Sixty-eight percent of the sample earned BR scores > 75 on the MCMI-II Antisocial scale. Most (77 of 88) of those in the non-ASPD group (those with MCMI-II BRs < 75) had "other disorders," according to MCMI-II classification criteria. Outcome analyses controlled for the presence of other MCMI-II Axis I and Axis II disorders for both the ASPD and non-ASPD groups. These analyses suggested no significant differences between the ASPD and non-ASPD groups in treatment retention, drug use at 19-month follow-up, or posttreatment arrests. These results parallel those obtained in an earlier study, in which Messina, Wish, and Nemes (1999) used the SCID-II to classify the same subjects as having ASPD ($n = 166$) or not ($n = 172$), in which no differences were found between the groups in treatment completion, drug use at 12-month follow-up, or postdischarge arrest.

Messina and colleagues caution that results of this investigation may not parallel those in other studies, because 98% of the sample was black and because participants both with and without ASPD had unusually extensive histories of both crime and drug dependence. Furthermore, the high rates of comorbidity in both the ASPD and non-ASPD groups may have confounded the distinction between the groups in ways that are difficult to appreciate. Despite this, the two studies by Messina's group using quite different methods of diagnosing ASPD contribute to a growing literature suggesting that those with this disorder benefit from various forms of therapeutic community treatment and aftercare as much as those without it.

Patient × Treatment Matching

Ball et al. (2004) examined the validity of two MCMI-III subtyping procedures in evaluating clinical status and treatment outcomes in recently detoxified opioid-dependent outpatients (74% male, 80% European American) participating in a 3-month randomized clinical trial. Potential participants were excluded if they presented with significant medical conditions, lifetime schizophrenia, or bipolar disorder, or if they had received addiction treatment in the previous 3 months. Participants were randomly assigned to one of three conditions, each of which involved a weekly coping skills group and naltrexone administered three times weekly: (1) no incentive voucher; (2) an incentive voucher linked with drug-free status and naltrexone compliance; and (3) the incentive voucher combined with relationship counseling.

Ball et al. (2004) suggested that guidance drawn from Millon's theoretical model might serve as a useful basis for predicting differential response of psychopathology subtypes to various substance use treatment combinations. For example, they argued that MCMI psychopathology subgroups (i.e., high psychiatric severity and affective/ neurotic) defined in part by unusual sensitivity to external contingencies, including need for attention, approval, and support from others, might show incremental benefit from the addition of incentive vouchers and relationship counseling to coping skills group and naltrexone treatment administered three times weekly. The addition of supportive behavior therapy in these MCMI subgroups was hypothesized to compensate for the loss of an important pharmacological means of affect regulation associated with naltrexone treatment. Ball et al. (2004) noted:

> By comparison, depressed, anxious, or otherwise psychiatrically distressed subtypes might be expected to require significant social support or engagement with others for sustained symptom reduction. Monetary incentives also may be helpful for these types of distressed patients to the extent that they increase the anticipation of pleasure rather than pain from the environment, improve behavioral mobility, or counteract hopeless or helpless beliefs about symptom improvement. Thus, reinforcement contingencies, coping skills, and relational support may provide differential benefit to subtypes based on Millon's biopsychosocial personality theory. (p. 700)

Previous research suggests that antisocial personality is not a risk factor for poor response to drug treatment (i.e., McMahon, 2001), particularly when incentive reinforcements are provided (Brooner, Kidorf, King, & Stoller, 1998; Silverman et al., 1998; Messina et al. 2003). However, there is some evidence that antisocial substance-abusing individuals may not be optimally matched with relationship-focused treatments (Kadden, Cooney, Getter, & Litt, 1989; Longabaugh et al., 1994). Ball et al. (2004) wrote:

> The possibility that antisocial/narcissistic individuals with substance abuse may be responsive to external contingencies involving immediate, personal gain (monetary incentives), but not requiring cooperative work with others (as in relationship counseling or an interactional group), is at least partly consistent with Millon's (1999) description of antisocial and narcissistic personality patterns. (p. 700)

Ball et al. (2004) used Calsyn, Fleming, Wells, and Saxon's (1996) profile-sorting approach and found that two-thirds of their sample met Axis I affective disturbance criteria. They found no other high-prevalence Axis I type. The only high-frequency Axis II subtype involved elevations on the MCMI-III Antisocial and Narcissistic scales, into which 46% of cases were classified. Because of the small number of individuals within most other Axis I and II categories, they limited their evaluation to validity of the affective disturbance (Axis I) and antisocial–narcissistic (Axis II) subtypes. They also conducted both hierarchical and nonhierarchical cluster analyses separately, based on the MCMI-III Axis I and Axis II scales. The clusters that emerged in separate Axis I and Axis II analyses were sufficiently closely related ($k = .78$) that they were used in subsequent analyses of cluster subtypes based on combined Axis I and II. Several clustering procedures (k-means and average linkage) yielded two clearly differentiated subtypes (i.e., high psychiatric severity and low psychiatric severity). The k-means solution was chosen because it yielded better cell sizes for subsequent cluster type × treatment analyses.

Highlighting the importance of the MCMI typing procedures was the find that those participants classified into each of the three psychopathology subtypes failed to demonstrate significant reductions in opiate use over the 12-treatment period. In contrast, the nonaffective, nonantisocial, and low-psychiatric-severity comparison groups did show significant decreases in opiate use over the same period. Several anticipated, and unanticipated but interesting, results emerged in MCMI-III subtype × treatment × time analyses. The affective disturbance subtype responded better in the incentive-voucher conditions than in the no-incentive-voucher condition with respect to naltrexone compliance and drug abstinence. Members of the nonaffective subgroup in the no-incentive-voucher condition demonstrated greater reduction in opiate use than did either their counterparts in the incentive-voucher conditions or members of the affective subgroup in the no-incentive-voucher condition. Participants in the antisocial–narcissistic subgroup demonstrated greater reductions in opiate use in the no-voucher condition than in the two voucher conditions. Surprisingly, however, antisocial–narcissistic individuals demonstrated greater opiate use reductions in the voucher + relationship counseling condition than in the voucher-alone condition. By contrast, the nonantisocial comparison group did better in the voucher-alone condition than in the voucher + relationship counseling condition.

Notably, those in the high-psychiatric-severity group did demonstrate significantly greater benefit from both voucher conditions, including the one that included relationship counseling, than did their counterparts in the no-voucher condition. In contrast, those in the MCMI-III low-psychiatric-severity subgroup showed greater reduction in alcohol use severity in the no-voucher condition than in the voucher conditions. Thus the highly touted voucher treatment, though generally effective, does not appear to provide uniform benefits for all.

Ball et al.'s (2004) findings are of considerable interest. The MCMI-III psychopathology subtypes identified by Ball and associates were linked with greater substance abuse severity at treatment entry and with no reduction in opiate use over 12 weeks of outpatient treatment. Furthermore, several MCMI-III subtype × treatment × time interaction effects are of particular interest. Those in the MCMI-III affective disturbance group demonstrated greater opiate reduction effects in both voucher conditions, whereas this effect was not found in the MCMI-III high-psychopathology group. The superiority of the incentive-voucher-enhanced version of treatment was hypothesized because naltrexone was considered to be likely to eliminate drug-use-related positive reinforcements (i.e., enhanced mood) and negative reinforcements (i.e., stress management benefits) upon which those with mood disturbance and high psychiatric severity might strongly depend. Additional behavioral interventions were considered likely to be especially important to provide alternative coping responses, reinforcements, or relational supports in these groups. It may be that the affective disturbance subgroup was better able to benefit from available incentives than those with more severe psychiatric disturbance.

Evidence was found that the MCMI-III nonaffective, low-psychiatric-severity, and antisocial–narcissistic subgroups did particularly well in the no-voucher condition compared with the voucher conditions. The greater antisocial–narcissistic response to the no-voucher condition appears to contrast with the findings of Messina et al. (2003), in which participants with ASPD in drug treatment demonstrated a superior response to voucher conditions that did not involve relationship counseling. Also surprising was that Ball et al. (2004) found that antisocial–narcissistic individuals demonstrated greater opiate use reductions in the voucher + relationship counseling condition than in the voucher-alone condition. Theory and previous research suggest that those with antisocial personalities may not benefit from relationship-focused interventions (i.e., Kadden et al., 1989). However, Ball and associates point out that those in their antisocial–narcissistic group obtained less elevated scores on the MCMI Antisocial and Narcissistic scales than comparably labeled groups in other studies. Also, those who had partners available for relationship counseling were perhaps unlikely to present with rigidly antisocial qualities.

Of further interest is that Ball's finding that the antisocial–narcissistic group did particularly well in the no-incentive-voucher condition appears to contrast with results from a series of studies in which methadone maintenance patients with antisocial personalities have done better when incentives are added to standard treatment (Brooner et al., 1998; Messina et al., 2003; Silverman et al., 1996, 1998). Ball et al. (2004) point out that the results of available studies are difficult to compare. Different methods of identifying antisocial personality may not be comparable (see Messina et al., 2003). Ball et al., (2004) also note that about half of the potential participants approached dropped out prior to, during, or immediately after treatment initiation. Moreover, their sample was better educated, was less impaired, was more likely to be employed, and had lower rates of intravenous heroin use than are typical in most methadone maintenance programs.

Despite its limitations, the Ball et al. (2004) study represents an important step in identifying subgroup differences in response to drug treatment approaches for which general efficacy has been established. Naltrexone use has been embraced in the treatment of cocaine-, opioid-, marijuana-, and alcohol-dependent patients in diverse settings. However, many do not benefit from this treatment approach, and use of the MCMI-III has provided an important beginning in the process of understanding patterns of treatment response and nonresponse.

Individual Case Analysis and Treatment Planning

At the beginning of this chapter, we have argued that examination of co-occurring psychiatric disorders and dimensions of psychopathology among well-defined groups with substance abuse holds promise for better understanding important clinical status characteristics and for developing more carefully tailored interventions. Indeed, the value of group research involving the MCMI may be most clearly revealed in its contribution to clarifying interactions among personality structure, symptom expression, and substance abuse in individual clinical cases. The case example of Andrew S. is offered to illustrate how careful examination of these relationships can be used to clarify the meaning of a pattern of substance abuse, and to reveal how treatment planning may be facilitated in this process.

Assessment Procedures

1. An individual interview and review of case notes provided information relevant to social background, personality functioning and symptom status, and current social environment.
2. The MCMI-III was administered to provide information relevant to the assessment of personality disorder and clinical symptom status. Andrew's MCMI-III BR scores are presented in Table 12.1.
3. The Life Experience Survey was administered to contribute to the assessment of the nature and impact of life event stressors.
4. The Perceived Social Network Inventory was used to assist in the evaluation of quantity and quality of perceived social support.
5. The BDI was used to assess current symptoms of depression. Andrew's score on the BDI was 34.

Social History

Andrew S. is a 29-year-old single European American male who was born in Newark, New Jersey, and raised in Fort Lauderdale, Florida. He currently resides with his 73-year-old father in the house in which he was raised. He has been seen for psychotherapy at a local community mental health center for approximately 5 years. Andrew believes that he achieved developmental milestones without difficulty, and reports that he has had no major medical illnesses. He remembers his early family environment as characterized by little cohesion and consider-

TABLE 12.1. MCMI-III Results for Andrew S.

MCMI-III scale	Base rate scores
Disclosure	78
Desirability	45
Debasement	80
Schizoid	69
Avoidant	82
Depressive	70
Dependent	68
Histrionic	11
Narcissistic	47
Antisocial	65
Sadistic (Aggressive)	57
Compulsive	48
Negativistic (Passive-Aggressive)	72
Masochistic (Self-Defeating)	68
Schizotypal	70
Borderline	66
Paranoid	68
Anxiety	72
Somatoform	68
Bipolar: Manic	46
Dysthymia	73
Alcohol Dependence	87
Drug Dependence	74
Post-Traumatic Stress Disorder	70
Thought Disorder	60
Major Depression	88
Delusional Disorder	56

able conflict. He recalls that his mother (now deceased) was consistently critical of his father, who worked inconsistently and failed to support the family adequately. She purchased the house in which the family lived, and she worked at what Andrew describes as "menial jobs" to make ends meet. Andrew believes that she hated her life and took her frustrations out on all family members. She was particularly vehement and relentless in her criticism of her husband. He remembers that his father seemed consistently demoralized and disengaged from the family. Andrew also found family life aversive and often retreated to his room when at home.

Andrew recalls rarely having children from school or the neighborhood over to his house. He remembers lacking confidence socially and having few friendships during his childhood. A younger brother appeared to have been less adversely affected by family influences, and Andrew admires his ability to have risen above it all. He reports that he was an average student in elementary school and was criticized by his mother for not living up to his potential.

In his high school years, Andrew remembers being slightly more socially active and dating occasionally. He cannot recall ever having a steady girlfriend during these years, however; Andrew remembers struggling with a deep fear that he would be devastated by a rejection. He attempted to become involved in sports, but recalls "never making the teams" and being selected last in intramural sporting activities. He experimented with alcohol and drugs (marijuana and cocaine) throughout high school and became rather heavily involved in drug use by his senior year. Although his grades deteriorated during this time, he graduated and entered a local community college. His use of alcohol and drugs eventually became habitual and periodically heavy. While in college, he became involved in some limited "drug dealing" to support his cocaine use. He eventually finished a 2-year college degree and entered a 4-year program in computer science at a local private university. He failed so many courses that he was asked to leave after a year. He received little support from his family and recalls not having the self-control to work, to study, or to attend classes consistently. He admits that his drug use contributed to his failure.

Andrew recalls that his failure in college was demoralizing and believes he has never really recovered from it. His family cut off his support, and he was on his own financially. After a period of living in his car and in inexpensive rooming houses, Andrew rented a room in the private home of a woman more than 20 years his senior. In exchange for reduced rent, he did repairs and home maintenance. A friendship and eventually a 2-year affair developed. Andrew remembers experiencing more acceptance and intimacy in this relationship than he ever had before. However, in retrospect, he regrets that this woman became "equal parts mother, therapist, and lover." He recalls that as he was unable to satisfy her needs, she became demanding and possessive. He began experiencing much anxiety over her demands for greater self-revelation, commitment, and intimacy. Andrew began drinking heavily during this time; he also often became verbally abusive, and the relationship ended badly. This experience was reportedly profoundly disillusioning and hurtful.

Andrew's work history has been inconsistent and fraught with frustration and failure. He does recall several short-lived successes. He started his own computer consultation business in which he built custom computers and did software troubleshooting. He recalls taking pride in his work and enjoying moderate success for a time. On one occasion, he extended himself financially in purchasing expensive computer components to fill a large order. The customer who had placed this order went out of business and defaulted on his obligation to Andrew. He was unable to recover financially from this setback, and his business failed. Another job involved selling computers and software at a local retail outlet. He remembers bitterly that although he was a top salesperson in the store, he was repeatedly passed over for promotions. Eventually, he quit in anger and frustration. Andrew repeatedly recalls these two events as of central importance in understanding his career frustrations. He has claimed that he will never subject himself to the humiliation of working for someone else again.

Andrew has been attempting to reestablish a home-based computer consultation business. For 3 years, he has worked to develop contacts, produce advertising brochures, and make a go of it. Despite exceedingly limited encouragement from potential customers, he has persisted in this effort. He has rigidly refused to seek even part-time employment elsewhere. He has reported working for hours in frustration, attempting to create professional-appearing advertising brochures on his personal computer and waiting for his business telephone to ring. Only recently has he concluded that this business will never succeed.

Despite persistent efforts to encourage greater social involvement by his last three therapists, Andrew has refused to initiate more than minimal contact with others. He believes that he would certainly be rejected by any woman he might meet, and that other men would have little understanding of his life circumstances and limited achievements. He has been supported entirely by his father for 4 years and has had little social contact other than with several family members and his therapist. For years, his father criticized his unwillingness to work and live on his own; recently, however, he seems to have abandoned this critical posture. Andrew believes that his father now recognizes that he benefits from Andrew's company and needs his help in keeping up with the house.

Andrew has experienced episodes of serious depression over the years and has periodically taken various antidepressant medications. He has been disturbed by side effects and has frequently sought and received his psychiatrist's approval to discontinue such medications. He has also received both residential and outpatient drug treatment in the past. He claims to have experienced the confrontation-oriented therapy groups as intolerable. He dropped out in less than a week from his last residential treatment program. Currently, Andrew reports moderate daily alcohol consumption and periodic marijuana use. He argues that drinking helps soothe his inner turmoil and allows him to sleep at night. Marijuana is reportedly used to cope with periods of high anxiety experienced in connection with business concerns and family conflicts. Although he is currently slightly overweight, no other significant medical problems are reported.

Case Conceptualization

Andrew displays a pervasive mistrust of others and an unwillingness to involve himself in close relationships. He appears compelled by the need to distance himself from social encounters, which are seen as likely to reawaken or reenact past disappointments. He has repeatedly stated that to extend himself socially would require risking more emotionally than he has to risk. He believes that any but the most predictable relationships represent a threat to his fragile adaptation. Andrew had demonstrated an acute sensitivity to verbal and nonverbal cues that carry even a hint of negative judgment. He has learned that even rather "minor" social setbacks call up disturbing memories of past rejections and awaken increased sensitivity to further rejection. Such events may result in distracting thoughts and disturbing feelings that interfere with efficient cognitive processing, reduce his ability to cope effectively with a variety of life demands, and often trigger episodes of substance abuse.

Andrew is harshly critical in self-evaluation. He is preoccupied with his limitations and failures, and frequently compares his own attainments with those he believes are typical of men his age: "Most men my age are established in careers, are married, and have started families. I have accomplished none of those things." To a large degree, he finds no basis for disputing the consistently negative evaluations made of him by his father, aunt, and brother. Unfortunately, these are the only three individuals he identifies as sources of social support. He is highly introspective and spends much time and energy ruminating about the misery and emptiness of his life. His most reliable escape has involved fantasies about how his life will fall into place upon his achieving great success in business. He has said often that women will notice him when he has made money. However, his fantasies have failed to provide consistent relief. Ultimately, they serve only to provide sharp contrast between what he has and what he desires. During these periods, he abuses alcohol to deaden his feelings of deep distress.

Andrew's consistently harsh self-criticism, pervasive fear of rejection, and unfulfilled needs for success and affection lead often to a mixture of anxious irritability, deflated self-esteem, and feelings of dejection and dysphoria. He uses alcohol daily to cope with these troubling thoughts and feelings. Periodic complaints of lethargy, weariness, and apathy appear to reflect his underlying depressed mood and residual alcohol withdrawal effects.

Andrew's avoidance of occupational activities requiring interpersonal contact, restraint in relationships due to a fear of being shamed, preoccupation with criticism or rejection in social situations, and feelings of social inadequacy and inferiority indicate that he clearly meets DSM-IV-TR (American Psychiatric Association, 2000) criteria for avoidant personality disorder. Further evidence for the prominence of avoidant personality features is found in his primary elevation (BR = 82) on the MCMI-III Avoidant personality scale.

It is never completely clear what developmental factors contribute to the formation of a pathological personality. However, in Andrew's case, family environment and early and ongoing alienation from peers seem important contributors. Andrew was exposed to considerable hostility and conflict over many years in his family. His mother was perceived as having been consistently and harshly rejecting of his father. Early and ongoing conflicts observed in this relationship have probably contributed to his deeply held belief that intimate relationships are dangerous and better avoided. His mother's consistent criticism of his school achievement and social behavior, and his father's apparent indifference, also influenced Andrew's sense of inadequacy and anticipation of rejection. Furthermore, Andrew recalls never having developed a sense of confidence and competence in the interpersonal arena. Few friendships were developed, efforts to compete in sporting activities were largely unsuccessful, and social anxieties were in evidence early. Requisite skills for dating in adolescence and the development of more intimate relations in later years were notably missing. Andrew recalls experiencing intense anxiety and conflict in his few heterosexual relationships. He recalls that the anticipation of rejection was more than he could tolerate. He recounts similarly disappointing relationships with his few male friends. As described previously, work relationships have been particularly troublesome. In recent years, he has been preoccupied with work failures. It is in this area that he has held some hope for the future. Recently, however, Andrew has concluded that his 3-year effort to establish a home-based computer consultation business will not succeed. This realization has been deeply discouraging.

Andrew laments that he is currently reenacting the pattern of failure that he watched his father live. He is living in his father's home and is totally dependent upon him for support. Although Andrew's father has recently reduced his criticism, Andrew has more than taken up the slack. He is harshly self-critical and finds his current circumstances humiliating. He continues to insist that he doesn't have the trust in others, the time, or the desire to establish a career involving work for others. At times he talks of attempting to start another business, perhaps in financial consultation. At other times, he displays a dejected hopelessness about any future prospects.

Andrew currently displays obvious symptoms of agitated depression. His responses to the MCMI-III Major Depression scale (BR = 88) and BDI (raw score = 34) reflect desperate unhappiness, feeling of failure, guilt, self-blame, irritability, loss of interest in others, indecisiveness, early morning waking, fatigue, and appetite disturbance. Scores on both the MCMI-III and BDI suggest current serious depression. He clearly appears to meet DSM-IV-TR criteria for major depressive disorder, recurrent. Symptoms of depressed mood, diminished interest or pleasure, insomnia, psychomotor agitation, and feelings of worthlessness have clearly been present for more than 2 weeks. Significant distress and impaired functioning are obvious. His symptoms, although aggravated by alcohol ingestion, are probably not primarily attributable to alcohol use. He has often experienced mood disturbance during periods of extended abstinence. Andrew also qualifies for the DSM-IV-TR diagnosis of alcohol dependence, as reflected in an obvious pattern of tolerance and withdrawal. He admits that his work efforts are frequently impaired due to alcohol use, and that his bouts of depression and irritability are often exacerbated by continued drinking. His MCMI-III BR score of 87 on the Alcohol Dependence scale supports this diagnostic impression.

Treatment Recommendations

Immediate Objectives

Currently, Andrew's serious depression and chronic alcohol abuse are interfering with his ability to involve himself productively in psychotherapy. Andrew has been strongly encouraged to seek an immediate psychiatric and substance abuse treatment reevaluation. Appropriate antidepressant medication and treatment for substance dependence might contribute significantly to Andrew's ability to face the rigors of psychotherapy. Andrew has found the demands for social participation, self-revelation, and interpersonal confrontation in residential drug treatment to be intolerable. Several studies have found that those with Andrew's personality and symptom profile are likely to drop out of residential treatment, respond poorly, and show early relapse (Fals-Stewart, 1992; McMahon, Kelley, & Kouzekanani, 1993; McMahon, 2001; Ball et al., 2004). He has never completed a full course of residential treatment, and he seems unlikely to be able to do so at this point. Ball et al. (2004) have found outpatient coping skills training combined with naltrexone and voucher reinforcement to be a promising treatment package for individuals with Andrew's profile. In his case, individual outpatient drug counseling (Mercer & Woody, 1999) might be preferable to a group approach, at least initially. This approach emphasizes the establishment of a therapeutic alliance and involves motivational enhancement in the process of abstinence goal setting. Andrew's anticipation of failure in substance abuse treatment, and his ambivalence regarding abstinence as a realistic goal, will be critical issues to deal with early in treatment. Importantly, individual substance abuse counseling addresses the impact of dysphoric mood on substance use and encourages development of non-substance-related coping strategies. It is frequently used in combination with psychotherapy and pharmacotherapy interventions. Individual drug counseling fits well with other substance abuse treatments because it was designed to be part of a comprehensive treatment package that includes, when necessary, medical and psychological assessments and treatments, detoxification, employment counseling, and self-help programming. It is often used in conjunction with pharmacotherapy approaches for substance dependence and other comorbid psychiatric conditions, including depression. Individual counseling has been used in combination with naltrexone for treatment of alcohol addiction (Mercer & Woody, 1999).

Longer Term Objectives

The recommendations for therapeutic intervention that follow should be implemented only after Andrew demonstrates a significant reduction in substance use and depressive symptoms, and enjoys a reasonable period of recovery. Supportive interventions should be emphasized until that time.

Andrew's pattern of social isolation has severely limited his opportunities for potentially corrective social learning experiences. Contributing to distancing from others is his belief that he cannot endure the negative affect he experiences in social situations. The psychotherapeutic relationship has been one of the few Andrew has been able to endure. This relationship may be used carefully to identify and counter maladaptive thoughts regarding personal relationships. Andrew has periodically shared negative thoughts about his therapists and about the therapy process. Beck et al. (1990) recommend that such thoughts may be elicited during therapy when there is a change from typical to more negative affect. As he realizes that the therapist will not reject him despite these expressions of criticism, Andrew should begin to modify his assumptions about the dangers of self-expression in other relationships as well.

It will also be important to explore more thoroughly the probable origins of Andrew's avoidant pattern. He has often demonstrated resistance to this work. His mother's criticism, his father's indifference, and his disappointing peer interactions have contributed to Andrew's fundamental beliefs about his own lack of acceptability. He tends to focus excessively on these experiences and on their most negative aspects. Discussions of these early relationships should lead to uncovering of dysfunctional thoughts that may be challenged and reworked. Andrew lists his father, brother, and uncle as his only sources of social support during times of stress. Unfortunately, he also describes these three individuals as being consistent sources of criticism. Although he has resisted such a proposal in the past, consideration should be given to family sessions, which might address both historical concerns and current family influences that contribute to Andrew's self-critical attitudes and avoidant behaviors.

Although Andrew is quite articulate, he lacks basic social skills such as friendliness, warmth, adequate focus on others in social encounters, and empathy. Deficits are also apparent in his nonverbal behaviors, including limited eye contact and awkwardness in use of gestures. Further problems are apparent in response timing and turn taking in social interactions.

A social skills deficit analysis and social skills training intervention should be considered. Treatment involves work on each deficient response—beginning with conversational abilities, followed by paralinguistic skills, and finally by nonverbal behaviors. *In vivo* practice will be required in order for newly acquired skills to generalize to the natural environment. In Andrew's case, considerable work in the relative safety of the therapeutic environment should precede efforts at application in the outside world. One preliminary step to encourage generalization might involve Andrew's participation in a supportive group that involves structured approaches to social skills building.

Therapy with Andrew will probably continue as a gradual process involving building trust, confidence, and feelings of self-adequacy. However, care should be taken not to allow Andrew to experience the therapeutic relationship as a permanent substitute for relationships outside therapy. There is clear potential for this, and his therapist must demonstrate determination in insisting on concrete goals and evidence of change in social behavior.

Summary

Clinical research studies involving the MCMI have been important in clarifying group relations among personality–psychopathology, clinical status, and treatment response among those presenting with substance dependence in a manner that facilitates treatment planning and clinical management. The MCMI has been useful in predicting such important treatment outcomes as dropout, recovery of employment functioning, HIV risk behavior, psychiatric symptom status, and substance use relapse. An important recent study has examined differential responsiveness of MCMI-III subtypes to carefully defined substance abuse treatment conditions in a manner coordinated with Millon's theory of personality and psychopathology. Because clinicians are ultimately required to understand and plan effective treatments for individuals, we have presented a case that illustrates the usefulness of the MCMI-III in carefully examining the coincidence of personality disorder, clinical symptom status, and substance dependence in individual clinical conceptualization and treatment formulation.

Note

1. Three editions of the MCMI have been published (MCMI-I, MCMI-II, and MCMI-III). Throughout the chapter, we use the label MCMI when the discussion applies to all versions of the test. In all other instances, we refer specifically to the MCMI-I, MCMI-II, or MCMI-III.

References

Abbott, P. J., Weller, S. B., & Walker, S. R. (1994). Psychiatric disorders of opioid addicts entering treatment: Preliminary data. *Journal of Addictive Disorders, 13,* 1–11.

American Psychiatric Association. (2000). *Diagnostic and statistical manual of mental disorders* (4th ed., text rev.). Washington, DC: Author.

Ball, S. A., Nich, C., Rounsaville, B. J., Eagan, D., & Carroll, K. M. (2004). Millon Clinical Multiaxial Inventory–III subtypes of opioid dependence: Validity and matching to behavior therapies. *Journal of Consulting and Clinical Psychology, 72,* 698–711.

Beck, A. T. (1967). *Depression: Clinical, experimental, and theoretical aspects*. New York: Harper & Row.

Beck, A. T., Freeman, A. M., & Associates. (1990). *Cognitive therapy of personality disorders*. New York: Guilford Press.

Brooner, R. K., Kidorf, M., King, V. L., & Stoller, K. (1998). Preliminary evidence of good treatment response in antisocial drug abusers. *Drug and Alcohol Dependence, 49*, 249–260.

Brownell, K. D., Marlatt, G. A., Lichtenstein, E., & Wilson, G. T. (1986). Understanding and preventing relapse. *American Psychologist, 41*, 765–782.

Cacciola, J. S., Alterman, A. I., & Rutherford, M. J. (1995). Treatment response and problem severity of antisocial substance abusers. *Journal of Nervous and Mental Disease, 183*, 166–171.

Calsyn, D. A., Fleming, C., Wells, E. A., & Saxon, A. J. (1996). Personality disorder subtypes among opiate addicts in methadone maintenance. *Psychology of Addictive Behaviors, 10*, 3–8.

Calsyn, D. A., Wells, E. A., Fleming, C., & Saxon, A. J. (2000). Changes in Millon Clinical Multiaxial Inventory scores among opiate addicts as a function of retention in methadone maintenance treatment and recent drug use. *American Journal of Drug and Alcohol Abuse, 26*, 297–309.

Carroll, K. M., Rounsaville, B. J., Gordon, L. T., Nich, C., Jatlow, P. M., Bisighini, R. M., et al. (1994). Psychotherapy and pharmacotherapy for ambulatory cocaine abusers. *Archives of General Psychiatry, 51*, 177–187.

Chen, E. Y., Brown, M. Z., Lo, T. T. Y., & Linehan, M. M. (2007). Sexually transmitted disease rates and high-risk sexual behaviors in borderline personality disorder versus borderline personality disorder with substance use disorder. *Journal ofNervous and Mental Disease, 195*, 125–129.

Compton, W. M., Cottler, L. B., Jacobs, J. L., Ben-Abdallah, A. B., & Spitznagel, E. L. (2003). The role of psychiatric disorders in predicting drug dependence treatment outcomes. *American Journal of Psychiatry, 160*, 890–895.

Compton, W. M., Cottler, L. B., Spitznagel, E. L., Ben-Abdallah, A. B., & Gallagher, T. (1998). Cocaine users with antisocial personality improve HIV risk behaviors as much as those without antisocial personality. *Drug and Alcohol Dependence, 49*, 239–247.

Corbisiero, J. R., & Reznikoff, M. (1991). The relationship between personality type and style of alcohol use. *Journal of Clinical Psychology, 47*, 291–298.

Corrigan, S. A., Thompson, K. E., Malow, R., & Sorensen, J. L. (1992). Psychoeducational approach to prevent HIV transmission among injection drug users. *Psychology of Addictive Behaviors, 6*, 114–119.

Craig, R. J. (1984). Can personality tests predict treatment dropouts? *International Journal of the Addictions, 23*, 115–124.

Craig, R. J., Bivens, A., & Olson, R. (1997). MCMI-III-derived typological analysis of cocaine and heroin addicts. *Journal of Personality Assessment, 69*, 583–595.

Craig, R. J., & Olson, R. E. (1988). Differences in psychological need hierarchy between program completers and dropouts from a drug abuse treatment program. *American Journal of Alcohol Abuse, 14*, 89–96.

Craig, R. J., & Olson, R. E. (1990). MCMI comparisons of cocaine abusers and heroin addicts. *Journal of Clinical Psychology, 46*, 230–237.

de Groot, M. H., Franken, I. H. A., van der Meer, C. W., & Hendriks, V. M. (2003). Stability and change in dimensional ratings of personality disorders in drug abuse patients during treatment. *Journal of Substance Abuse Treatment, 24*, 115–120.

Donat, D. C., Walters, J., & Hume, A. (1991). Personality characteristics of alcohol dependent inpatients: Relationship of MCMI subtypes to self-reported drinking behavior. *Journal of Personality Assessment, 57*, 335–344.

Fals-Stewart, W. (1992). Personality characteristics of substance abusers: An MCMI cluster typology of recreational drug users treated in a therapeutic community and its relationship to length of stay and outcome. *Journal of Personality Assessment, 59*, 515–527.

Gill, K., Nolimal, D., & Crowley, T. J. (1992). Antisocial personality disorder, HIV risk behavior and retention in methadone maintenance therapy. *Drug and Alcohol Dependence*, *30*, 247–252.

Gregoire, T. K., & Snively, C. A. (2001). The relationship of social support and economic self-sufficiency to substance abuse outcomes in a long-term recovery program for women. *Journal of Drug Education*, *31*, 221–237.

Haller, D. L., & Miles, D. R. (2004). Psychopathology is associated with completion of residential treatment in drug dependent women. *Journal of Addictive Diseases*, *23*, 17–28.

Haller, D. L., Miles, D. R., & Dawson, K. S. (2002). Psychopathology influences treatment retention among drug-dependent women. *Journal of Substance Abuse Treatment*, *23*, 431–436.

Hser, Y. I., Hoffman, V., Grella, C. E., & Anglin, M. D. (2001). A 33 year follow-up of narcotics addicts. *Archives of General Psychology*, *58*, 503–508.

Kadden, R. M., Cooney, N. L., Getter, H., & Litt, M. D. (1989). Matching alcoholics to coping skills or interactional therapies: Posttreatment results. *Journal of Consulting and Clinical Psychology*, *57*, 698–704.

Kalichman, S. C., Carey, M. P., & Carey, K. B. (1996). Human immunodeficiency virus (HIV) risk among the seriously mentally ill. *Clinical Psychology: Science and Practice*, *3*, 130–143.

Kelly, J. A., Murphy, D. A., Bahr, G. R., & Brasfield, T. R. (1992). AIDS/HIV risk behavior among the chronically mentally ill. *American Journal of Psychiatry*, *149*, 886–889.

Klerman, G. L., & Weissman, M. M. (1986). The interpersonal approach to understanding depression. In T. Millon & G. Klerman (Eds.), *Contemporary directions in psychopathology: Toward the DSM-IV*. New York: Guilford Press.

Longabaugh, R., Rubin, A., Malloy, P., Beattie, M., Clifford, P. R., & Noel, N. (1994). Drinking outcome of alcohol abusers diagnosed as antisocial personality disorder. *Alcoholism: Clinical and Experimental Research*, *18*, 410–416.

Matano, R. A., Locke, K. D., & Schwartz, K. (1994). MCMI personality subtypes for male and female alcoholics. *Journal of Personality Assessment*, *63*, 250–264.

McMahon, R. C. (2001). Personality, stress, and social support in cocaine relapse prediction. *Journal of Substance Abuse Treatment*, *21*, 77–87.

McMahon, R. C., & Davidson, R. (1985a). An examination of the relationship between personality patterns and symptom/mood patterns. *Journal of Personality Assessment*, *49*, 552–556.

McMahon, R. C., & Davidson, R. (1985b). Transient versus enduring depression among alcoholics in inpatient treatment. *Journal of Psychopathology and Behavioral Assessment*, *7*, 317–328.

McMahon, R. C., & Enders, C. (2005). *Predictors of recovery from employment problems after residential cocaine treatment*. Presentation at the 113th Annual Convention of the American Psychological Association, Washington, DC.

McMahon, R. C., Kelley, A., & Kouzekanani, K. (1993). Personality and coping styles in the prediction of dropout from treatment for cocaine abuse. *Journal of Personality Assessment*, *61*, 147–155.

McMahon, R. C., Malow, R. M., & Jennings, T. E. (2000). Personality, stress, and social support in HIV risk prediction. *AIDS and Behavior*, *4*, 399–410.

McMahon, R. C., Malow, R. M., & Penedo, F. J. (1998). Substance abuse problems, psychiatric severity, and HIV risk in Millon Clinical Multiaxial Inventory–II personality subgroups. *Psychology of Addictive Behaviors*, *12*, 3–13.

McMahon, R. C., & Richards, S. K. (1996). Profile patterns, consistency and change in the Millon Clinical Multiaxial Inventory–II in cocaine abusers. *Journal of Clinical Psychology*, *52*, 75–79.

McMahon, R. C., Schram, L., & Davidson, R. (1993). Negative life events, social support, and depression in three personality types. *Journal of Personality Disorders*, *7*, 241–254.

McMahon, R. C., & Tyson, D. (1990). Personality factors in transient versus enduring depression among inpatient alcoholic women: A preliminary investigation. *Journal of Personality Disorders*, *4*, 150–160.

Mercer, D. E., & Woody, G. E. (1999). *Individual drug counseling*. Rockville, MD: National Institute on Drug Abuse.

Messina, N., Farabee, D., & Rawson, R. (2003). Treatment responsivity of cocaine-dependent patients with antisocial personality disorder to cognitive-behavioral and contingency management interventions. *Journal of Consulting and Clinical Psychology, 71*, 320–329.

Messina, N., Wish, E., Hoffman, J., & Nemes, S. (2001). Diagnosing antisocial personality disorder among substance abusers: The SCID versus the MCMI-II. *American Journal of Drug and Alcohol Abuse, 27*, 699–717.

Messina, N., Wish, E., Hoffman, J., & Nemes, S. (2002). Antisocial personality disorder and TC treatment outcomes. *American Journal of Drug and Alcohol Abuse, 28*(2), 197–212.

Messina, N., Wish, E., & Nemes, S. (1999). Therapeutic community treatment for substance abusers with antisocial personality disorder. *Journal of Substance Abuse Treatment, 17*, 121–128.

Millon, T. (1981). *Disorders of personality: DSM-III, Axis II.* New York: Wiley.

Millon, T., & Davis, R. D. (1996). *Disorders of personality: DSM-IV and beyond.* New York: Wiley.

Schinka, J. A., Hughes, P. H., Coletti, S. D., Hamilton, N. L., Renard, C. G., Urmann, C. F., et al. (1999). Changes in personality characteristics in women treated in a therapeutic community. *Journal of Substance Abuse Treatment, 16*, 137–142.

Schuckit, M. (1983). Alcoholic patients with secondary depression. *Archives of General Psychiatry, 140*, 711–714.

Siegal, H. A., Li, L., & Rapp, R. C. (2002). Abstinence trajectories among treated crack cocaine users. *Addictive Behaviors, 27*, 437–449.

Silverman, K., Higgins, S. T., Brooner, R. K., Montoya, I. D., Cone, E. J., Schuster, C., et al. (1996). Sustained cocaine abstinence in methadone maintenance patients through voucher-based reinforcement therapy. *Archives of General Psychiatry, 53*, 409–415.

Silverman, K., Wong, C., Umbricht-Schneiter, A., Montoya, I., Schuster, C., & Preston, K. (1998). Broad beneficial effects of cocaine abstinence reinforcement among methadone patients. *Journal of Consulting and Clinical Psychology, 66*, 811–824.

Stark, M. J., & Campbell, B. K. (1988). Personality, drug use, and early attrition from substance abuse treatment. *American Journal of Drug and Alcohol Abuse, 14*, 475–485.

Tourian, K., Alterman, A., Metzger, D., Rutherford, M., Cacciola, J. S., & McKay, J. R. (1997). Validity of three measures of antisociality in predicting HIV risk behaviors in methadone maintenance patients. *Drug and Alcohol Dependence, 47*, 99–107.

Wills, T. A. (1990). Stress and coping factors in the epidemiology of substance abuse. In L. Kozlowski, H. Annis, H. Cappell, F. Glaser, M. Goodstadt, Y. Israel, et al. (Eds.), *Research advances in alcohol and drug problems.* New York: Plenum Press.

CHAPTER 13

Personological Assessment and Treatment of Older Adults

Lee Hyer
Victor Molinari
Whitney L. Mills
Catherine Yeager

In the context of aging, the general topic of personality and the specific theme of personality disorders (PDs) are complex. Perhaps the central question is whether such multifaceted and nebulous constructs can provide useful data. Hayflick (1988) says, "Ageing is a stochastic process that occurs after reproductive maturation and results from the diminishing energy available to maintain molecular fidelity." Millon notes that personality emerges out of a stochastic indeterminateness to provide order across time (Millon, 1990). As aging provokes variability in many domains, but ultimately represents ineluctable decline, and personality involves a consistency across the lifespan, how these two are clinically connected and understandable is the subject of our inquiry.

In this chapter, we map the importance of personality onto aging from several perspectives. First, we consider the construct of personality at late life in regard to the usual overall biopsychosocial changes that take place. Next, we provide a brief background on aging and PDs: the prevalence of PDs among elderly individuals in different settings and comorbidities, as well as a discussion of heterotypic continuity and of how this concept might be used to integrate the disparate findings. We then consider a special problem with aging: dementia. Next, we address general issues of personality assessment raised by the Millon model of PDs, and describe how this model assists in the formulation of care at late life. Finally, we attend to treatment, highlighting interventions at late life with an emphasis on personality. At the end of the chapter, we present a case that demonstrates the utility of the Millon measures for the assessment of this population. Throughout, we hover around and above the core personality constructs of personality traits and PDs, attempting to identify the issues characteristic of each in the context of aging.

Personality Psychology

Research on personality has made considerable progress in the past 30 years. The overall focus has been on trait consistency across the lifespan, its phenomenology, and ways to improve measurement. Regarding the lifespan, the broad outline of personality is now better understood (Caspi, Roberts, & Shiner, 2005; Helson, Kwan, John, & Jones, 2002; Jones & Meredith, 1996; McCrae & Costa, 2003; Mroczek & Spiro, 2003; Small, Herzog, Hultsch, & Dixon, 2003; Steunenberg, Twisk, Beekman, Deeg, & Kerkhof, 2005). Perhaps this is due to improved scales based on sound personality models (Millon, 1969, 1983), as well as to the actuarial data based on the five-factor model (Digman, 1990; McCrae, 2002). In addition, recent progress in the use of statistical methods has provided newer tools to examine longitudinal trajectories of personality traits. Structural equation modeling (Small et al., 2003), latent curve analysis (Jones & Meredith, 1996), and multilevel modeling approaches (Mroczek & Spiro, 2003; Steunenberg et al., 2005), including longitudinal hierarchical linear modeling (Helson et al., 2003), have been applied.

These developments in personality have special application for older adults. Mroczek and Sprio (2003), for example, followed a sample of 1,600 men from the Normative Aging Study for 12 years and found curvilinear slopes for neuroticism (N), which declined up to age 80, and an overall linear trajectory for extraversion (E) indicating no average change. E declined in subjects older than 80 years. As with many such studies, there were considerable intraindividual differences. Helson et al. (2002), too, found that measures of dominance and independence peaked in middle age and that measures of social vitality declined with age. Some measures of norm adherence, such as self-control, increased with age. In a recent study, Terracciano, McCrae, and Costa (2006) examined personality traits over a 42-year period by using data from the Baltimore Longitudinal Study on Aging (N = 2,359; individuals ages 17–98; data collected between 1958 and 2002). Hierarchical linear modeling analysis revealed cumulative mean-level changes averaging about 0.5 SD across adulthood. Scores on E showed distinct developmental patterns: Activity declined from ages 60 to 90 years, restraint increased, "ascendance" peaked at 60, and sociability declined slightly. Scales related to N showed curvilinear declines up to age 70 and increased thereafter. Agreeableness (A) and openness to experience (O) changed little. Masculinity declined linearly. Once again, there was significant individual variability in change. Men and women were similar in variability and death rates, as well as in attrition slopes.

One marker of personality is emotionality. At later life, this feature of personality exhibits both similarities to and differences from its manifestations at younger ages. Research typically shows that the emotion system maintains itself into old age, with the capacity to experience and express emotions (both positive and negative) remaining intact. Furthermore, research indicates that older adults experience better emotional well-being than younger adults, in that the incidence of negative emotional events and moods appears to decline with age, while positive mood states appear either to remain stable or to increase. Older adults report greater efforts to control the experience of emotion in their daily lives (Gross et al., 1997; Lawton, Kleban, Rajagopal, & Dean, 1992). It would seem that, with age, the emotional signatures tend to mellow. Research with community-dwelling older adults consistently finds mood profiles to be more positive (i.e., similar or better levels of positive affect and lower levels of negative affect) than those of younger and middle-aged adults (Gueldner et al., 2001). These findings, however, represent the outcome of the trans-action between an individual's environment and health status on the one hand, and his or her ability to actively select and develop adequate compensatory strategies on the other. When frailty occurs, lower levels of generally positive mood states are found for older residents, and these may reflect their increased need for security and consequent reduction in their ability to shape their environment proactively.

Finally, we suggest that personality might best be reconsidered, due to the many differences related to aging. Hooker and McAdams (2003) have outlined an aging research agenda that specifies several issues pertinent to personality in later life. They outline a structure and process model noting six foci of personality. This model includes traits (dispositional signatures), personal action constructs (goals or motiva-tions), and life stories (narrative reflections of self) as structural components, as well as short-term states such as within-person changes (emotions), self-regulation (pri-mary and secondary control processes or assimilative or accommodative procedures), and self-narration (remembering) as the parallel process constructs. These constructs are distinct from most research on younger adults and allow the clinician to assess how persons at late life "become increasingly like themselves" (Neugarten, 1964).

Personality Disorders

Up to this point, we have been discussing personality traits. A personality trait repre-sents a typical style, but does not necessarily result in disability in key life settings, at work, or in interpersonal relationships. Older people exhibit a mix of symptoms that are adaptive and maladaptive over time. But for a diagnosis of a PD, the construct requires a problem developing early in life (late adolescence) and persisting. The diagnosis of a PD requires that the maladaptive pattern be inflexible and persistent to the extent that the patient suffers significant distress or has functional impairment. A PD, then, requires an enduring pattern that must leave its mark in several settings. At late life, patients with PD generally present with an array of problems based on core *Diagnostic and Statistical Manual of Mental Disorders* (DSM) features (interactive, impulsive, affective, and cognitive), plus many components otherwise related to later life (medical illness, functional disability, psychosocial problems, etc.). To assess a PD at late life, then, one must carefully consider the relationship between aging and the PD. Sometimes a PD may not be obvious until later life, but, upon inspection of the phenomenology of the trait/disorder, it becomes evident that it has always been there. It is also possible that some personality traits do not become troublesome until later life.

PDs are best represented as polythetic, coming in many forms. That said, there are prototype markers for each PD, and these assert a rather strong influence over

TABLE 13.1. Importance of PDs in Later Life

PDs are intensifications of normal personality traits.

PDs are not homogeneous entities, but come in several subtypes.

PDs predispose individuals to particular clinical syndromes.

PDs are often subclinical expressions of psychopathological conditions.

PDs may not contribute to the pathogenesis of a clinical syndrome, but may influence the manner in which it is expressed.

PDs may be modified as a consequence of the effects of a clinical (Axis I) disorder.

Axis I problems. PDs (or traits) "suggest" the form of psychopathology as a result of stress, implying that Axis II and Axis I are cohabitators and share similar dimensions. Table 13.1 highlights the many features of the covariance structure of Axis II traits and Axis I symptoms.

Epidemiology of PDs

Community Samples

Estimates of the prevalence of PDs in community settings have varied widely, with rates ranging from 6.6% to 63%. Studies of community samples have indicated that, overall, lower rates of PDs have been reported in older adults than in younger adults. In particular, older adults have been found to score lower than younger adults on scales assessing antisocial, histrionic, narcissistic, borderline, and paranoid PDs, while scoring higher on scales measuring obsessive–compulsive and schizoid PDs (Cohen et al., 1994; Segal, Hook, & Coolidge, 2001).

Ames and Molinari (1994) administered the Structured Interview for Disorders of Personality—Revised (SIDP-R) to 200 older adults (mean age = 72 years) attending a senior center, yielding a 13% prevalence rate. This sample was compared with a group of 797 younger adults who had been administered the SIDP-R. Prevalence of PDs in the younger sample was 17.9%, indicating that the older adults had significantly lower rates of PDs. The study also found that no older adult met the criteria for more than one PD, and that there was no difference in frequency of PDs between genders.

In a study of 810 community-dwelling participants, Cohen et al. (1994) administered the semistructured Standardized Psychiatric Examination to determine levels of PDs in younger and older adults. The prevalence rate for the older adults (55 years and older) was 6.6%, versus 10.5% for the younger adults; older participants were thus significantly less likely to have PDs.

Segal and Coolidge (1998) found much higher PD prevalence rates in a study of 189 community-dwelling older adults (mean age = 76.2 years) attending a community center. Participants were self-administered the Personality Disorder Questionnaire—Revised (PDQ-R), which resulted in a 63% prevalence rate. These results may have been caused by the PDQ-R's high sensitivity to pathology. Another factor could have been the self-selection of participants, because persons with existing personality and interpersonal problems may have been more likely to seek out the services of the community center. The results of this study are in contrast to previous findings of decreased prevalence of PDs in older adults.

Most recently, Segal, Coolidge, and Rosowsky (2006) conducted a study of 681 community-dwelling participants ranging in age from 18 to 89. Prevalence was measured with the Coolidge Axis II Inventory (CATI) self-report, and participants were compared in two groups: older ($n = 114$, ages 60–89) and younger ($n = 567$, ages 18–59). The study found PDs in 11% of the older sample and 20% of the younger group. These results were similar to the findings of Abrams and Horowitz (1996), who conducted a meta-analysis of methodologically sophisticated studies of personality in older adults. The study revealed average PD prevalence rates of 10% for older adults (defined as 50 years and older) and 21% for younger adults. Previous findings of age effects were neither supported nor contradicted, although for certain PDs a decline in frequency and intensity with age was generally supported by the literature. Specifically, the "high-energy" DSM Cluster B PDs declined with age. This mellowing was attributed to the greater mortality rates in their younger years for those with Cluster B PDs. Lower rates of PDs in older age were also postulated to be related to the age-insensitivity of some DSM criteria for PDs and to the likelihood that PDs may be underdiagnosed in general, but particularly in older adults.

Mental Health Settings

Early studies of PDs in older adults in mental health settings found relatively low prevalence rates compared to later studies. Mezzich, Fabrega, Coffman, and Glavin (1987) conducted a retrospective chart review of older inpatients and outpatients and determined a 5.1% PD prevalence rate. Casey and Schrodt (1989) found a 7% prevalence rate among 100 consecutive admissions to a geriatric psychiatry unit, as determined by chart reviews of psychiatrist ratings. Research in mental health settings has shown great variation in estimates of PD prevalence between diagnoses by attending psychiatrists and diagnoses by structured interviews (Molinari, Ames, & Essa, 1994; Molinari & Marmion, 1993).

In a study of 36 geropsychiatric outpatients, Molinari and Marmion (1993) administered the SIDP-R and compared the findings with a sample of 298 young adult outpatients. Results indicated that 58% of the elderly population met criteria for a PD. When compared with the younger sample, the older sample exhibited a significantly lower prevalence of PDs, and significantly fewer persons met criteria for more than one PD. Compared with diagnoses determined by attending psychiatrists, the SIDP-R yielded a nearly statistically significant greater number of PD diagnoses.

Molinari et al. (1994) conducted a study with 200 geropsychiatric inpatients. Participants were administered the SIDP-R and found a 56.5% PD prevalence rate for older participants. A young comparison sample of 131 psychiatric inpatients revealed no significant difference in PD prevalence rates between the groups. Congruent with the findings of the Molinari and Marmion (1993) study, this investigation found that the SIDP-R yielded more PD diagnoses than did the attending psychiatrists.

In a cross-sectional study of changes in personality with age for individuals with PD, Molinari, Kunik, Snow-Turek, Deleon, and Williams (1999) administered a battery of tests to 392 psychiatric inpatients diagnosed with a PD. The battery included the Minnesota Multiphasic Personality Inventory (MMPI), Millon Clinical Multiaxial Inventory (MCMI), California Psychological Inventory, and Psychological

Inventory of Personality Styles. The study concluded that older adults with PDs were consistently less impulsive, paranoid, high-energy, antisocial, and irresponsible than their younger counterparts. These findings support the previous literature indicating a mellowing of PDs with age.

Long-Term Care Settings

PDs have not been well studied in long-term care settings, and no literature exists for PDs in assisted living facilities. Studies conducted in nursing homes have determined that 11% to 15% of that population meets criteria for a PD diagnosis (Margo, Robinson, & Corea, 1980; Teeter, Garetz, Miller, & Heiland, 1976). Margo et al. (1980) estimated that 15% of nursing home referrals were actually for personality problems. Clearly, one reason for this dearth of information is both the absence of an appropriate assessment tool; another is the absence of prototype markers of PD behavior in such a setting.

PDs and Comorbid Psychiatric Conditions

Comorbidities

PD comorbidity is the rule among younger adults (generally > 50%), but the extent to which this applies to older adults is less well known. The relationship in later life between Axis II and the Axis I disorders is also not known; however, several studies have suggested that comorbidity with Axis I disorders is high. Variations in PD prevalence estimates may be related to the influence of affective/mood disorders, especially depression. Studies of PD in mental health settings without consideration of comorbid affective/mood disorders have revealed lower prevalence rates (Mezzich et al., 1987; Casey & Schrodt, 1989) than later studies of PDs that include persons with such disorders have.

Thompson et al. (1988) determined that 33% of depressed older adults being treated with psychotherapy in a geropsychiatric outpatient clinic also met DSM-III PD criteria. Fogel and Westlake (1990) included 2,332 inpatients with major depression and found that 15.8% also met criteria for a PD. Kunik et al. (1994) evaluated depressed older adults as inpatients and found that 24% had a comorbid PD. Even higher rates have been reported. For example, Molinari and Marmion (1995) conducted a study of 24 geropsychiatric outpatients and 52 geropsychiatric inpatients with affective disorders who were administered the SIDP-R and found a 63% PD prevalence rate. The high comorbidity is problematic for at least two reasons; (1) Comorbidity causes even more complications with treatment; and (2) at least one-quarter of individuals with one PD will have other PDs (Segal, Coolidge, & Rosowsky, 2006).

Abrams and Horowitz (1996) examined the relationship between PDs and functioning in acutely depressed older psychiatric patients. This study determined that greater disability and increased impairment in social and interpersonal functioning were related to Axis II pathology. In their review of this literature, Agronin and Maletta (2000) concluded that Axis I pathology, especially major depressive disorder, is intrinsically related to PDs in later life.

Heterotypic Continuity

Longitudinal data find that PD features decline with age (Lenzenweger, Johnson, & Willett, 2004), but that significant problems remain (Moffitt, Caspi, Harrington, & Milne, 2002). The overall results suggest a mellowing of the "high-energy" Cluster B PDs with aging, and relative stability of the Cluster A (odd) and Cluster C (anxious) PDs. Two alternative explanations have been postulated. First, the mellowing of a PD is a true phenomenon (at least among Cluster B males) due to normal biological changes associated with aging, such as the reduction in testosterone. Older adults express less florid symptomatology by finally learning to harness their energy and control their impulses. Second, this mellowing also has been explained as an assessment artifact and methodological confound that skews toward a reduction in prevalence rates for this age group, because the DSM is age-insensitive and does not include developmentally appropriate criteria. From this viewpoint, manifestations of PDs in later life are not adequately identified by DSM, but nevertheless may cause significant psychosocial difficulties.

One way of making sense of the divergent PD literature described above is via the concept of "heterotypic continuity." Heterotypic continuity means that one's core personality remains basically unchanged, but is behaviorally expressed in developmentally congruent ways throughout the lifespan. Symptoms or behaviors that convey an older adult's basic character may thus be manifested via so-called "aging variants" (Rosowsky & Gurian, 1991; Sadovoy & Fogel, 1992; Segal, Hersen, Van Hasselt, Silberman, & Roth, 1996). In other words, negative personality traits may be reformed, sublimated, assuaged, or reexpressed in ways that are less troubling (Segal et al., 2006).

In summary, it appears that appropriate diagnostic criteria for older adults are lacking, and that the measures for such constructs in elderly persons leave this group vulnerable to misdiagnosis and poor treatment opportunities.

Dementia

One other area of concern for personality is cognitive decline, especially dementia. Dementia accrues dramatically in late life, building to estimated prevalence rates of up to 50% over age 85. Even if an older person does not have a degenerative disease, the insults of normal aging (benign senescent forgetfulness) or mild cognitive impairment of one type or another may be present (Jeste et al., 1999). Dementia (or cognitive decline) may cause changes in personality, either before or after obvious penetrance of problems. Organic brain changes alter a person's predominant personality traits—increasing, decreasing, or neutralizing them. As the disease progresses, personality traits may be exacerbated as the person tries to shut down or defend the self. Over time, there remains a vague awareness of the person; the person may become "a shadow of his or her former self."

When one develops dementia, whether the initial reaction is a generic response resulting from the disease or a guarded reaction of accommodation that follows the influence of premorbid traits is unclear. Personality in the context of dementia is generally addressed by distinctive models of complications in treatment (Abrams &

Horowitz, 1999). Research, for example, shows that agitation, depression, and aggression, as well as delusions or hallucinations, are present in over three-quarters of individuals at some point during the course of a dementia. To many, these manifestations are considered "personality." This applies to both major causes of dementia—Alzheimer's disease (Grossberg & Desai, 2003), and vascular dementia (Nussbaum, 1997).

The extent to which these dementia-related behavior changes are influenced by premorbid personality traits, however, has not been thoroughly considered. Some studies have found little evidence for the influence of personality (Abrams & Horowitz, 1999), while others suggest that premorbid personality may be helpful in understanding and predicting dementia-related behavior changes (Finkel, 1998). For example, Chatterjee, Strauss, Smyth, and Whitehouse (1992) found a correlation between premorbid personality characteristics and subsequent psychiatric symptoms in dementia. Patients exhibiting symptoms of depressed mood were rated as premorbidly more neurotic or less emotionally stable. Patients with paranoid delusions were rated as having been more hostile prior to the onset of dementia. Patients with hallucinations were reported as premorbidly more open, particularly in the facets of fantasy and aesthetics.

Gould and Hyer (2004) have suggested that, of patients with dementia, premorbid personality traits (e.g., neuroticism) have an impact on their behavior profile during the course of the illness. They assessed the influence of premorbid personality on the expression of behavioral disturbances among individuals with dementia. A total of 68 outpatients with a diagnosis of dementia were assessed for current cognitive functioning, premorbid personality traits, and new behavioral disturbances since dementia onset. The results of this study showed some evidence for the influence of personality on the expression of both irritability and withdrawal. Specifically, increased withdrawal and irritability after dementia onset were associated with an inhibited premorbid personality style. In addition, a premorbid independent personality style was associated with less withdrawal. This was a strict test to see whether personality variables would add to already known predictors of symptomatology. Statistically, they were not competitive with the more known variables. Results suggested that personality may be a "value-added" construct in the explanation of problem behaviors for those who are developing dementia. It would seem, then, that even under the worst of circumstances, when the brain is degenerating, personality asserts an influence.

Assessment

The critical assessment issues concerning PDs in younger age groups also apply in later life. These include (1) a high degree of comorbidity; (2) the instability of Axis II clinical manifestations over time; (3) a lack of discrete boundaries between individual PDs and PD clusters; (4) heterogeneity within diagnoses due to a polythetic classification system; (5) differing threshold levels of PDs; (6) redundant criteria for each disorder; and (7) nonweighted diagnostic criteria that vary from core to peripheral characteristics, with little specification of level of severity. In addition, as with any area of study, the many methodological problems inherent in personality research influence the nature of results. Confounds in personality research include differences in settings where samples are acquired; use of cross-sectional data; problems with the diagnostic criteria used (as noted earlier, heterotypic continuity of behaviors in a given personality is not adequately reflected in older age); differences in type of measurement (self-report vs. clinical interview); the nature of the cutoff between trait and disorder; and the masking of biological and cultural issues.

There is no "gold standard" for the measurement of PDs in late life. Indeed, no PD measures have been specifically developed for this age group. Structured interviews are more reliable than unstructured ones or self-report measures, but self-reports can be very helpful, as long as the problems of false positives and negatives can be clinically understood. Livesley (1998) specifies that a two-stage process for PD evaluation is preferable—an interview based on DSM to establish the PD category, and later a self-report scale to determine the severity of the PD. Paris (2003) adds that early diagnosis of a PD has a considerable clinical advantage: Necessary adjustments for care can be applied early in treatment.

It is ironic that such a case must be made for older adults, because assessment traditionally has been a hallmark of geropsychological practice (Segal, Coolidge, & Hersen, 1998). The dynamic interplay of comorbidities, medical problems, situational stressors, and functional decline provide an "agar jar" of confusion for the presence of a PD. In general, measurement of PDs at late life is made more difficult by the already hardened myths of aging as a period of brittle adaptation or developmental stagnation (Zweig & Agronin, 2006); by the absence of longitudinal data; and by unreliable measurement instruments.

That said, several suggestions can be made for the assessment of older adults in general (see Table 13.2). A multimethod package that includes chart/record review, clinical review with the patient, interview with informants, self-report objective personality inventories, and semistructured interviews is clearly best practice (Segal et al., 2006). This can be a daunting and time-consuming enterprise. However, given that the ability of clinicians to diagnose and treat older adults who may have a PD is suspect (Sadavoy, 1996), prudence and a certain amount of structure are important for accurate assessment.

As the rules of assessment apply to later life and PDs, it may be best to diagnose and treat from a "double-think" perspective. That is, the clinician uses both Axis II and Axis I considerations to assist in the case formulation and treatment. At the same time, the clinician respects cognitive problems, seeks parsimony in diagnoses,

---

TABLE 13.2. General Assessment Recommendations

Carefully assess for Axis I and Axis III problems (call the
    patient's primary care provider).
Screen for traits and PDs (see measures outlined in Table 13.4).
Use structured interviews initially.
Interview significant others.
Use Axis IV and Axis V as markers for functioning.
Use measures of PD that you are familiar with.
Assess neurocognitive status.
Assess age-related changes in the context of Axis I and Axis III.

TABLE 13.3. Differential Diagnosis Axioms

1. "Double-think" for assessment: Axis II and Axis I.
2. With older adults, comorbidity is the rule, not the exception.
3. Cognitive disorder trumps all other diagnoses.
4. Axis I symptomatology (i.e., irritable depression) could be mistaken for Axis II (e.g., borderline, dependent) pathology.
5. Priority is given to the disorder that has been present longest.
6. Apply the safety rule—be prudent with diagnostic implications.
7. Developmental history is essential.
8. Recent history is better than ancient history.
9. Crisis-generated data are suspect.
10. Collateral information is at least equal to history from the patient.
11. Objective assessments are better than subjective judgments.

respects more long-standing psychosocial problems as well as history (relative to recent behavior), and regards crisis-generated data with some skepticism. Collateral information and objective measures are also important to the systematic assessment of PDs; we believe that objective measures are chief in the understanding of late-life problems. Table 13.3 outlines these issues, and the case presentation at the end of this chapter echoes the need for objective assessment.

Several self-report measures and structured inventories exist (see Table 13.4 for descriptions). Most have not been applied carefully to older adults; exceptions involve the NEO-PI-R, PACL, SNAP, and SCID-II (see Table 13.4). However, we believe that all can be used clinically in the identification of late-life PDs, as they map onto the DSM or extant models of normal aging that are suitable for clinical care. Clinicians must exercise caution, however, when administering these measures to older adults for whom there is a question of cognitive decline. Our experience with this population suggests that patients in the early stages of dementia may not have the stamina or cognitive clarity to complete long personality inventories accurately. When in doubt, a brief measure, such as the PACL, should be used.

Millon's Model of Personality in Later Life

> To uproot a personality disorder, one must wrangle with the ballast of a lifetime, a developmental disorder of the entire matrix of the person, produced and perpetuated across years. By any reasoning, the pervasiveness and entrenched tenacity of the pathology, soaks up therapeutic resources, leading inevitably to pessimism and disaffection for therapists.
>
> —THEODORE MILLON

The Millon (1969, 1981, 1983) model has been discussed in other chapters of this book. The model is theory-based and anchored to the multiaxial system of the DSMs. Although it was not originally developed for late-life applications, it is still relevant in late life. To summarize, the model specifies a complete clinical science of personality—one that embodies theory, taxonomy, instrumentation, and intervention. As at younger ages, the makeup of the entire matrix of an older person's salient domains remains important (Millon & Davis, 1996). It encompasses the person's

TABLE 13.4. Personality Disorder Measures

Self-report measures

NEO-PI-R

The NEO Personality Inventory—Revised (NEO-PI-R) assesses the five-factor model of personality (neuroticism, extraversion, openness to experience, agreeableness, and conscientiousness), as well as the six facets or traits that encompass each domain, with 243 self-report items. The NEO-PI-R has been validated on a variety of populations, including older adults, but does not measure PDs formally (Costa & McCrae, 1992).

MMPI-2

The Minnesota Multiphasic Personality Inventory–2 (MMPI-2) is a widely used and researched assessment of psychopathology and PDs in adult populations. Symptom profiles, Axis I disorders, and personality traits can be assessed with the MMPI-2, but it is not a direct measure of the DSM-IV PDs (Butcher, Dahlstrom, Graham, Tellegen, & Kaemmer, 1989).

PACL

The Personality Adjective Check List (PACL) is a self-report measure of Millon's eight personality patterns consisting of 153 items. The PACL may be utilized in the assessment of PDs in general, as well as three severe personality patterns in particular: schizoid, cycloid, and paranoid (Strack, 1991).

MIPS *Revised*

The Millon Index of Personality Styles *Revised* (MIPS *Revised*) assesses normal personality styles. The index consists of 180 true–false items to measure three dimensions: Motivating Styles, Thinking Styles, and Behaving Styles (Millon, 2003).

MBMD

The Millon Behavioral Medicine Diagnostic (MBMD) aids clinicians in assessing patients with psychological problems and physical illnesses. The 165-item test includes response patterns, negative health habits, psychiatric indicators, coping styles, and stress moderators to help create successful treatment plans for patients (Millon, Antoni, Millon, Minor, & Grossman, 2001).

MCMI-III

The original Millon Clinical Multiaxial Inventory (MCMI) was one of the earliest standardized self-report assessments of personality disorders. The current version, the MCMI-III, is largely consistent with DSM-IV(-TR) criteria, but some differences do exist because the inventory is theoretically anchored on Millon's theory of personality. The 175-item true–false inventory consists of 14 Clinical Personality Patterns, three Severe Personality Pathology Scales, seven Moderate Clinical Syndrome Scales, and three Severe Clinical Syndrome Scales to assess PDs and clinical syndromes (Millon, 1997).

CATI

The Coolidge Axis II Inventory (CATI) is a 225-item self-report measure of all 10 standard DSM-IV(-TR) PDs, as well as depressive, passive–aggressive, self-defeating, and sadistic PDs. In addition, the CATI assesses neuropsychological dysfunction, executive function, and several Axis I disorders (Coolidge, 2000).

PDQ-4+

The Personality Diagnostic Questionnaire—Fourth Edition Plus (PDQ-4+) assesses the 10 standard DSM-IV(-TR) PDs and (as the plus indicates) passive–aggressive and depressive PDs. The questionnaire consists of 99 true–false items and has been associated with high false-positive rates (Bagby & Farvolden, 2004) indicating that it may not be most useful as a clinical assessment, but as a screening tool (Hyler, 1994).

(continued)

TABLE 13.4. *(continued)*

SNAP

The Schedule for Nonadaptive and Adaptive Personality (SNAP) is a 375 true–false item self-report assessment of trait dimensions of PDs. The instrument includes 12 trait scales (Mistrust, Manipulativeness, Aggression, Self-Harm, Eccentric Perceptions, Dependency, Exhibitionism, Entitlement, Detachment, Impulsivity, Propriety, and Workaholism); three temperament scales (Negative Temperament, Positive Temperament, and Disinhibition); and 13 diagnostic scales consistent with the 10 standard DSM-IV(-TR) PDs as well as passive–aggressive, sadistic, and self-defeating disorders (Clark, 1993).

Semistructured or structured interviews

There are a number of validated PD instruments tied to DSM criteria; however, none of these instruments have been validated on older adults.

IPDE

The two-module International Personality Disorder Examination (IPDE) was developed as an assessment of personality disorders utilizing both the DSM-IV(-TR) and ICD-10 criteria. The self-report IPDE Screening Questionnaire contains 77 DSM-IV(-TR) or 59 ICD-10 true–false questions that can be scored quickly to determine the need for the structured IPDE Interview to determine presence of specific PDs (Loranger, 1999).

SCID-II

The Structured Clinical Interview for DSM-IV Axis II Personality Disorders (SCID-II) was designed to diagnose the 10 standard DSM-IV(-TR) PDs as well as depressive PD, passive–aggressive PD, and PD not otherwise specified. The instrument characterizes the patient's inner experience through an overview of typical behavior, relationships, and capability of self-reflection (First, Gibbon, Spitzer, Williams, & Benjamin, 1997).

PDI-IV

The semistructured Personality Disorder Interview–IV (PDI-IV) diagnoses the 10 standard DSM-IV(-TR) Axis II PDs as well as passive–aggressive and depressive PDs. The scoring booklet allows clinicians to rank multiple diagnoses according to importance (Widiger, Mangine, Corbitt, Ellis, & Thomas, 1995).

SIDP-IV

The Structured Interview for DSM-IV Personality (SIDP-IV) assesses the DSM-IV(-TR) Axis II PDs as well as self-defeating PD, depressive PD, and negativistic PD. Patients are not assessed by individual disorder, but by investigating 10 groupings of "topical sections" (interests and activities, work style, close relationships, social relationships, emotions, observational criteria, self-perception, perception of others, stress and anger, and social conformity) to determine the presence of a PD (Pfohl, Blum, & Zimmerman, 1997).

DIPD-IV

The Diagnostic Interview for DSM-IV Personality Disorders (DIPD-IV) is a semistructured assessment of the DSM-IV(-TR) PDs and, in addition, passive–aggressive and depressive PDs. The interview contains 108 sets of questions to determine the presence or absence of PD on a disorder-by-disorder basis by evaluating typical thoughts, feelings, and behaviors in the past 2 years (Zanarini, Frankenburg, Sickel, & Yong, 1996).

SWAP-200

The Shedler–Westen Assessment Procedure–200 (SWAP-200) is a clinician Q-sort assessing personality and PDs. The 200 items are rank-ordered by the clinician, depending on their value as descriptions of the patient in order to elucidate indicators of personality dysfunction (Westen & Shedler, 1999a, 1999b).

biopsychosocial patterns and is predictive of adjustment, both psychosocial and medical (Ruegg & Frances, 1995). Even in late life, personality continues to influence the nature and severity of symptoms and overall adjustment of treatment-seeking patients. A comprehensive awareness of the structural integrity of this linked nexus (behaviors, thoughts, emotions, and interpersonal and biological patterns) serves the clinician well (Millon & Davis, 1996). If this theory is correct, the "methods of operation" of the personality provide necessary data for understanding the person—perhaps the most data currently possible.

According to the Millon theory, personality is akin to the immune system, the competence of which determines the reaction of the person, not the type or extent of the stressor. Core types of personality developed over time are based on three polarities: the nature of reinforcement (pain or pleasure), source of reward (self or others), and instrumental style (active or passive). Initially there were eight basic personality types. Two additional types (sadistic and self-defeating personality) were added to this model for consistence with DSM-III-R, and one more (depressive personality) for consistency with Appendix B of DSM-IV. Three severe personality types represent extensions or exaggerations of the basic eight personalities; these are schizotypal, borderline, and paranoid. In later writings, Millon (1988, 1990) brought evolutionary theory to bear on his reinforcement model.

As with younger clients, the clinician's tasks with a late-life client are as follows:

1. To establish the basic personality pattern(s) of the person across the lifespan.
2. To modify this information with elevations in the severe personality styles, if any.
3. To integrate the unique personality profile with the current clinical symptoms.
4. To formulate a case formulation of the person based on personological primacy.

Effectively, knowledge of personality reduces the heterogeneity of the person, as this isolates the critical dimensions that must be addressed to enable change to occur. Millon has identified two knowledge sources: the three polarities, and the functional and structural domains of personality. Pathology represents an excessive dependence on a reward–avoidance system or an imbalance of the polarities (see other chapters). Again, this model applies as well at late life as at other ages. Millon (1969) notes, "By framing our thinking in terms of what reinforcements the individual is seeking, where he is looking to find them, and how he performs, we may see more simply and more clearly the essential strategies which guide [his life]" (p. 193).

In addition to balancing the three polarities, a domain-based formulation of a PD allows the clinician to analyze the person at a closer level, at a prominent locus in the system where most change can unfold. There are four structural domains that are deeply embedded, quasi-permanent templates or features of a person, and four functional domains, designed to perpetuate the system. Functions are expressive modes of regulatory action and include expressive behaviors, interpersonal conduct, cognitive style, and functional mechanisms. As an example, the avoidant personality is believed to have similar modal features at early and late ages, with slight differences (see Table 13.5), such as an exacerbation of avoidant behaviors. The most salient domains in late life continue to be those in early life.

TABLE 13.5. Avoidant Personality Traits in Young Adulthood versus Older Age

Younger age	Older age
Expressive behaviors	Expressive behaviors
Expressively fretful	Avoidant/inactive
Anguished mood	Worrier
Interpersonal conduct	Interpersonal conduct
Aversive	Avoidant/stress-averse
Cognitive style	Polite
Cognitively distracted	Cognitive style
Alienated self-image	Alienated self-image
Vexatious objects	Distracted
Regulatory mechanisms	Impoverished
Fantasy mechanism	Regulatory mechanisms
Fragile organization	Excessive reminiscence
	Organizationally simple

The prototype of the personality (such as the one presented in Table 13.5), based on polarities and domains, allows the clinician to hone in on the particular points in the system that are especially sensitive to change. In effect, this model provides the components for a case formulation that is dynamic and can be altered as time and need dictate.

Treatment

Perhaps it is best to consider Axis II as a body of descriptive material collated across several perspectives. This formulation allows for modal criteria to define and diagnose a PD, but looser criteria to treat the PD. It therefore is not so much an explanatory model as a framework for guidance in understanding the person.

Research Findings on Late-Life Treatment

The research literature on the psychological treatment of older adults, while growing, is still small in comparison to the intervention literature in other populations. However, a number of general reviews are available for the treatment of depression in older adults (e.g., Gatz et al., 1998; Niederehe, 1996; Reynolds & Kupfer, 1999; Rubinstein & Lawton, 1997; Scogin & McElreath, 1994; Scogin, Welsh, Hanson, Stump, & Coates, 2005; Teri & McCurry, 2000).

In an early meta-analysis on cognitive-behavioral therapy (CBT), Dobson (1989) found suggestive evidence that age may predict a negative outcome in CBT for depression. The more recent literature suggests that CBT can be an efficacious treatment for late-life depression (Teri, Curtis, Gallagher-Thompson, & Thompson, 1994; Beutler et al., 1987; Gallagher & Thompson, 1981, 1982; Hyer, Swanson, Lefkowitz, Hillesland, et al., 1990; Hyer, Swanson, & Lefkowitz, 1990; McCarthy, Katz, & Foa, 1991; Thompson, Gallagher, & Breckenridge, 1987) and anxiety (Scogin, Rickard, Keith, Wilson, & McElreath, 1992). Moreover, CBT has been useful in the maintenance of treatment gains (Gallagher-Thompson, Hanley-Peterson, &

Thompson, 1990). Efficacy also has been shown in a wide variety of pathological areas (see Zeiss & Steffen, 1996) when CBT is combined with medication (Gerson, Belin, Kaufman, Mintz, & Jarvik, 1999; Thompson, Gallagher, Hanser, Gantz, & Steffen, 1991) or applied to more difficult psychopathology (Hanley-Peterson et al., 1990; Thompson et al., 1988). The same results apply (but to a lesser extent) to interpersonal psychotherapy (McReynolds, Garske, & Turpin, 1999).

Recently, treatments that share therapeutic components with CBT have also demonstrated efficacy for late-life depression, and bear mention here. These treatments include problem-solving therapy (Alexopoulos, Raue, & Arean, 2003), dialectical behavior therapy (Lynch, Morse, Mendelson, & Robins, 2003), interpersonal therapy (Karel & Hinrichsen, 2000; Miller, Frank, Cornes, Houck, & Reynolds, 2003), and behavioral activation (Teri, Logsdon, Uomoto, & McCurry, 1997), as well as a modified form of CBT for chronically and severely depressed older patients (McCullough, 2000). Problem-solving therapy addresses core action tendencies in a structured way, which reflects a core treatment component of CBT. Dialectical behavior therapy highlights elements of radical acceptance, mindfulness, distress tolerance, and assertiveness training. Interpersonal therapy addresses interpersonally relevant factors in a context of education, goal setting, and socialization. Behavioral activation uses traditional behavioral techniques, including mastery and pleasurable activities, graded task assignments, and goal setting. In addition, we note that the CBT elements of bibliotherapy (Jamison & Scogin, 1995) and wellness interventions in classroom and home settings for older adults, such as relaxation, cognitive restructuring, problem solving, communication, and behavior activation (Rybarczyk, DeMarco, DeLaCruz, & Lapidos, 1999), have been evaluated as efficacious. Finally, we note that combined pharmacotherapy and CBT for late-life depression has demonstrated efficacy (Gerson et al., 1999).

There is research demonstrating the effectiveness of CBT for other disorders in later life: sexual dysfunction (e.g., Zeiss, Delmonico, Zeiss, & Dornbrand, 1991), sleep problems (e.g., Lichstein & Johnson, 1993), and tension (e.g., Scogin et al., 1992). This is true for CBT applied individually (Thompson et al., 1987), with groups (Hyer, Hilton, Friedman, & Sacks, in press), and in various venues (e.g., Carstensen, 1988). Positive results also have been shown in regard to medical illness, including such factors as improved sense of control/choice (Burish et al., 1984; Wallston et al., 1991), reduced anxiety (Carey & Burish, 1985), increased relaxation (Burish, Snyder, & Jenkins, 1991; Burish, Vasterling, Carey, Matt, & Krozely, 1988; Carey & Burish, 1987), and amelioration of conditioned aversive responses (Burish & Carey, 1986; Burish, Carey, Krozely, & Greco, 1987). Finally, CBT has been associated with improved psychological functioning in patients undergoing chemotherapy (Arean et al., 1993; Carey & Burish, 1988; Nezu, Nezu, Friedman, Faddis, & Houts, 1998).

Therapy Adaptation

There exist few data on the exact methods of adapting therapy for older adults, or on the influence of such therapeutic alterations. We provide several in Table 13.6. These may change as the aging cohort changes. If adaptations are required, then we need to know whether this is due to developmental changes, cohort differences, or the envi-

TABLE 13.6. Alterations in Therapy for Older Adults

- Patient education is *critical*. Long socialization is necessary. Check expectations frequently.
- Patients need to be asked about their knowledge about therapy, as well as concerns.
- Bring in family members if needed.
- Make changes in information processing as needed: Go slowly. Repeat. Shorten. Check ("How are you hearing me?"). Use multiple channels. Cue and review. Repetition and summary during sessions, not just at end.
- Adjust treatment on the basis of social developmental stages. Social support must be selective.
- Use shorter sessions.
- Get permission and consult with patients' primary care providers.
- CBT alterations:
    Reframe before use of cognitive distortions.
    Focus on past more and generative issues.
    Use tapes, phone calls.
    Engage in case management—act as a social worker.
    Bring in the environment more (practical issues and family).
    Break down issues.
    Discuss the problem in depth.
    Use the Mimi-Mental State Exam frequently if needed.
    Use qualities representing relative strengths of older adults.
    Pace material more slowly.
    Employ multimodal training ("say it, show it, do it").
    Use memory aids (tapes, written assignment, notebooks).
    Use strategies for staying on track in session.
    Plan for generalization of training.
    Draw on patient's own knowledge of personal strengths and experience with handling
        past problems.

ronment in which the intervention occurs. Older adults have been shown to respond favorably to the present-focused nature of CBT and to enjoy its skill acquisition and educative components (Thompson, 1996). Thompson (1996) and others (e.g., Gallagher-Thompson & Coon, 1996) have advanced specific modifications to CBT for depression for use in older patient populations. These may have special application to older adults who exhibit cognitive decline (Snow, Powers, & Liles, 2006). In fact, the cognitive load of CBT on older adults does not have to be high.

In spite of the lack of solid information about which adaptations are most effective, researchers have identified the benefits of some stock CBT techniques for older adults. For example, the use of handouts and homework for older patients is particularly recommended, in order to facilitate learning and remembering. Good homework compliance has been shown to predict positive treatment outcome in CBT for late-life depression (Coon & Thompson, 2003). Zeiss and Steffen (1996) have urged clinicians using homework assignments with older adults to help clients find ways to "say it, show it, do it." For example, in teaching an older client communication skills, the clinician first explains one principle or tenet of effective communication. The clinician then role-plays the client employing this communication technique in a scenario relevant to the client's life. Next, the client is prompted to practice the technique (as him- or herself) in the same role play (Gallagher-Thompson & Coon, 1996). The clinician then gives the older client constructive feedback, and the sequence can be repeated through successive approximations. In addition, as in CBT for clients of all ages, the clinician can audiotape each session for the older adult to review between sessions, to facilitate the therapeutic and skill acquisition process. Last, to facilitate and maintain active engagement in the therapeutic process and enhance learning, the older adult is frequently prompted to summarize the material out loud during the session. Similarly, a brief review of the session's highlights to begin and conclude each session is particularly important in this patient population (see Thompson, Gallagher-Thompson, & Dick, 1995). As with the treatment of any psychiatric condition in late life, the active involvement of family members and other health care providers (especially physicians) is critical for effective CBT of late-life depression.

Personality Rules of Care in Therapy

The purpose is not to put persons in the classification system, but instead to reorient the system with respect to the person by determining how his or her unique, ontological constellation of attributes overflows and exceeds it. The classification thus becomes a point of departure for comparison and contrast, a way station in achieving total understanding of the complexity of the whole, not a destination in itself. When in the course of an assessment the clinician begins to feel that the subject is understood at a level where ordinary diagnostic labels no longer adequately apply, the classification system is well on its way to be falsified relative to the individual, and a truly idiographic understanding of the person is close at hand, ready to be approached in a comprehensive and systematic way therapeutically.

—THEODORE MILLON (p. 109)

The ravages of Axis I–Axis II interactions usually make treatment problematic. For over three decades, various hypotheses related to this interaction have been espoused—predisposition, subclinical or prodromal symptoms, life events, scarring, pathoplasty, or *forme fruste*. In addition, most "rules" of therapy addressing therapy type, severity, case mix issues, and interventions are just guides, as the complexity of such a case explodes in a therapy room.

Each person with a PD has a unique biopsychosocial etiology. The clinician is treating a person, not a disease. The consequences of failing to identify and attend to PDs can be troubling indeed. When PDs are not addressed up front, the results are almost always lengthier therapy, more frequent treatment failures, and unnecessary complications to the therapeutic relationship (Sadavoy, 1999). It is also important to be aware that those with PDs develop Axis I disorders earlier in life, have more symptoms, display longer episodes of these disorders, and have more frequent relapses. After treatment, those with PDs reveal greater residual problems, have greater levels of relapse, and experience lower quality of life. It is believed that the PD pattern is always present but becomes especially "noisy" in times of stress.

Given all this, the distinct components of treatment, delivery, receipt, and enactment require modification when a PD is present. The client must be presented with materials and tasks, receive them openly, and carry out assignments. Tracey and Ray (1984) have outlined a model of treatment for PDs that includes the processes of "engagement" (forming initial therapeutic alliance and identifying targets for intervention), "discrepancy" (challenging problematic patterns with novel insights and experiences), and "consolidation" (generalizing and internalizing initial changes). In Benjamin's (1993) model, too, a key task is that of establishing a collaboration. Benjamin notes that empathic processes may or may not be appropriate in this task; she stresses the importance of facilitating the patient's recognition of his or her interpersonal patterns of behavior. Equally significant are the tasks of "blocking maladaptive patterns" and addressing the patient's underlying fears and wishes. New learning should always be facilitated, to encourage the acquisition of interpersonal behaviors that are more adaptive and more gratifying than those previously employed. Personality work should be done in stages or stepwise (like the building of a NASA project), and multiple modes should be used. Behavior, mood, and cognitions (and biology) must "move together."

There are some therapy rules for PDs in late life that must be attended to, however. The older patient arrives in therapy with problems that are externalized, egosyntonic, and closed to change. In treatment, both the core features characteristic of all PDs and those unique to each one must be considered. As with therapy at any age, the more impaired the older adult, the more the intervention will require therapeutic support, family support, and environmental support. Behavioral activation, too, is a primary consideration for the older client. For the higher-functioning person, more interventions can be directed to problems at the "inner level" of the person.

In sum, adaptations in therapy such as the ones described above are appropriate but generally mild and can be increased with more impaired (e.g., "older old") elderly patients. Table 13.7 outlines various PD treatment axioms.

Therapy is best defined not by techniques, but by conceptualization. It is a model of care that has rules. In an older client with a PD, the "head" changes in therapy before the "gut." The person must experience the "sensation of the PD" and see that change is okay before change takes place. As a general rule, the clinician attacks the overall rigidity in the PD, to increase flexibility and to decrease self-defeating patterns. Zweig and Agronin (2006) outline several treatment rubrics. The core rubric involves taking a common-factors integrative approach that strives to employ a combination of therapeutic modalities tailored to individual treatment goals, uses both somatic and psychosocial approaches, and appreciates the psychodynamic influence of a PD. In effect, this approach is a case formulation with a PD element in the treat-

---

TABLE 13.7. PD Treatment Axioms in Late Life

1. Ensure unconditional acceptance and validate the patient as a person, but establish negative consequences for unacceptable behaviors.
2. Elucidate expectations for reasonable and responsible behavior, and the protection of personal boundaries for both you and the patient.
3. Consistency must be established so patients are aware that, despite their demands and behaviors, you will not give up on them. In order to allow gradual change, structure can be provided via a "holding environment."
4. Countertransference may determine treatment options by increasing understanding of patients and how they affect others. Careful not to respond impulsively or to "act out" against a patient in terms of unwarranted or premature assumptions or interpretations.
5. Use a coordinated team approach. Communication and regular meetings are necessary to prevent a patient from potentially dividing the team—causing members to "take sides," and destroying the necessary consistency, integration, and structure of the biopsychosocial approach the patient needs.

ment plan. In addition, the clinician applies therapeutic components as specified in CBT, and utilizes the family and the treatment team to advance treatment goals.

The case formulation, then, is requisite for an older adult. This allows for hypotheses about the case, as well as a structured plan for intervention. Persons (2005) has outlined a format for case formulation:

Identifying information
Problem list
Diagnostic list
Origins and history of problem behaviors
Beliefs
Current precipitants
Personality formulation
Hypothesis
Treatment plan
Obstacles
Strengths

As in the American Psychological Association's emphasis on evidence-based practice in psychology, the idea is to formulate an empirically based therapy on the basis of a person with a defined background. The case is then carefully formulated, and the PD rubric is applied to components of the person. Millon's model is a good place to start.

In treatment, personality change is probably more like a "punctuated equilibrium" than a slow, continuous process. Personality shows periods of some growth and then a reconfiguration into a new gestalt. Use of a particular mode of therapy is a function of therapist preference, type of training, and patient receptivity to a specific model and interventions. Also, cognitive, behavioral, psychodynamic, and interpersonal approaches may be effective at particular points of the therapeutic process. We provide several suggestions (see Table 13.8) based on CBT for a later-life client in the context of a PD. Medications are not addressed here. This particular intervention is best considered in connection with attempting to reduce the intensity and frequency of maladaptive behaviors, avoiding behavioral crises, and treating comorbid psychiatric disorders. Zweig and Agronin (2006) outline several suggestions for medication for more severe expressions of PDs.

The MBMD and the Case of Mr. N.

The Millon Behavioral Medicine Diagnostic (MBMD; Millon, Antoni, Millon, Minor, & Grossman, 2001) is a scale that has been helpful with older adults for several reasons, but mostly because this age group has a high preponderance of medical problems. The MBMD is based on Millon's belief that personality-mediated coping styles are powerful influences on the genesis and course of medical illness. The MBMD focuses especially on assessing (1) psychiatric factors in medical patients; (2) stress moderators that increase (e.g., spirituality) or decrease (e.g., lack of social supports) coping; (3) factors that have an impact on treatment prognostics, such as a

TABLE 13.8. Rules for PD Treatment

Getting started:

Remember that the conceptualization of a PD for a given person may alter over time.
Given the longer lifespan, more time is required to diagnose PDs in older adults.
Think on two levels—symptoms and personality.
Assess for PDs.
Educate patients about the nature of their disorders and the proposed type of treatment.
Elicit feedback from patients to show that you value their input and to emphasize the
    importance of their active participation in treatment.

If Axis II is present, then:

Be active—evaluate for medications, consult with treatment team, make appropriate referrals.

Apply Millon model:

Polarities (see text).
Domains (see text).

Rules of therapy:

Be clear and explicit with patients regarding your role and their role.
Get commitment to change and reinforce the importance of tolerating discomfort.

Encourage goal thinking around personality:

"What do you want from therapy?"
"How would you like to be different?"
"How do you get in your own way?"
"Imagine a year from now . . . "

Cognition:

Core beliefs → intermediate beliefs → automatic thoughts
    Attitudes
    Assumptions
    Rules
Several CBT techniques (Beck, 1999) can be used to expose the core beliefs:
    Downward arrow
    Core belief worksheet
    Early learning
    Education
Several CBT techniques (Beck, 1999) can be used to address the core beliefs:
    Advantages–disadvantages of beliefs
    Cognitive continuum
    Behavioral experiments
    Acting "as if"
    Role playing of emotional side and rational side
    Monitoring core beliefs
    Restructuring early memories
    Coping cards
    Imagery and rehearsal
    Subjective units of distress
    Disputation and rational reaction
    Debriefing
    Capsule summaries (used frequently).

(continued)

TABLE 13.8. *(continued)*

Stay present-focused and down-to-earth:

Role-play; use anxiety management training methods.
Remain data-centered.
Special techniques for cognitive restructuring:
    Identify and label automatic triggers.
    Dispute via challenges.
    Promote coping strategies.
    Challenge dysfunctional schemas.
    Conduct exposure to feared situations.
    Conduct experiments (expect patient to pass or use coping card).
    Teach diaphragmatic breathing and use of self-rewards.

Emotion:

Those with PDs are addicted to the "comfort" of their emotional patterns.
Respect affect: Affect recruits cognitions. Identify emotions and help the person tolerate
    previously unacceptable emotions. Attend to the role of imagery in emotions.

Address interpersonal style that leads to conflict with others:

Point out "now events."
"You seem to want me to . . . "
"Are you aware that . . . "
"Has it ever happened that you . . . "

Monitor client satisfaction:

Use symptom measures (gauge success in terms of both PD and Axis I symptom remission).
Monitor therapeutic alliance.

tendency to abuse medications or poor compliance with physician orders; and (4) lifestyle habits that have a negative effect on health, such as cigarette smoking. The MBMD also provides information on test validity and response style, and indicates whether psychiatric referral is recommended.

Mr. N. is a 71-year-old former police officer and independent private investigator who was referred by his family for neuropsychological assessment because of memory difficulties. His forgetfulness and increasing disorganization have reportedly contributed to business account-ing irregularities and a run-in with the Internal Revenue Service. He is at heightened risk for dementia because his mother died of complications secondary to Alzheimer's disease, and because he himself has suffered from cardiovascular disease for the past 10 years. There is no history of psychiatric illness.

Mr. N. was accompanied to the evaluation by his wife and adult children. He was an attractive, robust, trim man who looked younger than his chronological age. In spite of his apparent vitality, however, Mr. N. was generally inactive, preferring to stay at home or, at most, to visit his grandchildren who lived nearby. He had no hobbies and did not exercise. During the clinical interview, Mr. N. was surprisingly quiet, almost bland in his presentation. His mood appeared euthymic, and he showed little emotion during the evaluation, with the exception of smiling whenever a question was directed to him. Mr. N. did not initiate conver-sation and allowed his family members to answer the assessor's questions. When Mr. N. did respond to the assessor's inquiries, his answers tended to be clipped, although reasonably accurate. He was aware that he was experiencing some memory problems, but seemed uncon-cerned. Family members stated that Mr. N.'s personality had changed in the past 2 years; he was no longer the affable, gregarious man who took pride in his skills and talents. In other words, in years past, Mr. N. had been "his own man." His son bemoaned the change: "He used to be a presence." Indeed, the family worried that Mr. N. might be suffering from depres-sion.

Mr. N.'s Mini-Mental State Exam score was 26; this was of some concern, given his age and education (14 years), but was not clinically significant. Testing revealed that although Mr. N.'s performance was variable across neuropsychological domains, he demonstrated mild to severe impairment in the domains of attention, learning and memory, and cognitive flexibility. His neuropsychological test performance is presented in Table 13.9.

Mr. N. also completed self-report measures of depression (Beck Depression Inventory–II) and anxiety (Beck Anxiety Inventory); his scores on these were well within normal limits. However, his responses on the MBMD were revealing (see his Interpretive Report in Figure 13.1). First, as can be seen, Mr. N. has produced a valid clinical profile, although he tends to portray himself in a rather favorable light (see the Desirability indicator). As in other Millon personality measures, some of the MBMD clinical scales have been adjusted to account for this response style. The overall clinical profile shows a man who is in no acute psychological distress. Activity level is low, and he may be at risk of exacerbating his medical condition if he does not increase physical activity and exercise.

On the MBMD clinical scales, Mr. N. has presented himself as a very self-assured and easygoing individual who requires a fair amount of socialization and stimulation to feel con-tent. He becomes bored and inattentive when faced with routine, repetitive activities. He is

TABLE 13.9. Neuropsychological Test Performance of Mr. N.

Test	Percentile
Repeatable Battery for the Assessment of Neuropsychological Status (RBANS)	
Total Score	2nd
Attention Score	<1st
Visuospatial/Construction	1st
Language	30th
Learning/Immediate Memory	7th
Delayed Memory	14th
Wechsler Memory Scale–III	
General Memory Cumulative	13th
Working Memory Cumulative	13th
Immediate Memory Cumulative Score	9th
Visual Immediate Memory	34th
Auditory Immediate Memory	4th
Delayed Visual Memory	66th
Delayed Auditory Memory	6th
Auditory Recognition	9th
Controlled Oral Word Association Test	<10th
Trail-Making Test	
Trails A	25th
Trails B (4 errors)	<1st
Wisconsin Card Sorting Test (no categories completed)	<1st

Norms: General Medical   **Valid Profile**
Medical Problem(s):
Code: -// 5 ** 4 * // -**-* C E F B + // -**-* H I + //

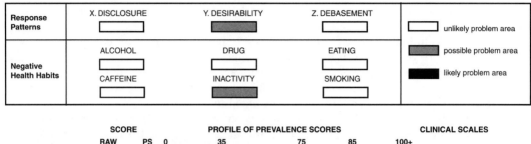

	SCORE		PROFILE OF PREVALENCE SCORES	CLINICAL SCALES

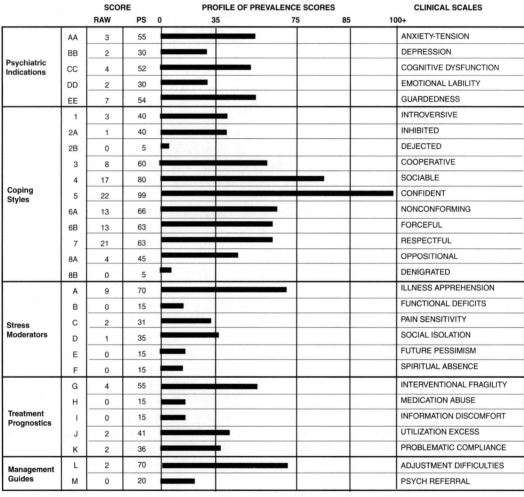

FIGURE 13.1. MBMD Interpretative Report for Mr. N.

every bit his own man, and desires to call his own shots and handle his own affairs. By his nature, he handles minor stressors well and may downplay medical problems initially. However, when a medical illness becomes more serious and/or chronic, Mr. N. is likely to become irritable and dramatic in an attempt to cope with his fears and frustrations. He also is likely to withdraw socially. Although he has been initially cooperative with his health care team, this will be short-lived as his illness becomes more worrisome. Mr. N. is likely to become dismissive and annoyed with doctors to cover up his anxiety. Indeed, he may show poor treatment compliance without firm instructions and frequent follow-ups by his health care team.

In terms of stress moderators, Mr. N. has endorsed a number of assets, including a strong sense of functional competence (which will motivate him to push through the burdens of his illness to return to his daily activities as soon as possible). He is also an optimistic individual who believes that his medical difficulties can be successfully managed. This attitude, as well as his strong spiritual faith, will probably enable Mr. N. to function better with chronic illness than other patients in similar circumstances. Finally, in terms of treatment prognostics, there is no indication that Mr. N. will overutilize the health care system or abuse medications. On the other hand, his treatment team should be mindful that Mr. N. will be initially difficult to engage successfully in treatment, and will require open communication and firm instructions to increase his compliance with medical interventions.

How does the information gleaned from the MBMD align with Mr. N.'s premorbid personality style? We now have a better understanding of the former police officer and detective whom the family has described as always "a presence" and "a man who doesn't take orders from anyone." According to MBMD personality indicators, this confident, self-possessed individual still exists, but he is no longer interacting energetically and enthusiastically with his environment. Are we seeing simply a mellowing of personality with age? Is his personality as spirited as ever, but is he withdrawing from social interactions in self-protection—or is he simply "biting his lip" in response to the prodding of annoying family members and doctors who wish to confront the possibility that he has a debilitating neurogenerative disease? Or are we seeing an attenuation of personality features because of the early stages of dementia? Although it may take time for the answer to reveal itself, we now have a much better understanding of the man before us and can tailor our interventions to utilize his strengths and accommodate to his defenses.

Conclusion

PDs are not diseases. They are complex but understandable reflectors of a person— habits that are rigid, and patterns that are often self-defeating. PDs are persistent, but decipherable. Health care providers seem to know when someone has a PD; often these patients are seen as willful and unpleasant.

In this chapter, we have addressed a forgotten arena—personality in later life. This is often thought to be an unimportant issue, as personality traits pale in comparison with other aging problems or, worse, that these traits are immutable throughout life. In reality, personality bends with age, but it does not break. It continues to assist in the sculpting of the ineluctable decline process of moving to late life. From another perspective, personality mediates the cohort-specific concerns of living. It is the key construct that influences the psychological health of the person, young or old. Therefore, the health-care provider ignores this at his/her own risk.

One of the leading writers on personality and meaning, Dan McAdams, has asked a critical question: "What do we know when we know a person?" We believe that personality is the most efficient and economical path to answering this question. It provides an understandable and human template for both clinical treatment and the human quest for meaning. Let us hope that future research will provide better measures and models for its understanding. In late life, when cognitive decline or dementia sets in, when Axis III problems abound, and when loss is persistent, personality remains and understated but clinically useful and relevant construct, one that provides direction for care.

References

Abrams, R. C., & Horowitz, S. V. (1996). Personality disorders after age 50: A meta-analysis. *Journal of Personality Disorders, 10*(3), 271–281.

Abrams, R. C., & Horowitz, S. V. (1999). Personality disorders after age 50: A meta-analytic review of the literature. In E. Rosowsky, R. C. Abrams, & R. A. Zweig (Eds.), *Personality disorders in older adults: Emerging issues in diagnosis and treatment* (pp. 55–68). Mahwah, NJ: Erlbaum.

Agronin, M., & Maletta, G. (2000). Personality disorders in late life: Understanding and overcoming the gap in research. *Journal of the American Geriatrics Society, 8,* 4–18.

Alexopoulos, G. S., Raue, P., & Arean, P. (2003). Problem-solving therapy versus supportive therapy in geriatric major depression with executive dysfunction. *American Journal of Geriatric Psychiatry, 11*(1), 46–52.

Ames, A., & Molinari, V. (1994). Prevalence of personality disorders in community-living elderly. *Journal of Geriatric Psychiatry and Neurology, 7,* 189–194.

Arean, P. A., Perri, M. G., Nezu, A. M., Schein, R. L., Christopher, F., & Joseph, T. X. (1993). Comparative effectiveness of social problem-solving therapy and reminiscence therapy as treatments for depression in older adults. *Journal of Consulting and Clinical Psychology, 61*(6), 1003–1010.

Bagby, R. M., & Farvolden, P. (2004). Personality Diagnostic Questionnaire–4 (PDQ-4). In M. Hersen (Series Ed.) & M. Hilsenroth & D. L. Segal (Vol. Eds.), *Comprehensive handbook of psychological assessment: Vol. 2. Personality assessment* (pp. 122–133). Hoboken, NJ: Wiley.

Beck, A. T. (1999). Cognitive aspects of personality disorders and their relation to syndromal disorders: A psychoevolutionary approach. In C. R. Cloninger (Ed.), *Personality and psychopathology* (pp. 411–429). Washington, DC: American Psychiatric Press

Benjamin, L. S. (1993). Every psychopathology is a gift of love. *Psychotherapy Research, 3*(1), 1–24.

Beutler, L. E., Mahoney, M. J., Norcross, J. C., Prochaska, J. O., Sollod, R. M., & Robertson, M. (1987). Training integrative and eclectic psychotherapists: II. *Journal of Integrative and Eclectic Psychotherapy, 6,* 296–332.

Burish, T. G., & Carey, M. P. (1986). Conditioned aversive responses in cancer chemotherapy patients: Theoretical and developmental analysis. *Journal of Consulting and Clinical Psychology, 54*(5), 593–600.

Burish, T. G., Carey, M. P., Krozely, M. G., & Greco, F. A. (1987). Conditioned side effects induced by cancer chemotherapy: Prevention through behavioral treatment. *Journal of Consulting and Clinical Psychology, 55*(1), 42–48.

Burish, T. G., Carey, M. P., Wallston, K. A., Stein, M. J., Jamison, R. N., & Naramore Lyles, J. (1984). Health locus of control and chronic disease: An external orientation may be advantageous. *Journal of Social and Clinical Psychology, 2*(4), 326–332.

Burish, T. G., Snyder, S. L., & Jenkins, R. A. (1991). Preparing patients for cancer chemotherapy: Effect of coping preparation and relaxation interventions. *Journal of Consulting and Clinical Psychology, 59*(4), 518–525.

Burish, T. G., Vasterling, J. J., Carey, M. P., Matt, D. A., & Krozely, M. G. (1988). Posttreatment use of relaxation training by cancer patients. *The Hospice Journal, 4*(2), 1–8.

Butcher, J. N., Dahlstrom, W. G., Graham, J. R., Tellegen, A., & Kaemmer, B. (1989). *Minnesota Multiphasic Personality Inventory-2 (MMPI-2): Manual for administration and scoring.* Minneapolis: University of Minnesota Press.

Carey, M. P., & Burish, T. G. (1985). Anxiety as a predictor of behavioral therapy outcome for cancer chemotherapy patients. *Journal of Consulting and Clinical Psychology, 53*(6), 860–865.

Carey, M. P., & Burish, T. G. (1987). Providing relaxation training to cancer chemotherapy patients: A comparison of three delivery techniques. *Journal of Consulting and Clinical Psychology, 55*(5), 732–737.

Carey, M. P., & Burish, T. G. (1988). Etiology and treatment of the psychological side effects associated with cancer chemotherapy: A critical review and discussion. *Psychological Bulletin, 104*(3), 307–325.

Carstensen, L. L. (1988). The emerging field of behavioral gerontology. *Behavior Therapy, 19,* 259–281.

Casey, D. A., & Schrodt, C. J. (1989). Axis II diagnoses in geriatric inpatients. *Journal of Geriatric Psychiatry and Neurology, 2,* 87–88.

Caspi, A., Roberts, B. W., & Shiner, R. L. (2005). Personality development: Stability and change. *Annual Review of Psychology, 56,* 453–484.

Chatterjee, A., Strauss, M., Smyth, K., & Whitehouse, P. (1992). Personality changes in Alzheimer's disease. *Archives of Neurology, 49*(5), 486–491.

Clark, L. A. (1993). *Schedule for Nonadaptive and Adaptive Personality.* Minneapolis: University of Minnesota Press.

Cohen, B. J., Nestadt, G., Samuels, J. F., Romanoski, A. J., McHugh, P. R., & Rabins, P. V. (1994). Personality disorder in later life: A community study. *British Journal of Psychiatry, 165,* 493–499.

Coolidge, F. L. (2000). *Coolidge Axis II Inventory: Manual.* Colorado Springs, CO: Author.

Coon, D. W., & Thompson, L. W. (2003). The relationship between homework compliance and treatment outcomes among older adult outpatients with mild-to-moderate depression. *American Journal of Geriatric Psychiatry, 11,* 53–61.

Costa, P. T., Jr., & McCrae, R. R. (1992). *Revised NEO Personality Inventory (NEO-PI-R) and NEO Five-Factor Inventory (NEO-FFI) Professional Manual.* Odessa, FL: Psychological Assessment Resources.

Digman, J. M. (1990). Personality structure: Emergence of the five-factor model. *Annual Review of Psychology, 41,* 417–440.

Dobson, K. S. (1989). A meta-analysis of the efficacy of cognitive therapy for depression. *Journal of Consulting and Clinical Psychology, 57,* 414–419.

Finkel, S. I. (1998). *Behavioral and psychological symptoms of dementia (module 2).* UK: Gardiner-Caldwell Communications.

First, M. B., Gibbon, M., Spitzer, R. L., Williams, J. B. W., & Benjamin, L. S. (1997). *Structured Clinical Interview for DSM-IV Axis II Personality Disorders (SCID-II).* Washington, DC: American Psychiatric Press.

Fogel, B. S., & Westlake, R. (1990). Personality disorder diagnoses and age in inpatients with major depression. *Journal of Clinical Psychiatry, 51*(6), 232–235.

Gallagher, D., & Thompson, L. W. (1981). *Depression in the elderly: A behavioral treatment manual.* Los Angeles: University of Southern California Press.

Gallagher, D., & Thompson, L. W. (1982). Treatment of major depressive disorders in older adult outpatients with brief psychotherapies. *Psychotherapy: Theory, Research, and Practice, 19*(4), 482–490.

Gallagher-Thompson, D., & Coon, D. W. (1996). Depression. In J. I. Sheikh & I. D. Yalom (Eds.), *Treating the elderly* (pp. 1–44). San Francisco: Jossey-Bass.

Gallagher-Thompson, D., Futterman, A., Hanley-Peterson, P., Zeiss, A., Ironson, G., & Thompson,

L. W. (1992). Endogenous depression in the elderly: Prevalence and agreement among measures. *Journal of Consulting and Clinical Psychology, 60*(2), 300–303.

Gallagher-Thompson, D., Hanley-Peterson, P., & Thompson, L. W. (1990). Maintenance of gains versus relapse following brief psychotherapy for depression. *Journal of Consulting and Clinical Psychology, 58*(3), 371–374.

Gatz, M., Fiske, A., Fox, L. S., Kaskie, B., Kasl-Godley, J. E., McCallum, T. J., et al. (1998). Empirically validated psychological treatments for older adults. *Journal of Mental Health and Aging, 4,* 9–46.

Gerson, S., Belin, T. R., Kaufman, A., Mintz, J., & Jarvik, L. (1999). Pharmacological and psychological treatments for depressed older patients: A meta-analysis and overview of recent findings. *Harvard Review of Psychiatry, 7*(1), 1–28.

Gould, S. L., & Hyer, L. A. (2004). Dementia and behavioral disturbance: Does premorbid personality really matter? *Psychological Reports, 95*(3), 1072–1078.

Gross, J. J., Carstensen, L. L., Pasupathi, M., Tsai, J., Skorpen, C. G., & Hsu, A. Y. C. (1997). Emotion and aging: Experience, expression, and control. *Psychology and Aging, 12*(4), 590–599.

Grossberg, G., & Desai, A. (2003). Management of Alzheimer's disease. *Journal of Gerontology, 58A*(4), 531–553.

Gueldner, S. H., Loeb, S., Morris, D., Penrod, J., Bramlett, M., Johnston, L., et al. (2001). A comparison of life satisfaction and mood in nursing home residents and community-dwelling elders. *Archives of Psychiatric Nursing, 15*(5), 232–240.

Hayflick, L. (1988). Aging in cultured human cells. In B. Kent & R. N. Butler (Eds.), *Human aging research: Concepts and techniques.* New York: Raven Press.

Helson, R., Kwan, V. S. Y., John, O. P., & Jones, C. (2002). The growing evidence for personality change in adulthood: Findings from research with personality inventories. *Journal of Research in Personality, 36*(4), 287–306.

Hooker, K., & McAdams, D. (2003). Personality reconsidered: A new agenda for aging research. *Journal of Gerontology, 58B*(6), 296–304.

Hyer, L., Hilton, N., Sacks, A., & Yeager, C. (in press). GIST: An efficient and effective cognitive behavioral therapy in long term care. *Clinical Gerontologist.* Manuscript submitted for publication.

Hyer, L., Swanson, G., & Lefkowitz, R. (1990). The use of a cognitive schema model with stress groups at later life. *Clinical Gerontologist, 9*(3/4), 145–190.

Hyer, L., Swanson, G., Lefkowitz, R., Hillesland, D., Davis, H., & Woods, M. G. (1990). The application of the cognitive behavioral model of two older stressor groups. *Clinical Gerontologist, 9,* 145–190.

Hyler, S. E. (1994). *Personality Diagnostic Questionnaire—Fourth Edition Plus (PDQ-4+.* New York: New York State Psychiatric Institute.

Jamison, C., & Scogin, F. (1995). The outcome of cognitive bibliotherapy with depressed adults. *Journal of Consulting and Clinical Psychology, 63*(4), 644–650.

Jeste, D. V., Alexopoulos, G. S., Bartels, S. J., Cummings, J. L., Gallo, J. J., Gottlieb, G. L., et al. (1999). Consensus statement on the upcoming crisis in geriatric mental health. *Archives of General Psychiatry, 56*(9), 848–853.

Jones, C. J., & Meredith, W. (1996). Patterns of personality change across the life span. *Psychological Aging, 11*(1), 57–65.

Karel, M. C., & Hinrichsen, G. (2000). Treatment of depression in late life: Psychotherapeutic interventions. *Clinical Psychology Review, 20,* 707–729.

Kunik, M. E., Mulsant, B. H., Rifai, A. H., & Sweet, R. A. (1994). Diagnostic rate of comorbid personality disorder in elderly psychiatric patients. *American Journal of Psychiatry, 151,* 603–605.

Lawton, M. P., Kleban, M. H., Rajagopal, D., & Dean, J. (1992). Dimensions of affective experience in three age groups. *Psychological Aging, 7*(2), 171–184.

Lenzenweger, M. F., Johnson, M. D., & Willett, J. B. (2004). Individual growth curve analysis illuminates stability and change in personality disorder features. *Archives of General Psychiatry*, *61*, 1015–1024.

Lichstein, K. L., & Johnson, R. S. (1993). Relaxation for insomnia and hypnotic medication use in older women. *Psychological Aging*, *8*(1), 103–111.

Livesley, W. J. (1998). Suggestions for a framework for an empirically based classification of personality disorder. *Canadian Journal of Psychiatry*, *43*, 137–147.

Loranger, A. W. (1999). *International Personality Disorder Examination: DSM-IV and ICD-10 Interviews*. Odessa, FL: Psychological Assessment Resources.

Lynch, T. R., Morse, J. Q., Mendelson, T., & Robins, C. J. (2003). Dialectical behavior therapy for depressed older adults: A randomized pilot study. *American Journal of Geriatric Psychiatry*, *11*(1), 33–45.

Margo, J. L., Robinson, J. R., & Corea, S. (1980). Referrals to a psychiatric service from old people's homes. *British Journal of Psychiatry*, *136*, 396–401.

McCarthy, P. R., Katz, I. R., & Foa, E. B. (1991). Cognitive-behavioural treatment of anxiety in the elderly: A proposed model. In C. Salzman & B. D. Lebowitz (Eds.), *Anxiety in the elderly*. New York: Springer.

McCrae, R. R. (2002). The maturation of personality psychology: Adult personality development and psychological well-being. *Journal of Research in Personality*, *36*(4), 307–317.

McCrae, R. R., & Costa, P. T., Jr. (2003). *Personality in adulthood: A five-factor theory perspective* (2nd ed.). New York: Guilford Press.

McCullough (2000). *Cognitive behavioral analysis systems of psychotherapy: Treatment of chronic depression*. New York: Guilford Press.

McReynolds, C. J., Garske, G. G., & Turpin, J. O. (1999). Psychiatric rehabilitation: A survey of rehabilitation counseling education programs. *Journal of Rehabilitation*, *65*(4), 45–49.

Mezzich, J. E., Fabrega, H., Coffman, G. A., & Glavin, Y. (1987). Comprehensively diagnosing geriatric patients. *Comprehensive Psychiatry*, *28*, 68–76.

Miller, M. D., Frank, E., Cornes, C., Houck, P. R., & Reynolds, C. F., III. (2003). The value of maintenance interpersonal psychotherapy (IPT) in older adults with different IPT foci. *American Journal of Geriatric Psychiatry*, *11*(1), 97–102.

Millon, T. (1969). *Modern psychopathology: A biosocial approach to maladaptive learning and functioning*. Philadelphia: Saunders.

Millon, T. (1981). *Disorders of personality: DSM-III, Axis II*. New York: Wiley.

Millon, T. (1983). *Millon Clinical Multiaxial Inventory manual* (3rd ed.). Minneapolis, MN: National Computer Systems.

Millon, T. (1988). Personologic psychotherapy: Ten commandments for a post-eclectic approach to integrative treatment. *Psychotherapy*, *25*, 209–219.

Millon, T. (1990). *Toward a new personology: An evolutionary model*. New York: Wiley-Interscience.

Millon, T. (2003). *Millon Index of Personality Styles Revised*. Minneapolis, MN: Pearson Assessments.

Millon, T., Antoni, M. H., Millon, C., Minor, S., & Grossman, S. (2001). *Test manual for the Millon Behavioral Medicine Diagnostic (MBMD)*. Minneapolis, MN: Pearson Assessments.

Millon, T., & Davis, R. D. (1996). *Disorders of personality: DSM-IV and beyond*. New York: Wiley.

Millon, T. (with Davis, R. D., & Millon, C.). (1997). *MCMI-III manual* (2nd ed.). Minneapolis, MN: National Computer Systems.

Moffitt, T. E., Caspi, A., Harrington, H., & Milne, B. J. (2002). Males on the life-course-persistent and adolescence-limited antisocial pathways: Follow-up at age 26 years. *Development and Psychopathology*, *14*, 179–207.

Molinari, V., Ames, A., & Essa, M. (1994). Prevalence of personality disorders in two geropsychiatric inpatient units. *Journal of Geriatric Psychiatry and Neurology*, *7*, 209–215.

Molinari, V., Kunik, M. E., Snow-Turek, A. L., Deleon, H., & Williams, W. (1999). Age-related personality differences in inpatients with personality disorder: A cross-sectional study. *Journal of Clinical Geropsychology, 5,* 191–202.

Molinari, V., & Marmion, J. (1993). Personality disorders in geropsychiatric outpatients. *Psychological Reports, 73,* 256–258.

Molinari, V., & Marmion, J. (1995). Relationship between affective disorders and Axis II diagnoses in geropsychiatric patients. *Journal of Geriatric Psychiatry and Neurology, 8,* 61–64.

Mroczek, D. K., & Spiro, A., III. (2003). Modeling intraindividual change in personality traits: Findings from the Normative Aging Study. *Journal of Gerontology, 58B,* P153–P165.

Neugarten, B. (1964). *Personality in middle and late life.* New York: Atherton Press.

Nezu, A. M., Nezu, C. M., Friedman, S. H., Faddis, S., & Houts, P. S. (1998). *Helping cancer patients cope: A problem-solving approach.* Washington, DC: American Psychological Association.

Niederehe, G. (1996). Psychosocial treatments with depressed older adults: A research update. *American Journal of Geriatric Psychiatry, 4*(Suppl. 1), S66–S78.

Nussbaum, P. (1997). *Handbook of the neuropsychology of aging.* New York: Plenum Press.

Paris, J. (2003). *Personality disorders over time.* Washington, DC: American Psychiatric Press.

Persons, J. B. (2005). Empiricism, mechanism, and the practice of cognitive-behavior therapy. *Behavior Therapy, 36,* 107–118.

Pfohl, B., Blum, N., & Zimmerman, M. (1997). *Structured Interview for DSM-IV Personality (SIDP-IV).* Washington, DC: American Psychiatric Press.

Reynolds, C. F., & Kupfer, D. J. (1999). Depression and aging: A look to the future. *Psychiatric Services, 50,* 1167–1172.

Rosowsky, E., & Gurian, B. (1991). Borderline personality disorder in late life. *International Psychogeriatrics, 3,* 39–52.

Rubinstein, R. L., & Lawton, M. P. (1997). *Depression in long-term and residential care: Advances in research and treatment.* New York: Springer.

Ruegg, R., & Frances, A. (1995). New research in personality disorders. *Journal of Personality Disorders, 9*(1), 1–8.

Rybarczyk, B., DeMarco, G., DeLaCruz, M., & Lapidos, S. (1999). Comparing mind–body wellness interventions for older adults with chronic illness: Classroom versus home instruction. *Behavioral Medicine, 24*(4), 181–190.

Sadavoy, J. (1996). Personality disorder in old age: Symptom expression. *Clinical Gerontologist, 16*(3), 19–36.

Sadavoy, J. (1999). The effect of personality disorder on Axis I disorder in the elderly. In M. Duffy (Ed.), *Handbook of counseling and psychotherapy with older adults* (pp. 397–413). New York: Wiley.

Sadavoy, J., & Fogel, F. (1992). Personality disorders in old age. In J. E. Birren, R. B. Sloane, & G. D. Cohen (Eds.), *Handbook of mental health and aging* (2nd ed., pp. 433–462). San Diego: Academic Press.

Scogin, F., & McElreath, L. (1994). Efficacy of psycho-social treatments for geriatric depression: A qualitative review. *Journal of Consulting and Clinical Psychology, 62,* 69–74.

Scogin, F., Rickard, H. C., Keith, S., Wilson, J., & McElreath, L. (1992). Progressive and imaginal relaxation training for elderly persons with subjective anxiety. *Psychological Aging, 7*(3), 419–424.

Scogin, F., Welsh, D., Hanson, A., Stump, J., & Coates, A. (2005). Evidence-based psychotherapies for depression in older adults. *Clinical Psychology: Science and Practice, 12*(3), 222–237.

Segal, D. L., & Coolidge, F. L. (1998). Personality disorders. In A. S. Bellack & M. Hersen (Eds.), *Comprehensive clinical psychology: Vol. 7. Clinical geropsychology* (pp. 267–289). New York: Elsevier Science.

Segal, D. L., Coolidge, F. L., & Hersen, M. (1998). Psychological testing of older people. In I. H. Nordhus, G. R. VandenBos, S. Berg, & P. Fromholt (Eds.), *Clinical geropsychology.* Washington, DC: American Psychological Association.

Segal, D. L., Coolidge, F. L., & Rosowsky, E. (2006). *Personality disorders and older adults: Diagnosis, assessment, and treatment*. New York: Wiley.

Segal, D. L., Hersen, M., Van Hasselt, V. B., Silberman, C. S., & Roth, L. (1996). Diagnosis and assessment of personality disorders in older adults: A critical review. *Journal of Personality Disorders*, 10(4), 384–399.

Segal, D. L., Hook, J. N., & Coolidge, F. L. (2001). Personality dysfunction, coping styles, and clinical symptoms in younger and older adults. *Journal of Clinical Geropsychology*, 7, 201–212.

Small, B. J., Hertzog, C., Hultsch, D. F., & Dixon, R. A. (2003). Stability and change in adult personality over 6 years: Findings from the Victoria Longitudinal Study. *Journal of Gerontology*, 58B, P166–P176.

Snow, L., Powers, D., & Liles, D. (2006). Cognitive-behavioral therapy for long-term care patients with dementia. In L. Hyer & R. Intrieri (Eds.), *Geropsychological interventions in long term care* (pp. 210–241). New York: Springer.

Strack, S. (1991). *Manual for the Personality Adjective Check List (PACL), Revised Edition*. Pasadena, CA: 21st Century Assessment.

Steunenberg, B., Twisk, J. W. R., Beekman, A. T. F., Deeg, D. J., & Kekhof, A. J. F. M. (2005). Stability and change of neuroticism in aging. *Journal of Gerontology*, 60B, P27–P33.

Teeter, R. B., Garetz, F. K., Miller, W. R., & Heiland, W. F. (1976). Psychiatric disturbances of aged patients in skilled nursing homes. *American Journal of Psychiatry*, 133, 1430–1434.

Teri, L., Curtis, J., Gallagher-Thompson, D., & Thompson, L. (1994). Cognitive-behavioural therapy with depressed older adults. In L. S. Schneider, C. F. Reynolds, B. D. Lebowitz, & A. J. Friedhoff (Eds.), *Diagnosis and treatment of depression in late life: Results of the NIH Consensus Development Conference*. Washington, DC: American Psychiatric Press.

Teri, L., Logsdon, R. G., Uomoto, J., & McCurry, S. M. (1997). Behavioral treatment of depression in dementia patients: A controlled clinical trial. *Journal of Gerontology*, 52B(4), P159–P166.

Teri, L., & McCurry, S. M. (2000). Psychosocial therapies with older adults. In C. E. Coffey & J. C. Cummings (Eds.), *Textbook of geriatric neuropsychiatry* (2nd ed., pp. 861–890). Washington, DC: American Psychiatric Press.

Terracciano, A., McCrae, R. R., & Costa, P. T., Jr. (2006). Longitudinal trajectories in Guilford–Zimmerman Temperament Survey data: Results from the Baltimore Longitudinal Study of Aging. *Journal of Gerontology*, 61B, P108–P116.

Thompson, L. W. (1996). Cognitive-behavioral therapy and treatment for late-life depression. *Journal of Clinical Psychiatry*, 57(5), 29–37.

Thompson, L. W., Gallagher, D., & Breckenridge, J. S. (1987). Comparative effectiveness of psychotherapies for depressed elders. *Journal of Consulting and Clinical Psychology*, 55(3), 385–390.

Thompson, L. W., Gallagher, D., & Czirr, R. (1988). Personality disorder and outcome in the treatment of late-life depression. *Journal of Geriatric Psychiatry*, 21, 133–146.

Thompson, L. W., Gallagher, D., Hanser, S., Gantz, F., & Steffen, A. (1991, November). *Comparison of desipramine and cognitive/behavioral therapy in the treatment of late-life depression*. Paper presented at the meeting of the Gerontological Society of America, San Francisco.

Thompson, L. W., Gallagher-Thompson, D., & Dick, L. P. (1995). *Cognitive-behavioral therapy for late life depression: A therapist manual*. Palo Alto, CA: Older Adult and Family Center, Veterans Affairs Palo Alto Health Care System.

Tracey, T. J., & Ray, P. B. (1984). Stages of successful time-limited counseling: An interactional examination. *Journal of Counseling Psychology*, 31(1), 13–27.

Wallston, K. A., Smith, R. A., King, J. E., Smith, M. S., Rye, P., & Burish, T. G. (1991). Desire for control and choice of antiemetic treatment for cancer chemotherapy. *Western Journal of Nursing Research*, 13(1), 12–23.

Westen, D., & Shedler, J. (1999a). Revising and assessing Axis II: Part 1. Developing a clinically and empirically valid assessment method. *American Journal of Psychiatry*, 156, 258–272.

Westen, D., & Shedler, J. (1999b). Revising and assessing Axis II: Part 2. Toward an empirically based and clinically useful classification of personality disorders. *American Journal of Psychiatry, 156*, 273–285.

Widiger, T. A., Mangine, S., Corbitt, E. M., Ellis, C. G., & Thomas, G. V. (1995). *Personality Disorder Interview–IV: A semistructured interview for the assessment of personality disorders (Professional manual)*. Odessa, FL: Psychological Assessment Resources.

Zanarini, M. C., Frankenburg, F. R., Sickel, A. E., & Yong, L. (1996). *The Diagnostic Interview for DSM-IV Personality Disorders (DIPD-IV)*. Belmont, MA: McLean Hospital.

Zeiss, A. M., & Steffen, A. (1996). Treatment issues with elderly clients. *Cognitive and Behavioural Practice, 3*, 371–389.

Zeiss, R. A., Delmonico, R. L., Zeiss, A. M., & Dornbrand, L. (1991). Psychologic disorder and sexual dysfunction in elders. *Clinical Geriatric Medicine, 7*(1), 133–151.

Zweig, R. A., & Agronin, M. E. (2006). Personality disorders. In M. E. Agronin & G. J. Maletta (Eds.), *Principles and practice of geriatric psychiatry* (pp. 449–470). Philadelphia: Lippincott Williams & Wilkins.

CHAPTER 14

Using the MCMI
in General Treatment Planning

Jeffrey J. Magnavita

The conceptualization, assessment, and treatment of personality dysfunction and co-occurring clinical syndromes are among the most exciting, challenging, and controversial issues in the field of psychology and personology. There are many influences that make personology an exciting field, as well as many that lead to controversy. There are issues regarding the validity of the construct of personality; criticism that personality testing has gained "cult status" and is inappropriately applied (Paul, 2004); and questions about the validity and usefulness (PDM Task Force, 2006) of the main current diagnostic nosology (American Psychiatric Association, 2000) used to guide clinical practice. In fact, there are various types of personality classifications each having its own proponents: (1) categorical, (2) dimensional, (3) structural, (4) prototypal, and (5) relational systems of classification each. There are even those who challenge the very use of personality disorder diagnostic labels, on the grounds that they run the risk of "reifying, pathologizing, and objectifying the individual" (Jordan, 2004, p. 130).

Despite these and many other issues and dangers, personality remains a vital construct central to the conceptualization of psychopathology, and essential to clinicians' ability to develop effective treatment strategies. Notwithstanding the controversies, clinicians search for comprehensive theories to organize the phenomenological, historical, and clinical data they are inundated with when faced with those who seek relief from suffering. Theoretical and diagnostic systems are essential forms of pattern recognition, which allow us to organize information, to develop hypotheses about the etiology of psychopathology, and to strategize treatment interventions. Whether the various systems meet the criteria of clinical science is debatable, however (Lilienfeld & O'Donohue, 2007). Since symptom complexes and relational dysfunctions arise from and mutually shape the personality system, clinical assessment of personality is the bulwark of clinical practice. Such assessment includes techniques of diagnostic interviewing and history taking, as well as selective use of psychometric instruments. Barlow (2007) states: "What seems apparent in the near future is that we are arriving at a new understanding of the relationship of personality and psychopathology that will influence our conceptions of psychopathology and systems of classification" (p. xi).

In this regard, various useful psychometric instruments have been developed over the past century. These can be divided into two major categories: projective and objective assessment. Essentially, projective techniques encourage the subject to engage in deciphering often vague stimuli configurations (e.g., inkblots), interpreting pictures of people in various scenes, or drawing human figures. Although questions about their validity remain open to debate, projective techniques are used extensively by psychologists and remain a bulwark of clinical assessment (Paul, 2004). Not relying on apperception, objective tests requires respondents to answer an array of questions; the statistically derived patterns that emerge from their answers are related to various personality traits, patterns, and clinical syndromes. Objective tests also have their limitations, one of which is that they rely on the respondents' honestly answering the questions. Sophisticated instruments attempt to deal with those who want to appear healthier than they actually are or to appear more disturbed by building in scales to measure these response sets. The Millon Clinical Multiaxial Inventory–III (MCMI-III; Millon, 2006) is one such standardized test, which has established itself as a major assessment instrument useful for diagnostic formulations and general treatment planning to enhance clinical efficacy (Magnavita, 2005c). This chapter focuses on the use of the MCMI-III in clinical practice and describes some of the ways in which it can be employed by clinicians to enhance treatment planning within a unified framework. The next section reviews the underpinnings of the MCMI, as well as the movement—in part spearheaded by Millon's theoretical and scientific advances (1969, 1981, 1990)—that has resuscitated personology from a moribund state to one of increased scientific study and clinical utility.

Personology: "The Comeback Kid"

Falling out of favor in the middle of the 20th century, the study of personality has made a comeback—some would say, to the detriment of society (Paul, 2004)—and there is evidence that personality is now strongly ensconced in the pantheon of clinical science and practice. The resurgence in scientific and clinical study of personality has led to a renewed interest in the centrality of personality in clinical psychology. Personality-guided therapy as espoused by Millon (1999) emerges in a new form from early psychoanalytic theory's emphasis on character type and structure as the central domain of psychoanalysis and source of psychopathology. Instead of viewing symptoms, relational disturbances, and clinical syndromes as unique phenomena, a personality-guided conceptualization seeks to understand how the unique configuration of symptoms emerges from the type and integrity of the personality system. Millon aptly uses the metaphor of the immune system to describe personality. Just as the human body's immune system when it is operating optimally can ward off patho-gens, a personality system that is functioning adaptively and effectively is capable of metabolizing the feelings, stresses/strains, and occasional traumas of modern life without developing symptoms such as anxiety, depression, substance abuse, and so forth. In the well-functioning personality system, if a strain or trauma does become too much, the symptoms that occur are transient and recede with support and brief treatment. When personality is not functioning optimally, or is dysfunctional, there is a greater likelihood that clinical symptom complexes will emerge and psychological treatment will be required. The increased awareness of the high prevalence of person-ality disorders in the general population, and the fact that over 50% of those who are receiving mental health services are diagnosed with a personality disorder (Weissman, 1993), have also fueled the resurgence in the study of personality disor-ders.

Whether the anecdotal reports of increases in patients with personality disorders are the results of clearer diagnostic nosology, or whether this factor is combined with the rapid social changes of the 20th century, it is clear from epidemiological findings and clinical observation that there is an epidemic of personality disorders in children, adolescents, and adults (Magnavita, 2007). Clinicians in practice are under severe pressure to diagnose and treat their patients in increasingly briefer treatment formats. Therefore more emphasis on rapid and accurate assessment is essential; otherwise, there is a real danger that in the rush toward effective but brief treatment, clinicians will miss information that is important for optimal treatment planning and interven-tion. Tools that can assist the clinician in efficiently gathering such information become popular, and others with less utility fall by the wayside. The MCMI in its various editions is an instrument that has become a mainstay of clinical practice for many clinicians, judging by the sheer numbers of them using it. I have used this instrument extensively in my own outpatient practice, as well as in a community mental health agency and inpatient unit. I have also utilized it for determining the fit-ness for duty of, and otherwise assessing impaired professionals.

Theoretical Developments in Personality, Psychopathology, and Psychotherapy

Assessment needs to be grounded in theoretical constructs that can illuminate the domain systems being assessed and their influence on the development and mainte-nance of psychopathology and dysfunction (Magnavita, 2005a). Millon (1981) has advanced the notion of personality as a central organizing system that is shaped by a variety of influences from multiple domain systems, such as the primary attachment system, the family unit, societal institutions, and cultural forces. Incorporating new theoretical and empirical findings from chaos and complexity theory, we may con-ceptualize personality as an emergent phenomenon that is greater than the sum of its parts and cannot be located in any one domain system (Magnavita, 2006). It is not in a single or even in multiple domains that personality emerges, but in the complex holistic network of multiple domain levels from the intrapsychic to the sociocultural.

Conceptualizing psychopathology and dysfunction in a holistic fashion allows us to be alert to the interrelationships among the structures and processes of human adaptation and functioning. Each of the multiple complex systems operating in the human ecosystem has its particular functions and structures, and when these are scientifically studied, they add to clinical science and inform clinical practice. For example, the study of infant–mother (dyadic system) interactions though the microanalysis of videotapes clearly demonstrates complex exchanges of vocal, facial, and kinetic communications that lead to synchronized interactions (Beebe, Knoblauch, Rustin, & Sorter, 2005). In mother–infant dyads where there is chronic dyssynchrony, there is a greater likelihood of disorganized attachment, which is a predictor of adult psychopathology. There is some evidence that this may be one of the pathways to adult borderline disturbances. Clinical syndromes and chronic personality dysfunction are phenotypic expressions of a confluence of neurobiological, psychological, social, family, and cultural forces. Over the past century, clinical theorists have mapped various subsystems in which psychopathology and personality is expressed, ranging from the micro to the molar levels.

Whether a system is impaired at the intrapsychic, dyadic, triadic, or sociocultural level, if the impairment is not addressed, it reaches a systemic tipping point resulting in a reorganization of this system at a level of dysfunction that can be considered "harmful." The notion of "harmful dysfunction," developed by Wakefield (1999), describes how psychopathology can be viewed as "failures of naturally selected functions and harm is judged by cultural values" (Wakefield, 2006, p. 423). A harmful dysfunction, at whatever level it occurs, represents a system that is not operating according to its evolutionary design.

As psychologists, we are empowered and privileged by society to diagnose and label harmful dysfunction, and in doing so we co-construct the phenomena we endeavor to measure and understand. This necessitates "a scientific perspective concerning psychopathology and its treatment" (O'Donohue, Lilienfeld, & Fowler, 2007, p. 3). The metrics that we use, although advancing rapidly, remain insufficient in providing a holistic representation of the complexity we are endeavoring to represent. Nevertheless, we are required to assess the system to the best of our ability, with the best available diagnostic tools, so as not to miss any relevant contributions to the dysfunction that we encounter in clinical practice. A multiperspective assessment is always superior to single-domain sampling, except of course when the sampling techniques themselves have little or no validity. As all social scientists and clinicians know, the human system is extraordinarily complex, and researchers have not been given the same resources and funding to decipher it as scholars of the human genome in biology or the atom in physics have. The results of decoding the human personality system may be as remarkable as these—but short of a full-scale attempt at deciphering the human system, we are forced to rely on mapping the complexity as best we can for our purposes, based on available instrumentation and theoretical constructs.

The Challenge of Conceptualizing the Complexity of the Human Personality System

It is clear to any clinician reading this volume that conceptualizing a system as complex as the human personality system is currently beyond the realm of our psychological science. Nevertheless, we must begin by building and developing frameworks within which to create meaningful treatment interventions and design treatment packages to deliver to those who seek our services for their suffering. In order to organize our assessment and intervention, the total ecological system of the person, couple, family, or social system we are examining must be conceptualized within the context in which each subsystem operates; we must also keep in mind the part–whole relationships that characterize human personality systems. Each type of assessment instrument—whether objective instrument, projective technique, sociogram, brain scan, electroencephalogram, or psychodiagnostic interview and history—is biased with regard to the subsystem domain or domains being sampled. All critical domains must be considered to form a comprehensive or holographic perspective. The data gathered from a particular perspective must also be considered in the context of the total system. For example, a patient who is tested after recovering from an episode of drug or alcohol use will not necessarily have a valid profile.

A hologram is a three-dimensional representation that emerges from various networks and can be viewed differentially from various perspectives. Each perspective offers a view of the totality, but can never come close to capturing the complexity and the ever-shifting and evolving nature of the phenomena observed at any one point or multiple points in time. A single observation may be extremely important: When second-by-second interactions between infants and mothers are being microanalyzed, a 1-second frame may contain vital information, as in the case of a mother who is seen snarling at her child when attempting to calm the distressed infant (Beebe et al., 2005). But such information must always be considered in relation to the whole system. Sophisticated clinicians are aware of the limitations of any psychometric technique and consider it a means of sampling a complex, multifaceted organism embedded in various levels of interconnected biopsychosocial subsystems.

The self is in its essence relational, having its origins in evolutionarily fueled needs for robust attachment bonds, which enabled *Homo sapiens* to develop cultural systems (Magnavita, 2002). Personality is an emergent phenomenon that is formed by a complex network of interrelated domain systems and is shaped by our genetic predispositions and relational experience. Accumulating findings from neuroscience, developmental psychopathology, clinical science, and other disciplines have inspired a multidisciplinary model of convergent processes, which has been termed "personality systematics" (Magnavita, 2006). Personality systematics utilizes systems and complexity theories to decipher how the human personality system operates and functions, based on certain unifying principles.

Within a unified framework, we can view the levels of personality from various perspectives as they are embedded in the relational system. Relationships are the processes by which individuals are shaped and social systems develop and evolve. The evolution of *Homo sapiens* necessitated the development of increasingly complex relational tools, such as language, proxemics, and consciousness, to allow individuals to survive a harsh environment that was not hospitable to loners. A unified framework must allow for the interrelationships among all the empirically and theoretically relevant domain systems of human relationships. Systems theory (von Bertalanffy, 1968) and chaos theory (Gleick, 1987) are essential to understand the feedback mechanisms within any complex system. Drawing from the ecological work of Bronfenbrenner (1979), we can imagine the domains as nested structures that are embedded in larger structural networks. In previous works, I have moved toward an increasingly unified theoretical model of these domains and feedback mechanisms (Magnavita, 2005b, 2006).

At the microscopic level, we can observe and assess the interrelated domains that are conceptualized as biological/intrapsychic. For heuristic purposes, this level can be conceived as what occurs within an individual; it includes the interrelationship among neurobiology, affect–cognition–defense networks, and anxiety, for example. There has been abundant empirical and clinical evidence of the importance of these domains for the development of an individual's personality structure.

If we widen our perspective, we view the interpersonal/dyadic level of operation, or simply what occurs between two people. Advances in infant research are demonstrating the essential nature of the infant–mother dyad as the basis of all self–other relationships; this basic attachment system is used in later development to guide relationships. Again widening the perspective, we can now introduce the level of relational/triadic processes. Infant–mother pairs almost immediately have to deal with a third other. The term "triangulation" refers to what occurs when there is a third person involved in an unstable dyadic configuration. It has been well established that unstable dyads seek stabilization with a third party or triangle (Bowen, 1978).

These intrapsychic, dyadic, and triadic configurations are the building blocks of family and social groups and structures. These first three levels are embedded in the sociocultural/family system, which represents the fourth level of this unified framework. Clinicians operate within all four of these systems, but they are generally most comfortable assessing and intervening at the system level congruent with their training. Psychodynamic clinicians are concerned with intrapsychic processes and often don't feel comfortable in other realms; family-oriented clinicians often eschew the intrapsychic realm; and so forth. Each overlooked realm, however, is a source of important data about processes and functions. This may not be realized without an understanding of how these domains operate in a coordinated fashion—or, in the case of dysfunction, how uncoordinated action patterns predominate.

The Importance of Understanding the Level of Substrate Assessment

It is imperative to understand the unique nature of the assessment instrument that is being utilized, as well as its strengths and limitations, considering the personality system with its operating principles holistically. For example, a depression inventory may sample the biological/intrapsychic domain, but tell nothing about the interpersonal patterns that are reinforcing the depressed operating system. What is critical is to be mindful of the system and never to assume that one perspective fully represents the patient's reality. It is far beyond the scope of this chapter to present a comprehensive overview of the variety of assessment instruments used in clinical practice, but, broadly, they include standardized instruments such as the MCMI and Minnesota Multiphasic Personality Inventory (MMPI), to name the most popular; projective techniques such as the Rorschach, Thematic Apperception Test (TAT), House–Tree–Person (HTP), and Draw-a-Person; and clinical interviewing and history, the mainstays of clinical practice. Each form of assessment and specific techniques gather

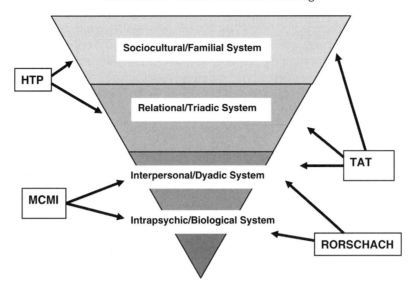

FIGURE 14.1. The total biopsychosocial system's four substrates and foci of assessment.

information from various levels of the patient's total ecological system, from the intrapsychic/biological to the sociocultural/familial (see Figure 14.1).

When considering instruments and standard interviewing and history-taking techniques, the clinician must seek to balance the tension that exists between the cost and time needed to administer and score a particular test or battery of tests, and the potential advantages of increased information and increased efficiency with which it is gathered. Thus the clinician should attempt to utilize the psychodiagnostic techniques that are best suited to the unique requirements of each case. More complex cases generally benefit from more assessment, which can better tease out the nature of the dysfunction. The next section discusses the use of the MCMI-III and its role in treatment planning.

The Clinical Utility and Role of the MCMI-III in Treatment Planning

Treatment planning is based on solid assessment and requires specialized training in psychopathology, psychodynamics, developmental psychopathology, family systems, diagnostic interviewing, and grounding in theories of change and methods of psychotherapy. When presented with a suffering person or persons, how do we clinicians proceed, and what do we do first? According to Millon (2006), "the initial focus should be on helping the client gain some relief from troubling symptoms" (p. 149). Depending on the context, this necessitates developing a therapeutic alliance. The optimal therapeutic alliance activates hope in the patient and gives him or her confidence in the clinician and the clinical process. Concomitantly, the clinician must be able to enter into a collaborative relationship that allows the patient to feel understood, while gathering the data necessary to make diagnostic formulations and develop hypotheses about the etiology and maintenance of the symptoms. Where possible, the optimal choice is restructuring the personality, so that intrapsychic and interpersonal functioning can be maximized and resiliency enhanced (Magnavita, 1997). Restructuring personality requires a systematic enhancement of vital personality functions such as affect regulation, defensive structure, relational schemas, and cognitive beliefs, as well as capacity for intimacy and closeness. The MCMI-III is a method of rapidly assessing clinical symptom clusters, as well as the personality configuration from which they emerge; it thus allows the clinician to focus more intensively on the major structural deficits and dysfunctional domain systems, while identifying and capitalizing on strengths. The MCMI-III is similar to other objective measures used in medicine and psychology. Just as an electrocardiogram provides a physician with a sample of cardiac functioning, the MCMI-III provides a clinician with a profile of vital functions of the personality system and the level at which it is adapting.

Assessing the Personality Configuration

More specifically, the MCMI can provide a coherent map of the individual's personality configuration, together with essential information about the relationship between the personality system and the clinical syndromes that emerge from it. When the personality system is functional, there is either transient or little evidence of clinical syndromes (anxiety, depression, substance abuse, etc.). However, when the personality system is dysfunctional, and depending on the severity of this dysfunction, various comorbid disorders are likely to make treatment planning and intervention complex. Generally speaking, the greater the degree of comorbid symptom expressions, the higher the level of psychopathology present. Although disturbances in interpersonal relationships are not assessed directly on the MCMI Clinical Syndrome Scales, difficulties in the interpersonal realm are inherent in Millon's personality configurations. Much useful information can also be derived from each personality pattern's characteristic interpersonal styles and representational systems. It therefore behooves the clinician to know the type and structure of the personality organization before intervening.

For example, a patient who scores high on the MCMI Avoidant personality scale and also suffers from anxiety is typically going to be someone whose inability to bear anxiety has fueled the avoidant pattern. Therefore, anxiety management is going to be a key element of treatment planning, along with enhancing interpersonal efficacy and self-esteem. Also, this should alert the clinician to family dynamics that may have played a role in these patterns. Avoidant personality traits are characteristic of developmentally delayed families, where separation and individuation are discouraged because they are too threatening to the parental subsystem (Magnavita, 2000). Assessing the family system and involving family members in treatment are key to restructuring this system, and thus enhancing autonomous functioning of the individual. A holographic representation can be developed once there is an understanding of how the personality system is organized and operates and what interpersonal patterns and symptom expressions are likely. This holographic view will include the individual, couple, family, and culture processes that interact to create the unique phenomenology of the patient and his or her multiple subsystems in which they operate.

Although each individual is unique, certain patterns are commonly seen in clinical practice. To return to the example of an individual with an avoidant personality who is operating at a borderline level of dysfunction, this person may show signs of generalized or free-floating anxiety, agoraphobia, and/or social phobia (depending on the family functioning), as depicted in the holographic diagram in Figure 14.2.

The MCMI is particularly well suited for rapidly obtaining information about an individual's personality functioning. It is similar to the use of an X-ray or magnetic resonance imaging by an orthopedic surgeon who wants to ferret out the structural problems that are impairing physical functioning. It is imperative for the clinician when addressing the clinical symptom patterns or Axis I diagnoses to determine how the unique personality configuration of the individual will either promote therapeutic progress or (more likely) hinder it. For example, when a patient has a high score on the Borderline scale, this should alert the clinician to the fact that first-line treatment approaches to an anxiety disorder may be problematic. A borderline patient is typically trying to establish intrapsychic and interpersonal coherence, and is in need of a stabilizing relationship with a secure attachment figure. First-line treatments for anxiety may actually destabilize such a patient, who may feel that he or she is not really "understood" by the clinician (which may be retraumatizing). Another patient with anxiety, who is high on obsessive–compulsive traits, may be a good candidate for cognitive-behavioral therapy because of the likelihood that he or she will adhere to a standard treatment protocol that requires practicing relaxation procedures or keeping a record of thoughts throughout the day.

Even though any test represents only one point in time–space relations, reading the MCMI profile with practice becomes a rapid form of pattern recognition from which motion and process can be inferred. For example, a high Borderline score in someone who appears stable may be a useful predictor of the likelihood of future

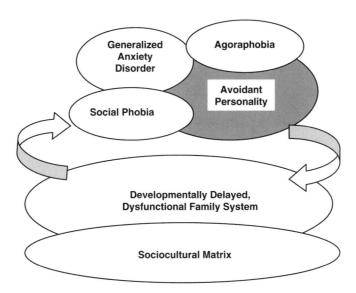

FIGURE 14.2. Holographic diagram of personality organization and emergent clinical syndromes interacting with the sociocultural/family matrices.

chaotic states characterized by emotional dysregulation and perceptual distortion, leading to all types of family and interpersonal conflicts. The clinical interview and psychotherapy process will allow the clinician to see how the pattern operates and what needs to be modified to enable more functional adaptation. Extrapolation from the profile becomes easier as the clinician comes to understand the basics of personality systematics and personality-guided principles of assessment and psychotherapy.

Comprehensive Assessment in Complex Cases

Patients who present with treatment-refractory conditions or complex issues that are not readily comprehended by the clinician are often good candidates for comprehensive assessment, which can include a battery of tests and procedures offering multiple samples and perspectives. Treatment-refractory cases include individuals who have seen multiple mental health professionals and report a lack of progress, have multiple hospitalizations, exhibit chronic suicidality, or are highly resistant to treatment. Often with patients who meet these criteria, a focal assessment can be invaluable for corroborating clinical impressions and initial formulations. The accumulated data can then be used to further refine a holistic picture of the various central domain systems and processes. Each assessment instrument or battery should be based on the referral questions asked, and matched to provide samples and corroboration of various domains of functioning. As advances in neuroscience and neuropsychology occur, more patients are administered tests that assess brain–behavior functions. These neuropsychological findings can be enhanced by understanding the dynamic organization and processes of the personality system. A neuropsychological perspective can be critical in understanding the unique processing patterns and channels each person utilizes. It is also imperative for those who specialize in neuropsychological assessment to assess the personality configuration and overall psychosocial functions, so that findings can be meaningfully integrated and holistically interpreted.

Clinical Uses and Range of Application in Practice

The MCMI-III can be used in a variety of ways that can enhance diagnostic clarity and focus treatment planning more precisely. The MCMI-III is a well established standardized instrument for differential diagnosis, which is a necessity for effective clinical practice. Although diagnostic systems all have their strengths and limitations, the MCMI-III offers the categorical sorting of syndromes and personality types/disorders of the *Diagnostic and Statistical Manual of Mental Disorders* (DSM), with the addition of placing these on a continuum of severity. Settings where the MCMI can be easily adopted include psychiatric hospitals, private practices, community mental heath agencies, general hospitals, forensic settings, or just about any place where an individual is able to complete the instrument and is not under undue duress (e.g., in an active theater of war). The rapid scoring available makes it possible to have the results of the testing available in some cases before the patient is seen. One of the problems that clinicians tend to deal with is the often extended turnaround time for a standard battery with projective testing, which is labor-intensive to score and interpret. Psychometric data are only useful if they are delivered in a timely fashion— especially in today's health care system, where brief treatment and short hospital stays are common. Few things are more frustrating to a clinician than receiving a valuable report after the treatment is well underway or the patient has terminated. My personal experience of using the MCMI-III as part of a comprehensive psychodiagnostic battery or as a stand-alone assessment with over 100 individuals for a variety of purposes and in various settings has made this instrument a mainstay of assessment in my clinical practice. I have repeatedly been amazed at how this 175-item true–false questionnaire has captured the personality system of the person I have assessed. This observation has been corroborated by the high number of patients who have expressed wonder that this instrument captured them so effectively. Clearly, the MCMI-III is best at differentiating pathology from the moderate to severe levels. With this in mind, clinicians should elect to use this instrument when they need greater clarification of clinical hunches or are stymied about the personality structure of an individual they are assessing or seeing for psychotherapy.

The Basics of Treatment Planning

In order to plan treatment effectively, the clinician must be conversant with the range of therapeutic approaches, modalities, and treatment formats available to him or her. The development of differential therapeutics in clinical psychology was a major advance in the field (Frances, Clarkin, & Perry, 1984). Prior to this development, there was very little consideration of the possibility that all treatments and formats are not equally effective. If certain treatments are not within a clinician's personal area of competence, the clinician should at least attain a basic understanding of how they work and the evidence base that exists to support each approach. In treatment planning, decisions must be made about the following components of a treatment plan:

1. *Type of therapy:* Psychopharmacological, psychoeducational, cognitive, cognitive-behavioral, psychodynamic, relational, integrative, unified, and so on. For each type of therapy an individual clinician uses, there is (or should be) a theory of personality and psychopathology, which explains how dysfunction occurs and how developmental factors can lead to personality disturbance and clinical syndromes.

2. *Modality of treatment:* Individual, couple, family, group, multifamily, ecological, and so on (or multiple modalities of therapy). Each modality of treatment has a specialized set of methods and techniques to restructure or modify process and structural components of the personality system.

3. *Treatment format:* Length of sessions, frequency of sessions, and intervals between sessions (Magnavita, 2005c, pp. 171–172).

In the following section, I present two cases of different degrees of complexity and describe how the MCMI-III was utilized in each treatment-planning process.

Case Examples

Confirming Diagnostic Impressions and Formulating a Treatment Plan

The patient came to treatment after having seen a number of psychotherapists and trying a variety of approaches to psychotherapy. The patient was a 23-year-old male who was living with his girlfriend and her daughter. She had asked him to leave her house because of his emotional problems but, wanted him to get help. The clinical interview revealed a young man of above-average to superior IQ, with good verbal ability and a coherent explanation of what was occurring in his relationship with his partner. He was accompanied by his partner to the first interview, and they both described how he became disconsolate and childlike, often having "temper tantrums" and acting in a passive–aggressive manner. They had done research on the Internet and wondered whether he had borderline personality disorder. The developmental history was consistent with a trajectory that someone with borderline pathology might exhibit. In this case, the patient reported traumatic treatment (i.e., emotional abuse by both parental figures). During the first session, the option of completing the MCMI-III was offered, and the patient was eager to comply in order to gain a clearer picture of his difficulties and to help focus the treatment.

His MCMI-III (see Figure 14.3) revealed elevations in both Disclosure and Debasement (base rate [BR] > 75), indicating that his response set might be an exaggeration of his distress and symptom constellations. Further examination of his profile showed elevations on the following Clinical Personality Patterns (BR > 75): Depressive, Dependent, Negativistic, and Masochistic. It also revealed an elevation in the Severe Personality Pathology category on the Borderline scale. An examination of the Clinical Syndromes showed an elevation on the Anxiety scale. In spite of the elevations and this patient's potential to exaggerate his difficulties, the results of the evaluation were highly consistent not only with his self-report in the interview and history, but with the observations of his significant other.

On the biological/intrapsychic level, the interpretive report captured the dynamic interplay: "Defective psychic structures suggest a failure to develop adequate internal cohesion and a less than satisfactory hierarchy of coping strategies." This statement speaks to the need in treatment planning for an approach that would begin to restructure and enhance his defensive functioning by providing a carefully titrated introduction to his defenses and helping him develop an awareness of their problematic nature. The interpretive report also identified some of his defenses, such as his negativism, explosive discharge of affect, stubbornness, acting out, and passive aggression, as well as his character patterns of self-sabotage and self-defeat. Concomitantly, working with basic skills to enhance emotional regulation would be necessary.

On the interpersonal/dyadic level, the report provided a picture of this patient's attachment style and interpersonal schema that suggested another aspect of the treatment focus: "He may permit himself to experience being exploited and abused. He may frequently anticipate being disillusioned with others, and for this reason may behave obstructively, thereby creating the expected disappointment." Further descriptive analysis of his pattern was provided: "Though seeking a measure of support and nurturance, he may be deeply untrusting, fearful of domination, and suspiciously alert to efforts that might undermine his self-determination and autonomy." This information would be indispensable in helping the clinician develop a strategy for creating a therapeutic alliance, which was all too likely to became problematic as the patient reenacted these patterns with the clinician, making it difficult to establish a collaborative partnership. His personal hostility would tend to stimulate the very rejection that he anticipated, and thus the psychotherapist would need seek to point out these patterns in a gentle way when they occurred and offer another model of relating.

As previously discussed, the MCMI-III provides important information about the intrapsychic and interpersonal levels of functioning. However, at the relational/triadic level, one can extrapolate. This patient's profile, which are high on borderline pathology, suggested that this individual would tend to engage in triangular relationships where he would seek to modulate his anxiety by drawing a third person into his conflicts. In fact, this was reported to be true. In regard to treatment planning, it would be important to enhance differentiation and develop a greater capacity for intimacy without activating his abandonment/engulfment.

I reviewed the report and then during the second session discussed it with the patient, using a format that I have refined with a series of patients. I inform the patient: "I will be

MILLON CLINICAL MULTIAXIAL INVENTORY - III
CONFIDENTIAL INFORMATION FOR PROFESSIONAL USE ONLY

Valid Profile

PERSONALITY CODE: 8A ** 3 8B 2B * 2A 6A 1 6B + 5 " 4 7 ' ' // - ** C * //

SYNDROME CODE: A ** - * // - ** - * //

DEMOGRAPHIC: 048761190/OT/M/22/W/N/15/MA/SC/-----/--/-----/

CATEGORY		RAW	BR	PROFILE OF SR SCORES	DIAGNOSTIC SCALES
MODIFYING INDICES	X	142	82		DISCLOSURE
	Y	11	51		DESIRABILITY
	Z	20	77		DEBASEMENT
CLINICAL PERSONALITY PATTERNS	1	7	60		SCHIZOID
	2A	12	73		AVOIDANT
	2B	14	78		DEPRESSIVE
	3	16	79		DEPENDENT
	4	12	34		HISTRIONIC
	5	16	53		NARCISSISTIC
	6A	13	68		ANTISOCIAL
	6B	13	60		SADISTIC
	7	10	31		COMPULSIVE
	8A	19	87		NEGATIVISTIC
	8B	15	79		MASOCHISTIC
SEVERE PERSONALITY PATHOLOGY	S	7	61		SCHIZOTYPAL
	C	17	81		BORDERLINE
	P	3	31		PARANOID
CLINICAL SYNDROMES	A	10	85		ANXIETY
	H	3	57		SOMATOFORM
	N	10	64		BIPOLAR: MANIC
	D	10	74		DYSTHYMIA
	B	9	74		ALCOHOL DEPENDENCE
	T	5	57		DRUG DEPENDENCE
	R	6	58		POST-TRAUMATIC STRESS
SEVERE CLINICAL SYNDROMES	SS	9	62		THOUGHT DISORDER
	CC	8	62		MAJOR DEPRESSION
	PP	0	0		DELUSIONAL DISORDER

Profile scale markers: 0   60   75   85   115

FIGURE 14.3. MCMI-III Profile Report for a 23-year-old male.

reviewing the results of the evaluation. In some instances the findings will fit and be quite accurate, and in others they may not accurately depict you." I further tell the individual (or couple) that I expect we will stop and discuss and explore the statements as we proceed. This allows the information to be defended against if it feels ego-alien. Generally, this approach allows us to view the findings as one source of feedback with which to get a better under-standing of the person's difficulties, and then to focus the treatment more effectively on the important issues. In most cases, the patient allows me to act as the filter and deliver the infor-mation without having to read the report. Others have asked whether they could read and digest the information, which I will arrange. One man with severe personality pathology was able to use the report to focus actively on his chronic character issues, which were destroying his relationships and career. The important point is that a clinician must use this information in a clinically sensitive way, based on the patient's capacities and adapted to his or her ways of processing emotionally laden information.

To return to the present case, the report was summarized (at times read word for word and at other times paraphrased, skipping terms or phrases that were not relevant or might be harmful) to the patient, and we worked together at deriving the meaning of the material and determining how close to his perception of himself it was. He reported that the information seemed very accurate; it felt as if it really described his struggles in relationships and with self-coherence in general, and more specifically with cognitive and emotional regulation. He expressed a sense of relief that the difficulties he was having were understood and accurately characterized in the report. This led to a feeling of hopefulness that he was not the only one suffering with this type of clinical manifestation, and he was clearly relieved when I said that there were various evidence-based treatment approaches available. This frank discussion also afforded us the opportunity to hypothesize about the roots of his struggles—especially the fact that his parents were unable to provide him with structure and stability because of the chaos in their lives. He was an only child, and they had looked to him for emotional affirmation.

As a result of the history, interview, and review of the MCMI-III, it was decided that the patient would enter a local partial hospital program that offered dialectical behavior therapy (DBT; Linehan, 1993), a well-established treatment for borderline personality disorder. In addition, he would see me for psychotherapy to address his problems with personality dys-function (manifested in his overdependence on his girlfriend, as well as in his other ineffective interpersonal patterns and self-defeating behavior). Finally, he agreed to a psychopharmaco-logical consultation and was prescribed an atypical antipsychotic medication to reduce his emotional dysregulation, regressive behavior, and concomitant perceptual distortion (which occurred when he became extremely anxious). These initial treatment interventions—combining individual psychotherapy, DBT in a partial hospital program, and psychopharma-cological intervention—led to rapid stabilization and longer-term treatment.

Complex Case Consultation

The MCMI-III can be a vital tool to assist in complex case consultation. Complex cases are generally ones where there are multiple and/or severe comorbid conditions, which place inordinate demands on mental health professionals. These conditions may include psychotic or major mood disorders, severe personality disorders, psy-choactive substance abuse/dependence, posttraumatic stress disorder, neurocognitive deficits, and others. Working with a community mental health agency, I developed a case consultation protocol that incorporates the MCMI-III. In many of these cases, the residential staff members who spend the majority of the time with the patients are often the least trained and experienced. Problems with recurring patterns of provoca-tive interpersonal behavior are often responded to by the staff in positive feedback loops, whereby the behavior escalates. Abusive patients can activate strong feelings in staff members, who may have few options other than calling the police or becoming punitive by taking away privileges. The staff can often feel under siege and powerless to relate effectively to some of these patients.

In one such case, the staff was experiencing a significant degree of frustration with a 20-year-old male who violated the basic rules of the residential program. He associated with troubled youth from the community and, against the residential rules, invited them into his housing unit. When limits were set, he responded with a fusillade of emotional abuse aimed at a particular female staff member who was his residential care worker. She was feeling abused and angry, but felt that she had little recourse; he seemed to sense intuitively this and go after her even more aggressively, often verbally abusing her.

One of the major challenges for this particular agency is that it is state-mandated to provide certain services for severely mentally ill patients, so in a sense the staff at times feels disempowered to set limits that would bar such an individual from receiving service. The case consultation protocol that has been developed for this agency is a flexible one, based on the needs of the staff and particulars of the case. The following components of the complex case consultation model and process are generally followed and modified where appropriate:

1. Staff consultation concerning the issues they are concerned about and the case background.
2. Review of medical records.
3. Inviting the patient to be part of the consultative process, which empowers the individual to become part of the solution.
4. Interviewing the patient and, when authorization is provided, videotaping the interview. Making a videotape for review with the staff can provide a vital learning opportunity and in many cases can allow for a more empathic response. When the patient is relating to the interviewer in a less hostile and more vulnerable manner, the staff can see the effects of the trauma that the patient has typically endured, and can be sensitized to and understand better the function of the patient's behavior.
5. Additional assessment to elucidate issues further and clarify diagnostic considerations. The MCMI-III is an excellent choice for this, because of its ease of administration and relevance to findings to treatment planning.
6. Conducting a team meeting with all those from the agency who participate in the patient's treatment and residential care, and developing a strategy to address the systemic issues that are being expressed.
7. Inviting the patient into the team meeting and empowering him or her to be part of the treatment-planning process. During this meeting, the staff and patient brainstorm about specific treatment options, which are then discussed with the patient as collaborator.
8. Modifying the treatment plan and creating clear expectations about choices available to the team and patient.
9. Follow-up consultation to adjust the plan where needed.

The 20-year-old patient described above agreed to participate in the complex case consultation, and agreed to allow me to interview him and videotape the interview. He was transported to the office by the residential care worker who was experiencing the greatest difficulty with the patient. This worker was interviewed first, and her perspective was taken and specific concerns explored. She reported feeling emotionally abused, frustrated, and impotent. She said, "When he gets angry, he yells, and that is what he learned to do." She reported an escalating pattern of emotional dysregulation when she attempted to set limits with him. She said that he had had a bad childhood, but was indulged and not parented by his grandmother. The residential worker also expressed a feeling of hopelessness that whatever approach she took seemed to result in the same escalating emotional spiral, where she felt emotionally beaten up and ineffective. After this, the patient was interviewed.

The patient presented as a highly anxious young man who became visibly upset with the video camera and asked how the tape would be used. His anxiety increased to the point of having some difficulty thinking and expressing himself, and thus it was decided to discontinue the videotaping. Once the issue of the videotape was resolved, however, his anxiety went down; his cognitive functions seemed to improve, and he related more coherently.

The patient made it clear at the beginning of the interview that he had "behavioral problems but no severe mental problems," and was "misdiagnosed" as suffering from a bipolar disorder. He had been maintained on a regimen of both a mood stabilizer and an antipsychotic for about the past 7 years, but was often noncompliant with the medications. He also reported that he had been diagnosed as a child with attention-deficit/hyperactivity disorder, oppositional defiant disorder, and Tourette's syndrome. He reported a sporadic work record at fast-food restaurants and some construction jobs, but stated, "I just quit. I get tired of it." He was once involved in a Job Corps program where he was learning how to do construction, but had a fight with another client and was asked to leave. He denied any head injuries, although it seemed from his speech and way of relating that neurocogntive deficits were likely. He reported a chaotic early childhood and said that his mother had been verbally abusive. He was sent to a series of group homes, shelters, and hospitals. He had never met his father, who was in prison. He reported being molested when he was "little" by a caretaker who would cut his knees with a razor blade and make him kneel in Epsom salts.

He was asked what his goals were, and he responded, "I want to become a loving father and have a car." He identified that he needed a full-time job and acknowledged that he had low self-esteem. He denied any drug or alcohol problems.

Following the interview, this patient agreed to take the MCMI-III, and the profile is depicted in Figure 14.4. His elevated Desirability scale (BR > 75) indicated his minimization of his difficulties and desire to present himself in an overly favorable light. This was consistent with the findings from the interview, where he minimized his psychiatric difficulties, denying that he suffered from a bipolar disorder (with which he believed he was misdiagnosed). In the Clinical Personality Patterns, there was an elevation of the Histrionic scale, suggestive of an individual who (according to the interpretive profile) "is typified by emotionality, resentful and demanding attitudes, a whiny tone, and a talent for making those around him miserable. He may also exhibit a high degree of lability, short periods of impulsive acting out, complaints, and sulking." The results suggested the following personality configuration: histrionic personality traits with paranoid personality features and negativistic (passive–aggressive) personality features. This was highly consistent with feedback from the staff members who worked with him in his residential unit. This highly resistant young man presented to the staff with a feeling of angry entitlement and demonstrated irresponsible behavior that was threatening his housing status in the program. His low scores on the Severe Personality Pathology Scales were probably the results of his symptoms' being effectively managed with pharmacological agents, as well as his desire to minimize his symptoms and appear healthier than his history indicated.

As part of the consultation process, a team meeting was held initially without the patient, and the staff members aired their considerable frustration over this young man's treatment-sabotaging behavior. A discussion of his issues and interpersonal patterns led to a greater understanding of how futile it was to enter into power struggles that this patient continually reenacted, leaving the staff feeling abused and demoralized. Later, the patient was invited into the team meeting; he expressed his desire to have his own apartment, in spite of the fact that

MILLON CLINICAL MULTIAXIAL INVENTORY - III
CONFIDENTIAL INFORMATION FOR PROFESSIONAL USE ONLY

Valid Profile

PERSONALITY CODE:　　8A ** 3 8B 2B * 2A 6A 1 6B + 5 " 4 7 ' ' // - ** C * //

SYNDROME CODE:　　A ** - * // - ** - * //

DEMOGRAPHIC:　　048761190/OT/M/22/W/N/15/MA/SC/-----/--/-----/

CATEGORY		SCORE		PROFILE OF SR SCORES				DIAGNOSTIC SCALES
		RAW	BR 0	60	75	85	115	
MODIFYING INDICES	X	75	49					DISCLOSURE
	Y	19	89					DESIRABILITY
	Z	2	38					DEBASEMENT
CLINICAL PERSONALITY PATTERNS	1	2	24					SCHIZOID
	2A	1	12					AVOIDANT
	2B	1	20					DEPRESSIVE
	3	5	50					DEPENDENT
	4	22	81					HISTRIONIC
	5	14	57					NARCISSISTIC
	6A	7	52					ANTISOCIAL
	6B	6	51					SADISTIC
	7	13	46					COMPULSIVE
	8A	8	60					NEGATIVISTIC
	8B	1	20					MASOCHISTIC
SEVERE PERSONALITY PATHOLOGY	S	0	0					SCHIZOTYPAL
	C	5	40					BORDERLINE
	P	6	62					PARANOID
CLINICAL SYNDROMES	A	0	0					ANXIETY
	H	0	0					SOMATOFORM
	N	3	36					BIPOLAR: MANIC
	D	3	60					DYSTHYMIA
	B	5	65					ALCOHOL DEPENDENCE
	T	3	45					DRUG DEPENDENCE
	R	0	0					POST-TRAUMATIC STRESS
SEVERE CLINICAL SYNDROMES	SS	0	0					THOUGHT DISORDER
	CC	0	0					MAJOR DEPRESSION
	PP	0	0					DELUSIONAL DISORDER

FIGURE 14.4. MCMI-III Profile Report for a 20-year-old male.

he did not work and had very little motivation to attain basic functional job skills. His need for drama and ability to elicit negative attention were clearly demonstrated in his interaction with the team during the meeting. He seemed most familiar with engaging in these power struggles, which were likely to have been adaptive patterns from his early history of abuse and dislocation. The consultant (myself) modeled how not to get caught in the fractious power struggle that the patient attempted to elicit by remaining nonreactive and attempting to make choices and consequences clear.

The team decided that the patient could choose either to stay in the program and comply with the residential house rules, or to leave and seek out alternative housing (which he had been threatening to do). If he decided to stay in order to help him reach his stated goal of independence, he was also invited to participate in ongoing psychotherapy, take his medications, and participate in a vocational rehabilitation plan. He attempted to engage in a power struggle by changing the topic, but the staff held firm about the choice, which was clearly his to make. He then suggested that another option would be to apply for Social Security Disability Insurance and use that to live on. This option was explored, and the time frame was explained, as well as the amount of income he could expect (which was too low to sustain himself outside of shelters). It became clear to the team that this young man suffered from what we termed "institutional syndrome": He was entirely dependent on, and yet resistant to taking advantage of, the rehabilitative services offered.

As in many complex and treatment-refractory cases, there were a number of interacting systemic-level dysfunctions. In this case, multiple factors at all four domain levels led to and served to maintain his low level of adaptive functioning. His history of neglect, abuse, and institutional care, along with neurobiological vulnerabilities and family dysfunction, had led to chronic patterns of maladjustment. In this case, the MCMI-III was incorporated as one part of a comprehensive and cost-effective treatment consultation, which was useful in corroborating impression and focalizing treatment issues. It was also suggested that a neuropsychological evaluation would be useful, but this type of service was unavailable.

Comparison of the Two Cases

The two cases presented in this chapter are worthy of comparison. Both cases selected were of males in their early 20s who suffered from ongoing and chronic disturbances in the personality system, as well as various clinical symptom expressions. In the first case, the young man, seen as an outpatient, was motivated to seek private treatment and was employed. He was assessed to have a superior IQ. He had almost completed college and attained mostly A's and was contemplating and being encouraged by his professors to seek a PhD. He followed recommendations and seemed to have an initial positive response to treatment. Reviewing the MCMI-III with him was a valuable process, which provided multiple opportunities to comprehend and address his issues.

In comparison, the patient in the second case was not highly motivated for treatment and had been resisting his agency's recommendation to enter into regular psychotherapy. His problems were historically more severe, he had fewer resources, and he minimized his psychiatric problems. In this case, the MCMI-III was not reviewed with the patient, but was utilized by the treatment team to achieve a better understanding of the patient's personality system and how to treat him more effectively. One can see that a clinician needs a great deal of flexibility to be able to respond to the demands of such clinical situations as these two. In some cases it is beneficial to review the findings directly with the patient, and in others this may be damaging or more than the patient can bear.

Summary

This chapter presents advances in the art and science of psychometrics and clinical practice. A brief review of the field of personology and development of clinical assessment issues is provided, and the need to achieve a comprehensive holographic picture of each patient at four levels of functioning is emphasized. The MCMI-III offers an excellent psychometric instrument with which to gather important information rapidly and efficiently about a patient's personality configuration and the clinical syndromes that emanate from these. With the increased emphasis on short lengths of treatment in managed care, treatment needs to be more focused. In order to focus treatment effectively, clinicians need instruments with proven validity that are based on a scientific approach to psychometrics. The information provided by the MCMI-III can be essential to treatment planning, especially in difficult or treatment-refractory cases. The information can also be used to corroborate the clinician's diagnostic impressions and to determine what type and format of treatment is most appropriate. Two cases of men in their early 20s in two different treatment settings are offered. The first was seen in an outpatient practice, and the second in a consultation at a community mental health agency. The various ways in which the MCMI-III can be utilized are discussed, with the caveat that the clinician needs to be able to modify the approach flexibly to maximize the benefit and do no harm to the patient.

References

American Psychiatric Association. (2000). *Diagnostic and statistical manual of mental disorders* (4th ed., text rev.). Washington, DC: Author.

Barlow, D. H. (2007). Foreword. In S. O. Lilienfeld & W. T. O'Donohue (Eds.), *The great ideas of clinical science: 17 principles that every mental health professional should understand* (pp. ix–xi). New York: Routledge.

Beebe, B., Knoblauch, S., Rustin, J., & Sorter, D. (2005). *Forms of intersubjectivity in infant research and adult treatment*. New York: Other Press.

Bowen, M. (1978). *Family therapy in clinical practice*. New York: Aronson.

Bronfenbrenner, U. (1979). *The ecology of human development: Experiments by nature and design*. Cambridge, MA: Harvard University Press.

Frances, A., Clarkin, J., & Perry, S. (1984). *Differential therapeutics in psychiatry: The art and science of treatment selection*. New York: Brunner/Mazel.

Gleick, J. (1987). *Chaos: Making a new science*. New York: Viking Press.

Jordan, J. V. (2004). Personality disorder of relational disconnection? In J. J. Magnavita (Ed.), *Handbook of personality disorders: Theory and practice* (pp. 120–134). Hoboken, NJ: Wiley.

Lilienfeld, S. O., & O'Donohue, W. T. (Eds.). (2007). *The great ideas of clinical science: 17 principles that every mental health professional should understand*. New York: Routledge.

Linehan, M. M. (1993). *Cognitive-behavioral treatment of borderline personality disorder*. New York: Guilford Press.

Magnavita, J. J. (1997). *Restructuring personality disorders: A short-term dynamic approach*. New York: Wiley.

Magnavita, J. J. (2000). *Relational therapy for personality disorders*. New York: Wiley.

Magnavita, J. J. (2002). *Theories of personality: Contemporary approaches to the science of personality*. New York: Wiley.

Magnavita, J. J. (2005a). *Personality-guided relational therapy: A unified approach*. Washington, DC: American Psychological Association.

Magnavita, J. J. (2005b). Systems theory foundations of personality, psychopathology, and psychotherapy. In S. Strack (Ed.), *Handbook of personology and psychopathology* (pp. 140–163). Hoboken, NJ: Wiley.

Magnavita, J. J. (2005c). Using the MCMI-III for treatment planning and to enhance clinical efficacy. In R. J. Craig (Ed.), *New directions in interpreting the Millon Clinical Multiaxial Inventory–III (MCMI-III)* (pp. 165–184). Hoboken, NJ: Wiley.

Magnavita, J. J. (2006). In search of the unifying principles of psychotherapy: Conceptual, empirical, and clinical convergence. *American Psychologist, 61*(8), 880–892.

Magnavita, J. J. (2007). A systemic family perspective on child and adolescent personality disorders. In A. Freeman & M. Reinecke (Eds.), *Handbook of personality disorders in children and adolescents* (pp. 131–181). Hoboken, NJ: Wiley.

Millon, T. (1969). *Modern psychopathology: A biosocial approach to maladaptive learning and functioning.* Philadelphia: Saunders.

Millon, T. (1981). *Disorders of personality: DSM-III, Axis II.* New York: Wiley.

Millon, T. (1990). *Toward a new personology: An evolutionary model.* New York: Wiley.

Millon, T. (Grossman, S. D., Meagher, S. E., Millon, C., & Everly, G.). (1999). *Personality-guided therapy.* New York: Wiley.

Millon, T. (with Millon, C., Davis, R., & Grossman, S.). (2006). *Millon Clinical Multiaxial Inventory–III (MCMI-III)* manual (3rd ed.). Minneapolis, MN: Pearson.

O'Donohue, W. T., Lilienfeld, S. O., & Fowler, K. A. (2007). Science is an essential safeguard against human error. In S. O. Lilienfeld & W. T. O'Donohue (Eds.), *The great ideas of clinical science: 17 principles that every mental health professional should understand* (pp. 3–27). New York: Routledge.

Paul, A. M. (2004). *The cult of personality: How personality tests are leading us to miseducate our children, mismanage our companies, and misunderstand ourselves.* New York: Free Press.

PDM Task Force. (2006). *Psychodynamic diagnostic manual.* Silver Spring, MD: Alliance of Psychoanalytic Organizations.

von Bertalanffy, L. (1968). *General system theory: Foundations, development, applications.* New York: Braziller.

Wakefield, J. C. (1999). Evolutionary versus prototype analyses of the concept of disorder. *Journal of Abnormal Psychology, 108,* 374–399.

Wakefield, J. C. (2006). Are there relational disorders?: A harmful dysfunction perspective: Comment on the special section. *Journal of Family Psychology, 20*(3), 423–427.

Weissman, M. M. (1993). The epidemiology of personality disorders: A 1990 update. *Journal of Personality Disorders, 7,* 44–62.

CHAPTER 15

Using the MCMI in Treating Couples

A. Rodney Nurse
Mark Stanton

The importance of assessing and treating couples is increasing, as is the recognition that personality plays an important role in couple dynamics (MacFarlane, 2004; Magnavita, 2005; Nurse, 1999). The primary thesis of this chapter is that couple therapy may be enhanced by the use of information provided by the Millon Clinical Multiaxial Inventory–III (MCMI-III, or simply MCMI). Using MCMI-III results can be helpful both to couple therapy designed to alleviate relationship distress in the absence of well-delineated individual psychopathology, and to couple therapy intended to alleviate couple interactions causing or aggravating well-defined individual psychopathology.

There is a complex, interactive dynamic between relationship problems and psychological disorders, including personality disorders. "The literature linking adult intimate relationships to mental health outcomes is substantial. There are documented connections between relational processes and the etiology, maintenance, relapse, and optimal treatment of many disorders" (Beach, Wamboldt, Kaslow, & Heyman, 2006, p. 360). Although most research on these connections currently focuses on Axis I disorders (e.g., depression), personality factors play a significant role in relational processes and may contribute to the vicious cycles that maintain or exacerbate psychological distress and disorders. The need to consider the relationship between relational disorders and personality disorders in the development of DSM-V has been recognized—an indication of the growing awareness that personality and relationship disorders are interwoven and deserve attention (First, Bell, & Cuthbert, 2002).

Perceptions of marital relationship quality and satisfaction are related to the personalities of the partners (Spotts et al., 2005). Although genetic influences and nonshared environmental factors may influence perceived relationship well-being, research indicates that personality (especially the wife's personality) explains a great deal about feelings of satisfaction or dissatisfaction with a relationship. In fact, one person's personality may influence both partners' perceptions of relationship quality. These findings argue for couple therapy interventions that adjust behaviors and perceptions in the relationship.

Reiss (1996, pp. x–xi) has described four categories for classifying the nature of relationships and individual disorders: (1) well-delineated disorders of relationships themselves; (2) well-defined relationship problems that are associated or interacting with individual disorders; (3) disorders that require relational information for valid diagnosis or treatment; and (4) individual disorders whose evocation, course, and treatment are strongly influenced by relationship factors (in such a case, the individual disorder is the main focus of treatment, but treatment of the relational group is necessary to promote positive treatment outcomes). All four types may include couple therapy, but the first two and the last may reasonably involve personality-guided couple therapy, as the personality-guided approach can benefit interventions in those domains.

Millon and Davis (1996) note the usefulness of couple therapy when personality disorders are present in the relationship. They suggest that the couple environment may actually encourage existing patterns, and that interventions are necessary to facilitate individual change in the couple relationship. It is necessary to confront "the complementarity of the partners' patterns" and secure collaboration from both partners (p. 425). For instance, they cite the typical dominating behaviors of compulsive individuals in relationships, as frequently evidenced by power struggles in the sexual arena. They recommend sex therapy that includes prescribed exercises (which fit the compulsive drive to follow protocols), consisting of yielding control to the partner, as a means of facilitating more positive sexual interaction. Another case in point would be concrete reallocation of household responsibilities for a narcissist–dependent couple, requiring the narcissistic partner to relinquish the entitled position commonly assumed.

Magnavita and MacFarlane (2004) review the role of such psychosocial factors as family dysfunction and relationship adversity in the etiology of personality disorders, as well as the impact of personality-disordered individuals on family members. They note that "personality-disordered individuals demonstrate disturbances in the relational matrix" (p. 27), and that they need assistance to create healthier intimate relationships. They suggest the importance of including family members, such as spouses or partners, in treatment; they also stress the need to adopt a systemic perspective to address the complex, multifaceted nature of personality disorders.

Personality-guided couple therapy is based on the assumption that personality contributes to the initial attraction of each partner for the other. It is likely that this attraction involves both similarities and differences in personality. The similarities provide common ground and a shared perception of life. They may most often be manifested in secondary personality styles (e.g., a narcissistic and a dependent partner who share secondary compulsive traits). The differences are often compensatory and function in a complementary fashion to address consciously or unconsciously perceived deficits in each partner's personality. For instance, it is common for an insecure dependent person to be attracted to the apparent self-confidence of a narcissistic individual, while the narcissistic partner appreciates the easy accommodation of the dependent person to his or her superordinate desires. These compensatory differences may create a relationship balance between two individuals who manifest individual deficits. Although this is a kind of "sick fit" between the two individuals, it accords with their existing personality styles, and it provides an initial sense of attraction and a conviction that they have found their perfect match.

However, as the relationship proceeds, it is likely that one or both of the partners will begin to chafe at some of the differences between them. The very characteristics that have initially attracted them to each other now serve to irritate and create friction. Couple therapists observe that personality traits of each person seem to "pull" negative personality manifestations from the other, in a kind of escalating reciprocal interaction. This cycle of destructive, unhealthy personality interaction patterns may create relationship problems on its own, but it can be especially destructive when combined with other individual disorders (e.g., depression, anxiety) or life circumstances (e.g., a medical condition or occupational distress). Couples may present for psychotherapy due to problems with intimacy, sexual relations, finance management, parenting, extended family relations, or joint problem solving, but these issues may be only symptoms of the troubled personality interaction patterns between them. Therapeutic intervention at the level of the personality interaction may alleviate much of the distress in the presenting problem arenas.

The MCMI-III provides relevant personality information in a concise, easy-to-access format. The assessment is easy to introduce and administer, and there are many sources of information for interpretation of the individual results. The personality-guided couple therapist can use the information to conduct a treatment process that addresses any problems in the personality interaction (see "Therapeutic Process," below).

It is also important for the personality-guided couple therapist to consider the presence of *Diagnostic and Statistical Manual of Mental Disorders*, fourth edition, text revision (DSM-IV-TR) Axis I disorders. The MCMI-III provides information about a range of clinical syndromes that may be addressed in the context of couple therapy (e.g., depression, anxiety, alcohol abuse, or drug abuse). For instance, substantial research finds that depressive symptoms are frequently present in one or both partners when a couple relationship is troubled (Gupta, Beach, & Coyne, 2005). Couple therapy is an appropriate venue to alleviate such depressive symptoms, and personality factors may inform that treatment. Substance abuse identified on the MCMI-III Drug Dependence or Alcohol Dependence scale may alert the therapist to consider further assessment of current use or abuse of these substances. There appears to be a reciprocal influence between couple discord and substance abuse (Birchler, Fals-Stewart, & O'Farrell, 2005), and each can be an antecedent to the other. Couple therapy has been demonstrated to be effective for the treatment of substance use disorders (Fals-Stewart, O'Farrell, & Birchler, 2005), and personality factors in the couple relationship may play a part in reinforcing abuse patterns or facilitating treatment interventions (Stanton, 2005). Birchler, Fals-Stewart, and O'Farrell (2005) suggest that the crucial dimension is the nature of compatibility on personality dimensions (e.g., desire to socialize). For example, if both partners enjoy or dislike social activity, it will be less problematic than if one is solitary (schizoid or avoidant) and the other is socially active (histrionic). A variety of treatment interventions for specific disorders may be readily amenable to the inclusion of personality-guided or personality-informed psychotherapy. For instance, Epstein and Baucom (2002) have developed an enhanced cognitive-behavioral model that includes the individual characteristics of each partner, in order to refine the cognitive-behavioral interventions to the specific needs of a couple.

Finally, it must be clear that personality-guided couple therapy recognizes the importance of the same core tasks found in other treatment models, such as the development of a therapeutic alliance and conveyed empathy (Norcross, 2002). These aspects of the therapeutic relationship are essential to addressing the personality dynamics that exist in couple relationships. The couple therapist must establish a working relationship that manifests trust, openness, and honest communication. The partners must believe that the therapist genuinely desires to help them *as a couple*, because the couple is the identified patient in this process. This requires an ability to align with both partners, and to challenge both partners.

Presented here is a plan for personality-guided couple therapy, including the administration of the MCMI-III; the interpretation of results (including response styles, contextual factors, individual personality, and couple personality interaction); options for interpreting the results with the partners (i.e., individual and conjoint approaches); and the therapeutic process one may follow with the couple.

Administration of the MCMI

In our experience, the MCMI is best introduced toward the end of the intake session in couple therapy. It is important to join the couple dynamics and build rapport with both partners before recommending completion of the MCMI. After listening carefully to the presenting issues and observing the couple interactions in the conjoint session, the personality-guided therapist is likely to have initial ideas about the personality characteristics of the two individuals and the nature of the interaction between their personalities, as well as hypotheses about any Axis I considerations or diagnoses.

It is important to present a clear rationale for completing the MCMI. After summarizing his or her understanding of the issues they have presented, the therapist should explain the approach to couple relationships from a personality perspective—one that recognizes the importance of the similarities and differences between the partners' personalities as they interact. A brief definition of personality may help the partners understand personality patterns, but the therapist should not provide too much input about his or her perceptions of them at this point, in order to avoid contaminating their responses to the MCMI items. Couples need to see that the therapist values the information from the assessment and that it will be worth their time to complete it. The idea of assessment may have been introduced in the first telephone contact with a couple, or assessment information may be included in the intake documentation, but most people need to understand that the assessment information facilitates rapid understanding of their couple patterns of interaction. The fact that the MCMI may be completed in approximately 30–40 minutes often allows the couple to complete it immediately following the intake session, since many people have that much flexibility in their schedules. Occasionally couples may need to schedule another time for the test, but it is helpful to have the results quickly in the treatment process.

Interpretation of Results

Once scored, the individual profiles should be reviewed for validity, response style, and overall meanings of significant scores; the interpretive approaches described elsewhere (Craig, 2005; Millon & Davis, 1996) may be used. It is important to recognize that response styles on the Modifying Indices of the MCMI (Disclosure, Desirability, Debasement) may reflect some response bias, such as underreporting or overreporting—not only because of reflection of the personality disorder itself or the impact of an Axis I disorder (e.g., depression) but also, due to the conjoint nature of the assessment context (Bagby & Marshall, 2005). For instance, some individuals may "fake good" in order to protectively establish the focus of treatment on the partner at the very beginning of treatment; other individuals may be so distressed by relationship dynamics that they present in more extreme fashion. It is not unusual to find lower Disclosure scores, or higher Desirability than Debasement scores, when the MCMI is used in couple assessment. This is especially important if evident in one partner, but not the other.

Contextual Factors

The individual profile should be compared for consistencies or inconsistencies with other available information, such as presenting complaints, socioeconomic levels, ethnicity, and occupational history.

Couple therapists also recognize the importance of each individual's family of origin, history of relationships for each partner, couple relationship history, lifespan, and life cycle dynamics as context for the interpretation of the MCMI-III profiles. Basic information about these factors may readily be gathered through completion of a simple couple's genogram (McGoldrick, Gerson, & Shellenberger, 1999). This process takes only minutes to complete, and it can be incorporated easily into the intake session, following the couple's explanation of the presenting issues. Gathering the information for the genogram often increases individual awareness of unresolved issues that may be having an impact on current relationship functioning. This information informs the MCMI-III results.

Individual Factors

Next, the individual characteristics on the personality and clinical dimensions may be reviewed and summarized. We have found it helpful to use the MCMI-III manual (Millon, 2006) for summary descriptions of each individual's highest personality score(s) and clinical syndromes. The charts in the manual (e.g., Table 2.2, Expression of Personality Disorders across the Functional and Structural Domains of Personality—Overview and Prototypes) provide key terminology and descriptions of Millon's functional and structural domains, which may be used to help partners understand their own and each other's personalities.

In addition, Millon and Davis (1996) provide detailed descriptions of each personality style measured by the MCMI. This is an incomparable resource for the clinician seeking an enhanced view of a particular disorder. The clinician can take into consideration for each disorder its fundamental (evolutionally based) polarity balance of pleasure–pain, active–passive, and self–other dimensions, in order to determine the needed overall direction for rebalancing of polarities and improved functioning. For each disorder, the authors have included a summary table that provides a description of the disorder's clinical domains, which cover the behavioral, phenomenal, intrapsychic, and biophysical levels. These tables can serve as tools for reasoning and reminders of the complexity of each particular disorder; as such, they can sharpen the thinking and increase the thoroughness of evaluation and therapy of even the busiest of clinicians.

The recent development of the Grossman Facet Scales (Grossman, 2005) enhances the focus on the specific domains relevant to each primary personality style. The third edition of the MCMI-III (Millon, 2006, pp. 111–117) includes a handy description of the Grossman Facet Scales (see also Grossman, Chapter 6, this volume). Strengths and potential weaknesses of each personality may be noted for review with the couple. An initial judgment may be made about the level of personality health or pathology.

Couple Personality Interaction

Once each individual partner's profile has been considered, it is important to look at the two profiles together to determine the nature of the personality interactions within the couple. An individual's personality may be functional when viewed independently, but dysfunctional in a relationship with another person's particular personality. As an example, an actor's histrionic–narcissistic disorder may be quite functional occupationally, or even career-enhancing. The compulsive disorder of the actor's partner may be occupationally helpful in the field of accounting. Although initially the couple's styles might have drawn them together (her to his excitement, him to her stability), as the marriage progresses their styles may no longer be functional in relation to each other. Instead, they may become problematic and conflicted in parenting and household management. What was originally an attraction now serves to repel and each partner from the other to erode the relationship.

It may also be that life cycle changes have altered the nature of the personality fit between the partners. For example, an avoidant–compulsive wife may have enjoyed the social stimulation and excitement provided by her histrionic husband in the early days of their relationship, but once children are born into the family, she may expect that he will "calm down" and "grow up" into the responsibilities she feels he should assume. However, he may resent the limitations the children place on their freedom as a couple, and he may dislike her attempts to control him. The differences have been tolerable until the change in conditions. Or it may be that one partner's personality has evolved over time, modified by occupational or situational demands. Sometimes one person adjusts his or her personality through individual psychotherapy in an effort to avoid some of the ego-dystonic or interpersonal problems the partner is experiencing in another environment (e.g., the workplace), only to find that this causes imbalance in the couple relationship. For instance, a husband with dependent traits may recognize the necessity to increase his level of assertion and his ability to manage conflict in order to advance at work. However, these adaptations may increase the level of conflict at home when he stands up more to the entitled and exploitive behaviors of his wife with narcissistic traits. These changes may leave the other partner wondering, "Where is the person I married?"

Knowledge of common personality combinations in couple relationships facilitates accurate understanding of typical couple dynamics. In our experience, some of the combinations manifest complementarity on the polarities noted by Millon (pleasure–pain, self–other, and active–passive). For example, the antisocial–dependent couple demonstrates the self–other reinforcement polarity: The person with antisocial traits evidences high self and low other, while the person with dependent traits evidences low self and high other (Davis & Millon, 1997). This manifests itself in the relationship as excessive submission by the person with dependent personality traits to the autonomous desires and irresponsible behaviors of the person with antisocial traits. Analysis of this couple on the active–passive polarity notes that the antisocial style is active and the dependent style is passive, so the partners also differ in primary orientation to adapting to their environment. The person with antisocial traits may enjoy the passive accommodation of the person with dependent traits to his or her impulsive acting out in social contexts, but it creates real difficulty if the passivity of the dependent partner in interaction with other people restricts or confines the person with antisocial traits (e.g., dependent behaviors toward a boss at work may lead to intense or unrestricted anger by the antisocial partner, who resents any restrictions that the work relationship places on his or her freedom). Some couples evidence similarity on some polarities, but differences on others (e.g., a narcissistic–dependent couple will differ on the self–other polarity, creating complementarity, but will share the passive adaptation style). The couple relationship may reinforce individual imbalance by creating a complementary couple dynamic, but this is essentially unhealthy for the individuals and problematic for the couple relationship over time. The purpose of couple therapy is to rebalance the polarities that exist in the couple relationship, in order to address individual deficits and enhance individual and couple satisfaction. The therapist can intervene to strengthen the weaker polarities and to lessen the impact of the stronger ones by reinforcing any action by one partner that helps balance the weaker polarities of the other partner, in addition to directly helping the first person to strengthen his or her own weaker polarities. For instance, couple therapy may increase the self orientation for the dependent partner, while increasing the other orientation of the narcissistic partner in concert, by encouraging increased self-awareness and assertion on the one hand and increased empathy on the other.

Another analysis of couple combinations is based on the primary and secondary personality characteristics of each individual united in the couple. Some couples with two-point personality types match on one style, but differ on another (e.g., a couple with a narcissistic–histrionic partner and a histrionic–dependent partner). Craig and Olson (1995), studying the MCMI-II, described three-point pairings that were likely to seek couple therapy (e.g., the conflictual relationship of a narcissistic–sadistic–histrionic partner and a negativistic–sadistic–borderline partner, or the overadequate–underadequate relationship of a narcissistic–sadistic–histrionic partner and a dependent partner). The couple therapist will develop an archive of examples and stories over time that can be used, with appropriate camouflage of details, to illustrate common couple combinations. Some common combinations include (1) compulsive with histrionic, (2) narcissistic with dependent, (3) compulsive with negativistic, (4) histrionic with schizoid or avoidant, (5) antisocial or sadistic with dependent or histrionic, and (6) narcissistic with borderline. Each of these combinations may become more complex when secondary personality characteristics are evident for either or both partners.

The clinician can conduct an in-depth analysis of the personality dynamics by referring to the clinical domains of each person's highest significant personality pattern score(s). As mentioned above, Millon and Davis (1996) characterize these at four levels: behavioral, phenomenological, intrapsychic, and biophysical. Each of these can have implications for couple therapy, but the behavioral level (expressive and interpersonal aspects) is immediately relevant to couple therapy (Nurse, 1999). Understanding the prototypal behavioral characteristics of each personality style provides the theoretical foundation for predicting the likely interpersonal dynamics between two personality types. These hypothetical interactions may be tested with the couple in the session when the assessment results are discussed.

For those profiles indicating more severe personality disorders (i.e., schizotypal, borderline, and paranoid), a more generally dysfunctional pattern is anticipated. These couples may require a more complex, in-depth evaluation with additional methods (such as the Rorschach), as well as a more complex treatment intervention.

Options for Discussing Results

There are two approaches to discussing the results of the MCMI with couples. Each has its rationale, including pros and cons for consideration by the therapist. One approach involves individual sessions with each partner to review his or her personal results. This method may be important in high-conflict relationships, where individuals are so guarded that they cannot receive assessment results without extremely defensive reactions, or there is the likelihood that one or both partners will use assessment results against the other partner in an attacking fashion. This approach may also be important if the therapist senses that he or she has not connected equally with the partners, or that one partner feels as if the therapist relates better to the other partner. An individual session can provide an opportunity to deepen the therapeutic relationship and demonstrate empathy for each person without fear of alienating the other. In addition, individual time can be important if the therapist needs to process other individual issues (e.g., childhood abuse, relationships outside the couple that influence couple dynamics) noted during the intake session. Some personality factors may argue for separate time (e.g., high Antisocial, Sadistic, or Dependent scores). The individual session provides more safety for each person to process his or her own results and allows open communication about the results, but the therapist must establish clear expectations about confidentiality and the use of information revealed in individual sessions in conjoint sessions (Gottlieb, 1995).

In the individual session, after the therapist has discussed the meaning of the results for the individual and to some extent considered possible meanings for the couple relationship, one additional step can often be useful: suggesting that the individual think about what he or she would chose to share most with the spouse. Both spouses should wait until the next couple session to begin sharing any test results. This delay is useful so that the therapist can facilitate shaping their discussions about results in terms of the couple's system, yet can maintain a balance between the couple system and each person's intrapersonal system, all with some awareness of the context of the overall social/cultural context within which the couple lives—similar to what Magnavita (2005) refers to as the "relational matrix." Talking about the results in this way allows room in this and future sessions for the therapist to pay attention to the unique aspects each individual contributes to the relationship, even while focusing on shifting the couple system for the better.

A variation on this approach is possible if the therapist is conducting treatment with a cotherapist of the opposite gender. It is possible to assign each spouse to the therapist of the same gender for the individual discussion of the results of the assessment. This allows each cotherapist to enhance the individual therapeutic relationship and to experience one partner in the absence of the influence and behavior of the other partner. Each cotherapist may then provide support to the same-sex couple partner in the conjoint sessions.

Another approach is to discuss the assessment in a conjoint session. This method recognizes the value of including both partners in the explanatory process, but it requires more caution and a clear agreement by the individuals that they will not use the terms or ideas against each other. In a conjoint session, the therapist is able to model personality understanding and accurate empathy for each partner, building the therapeutic alliance with the couple. Careful depiction of likely perceptions, thoughts, feelings, and behaviors allows each person to verify or discard personal applicability of each proposed personality stereotype to his or her real-life experience. Both individuals are invited to share personal examples in which they recognize the personality style(s) in their lives, and they are encouraged to discuss how the individual personality style(s) may relate to the presenting issue(s). Because each partner is present, he or she may be able to provide examples of the personality characteristics that the other individual did not easily recognize. If this is done in a friendly, collaborative, and constructive fashion, it actually begins the couple therapeutic process. For instance, one partner may provide illustrations of compulsive behaviors (e.g., moral superiority), because that partner felt the intensity of the experience, while the compulsive individual may tend to discount the force of that behavior in the relationship. On some occasions, the therapist may ask, "How does it feel when he [or she] does that?" to clarify the impact of the behavior on the relationship. Then the therapist briefly introduces some of the dynamics around the personality fit between the two partners in the couple relationship. It is possible to provide an overview of individual results and a brief description of couple personality interactions in one session, and thus to lay the groundwork for the treatment process.

Therapeutic Process

The first goal specific to personality-guided couple therapy is to increase both individuals' knowledge and awareness of personality factors in their relationship. Discussion of personality tendencies should emphasize both the positive and the potentially negative aspects of each person's personality. This starts in the assessment discussion session, but it usually is necessary to ask the couple to pay attention to key factors that have been identified and to record illustrations of personality traits observed in interactions between sessions. For instance, a histrionic husband may begin to see how strongly he reacts to situations and circumstances, escalating emotions and precipitating negative interaction. The compulsive wife may begin to recognize her controlling responses and her assumption of the moral high ground for her viewpoint on issues. As they do this, they begin to recognize the patterns of interaction generated by their personality mix. Patterns are frequently identified in key relationship arenas, such as finances, problem solving, and sex.

Over time, the exploration of personality tendencies often leads to personal and couple insight into their personality factors, and the partners are able to recount situations in which they recognized perceptions, thoughts, feelings, and behaviors driven by their personalities. Recognition of personality tendencies moves them to the conscious realm, where they may be managed by the individuals.

The next step is the development of interpersonal empathy around personality dynamics. This can happen in several ways. By sharing examples of personality-motivated behaviors, the partners may begin to enter each other's lived experience. As each sees the world through the personality filter of the other partner, the behaviors begin to make more sense to both. For instance, when a histrionic partner understands the low interpersonal drive of a schizoid partner, the interpretation of the lack of affection or sexual advances may shift from feelings of personal rejection to a more neutral recognition of that personality style. Alternatively, when a partner understands and empathizes with the intense drive of the compulsive partner, the compulsive behaviors seem less controlling. Often it is necessary to remind each partner of the unconscious manner and intensity in which his or her own personality evidences itself, in order to illustrate the experience of the other partner.

The third treatment goal is for each partner to recognize the perceptions, thoughts, feelings, or behaviors that create the most difficulty in the current relationship, and to make efforts to reduce or manage those personality characteristics. An important caveat that facilitates these efforts is the understanding that each partner has chosen the other for specific reasons, and that love for the other partner should motivate efforts to enhance the relationship satisfaction for that partner. So these efforts are founded on relationship commitment; if one or both partners are not truly committed to the relationship, it may become apparent at this point. If both are committed, this will enhance motivation for mutual need satisfaction in the relationship. When empathy and personality management happen in reciprocal form (each empathizing with the other and making efforts to minimize offensive behaviors), some of the friction and tension in the relationship will dissipate.

For instance, each partner usually becomes aware more quickly of his or her own personality patterns and the unconscious manner in which these patterns evidence themselves. This provides the foundation for understanding that the perceptions, thoughts, feelings, and behaviors of the other partner may not be premeditated, and that some of the acts that had previously seemed deliberately attacking, critical, negative, or mean-spirited may be better understood as personality-driven. In addition, as the partners recognize each other's efforts to manage problematic personality characteristics, they feel that their own perspectives and needs are valued. In our experience, this awareness often leads to the fourth treatment goal: decreased negative reactions to each other's personality-driven behaviors. Each partner is able to detach more and let go of some of the things that had previously caused tension, because he or she understands and empathizes with the other partner.

This mutual understanding, empathy, personality behavior management, and decreased reactivity may then lead to constructive relationship processes, such as conjoint problem solving. A generic focus on this goal is beneficial to the variety of issues and concerns reported by specific couples. Problems may surface in many different areas of the relationship (e.g., extended family, sexual relations, finances, communication, affective display), but treatment that improves the partners' ability to manage the personality interaction between them as they address specific problems or concerns is a skill that transfers from one issue to another.

Finally, the sixth desired treatment outcome is each partner's appreciation of the other's style as a counterbalance or compensation for the partner's own style. As both partners come to comprehend personality dynamics, it may be possible to frame differences as corrective mechanisms for one individual's deficits (e.g., a histrionic partner may help a compulsive partner become be a little more spontaneous). It is likely that this compensatory element was part of each partner's initial attraction to the other, but what was appealing soon became threatening or difficult. An understanding of the way in which each person assists the other can strengthen the relationship and increase relationship satisfaction.

The treatment process can be summarized as follows:

Couple: Describes presenting problem(s) in conjoint intake session.
Therapist: Begins developing therapeutic alliance, conducts intake evaluation, and explains rationale for completing the MCMI.
Therapist: Interprets response style and likely impact of individual results on couple interaction.
Therapist: Determines option for incorporating results into treatment (individual, conjoint).
Therapist: Develops therapeutic alliance, and models accurate empathy for both individuals.
Couple: Increases knowledge and awareness of each partner's personality styles.
Each individual: Develops insight into perceptions, thoughts, feelings, and behaviors driven by own personality.
Couple: Increases interpersonal empathy for each partner's personality.
Each individual: Makes efforts to manage or minimize personality-driven behaviors that offend the other partner.
Each individual: Decreases negative reactions to other partner's personality-driven behaviors.
Couple: Engages in conjoint problem solving that involves personality management in the process.
Each individual: Develops appreciation of other partner's style as counterbalance.

The MCMI-III results for one couple are presented in the next section. The case example is presented in a format that provides a pattern for interpreting MCMI-III couple profiles in general and for designing specific therapeutic strategies and interventions. This example is a composite of several couples; the couple dynamics remain true to the commonalities among them. The process of the couple assessment and therapy reflects an approximation of the six-part therapy model described above. As such, it shows a couple clearly able to make good use of the assessment/couple therapy model.

Rick and Jane: Dependent–Depressive

Couples don't always arrive at the therapist's doorstep presenting straightforward problems of relationship discord. Particularly in clinic settings, they show up burdened with the baggage of multiple, interweaving intrapersonal and interpersonal family-focused problems of long standing, and often with flawed ability to handle their social and/or work environment pressures as well.

Couple therapy has been used and evaluated as a treatment for mental health problems, writes Whisman (2006). In a section of this article, he includes a review of couple therapy for psychiatric disorders, citing three promising areas studied so far: depression, substance use disorders, and panic disorder with agoraphobia. The partners in the couple presented here had multiple problems, including depressive symptoms and substance abuse along with their dependent and depressive personality disorders. The assessment of the spouses and their couple therapy were aimed toward improving the spouses' individual and relationship functioning, so they could take more control over their lives and over parenting their children.

Background

Rick, age 47, with 2 years of college, was a periodically successful organizer/promoter for service businesses. Jane, 42, with 1 college year, had focused on raising a daughter, 16, and a son, 13. She had worked as a part-time retail clerk early in the marriage. They had married 17 years ago after meeting in a drug rehabilitation program. In past months, Rick's history of periodic alcohol abuse had worsened—he believed, stimulated by the socialization required in his work. Recently he had proclaimed that he was "now sober" and attending Alcoholics Anonymous (AA) regularly "to find out if I'm an alcoholic." The spouses stated that their daughter was "out of control": She was in juvenile hall again, but due out soon, and they might need to send her to a group home because the juvenile workers had told them that their daughter had been reacting to all the conflict at home culminating in the spouses' recent separation. Although their son seemed to be staying out of serious trouble, they were worried that some of his new friends might be "troublemakers." Rick announced to Jane that he was thinking of divorce, because he had met a woman at AA who seemed to meet his dreams and they had been spending long weekends together. Jane was devastated. Rick agreed to make one last try to work on their marital relationship, because he feared that Jane might make another suicide attempt.

Rick's MCMI-III Profile and Facet Scales

Rick's validity scores are acceptable (see Figure 15.1). The Clinical Personality Patterns suggest a distinctive combination of characteristics. The scores point to dependent personality

MILLON CLINICAL MULTIAXIAL INVENTORY - III
CONFIDENTIAL INFORMATION FOR PROFESSIONAL USE ONLY

PERSONALITY CODE: 3 ** <u>2A 8B</u> * 2B + 5 <u>6A 8A 6B</u> 7 4 1 " - ' ' // - ** - * //

SYNDROME CODE: - ** B * // -**-* //

DEMOGRAPHIC: 100207768/OT/M/47/W/S/14/--/--/-----/10/------/

CATEGORY		SCORE		PROFILE OF SR SCORES				DIAGNOSTIC SCALES
		RAW	BR 0	60	75	85	115	
MODIFYING INDICES	X	96	61					DISCLOSURE
	Y	12	55					DESIRABILITY
	Z	4	45					DEBASEMENT
CLINICAL PERSONALITY PATTERNS	1	3	48					SCHIZOID
	2A	8	78					AVOIDANT
	2B	6	73					DEPRESSIVE
	3	16	87					DEPENDENT
	4	11	40					HISTRIONIC
	5	15	59					NARCISSISTIC
	6A	7	52					ANTISOCIAL
	6B	8	51					SADISTIC
	7	14	47					COMPULSIVE
	8A	7	52					NEGATIVISTIC
	8B	8	78					MASOCHISTIC
SEVERE PERSONALITY PATHOLOGY	S	3	60					SCHIZOTYPAL
	C	4	40					BORDERLINE
	P	3	38					PARANOID
CLINICAL SYNDROMES	A	3	60					ANXIETY
	H	0	0					SOMATOFORM
	N	1	12					BIPOLAR: MANIC
	D	2	40					DYSTHYMIA
	B	10	81					ALCOHOL DEPENDENCE
	T	4	60					DRUG DEPENDENCE
	R	2	30					POST-TRAUMATIC STRESS
SEVERE CLINICAL SYNDROMES	SS	3	45					THOUGHT DISORDER
	CC	1	20					MAJOR DEPRESSION
	PP	1	25					DELUSIONAL DISORDER

FIGURE 15.1. MCMI-III Profile Report for Rick.

disorder accompanied by traits of avoidance and self-defeating qualities, with underlying depressive features.

A dependent individual like Rick has a fundamental need reflected in his polarity score emphasis (not shown) on nurturance of others to seek support, attention, and affection from others, and at the same time to guide and show them how and when to achieve these security goals.

When these needs are met, a dependent personality such as Rick can function relatively well for a significant period of time. For Rick, his work provides a rewarding avenue for reaching out toward others, who often reciprocate his warm social style in the work patterned context. He gains considerably in relationships in this setting, where his lack of connection with his genuine reactions is hidden from himself or denied, and therefore unseen by others generally. But in this social/work context, truly personal, genuine reactions are typically not expected.

Intimate relationships are his potential downfall. His emphasis on others may seem an admirable quality, but without sufficient attention to his own needs as an individual, it causes problems. The Facet Scale results (see Figure 15.2) suggest that a major behavioral aspect of his dependency is his interpersonal submissiveness. He tends automatically to go along with another in a close relationship. Focusing on another and being submissive interpersonally reinforce his avoidant traits and become manifest in his alienated self-image, the content of another Facet Scale.

Rick's Alcohol Dependence scale score falls in the significant range. It is easy to imagine how pressure builds, broken momentarily by an episode of alcohol abuse characterized by inappropriate expression of anger—followed by contrition, statements of "never again," or denial that his behavior has been as bad as others may tell him. He tends then to revert to his warm side. With his warmth coupled with practiced social skills, Rick may appear to be simply focused again on making and maintaining positive connections with others; yet at a deep level he may also be spurred by his fear of rejection and separation. So he has an unease underneath his surface, a personal sense of disconnection within himself, experienced as hollowness. As he comes to feel alienated and angry, his tension builds and he cycles into problem drinking again, adding to his sense of inadequacy and mounting depression. He finds himself stuck in a pattern of self-defeating thoughts.

Rick and others may believe that his bouts of alcohol abuse come about solely because he is addicted and simply needs to stop drinking. Physically addicted he may be, but his personality problems and the cycle described above certainly contribute to episodes of alcohol abuse, if not alcohol dependence. The cycle is much more engrained than Rick would like to believe.

Jane's MCMI-III Profile and Facet Scales

Jane's scores fall within acceptable ranges for validity (see Figure 15.3). Her Debasement score, however, points to her very open presentation of troublesome negative emotional and personal difficulties. Her Clinical Personality Patterns scores center on the Depressive personality scale. Her significantly depressed, moody appearance may create a gloomy mood in those around her and/or call out for protection and affection. This melancholy sense about her, while pushing some away, calls out to others to cheer her up, take care of her, and never abandon her. Unfortunately for her, she does not offer much positive back to those attracted to her. In fact, her moods shift erratically from this depressed state to moments of a variety of emotions, such as anger, resentment, anxiety, or excitability (see the Facet Scale scores in Figure 15.4). These demonstrated mood fluctuations reflect an inner immaturity and lack of structural development that put people off. She feels trapped, and her impulsiveness leads to self-

MILLON CLINICAL MULTIAXIAL INVENTORY - III
CONFIDENTIAL INFORMATION FOR PROFESSIONAL USE ONLY

FACET SCORES FOR HIGHEST PERSONALITY SCALES BR 65 OR HIGHER

HIGHEST PERSONALITY SCALE BR 65 OR HIGHER: SCALE 3 Dependent

SCALE	SCORE		PROFILE OF BR SCORES						FACET SCALES
	RAW	BR	0	60	70	80	90	100	
3.1	4	66							Inept Self-Image
3.2	6	83							Interpersonally Submissive
3.3	0	0							Immature Representations

SECOND HIGHEST PERSONALITY SCALE BR 65 OR HIGHER: SCALE C Borderline

SCALE	SCORE		PROFILE OF BR SCORES						FACET SCALES
	RAW	BR	0	60	70	80	90	100	
2A.1	1	23							Interpersonally Aversive
2A.2	5	77							Alienated Self-Image
2A.3	3	54							Vexatious Representations

THIRD HIGHEST PERSONALITY SCALE BR 65 OR HIGHER: SCALE 3 Dependent

SCALE	SCORE		PROFILE OF SR SCORES						FACET SCALES
	RAW	BR	0	60	70	80	90	100	
8B.1	1	30							Discredited Representations
8B.2	6	87							Cognitively Diffident
8B.3	4	66							Undeserving Self-Image

FIGURE 15.2. MCMI-III Facet Scale scores for Rick.

destructiveness. She has admitted to a suicide attempt, and she could be at risk again. Her overall depressiveness is woven together and is reinforced by her fatalistic cognitive style (again, see Figure 15.4); she is not only depressed, but she heaps depression on herself with her self-denigrating cognitions. She fears abandonment, yet her depressive attitude is laced with an unpredictable variability of moods that elicit that abandonment.

In fitting the depressive prototype picture indicated by a consideration of basic polarities, she appears to be living a life of suffering, essentially giving up to this inevitability. The best she can do, consistent with her avoidant aspects as well, is to be insensitive to seeking the possible pleasures in life. She tolerates life as she passively goes along with what happens to her, missing opportunities to take action, instead waiting—but she may not know for what.

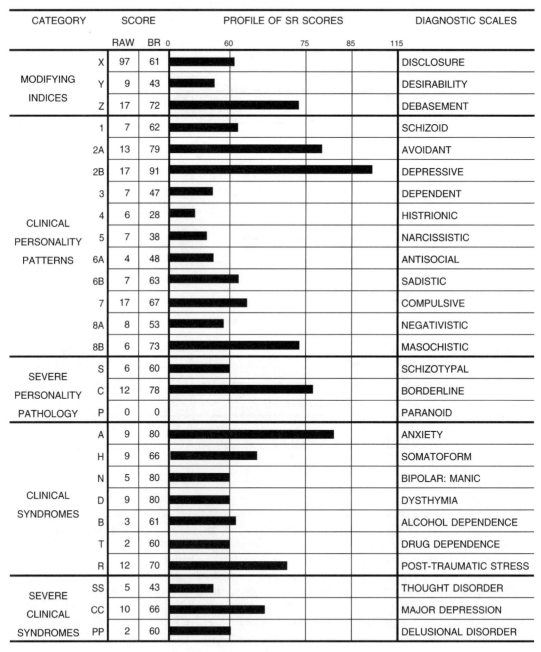

MILLON CLINICAL MULTIAXIAL INVENTORY - III
CONFIDENTIAL INFORMATION FOR PROFESSIONAL USE ONLY

Valid Profile

PERSONALITY CODE:　　2B ** 2A * 8B 7 <u>6B 1</u> + 8A <u>6A 3</u> 4 " 4 ' ' // - ** C * //

SYNDROME CODE:　　　- ** A * // - ** - * //

DEMOGRAPHIC:　　　100175961/OT/F/42/W/S/13/MA/LO/-----/10/-----/

CATEGORY		SCORE		PROFILE OF SR SCORES				DIAGNOSTIC SCALES
		RAW	BR 0	60	75	85	115	
MODIFYING INDICES	X	97	61					DISCLOSURE
	Y	9	43					DESIRABILITY
	Z	17	72					DEBASEMENT
CLINICAL PERSONALITY PATTERNS	1	7	62					SCHIZOID
	2A	13	79					AVOIDANT
	2B	17	91					DEPRESSIVE
	3	7	47					DEPENDENT
	4	6	28					HISTRIONIC
	5	7	38					NARCISSISTIC
	6A	4	48					ANTISOCIAL
	6B	7	63					SADISTIC
	7	17	67					COMPULSIVE
	8A	8	53					NEGATIVISTIC
	8B	6	73					MASOCHISTIC
SEVERE PERSONALITY PATHOLOGY	S	6	60					SCHIZOTYPAL
	C	12	78					BORDERLINE
	P	0	0					PARANOID
CLINICAL SYNDROMES	A	9	80					ANXIETY
	H	9	66					SOMATOFORM
	N	5	80					BIPOLAR: MANIC
	D	9	80					DYSTHYMIA
	B	3	61					ALCOHOL DEPENDENCE
	T	2	60					DRUG DEPENDENCE
	R	12	70					POST-TRAUMATIC STRESS
SEVERE CLINICAL SYNDROMES	SS	5	43					THOUGHT DISORDER
	CC	10	66					MAJOR DEPRESSION
	PP	2	60					DELUSIONAL DISORDER

FIGURE 15.3. MCMI-III Profile Report for Jane.

MILLON CLINICAL MULTIAXIAL INVENTORY - III
CONFIDENTIAL INFORMATION FOR PROFESSIONAL USE ONLY

FACET SCORES FOR HIGHEST PERSONALITY SCALES BR 65 OR HIGHER

HIGHEST PERSONALITY SCALE BR 65 OR HIGHER: SCALE 2B Depressive

SCALE	SCORE		PROFILE OF BR SCORES	FACET SCALES
	RAW	BR	0 60 70 80 90 100	
2B.1	3	50		Temperamentally Woeful
2B.2	4	63		Worthless Self-Image
2B.3	6	77		Cognitively Fatalistic

SECOND HIGHEST PERSONALITY SCALE BR 65 OR HIGHER: SCALE C Borderline

SCALE	SCORE		PROFILE OF BR SCORES	FACET SCALES
	RAW	BR	0 60 70 80 90 100	
2A.1	2	42		Interpersonally Aversive
2A.2	4	53		Alienated Self-Image
2A.3	6	87		Vexatious Representations

THIRD HIGHEST PERSONALITY SCALE BR 65 OR HIGHER: SCALE 3 Dependent

SCALE	SCORE		PROFILE OF SR SCORES	FACET SCALES
	RAW	BR	0 60 70 80 90 100	
C.1	8	90		Temperamentally Labile
C.2	1	18		Interpersonally Paradoxical
C.3	4	57		Uncertain Self-Image

FIGURE 15.4. MCMI-III Facet Scale scores for Jane.

Rick and Jane's Relationship

In some ways Rick and Jane were made for each other, as they often said to others early in their marriage. As indicated above, they had met in a drug rehabilitation program. Rick was turning 30, and Jane was just reaching her mid-20s. Both were ready to "settle down" after their drug-using period. Both were relatively slender, although Jane failed at the time to let Rick know that her bulimia was one reason. Obviously depressed, she tearfully expressed her neediness and wish for a relationship in the program's atmosphere of openness. Rick was a quick comforter. In fact, someone in a support group described Rick as riding in on his white horse to rescue the ready, willing, and beckoning damsel. This description was not rejected by the newly joining young couple. They experienced a romantic time in and then out of the program as they vowed to help each other stay clean and spend their lives together. Jane became pregnant, and they married. Rick at first attributed the very erratic ups and downs of Jane's moods to her pregnancy, during which she experienced his protectiveness and he liked being the protector.

Once the baby was born, though, the shift to a triad from a dyad was difficult for both spouses. By this time Rick was beginning to drink excessively episodically, and after the birth Jane was extremely melancholy, which they both attributed to the "baby blues"; however, her depression was punctuated by fits of erratic moods characterized by anger and crying, long past when her mood difficulties might have been expected to moderate.

Although they did begin to settle down as they had planned, things were gloomy at home. Jane tried clerking—it didn't help. They thought maybe a second child might; it helped briefly, then not at all, and things were worse. She cared less about herself, continuing to gain weight. She stated gloomily that her "fate" was to be a "brood mare." Rick gained satisfaction as he perfected his accommodation-oriented, genial, and warm (but fragile) persona and progressed at work. The couple's intimate relationship had by now cooled. Jane was hospitalized after a suicide gesture, diagnosed with major depression, and prescribed antidepressant medication. When their older child, a girl, reached adolescence, as Rick told the intake person later, "all hell began to break out—mother–daughter fights, rebellious and angry shouts and tears." Rick and Jane both felt alone, as indeed psychologically they were. Rick's alcohol excesses worsened, and he suspected that Jane might be addicted to some sort of pills. Trying AA, he got involved with a young woman, which turned out to be a ticket for the couple to seek assistance for themselves and their chaotic lives. Jane felt destroyed when she found out about the affair, saying that she had expected this all along.

Strategy and Tactics for Couple Therapy

When the couple sought help, it was as if each spouse was calling out for a life preserver. Jane's moods had become increasingly erratic. In Rick's (at least temporary) state of sobriety, he was fluctuating in his moods (though not as badly as she was); he was also drowning in her gloomy moods, saying that he could no longer help her and needed to leave for the woman he had found at AA. Although Jane was pessimistic about the outcome, Rick did push for trying to improve their marriage, and he was concerned about their daughter. They both wondered whether they should have family therapy.

Before couple therapy could begin, the family situation needed stabilizing. The daughter had by then her own individual therapist, who agreed with her teen patient that individual therapy plus a mandatory outpatient group and a switch to a General Equivalency Diploma program would be the plan. Rick and Jane were both prescribed antidepressants by their physician, and a mood stabilizer was added for Jane. They would be closely medically monitored. Rick would join an interpersonally oriented therapy group for people with a variety of diagnoses, to help him gain more understanding of his impact on others and develop confidence that he could stay more with his authentic reactions and not have to maintain his accommodating and persuasive front all the time. Jane would begin cognitively oriented individual therapy, anticipated to last for a considerable length of time as she struggled to gain more accurate ways of thinking and managing her internal processes in the shelter of a maternal therapist who encouraged optimism realistically. The parents and children met with the cotherapy team once to discuss the plan for help, adding that as things improved for all, they would at some point have family therapy. However, as one of the cotherapists said, the parents had to "get their act together first." It was not the job for either of the children to rescue the parents.

Once they had made a little progress in their other treatments, Rick and Jane entered weekly couple therapy with the male–female cotherapist team. Rick agreed to put aside his outside amorous relationship for a while, and managed to abide by this commitment—aided by the fact that after a time his paramour turned out (no surprise) to have variable moods similar to Jane, although not so depressive. She also demonstrated an instability of relatedness that drove her to find other romantic partners. Rick agreed to give AA a more consistent effort than he had heretofore. The couple did agree to concentrate on providing more emotional support to their children during these next months.

In couple therapy, the patients agreed to work on their destructive communication patterns first, at the insistence of the therapists. The basis for the work was the structured, well-researched book *Core Communication* (Miller & Miller, 1997). For Rick, this work served to target his cognitively diffident quality, noted on his third highest MCMI-III personality scale, Masochistic (Self-Defeating). It was focused on his alienated self-image, his false front. In this communication context, the therapists helped him venture to bring forth more genuine expression of his own needs without regard for what he believed to be Jane's needs. Whenever this happened, the therapists gave him warm responses for these gains, and at the same time would not let him back away from these gains by using self-deprecating language.

For Jane, the structured focus and activity were forced to a greater extent by the therapists. Several individual contacts initially with the female cotherapist helped her develop an alliance for the couple therapy. These contacts, together with her individual therapist contacts separate from the cotherapy process, enabled her to adjust to a mood stabilizer and to change to another antidepressant. As Jane worked to learn a new communication pattern with her husband, she interpreted his gains in contrast to her struggles as further evidence of her inevitable ineffectiveness interpersonally. The therapists did not dwell on her despondency, but instead simply helped with the effectiveness she did demonstrate as she and Rick worked on their communication patterns.

As the spouses settled into more direct communication about helping their struggling daughter and looking constructively to assist their son in his athletic and school activities, and as they (especially Jane) developed more inner stability, they seemed to experience a more reasonable coexistence that had moments of authentic connection. They also appeared to weather the practical difficulties that occurred when Rick was let go from work because his company was downsizing and he had to take another job with less pay. They ordered their priorities and put their daughter's therapy and their medication necessities first. Jane switched to a therapy group run by her individual therapist. They chose to leave the couple therapy, and made an appointment to return for a "checkup" in 3 months. There were more routine activities in their lives, and Rick's income would probably improve. In the meantime, Jane had begun part-time work in a nearby store—not too stressful, with some social contacts, additional structure, and some income. At least one family therapy session was still anticipated.

Reflecting on the work with Rick, Jane, and their overall severe family trouble makes it clear that its very complexity called for an equally complex diagnostic and treatment planning approach. The cotherapists established a beginning alliance so that the couple could trust them enough to accept their recommendations. The therapists quickly focused on the spouses' personalities (informed by the MCMI), and obtained a sense of their dyadic relationship (couple personality interaction patterns). They also considered the couple's nested position within the family triangles. It was important as well to obtain a sense of the couple's broader work and social systems (e.g., work, AA, school, juvenile justice, etc.). The cotherapists' judgment was that the daughter was receiving her needed professional attention apart from them at that point in time, but that the children and the parents would need to be seen together in some later sessions; however, it was much too early for this to take place. The parents first had to be able to work adequately together in their parenting abilities. They needed to reach a higher level of empowerment to be able to function well enough as parents raising two adolescents. To do this, they required couple therapy (informed by the MCMI-III results as described above) and different additional collateral forms of assistance: Both adults needed medication review and medication; Jane needed cognitively oriented individual therapy; and Rick could continue in AA, which fitted his personality dynamic and helped him in avoiding alcohol abuse. Taking these steps had to be mutually agreed upon with the parents. Explaining the logic for simultaneous therapeutic actions (potentiated pairings or groupings) helped with their "buy-in" to the combination approaches. This helped convey the cotherapists' confidence that the spouses could learn to manage their relationship and family responsibilities more effectively. They were also able to understand that for the overall changes to be helpful, they had to take place in a planned order (catalytic sequencing). Not only did Rick and Jane have to understand this structuring, but the children needed to learn this through the family session and see the opportunity for improvement of all their lives.

The Future for Using the MCMI with Couples

The field of couple and family psychology is growing and serves to connect research and practice with couples and families. This connection is facilitated by the activities of the American Psychological Association Division of Family Psychology, including its bulletin and journal. Those who are skillful in helping couples (and families) can through an examination become board-certified with the American Board of Couple and Family Psychology, one of 13 specialties of the American Board of Professional Psychology. The examination requires submission of two practice samples, one of couple or family assessment and one of intervention. The MCMI is one tool used in a number of assessment submissions, often coupled with a genogram, as mentioned earlier in this chapter. Use of the MCMI with couples by practitioners identified with high-quality work will encourage its use, so that it becomes as automatic a consideration with couples as the MCMI is now with full individual assessment batteries.

A second trend is the increasing emphasis in psychology on interrelationships. For instance, Magnavita's (2005; Magnavita & MacFarlane, 2004) theorizing balances the intrapersonal focus of Millon and Davis (1996) with the dyadic (couple) system, which in turn is embedded within the triadic constellations of the family, nesting itself within the broader societal context (see also Magnavita, Chapter 14, this volume). His "relational matrix" not only features horizontal systemic relationships, but also incorporates the couple's triangular relationships with children and the other triangular relationships with parents. This broader theorizing helps avoid sometimes overly simplified theoretical explanations. Work with couples can be viewed in this more complex way, and the MCMI can be used with a couple at the same time as the other relationships can be more easily kept in mind because of Magnavita's conceptualizations.

Third, there is a general movement in psychology toward the psychology of the "normal." The best examples consist of the individually oriented positive psychology spearheaded by Seligman (2004), the identification of what makes organizations flourish by Fredrickson and Losada (2005), and the organizational development process of the process of "appreciative inquiry" (Whitney & Trosten-Bloom, 2003). Gottman's (1994) research with couples parallels these developments in his discovery of what makes marriages successful. Perhaps in the future an inventory will be developed from the personality disorder measurements of the MCMI and combine with the approach of the Millon Index of Personality Styles (MIPS) to focus on effective personality qualities, all under the broader umbrella of Millon's Principle 5: "Personality exists on a continuum; no sharp division is possible between normality and pathology" (Millon & Davis, 1996, p. 12). In the meantime, it may be helpful for the skilled clinician to use the MCMI and the MIPS together with couples, provided that the clinician remains mindful of the distinctly different databases.

References

Bagby, R., & Marshall, M. (2005). Assessing response bias with the MCMI modifying indices. In R. Craig (Ed.), *New directions in interpreting the Millon Clinical Multiaxial Inventory–III* (pp. 227–247). Hoboken, NJ: Wiley.

Beach, S., Wamboldt, M., Kaslow, N., & Heyman, R. (2006). Describing relational problems in DSM-V: Toward better guidance for research and clinical practice. *Journal of Family Psychology, 20,* 359–368.

Birchler, G., Fals-Stewart, W., & O'Farrell, T. (2005). Couples therapy for alcoholism and drug abuse. In J. Lebow (Ed.), *Handbook of clinical family therapy* (pp. 251–280). Hoboken, NJ: Wiley.

Craig, R. (Ed.). (2005). *New directions in interpreting the Millon Clinical Multiaxial Inventory–III (MCMI-III).* Hoboken, NJ: Wiley.

Craig, R., & Olson, R. (1995). MCMI profiles and typologies for patients seen in marital therapy. *Psychological Reports, 76,* 163–170.

Davis, R., & Millon, T. (1997). The Millon inventories: Present and future directions. In T. Millon (Ed.), *The Millon inventories: Clinical and personality assessment* (pp. 525–537). New York: Guilford Press.

Epstein, N., & Baucom, D. (2002). Why couples are the way they are: Individual influences. In N. Epstein & D. Baucom (Eds.), *Enhanced cognitive-behavioral therapy for couples: A contextual approach* (pp. 105–143). Washington, DC: American Psychological Association.

Fals-Stewart, W., O'Farrell, T., & Birchler, G. (2005). Behavioral couples therapy for alcoholism and drug abuse: Where we've been, where we are, and where we're going. *Journal of Cognitive Psychotherapy, 19,* 229–246.

First, M. B., Bell, C., & Cuthbert, B. (2002). Personality disorders and relational disorders: A research agenda for addressing crucial gaps in DSM. In D. J. Kupfer, M. B. First, & D. A. Regier (Eds.), *A research agenda for DSM-V* (pp. 123–199). Washington, DC: American Psychiatric Association.

Fredrickson, B. L., & Losada, M. F. (2005). Positive affect and the complex dynamics of human flourishing. *American Psychologist, 60,* 678–686.

Gottlieb, M. (1995). Ethical dilemmas in change of format and live supervision. In R. Mikesell, D.-D. Lusterman, & S. McDaniel (Eds.), *Integrating family therapy: Handbook of family psychology and systems theory* (pp. 561–569). Washington, DC: American Psychological Association.

Gottman, J. (1994). *What predicts divorce?: The relationships between marital processes and marital outcomes.* Hillsdale, NJ: Erlbaum.

Grossman, S. (2005). The MCMI-III Facet Subscales. In R. Craig (Ed.), *New directions in interpreting the Millon Clinical Multiaxial Inventory–III* (pp. 3–31). Hoboken, NJ: Wiley.

Gupta, M., Beach, S., & Coyne, J. (2005). Optimizing couple and parenting interventions to address adult depression. In J. Lebow (Ed.), *Handbook of clinical family therapy* (pp. 228–250). Hoboken, NJ: Wiley.

MacFarlane, M. (Ed.). (2004). *Family treatment of personality disorders: Advances in clinical practice.* New York: Haworth Press.

Magnavita, J. (2005). *Personality-guided relational psychotherapy.* Washington, DC: American Psychological Association.

Magnavita, J., & MacFarlane, M. (2004). Family treatment of personality disorders: Historical overview and current perspectives. In M. MacFarlane (Ed.), *Family treatment of personality disorders: Advances in clinical practice* (pp. 3–39). New York: Haworth Press.

McGoldrick, M., Gerson, R., & Shellenberger, S. (1999). *Genograms: Assessment and intervention.* (2nd ed.). New York: Norton

Miller, S., & Miller, P. (1997). *Core communication: Skills and processes.* Littleton, CO: Interpersonal Communications Programs.

Millon, T., & Davis, R. (1996). *Disorders of personality: DSM-IV and beyond* (2nd ed.). New York: Wiley.

Millon, T. (with Millon, C., Davis, R., & Grossman, S.). (2006). *Millon Clinical Multiaxial Inventory–III: Manual* (3rd ed.). Minneapolis, MN: Pearson Assessments.

Norcross, J. C. (2002). Empirically supported therapy relationships. In J. C. Norcross (Ed.), *Psychotherapy relationships that work: Therapist contributions and responsiveness to patients* (pp. 3–16). New York: Oxford University Press.

Nurse, A. R. (1999). *Family assessment: Effective uses of personality tests with couples and families.* New York: Wiley.

Reiss, D. (1996). Foreword. In F. Kaslow (Ed.), *Handbook of relational diagnosis and dysfunctional family patterns* (pp. ix–xv). New York: Wiley.

Seligman, M. (2004). *Authentic happiness.* New York: Free Press.

Spotts, E., Lichtenstein, P., Pedersen, N., Neiderhiser, J., Hansson, K., Cederblad, M., et al. (2005). Personality and marital satisfaction: A behavioural genetic analysis. *European Journal of Personality, 19,* 205–227.

Stanton, M. (2005). Couples and addiction. In M. Harway (Ed.), *The handbook of couples therapy* (pp. 313–336). Hoboken, NJ: Wiley.

Whisman, M. (2006). Relationship discord and the onset, course, and treatment of psychiatric disorders and other clinically significant outcomes. *The Family Psychologist, 22,* 14–17.

Whitney, D., & Trosten-Bloom, A. (2003). *The power of appreciative inquiry.* San Francisco: Berrett-Koehler.

CHAPTER 16

The Adaptation of the MCMI-III in Two Non-English-Speaking Countries

State of the Art of the Dutch Language Version

Gina M. P. Rossi
Hedwig V. Sloore
Jan J. L. Derksen

The Dutch translation project for the Millon Clinical Multiaxial Inventory–III (MCMI-III) was described by Sloore and Derksen (1997) and compared with guidelines for test translation that were being developed at that time (Hambleton, 1994). Since then, these guidelines have been finalized and are available on the website of the International Test Commission (ITC, 2000).

The ITC's first principle of test development and adaptation involves taking into account the possible linguistic and cultural differences between the populations for whom the original and translated versions are intended. In translating the original English version of the MCMI-III into Dutch/Flemish, we encountered a double problem: We needed to take into account not only cultural differences between the United States and Europe, but also differences between The Netherlands and Flanders, the Flemish/Dutch-speaking part of Belgium. The Dutch language is officially spoken in The Netherlands and in Flanders. As such, it was logical to develop a Dutch translation that could be used in both countries. Although both countries share one official Dutch spelling system and thesaurus, there are some region-specific differences in word use and pronunciation. Just to give one example, people in Belgium are "walking in" the streets, while people in The Netherlands are "running through" the streets.

A committee approach, with two teams of bilingual translators, was adopted. In Belgium and The Netherlands, the two teams independently followed the same procedure: Two psychologists in each team, working independently of each other, made translations of all the original MCMI-III items. In the next step, each team tried to reach a consensus on the basis of discussion, so that one translation for each country was present. Then the teams jointly evaluated these translations in order to formulate a final translation that would be applicable in both countries. In cases of doubt about the exact meaning of an item, the advice of Theodore Millon was asked. In the next stage of the translation process, the questionnaire was given to several "ordinary" people, in order to check whether the item content was clear for most people (the ITC's [2000] second and fourth principles). Finally, a native English speaker who was also fluent in Dutch was asked to make a back-translation (without having knowledge of the original MCMI-III and its purpose). This back-translation was sent to Millon. Suggestions from Millon were reviewed by the translation committee, and most of them were integrated into the Dutch language research form (Sloore, Derksen, & De Mey, 1994).

A Short History of Research within Belgium

The first research project using a Dutch translation of the MCMI was started by Hedwig Sloore in the mid-1980s. The MCMI was administered to 427 patients in different clinical settings all over the Flemish/Dutch-speaking part of Belgium. Clinical evaluations ($n = 358$) were made, on the same basis as they were in the Millon (1982) study. The research results clearly demonstrated the robust structure of the MCMI. Although the absolute values of intercorrelations between scales were higher than the American values, the patterns observed between the personality disorder and clinical syndrome scales were the same. Principal-components analysis with varimax rotation resulted in four factors with eigenvalues larger than 1.00 (Sloore & Derksen, 1997). Similar factor structures were found in several American studies (Choca, Peterson, & Shanley, 1986; Choca, Shanley, & Van Denburg, 1992; Greenblatt, Modzierz, Murphy, & Trimakas, 1986; Lewis & Harder, 1990; Millon, 1982; Piersma, 1986). At that time, we also tried to calculate our own base rates (BRs). The procedure described by Millon (1982) for calculating BRs was used. However, this procedure proved to be problematic: Most of the median values of the BR 85 anchor point group were lower than the median values of the BR 75 anchor point group. As a consequence, this translation of the MCMI was never used in clinical practice.

Iris Van den Brande (2002) was the first Belgian researcher to work with the MCMI-III (Millon, 1994, 1997). She examined whether BRs for different disorders were similar in Belgium and the United States. This cannot be taken for granted across different cultural groups (Van de Vijver & Tanzer, 1997), although both U.S. culture and the cultures of most European countries (including Belgium and The Netherlands) are considered to be Western cultures. The similarity is often accepted without question, and American standardization norms are often applied in Belgium. Nevertheless, the research results of Van den Brande (2002) made clear that there was an absolute need for local BRs. The application of American BRs clearly posed several problems.

Gina Rossi (2004), for her doctoral dissertation, was working on the standardization of the Dutch language version of the MCMI-III (hereafter referred to as the

MCMI-III-D). She evaluated the advantages of criterion referencing over norm referencing (Rossi & Sloore, 2005), and concluded that in the case of disorders, criterion referencing should be used. However, when the original American system (Millon, 1997) that anchored scale elevations to the exact prevalence rates of disorders was applied in a Belgian sample, a direct connection of scores to prevalence percentages yielded problems for some scales (just as it did for the first MCMI Dutch version). For this reason, Rossi decided to explore construct equivalence between the Dutch and the original MCMI-III, and to develop a new rationale for Belgian BRs.

Rossi (2004) collected MCMI-III-D profiles of 1,235 Dutch-speaking patients and inmates of European descent. Institutions (N = 39) that volunteered to participate in the study were selected on the basis of the social map of Belgium (Mertens, Baert, & Clara, 1991), in order to cover a wide range of different institutions: ambulatory clinical settings, psychiatric hospitals, psychiatric departments in general hospitals, therapeutic communities, forensic guidance centers, and prisons. The MCMI-III-D was administered by experienced psychologists/psychiatrists during psychodiagnostic evaluation. The sample was heterogeneous in pathology, because all patients and convicts consecutively admitted between 1999 and 2003 were tested, provided that they volunteered to participate. All participants were informed and asked for their consent. Inmates were assured that participation in the project would have no effect on their status within the correctional system. MCMI-III-D profiles were scored with the Microtest Q Assessment System (Pearson Assessments, 2004). Profiles were considered valid if the total number of omitted or invalid responses (e.g., both a "yes" and a "no" response to a single item) was less than 12, if the Validity Index was less than 2, and if the raw score on scale X (Disclosure) was within the range of 34–178 (Millon, 2006). The profiles of 1,210 subjects were valid and used for the analyses reported in the current chapter. There were 471 females (39%) and 739 males (61%). The majority of the subjects (n = 828; 68%) were clinical patients: 643 inpatients and 185 outpatients. The remainder of the subjects (n = 382; 22%) came from forensic settings. Age varied from 18 to 74 years (M = 36.6 years; SD = 11.3). The range of Cronbach's alpha values for all MCMI-III-D scales (.67–.94) was similar to the range of values (.66–.95) for the American cross-validation sample (Millon, 2006, p. 58) (see Table 16.1).

Construct Equivalence between the Dutch and Original MCMI-III

A psychologist in Belgium or The Netherlands who administers the MCMI-III-D should be measuring the same traits as his or her counterpart in the United States who uses the original American version. This necessary condition is known as "construct equivalence" and can be operationally defined as factor invariance (e.g., Ten Berge, 1986). A similar factor structure for different language versions of the same instrument (the ITC's [2000] seventh principle) suggests that the underlying dimensions are the same, whereas a different factor structure suggests that the instrument measures different traits in these versions (Finn, 1984). Since the American BR scores are anchored to the exact prevalence percentages of disorders, which can differ across countries, analyses were carried out on raw scores. Calculations were based on the 1,210 valid MCMI-III-D profiles from the sample of Rossi (2004). Details on

TABLE 16.1. Internal Consistency (Cronbach's Alpha) of the MCMI-III Scales

Scale	MCMI-III-D	American cross-validation sample (Millon, 2006)
1—Schizoid	.72	.81
2A—Avoidant	.86	.89
2B—Depressive	.88	.89
3—Dependent	.82	.85
4—Histrionic	.80	.81
5—Narcissistic	.67	.67
6A—Antisocial	.72	.77
6B—Sadistic (Aggressive)	.76	.79
7—Compulsive	.68	.66
8A—Negativistic (Passive–Aggressive)	.78	.83
8B—Masochistic (Self-Defeating)	.84	.87
S—Schizotypal	.84	.85
C—Borderline	.82	.85
P—Paranoid	.80	.84
A—Anxiety	.86	.86
H—Somatoform	.84	.86
N—Bipolar: Manic	.70	.71
D—Dysthymia	.88	.88
B—Alcohol Dependence	.75	.82
T—Drug Dependence	.84	.83
R—Post-Traumatic Stress Disorder	.88	.89
SS—Thought Disorder	.86	.87
CC—Major Depression	.90	.90
PP—Delusional Disorder	.74	.79
Y—Desirability	.86	.86
Z—Debasement	.94	.95

the method used and interpretation of the factors can be found in Rossi, van der Ark, and Sloore (2007). The most important conclusion was the striking stability of the factor solution (all congruency coefficients were above .90).

• In spite of linguistic differences, the structure of the MCMI-III was similar across different cultures: The MCMI-III-D three-factor structure was congruent with the factor structure of American factor-analytic studies of the MCMI-III (Craig & Bivens, 1998; Haddy, Strack, & Choca, 2005).

• The factor structure of the MCMI-III-D was stable over methodological decisions: Neither the spurious correlations between the linearly dependent scales (vs. the use of nonoverlapping scales with only prototypal items) nor the application of principal-factors analysis followed by a direct oblimin rotation (vs. principal-components analysis with varimax rotation) affected the factor structure.

• The factor structure was also invariant across the sample characteristics of gender and setting: It was similar for males and females, and for clinical and forensic settings.

The number of factors was determined by parallel analysis, and the following four factors were identified for the MCMI-III-D ($N = 1,210$):

- Factor 1, labeled General Maladjustment, had positive loadings (pattern matrix) on these scales: Depressive (.79), Dependent (.72), Negativistic (.46), Masochistic (.61), Schizotypal (.45), Borderline (.76), Anxiety (.90), Somatoform (.90), Bipolar: Manic (.54), Dysthymia (.88), Post-Traumatic Stress Disorder (.81), Thought Disorder (.88), and Major Depression (.95).
- Factor 2, labeled Aggression/Social Deviance, had high positive loadings on the Antisocial (1.02), Sadistic (Aggressive) (.60), Alcohol Dependence (.61), and Drug Dependence (.73) scales, and a negative loading on the Compulsive (–.65) scale.
- Factor 3, labeled Paranoid/Delusional Thinking, had fair-sized positive loadings on the Paranoid (.90) and Delusional Disorder (.79) scales.
- Factor 4, labeled Emotional Instability–Detachment, had positive loadings on the Histrionic (.94) and Narcissistic (.65) scales, and negative loadings on the Schizoid (–.59) and Avoidant (–.65) scales.

The first factor, General Maladjustment, is identical to the first factor, Depression and Anxiety, that Sloore and Derksen (1997) found by factor analysis based on the MCMI. The factor is congruent with the expectations of Millon (2006), who considers a broad general maladjustment factor to be important. The second factor, Aggression/Social Deviance, corresponds to the Acting Out factor of Sloore and Derksen (1997); however, in the MCMI-III-D factor analysis, resulted clearly in a bipolar factor of social deviance versus conformity (see the high negative loading on the Compulsive scale). As such, it can be identified as the personality domain that McCrae and Costa (1999) defined as Conscientiousness. The third factor, Paranoid/Delusional Thinking, was labeled Delusional Cognitions by Sloore and Derksen (1997). This factor has also been described as the Psychotic factor (Craig & Weinberg, 1993). The fourth bipolar factor, Emotional Instability–Detachment, differs from the Dependence versus Dominance factor of Sloore and Derksen (1997). The detachment aspect still corresponds to dependence or social restraint on one side, but on the other side it represents emotional dysfunction rather than dominance and rebellious behavior.

Rationale for and Development of Belgian BR Scores

Although factor invariance confirmed the construct equivalence between the American and Dutch versions of the MCMI-III, this does not imply scalar equivalence. Scalar equivalence presumes, for instance, that a BR score of 85 on the Compulsive scale indicates the same degree of compulsiveness in different countries. However, when the American BR was used in the Belgian sample (Rossi, 2004), the sensitivity of this scale was only .07. Sensitivity values of all scales were problematic when American BR scores were used (mean = .28; range = .05–.66). There was a clear need for local Belgian BR scores.

In the case of criterion referencing, diagnostic decision making by clinicians was a crucial consideration. Therefore, several precautions were taken to guarantee reliable diagnoses. All clinicians involved in the standardization research were experienced in making clinical evaluations. In order to be allowed to make a *Diagnostic and Statistical Manual of Mental Disorders*, fourth edition, text revision (DSM-IV-

TR) diagnosis (American Psychiatric Association [APA], 2000) several inclusion criteria had to be fulfilled. A clinician had to have seen a patient for at least 4 hours of clinical contact, and a diagnosis was preferably made at the end of the assessment process. It was hoped that in this way, the clinician would have as complete an understanding of the patient's personality as possible. Clinicians made diagnostic ratings independently of the MCMI-III-D test results. Standardized semistructured interviews were recommended, and clinicians engaged in a "Longitudinal Expert evaluation that uses All Data" (LEAD; Spitzer, 1983).

The clinical evaluation process was standardized by using a rigorous and systematic rating system (for more detailed descriptions, see Rossi, Hauben, Van den Brande, & Sloore, 2003; Rossi, 2004; Rossi & Sloore, 2005). If no pathology was present, a score of 0 was assigned. If there was evidence of pathology, clinicians quantified this evidence by a score indicating the degree to which the symptoms for each personality disorder or clinical syndrome were present. If a personality disorder pattern was present, the clinician evaluated the degree to which the traits were present on a scale from 1 to 9 (1 = "traits," 3 = "style," 5 = "disorder," 7 = "marked disorder," 9 = "extreme disorder"). In the same way, the severity of clinical syndrome symptoms was evaluated on a scale from 1 to 9 (1 = "slight symptoms," 3 = "mild symptoms," 5 = "syndrome," 7 = "marked syndrome," 9 = "extreme syndrome"). The scale anchor points were clearly defined on the basis of the descriptions provided in the second edition of the MCMI-III manual (Millon, 1997). The definition of 5 = "syndrome," for example is as follows (Millon, 1997, p. 90): "Symptoms are sufficiently problematic to justify a clinical syndrome diagnosis. Difficulties in social, occupational, and/or family functioning are clearly present and treatment is advisable." In this way Rossi (2004) collected clinical ratings, in addition to the MCMI-III-D profiles. The final BR data set consisted of 524 patients (255 males and 269 females; average age = 36.6 years). Since the MCMI-III and MCMI-III-D were developed for use with adults who are seeking mental health treatment, the majority of subjects in the BR data set came from different clinical settings (n = 438). A smaller group came from forensic settings (n = 86).

In contrast to the procedure followed for the American MCMI-III (Millon, 1997, 2006), the transformation of raw scores into BR scores was not based on anchoring cutoff scores (BR = 75 or 85) for each scale to the real prevalence ratio of the characteristic in a specific population. On the contrary, the Belgian BRs were assigned on the basis of receiver operating characteristic (ROC) curve analyses. The method is described in detail in Rossi and Sloore (2005). The main advantages of the application of ROC BRs were as follows:

- ROC analysis has been recommended in recent clinical literature (e.g., Hsu, 2002; McNiel, Lam, & Binder, 2000; Swets, Dawes, & Monahan, 2000) and has been applied to develop clinical screening instruments (Nurnberg et al., 2000).
- This method of criterion referencing was useful for clinical decisions. The associated curves represent ratios of sensitivity and specificity, which are fundamental diagnostic efficiency statistics.
- In the Belgian sample, BRs derived via ROC analyses clearly performed better than prevalence BRs. The sensitivity of ROC BRs was markedly higher than the sensitivity of prevalence BRs (significant at p < .01 for 15 out of 24 scales at BR = 75,

and significant at $p < .01$ for 18 out of 24 scales at BR = 85; see Rossi & Sloore, 2005, p. 156, Table 6.6).
   • The ratios of sensitivity to specificity, or the impact of false negatives versus false positives, could be partially controlled.

This last aspect changed interpretation of MCMI-III-D results in an important way. The general principle for the MCMI-III-D was to optimize the ratio between sensitivity and specificity by choosing anchor points so that both sensitivity and specificity were above 70%. When such optimization was not possible, priority was given to sensitivity, or avoiding false negatives. When Rossi and Sloore (2005) compared the mean diagnostic validity statistics of Rossi (2004) with those of the American validation studies, the statistics for the Belgian sample were (as expected) generally weaker than those in the Millon (1997) study and stronger than those in the Millon (1994) study. However, sensitivity was higher and specificity was lower in the Belgian validation study than in either American validation study (see Rossi & Sloore, 2005, Table 6.7). Based on these results, Rossi and Sloore concluded that the MCMI-III-D was an excellent screening device (mean sensitivity = .71), but that its diagnostic utility was constrained (mean specificity = .56).
   Some more conclusions can be drawn on the basis of the mean diagnostic validity statistics. The probability that a trait/symptom is absent, given that the test is negative (negative predictive power [NPP] = .87), was higher than the probability that a trait/symptom is present, given that the test is positive (positive predictive power [PPP] = .28). Mean statistics of measures of incremental validity (increasing PPP = .07, increasing NPP = .08), chance-adjusted efficiency measures (Cohen's k = .16), and cutoff score independent measures (Cohen's d = .57) consistently showed that the MCMI-III-D performed better than chance and discriminated in the right direction.
   Later in this chapter we will describe two case studies: a woman with compulsive behavior patterns, and a man with posttraumatic stress symptoms. Therefore we provide, as examples, the detailed diagnostic validity statistics for the Compulsive and Post-Traumatic Stress Disorder scales of the MCMI-III-D at BR = 75 (anchored to a clinical rating of 1 = "traits" of a personality disorder pattern or "slight symptoms" of a clinical syndrome) in Table 16.2. As the table indicates, the MCMI-III-D seems to be an excellent device to screen for compulsive traits or symptoms of posttraumatic stress: Negative test results corresponded to a high probability that the trait/symptom was absent (NPP values), and sensitivity to the presence of traits/symptoms was adequate (sensitivity values). However, the scales should not be used to make diagnostic decisions: Positive test results remained highly hypothetical (PPP values) at the trait/symptom level.

Convergent Validity

Rossi (2004) collected 1,210 valid MCMI-III-D profiles. For 578 of these subjects, the Dutch language version of the Minnesota Multiphasic Personality Inventory–2 (MMPI-2) (Sloore, Derksen, Hellenbosch, & de Mey, 1993; Derksen, De Mey, Sloore, & Hellenbosch, 2006) was also administered. All MMPI-2 profiles met the

TABLE 16.2. Diagnostic Validity Statistics (BR = 75) for the MCMI-III-D Compulsive and Post-Traumatic Stress Disorder Scales (N = 524)

	MCMI-III scale	
Measure	Compulsive	Post-Traumatic Stress Disorder
Sensitivity	.79	.74
Specificity	.46	.53
PPP	.18	.33
NPP	.94	.87
Increasing PPP	.05	.09
Increasing NPP	.07	.11
Cohen's k	.10	.19
Cohen's d	.48	.59

validity criteria defined by Butcher et al. (2001): number of items omitted < 30, F < 100T, Fb < 110T, L < 80T, K < 65T, VRIN < 80T, TRIN < 80T, and S < 70T. Correlations between all MCMI-III-D scales and the Dutch MMPI-2 clinical scales were calculated. Due to the large number of tests, a Bonferroni correction was applied, and correlations were considered significant at $p < .0002$ (.05/240; 24 MCMI-III-D scales multiplied by 10 Dutch MMPI-2 clinical scales).

Table 16.3 shows the correlations of the MCMI-III-D Clinical Syndrome Scales with the Dutch MMPI-2 clinical scales. Since significant correlations were found between most of these MCMI-III-D and these MMPI-2 scales, we limit our discussion to the high correlations ($r \geq .60$). In general, the pattern of correlations corresponded to the pattern found by Millon (1997) between the respective MCMI-III and MMPI-2 scales. MMPI-2 scale 1, Hs (Hypochondriasis), had its highest correlation with the MCMI-III-D Somatoform scale; this is logical, since both scales measure aspects of somatization. Furthermore, scale Hs had high correlations with the MCMI-III-D Major Depression, Dysthymia, and Thought Disorder scales. Millon (1997) attributed the interrelationship of somatization and depression to shared vegetative features. MMPI-2 scale 2, D (Depression), had the highest correlations with the MCMI-III-D Dysthymia, Major Depression, and Somatoform scales. MMPI-2 scale 7, Pt (Psychasthenia), showed significant correlations with the MCMI-III-D Dysthymia, Thought Disorder, Anxiety, Somatoform, Major Depression, and Post-Traumatic Stress Disorder scales. The common theme captured by these scales seems to be anxiety. Although MMPI-2 scale 8, Sc (Schizophrenia), had (as could be expected) the highest correlation with the MCMI-III-D Thought Disorder scale, there were also strong correlations with the Post-Traumatic Stress Disorder, Anxiety, Major Depression, and Somatoform scales. Correlations with the subscales of scale Sc indicated that the Post-Traumatic Stress Disorder scale probably measured in the first place the social alienation aspect of schizophrenia (r Sc$_1$ = .63). The Anxiety scale seemed to go together with lack of ego mastery, defective inhibition (r Sc$_5$ = .65), whereas the Major Depression and Somatoform scales mainly represented lack of ego mastery, conative (r Sc$_4$ = .68 and .66, respectively).

The convergent validity of the MCMI-III-D personality disorder scales and the Dutch MMPI-2 scales has been examined in detail by Rossi, Van den Brande, Tobac,

TABLE 16.3. Correlations of the MCMI-III-D Clinical Syndrome Scales with the Dutch MMPI-2 Clinical Scales (*n* = 578)

MCMI-III-D scale	Hs	D	Hy	Pd	Mf	Pa	Pt	Sc	Ma	Si
A	.59	.54	.37	.40	.38	.51	**.74**	.70	.27	.50
H	**.66**	.67	.51	.34	.38	.46	**.74**	.69	.20	.49
N	.31	.14*	.08*	.31	.15*	.30	.44	.47	.45	.07*
D	**.62**	.68	.47	.40	.42	.48	**.77**	.73	.17	.54
B	.14*	.05*	−.06*	.39	−.02*	.12	.25	.33	.37	.06*
T	−.09*	−.21	−.19	.28	−.16	−.01*	.01*	.10*	.34	−.17
R	.55	.55	.36	.44	.41	.49	**.71**	.71	.26	.50
SS	.60	.59	.40	.39	.40	.49	**.76**	.74	.28	.48
CC	**.63**	.68	.50	.37	.42	.47	**.74**	.70	.19	.50
PP	.22	.05*	.01*	.34	−.01	.22	.05*	.01*	.34	−.01

Note. A, Anxiety; H, Somatoform; N, Bipolar: Manic; D, Dysthymia; B, Alcohol Dependence; T, Drug Dependence; SS, Thought Disorder; CC, Major Depression; PP, Delusional Disorder; Hs, Hypochondriasis; D, Depression; Hy, Hysteria; Pd, Psychopathic Deviate; Mf, Masculinity/Femininity; Pa, Paranoia; Pt, Psychasthenia; Sc, Schizophrenia; Ma, Hypomania; Si, Social Introversion. Correlations in bold face are *r* ≥ .60. Correlations marked * are *not* significant at *p* < .0002.

Sloore, and Hauben (2003). Their results and conclusions have been confirmed by Rossi (2004). Therefore, these correlations are not tabulated here; only the main conclusions are discussed:

- Better convergence was obtained than with previous versions of the MCMI, which means that all MCMI-III-D scales showed higher correlations with corresponding MMPI-2 scales.
- Correlations with the clinical and content MMPI-2 scales reflected logical and expected relationships.
- Concurrent validity was high with two sets of corresponding MMPI-2 personality disorder scales (set 1 of Morey, Waugh, & Blashfield, 1985; set 2 of Somwaru, 1994, & Ben-Porath, 1995).
- The only exception was the MCMI-III-D Compulsive scale, which showed negative correlations with corresponding scales.

Recent research (e.g., Craig, 2005) has suggested an alternative interpretation for the Compulsive scale of the MCMI-III. Elevated scores on this scale are often obtained by persons with healthy functioning, and elevated scores in clinical groups tend to be associated with less pathology. For this reason, the psychometric properties and the content validity of the MCMI-III-D Compulsive scale were extensively evaluated.

An Extensive Empirical Evaluation of the Compulsive Scale

The current study used the valid MCMI-III-D profiles (*N* = 1,210) and the clinical ratings (*N* = 540) that were available for validation research from the sample of Rossi (2004). Among these 540 patients, 69 showed compulsive traits (clinical rating ≥ 1).

In general, once a test has been published, scales are seldom modified. Consequently, research to improve construct representation is rare. Nevertheless, it is important to pay attention to the psychometric properties of scales so that instrument refinement is possible. An empirical evaluation should be done for all scales. As an illustration, the current study focused on the Compulsive scale (in both of the case studies presented later in this chapter, compulsive traits were present).

The current empirical evaluation of the Compulsive scale was based on the guidelines of Smith and McCarthy (1995) and tested with classical test theory procedures:

- A scale should measure a unidimensional construct and should be internally consistent. Therefore, Cronbach's alpha for the total scale, corrected item–total correlations, and alpha if an item was deleted were calculated. Cronbach's alpha is the most commonly used index of internal consistency and should be above .70 (Nunnally & Bernstein, 1994; see also West and Finch, 1997). A rule of thumb is that corrected item–total correlations should preferably be .30 or higher.
- It is important to examine the item difficulty and discriminative power of items for different subpopulations. Item endorsement frequencies were calculated for persons with and without compulsive traits. Items with an endorsement percentage below 15% or above 85% lack discriminative power (Kendell & Brockington, 1980). Item difficulty was evaluated by the proportion of individuals answering the item in the expected direction (Nunnally & Bernstein, 1994).

The Compulsive scale had a Cronbach's alpha of .68, which is lower than the lower-bound criterion of .70. However, this value is similar to the values provided in the MCMI-III manual for the American normative sample (Millon, 2006, p. 58: $\alpha = .66$), and the Cronbach's alpha based on standardized items was .71. Table 16.4 displays the corrected item–total correlations and Cronbach's alpha if an item was deleted. The deletion of item 29, "People usually think of me as a reserved and serious-minded person," would result in a higher Cronbach's alpha value for the total scale. This is remarkable, since this is a true prototypal item. Moreover, this item and item 41 ("I've done a number of stupid things on impulse that ended up causing me great trouble") had a very low corrected item–total correlation. Except for these two items, corrected item-total correlations ranged from .27 to .46 (mean = .32). The items met the rule of thumb that such correlations should be .30 or higher. Items with correlations above .35 were item 2 ("I think highly of rules because they are a good guide to follow"), item 82 ("I always make sure that my work is well planned and organized"), item 137 ("I always see to it that my work is finished before taking time out for leisure activities"), and the reverse-scored item 14 ("Sometimes I can be pretty rough and mean in my relations with my family"). The central content of the scale seemed to go together with rigidity, preoccupation with rules, organization, and conscientiousness. Except for two items, therefore, the Compulsive scale appeared to be a unidimensional construct and an internally consistent scale.

Table 16.5 shows the item endorsement frequencies for persons with and without compulsive traits. All items had some discriminative power: There were no item endorsement percentages below 15% or above 85%. The item difficulty level was

TABLE 16.4. Corrected Item–Total Correlations and Cronbach's Alpha if Item Deleted for the Compulsive Scale (N = 1,210)

Item	Corrected item–total correlation	Cronbach's alpha if item deleted
2*	.38	*.65*
29*	*.02*	*.70*
59*	**.33**	*.66*
82*	**.46**	*.64*
97*	.29	*.66*
114*	.26	*.67*
137*	**.41**	*.64*
172*	.28	*.66*
7**	.27	*.67*
14**	**.35**	*.66*
22**	**.32**	*.66*
41**	*.09*	*.68*
53**	.29	*.67*
72**	.27	*.67*
101**	.28	*.67*
139**	.29	*.66*
166**	.28	*.67*

Note. *True prototypal item. **False (reverse-scored) item. Cronbach's alpha values higher than .68 (the total scale Cronbach's alpha) and item–total correlations below .10 are given in italics. Corrected item–total correlations above .30 are given in boldface.

adequate: All items were responded to in the expected direction. For all true proto-typal items, endorsement frequencies (% true responses) were higher for persons with compulsive traits, and on reverse-scored items, endorsement frequencies (% true responses) were higher for persons without compulsive traits. Nevertheless, not all endorsement frequencies were significantly different for persons with and without compulsive traits. Based on the results of classical test theory, the omission of item 29 seems advisable: Endorsement frequencies were not significantly different for persons with and without compulsive traits; it had a low corrected item–total correlation; and the total scale Cronbach's alpha value would be higher if the item were deleted from the scale.

The next step in exploring possibilities for scale refinement and improvement of construct representation was the evaluation of the content validity and specificity of the items. The content validity was rated independently by three psychologists with expertise in test validation and personality disorders. They evaluated content homo-geneity in terms of content adherence to DSM-IV-TR criteria (APA, 2000). Millon (1997, pp. 39–40) described the correspondence between the MCMI-III prototypal items and the DSM criteria. The expert raters had no prior knowledge of the classifi-cation of Millon (1997). Only DSM-IV-TR criteria that corresponded with a certain MCMI-III-D item according to all experts were reported. Item specificity was judged on a 4-point rating scale:

TABLE 16.5. Item Endorsement Frequencies Expressed in Percentages of Groups with (*n* = 69) and without (*n* = 471) Compulsive Traits

Item	% true responses		χ^2 two-sided	% false responses	
	With traits	Without traits		With traits	Without traits
2*	69.6	54.6	**.019**	30.4	45.4
29*	47.8	43.1	.460	52.2	56.9
59*	72.5	65.2	.233	27.5	34.8
82*	78.3	68.2	.089	21.7	31.8
97*	47.8	42.7	.420	52.2	57.3
114*	78.3	76.9	.796	21.7	23.1
137*	76.8	59.4	**.006**	23.2	40.6
172*	68.1	51.4	**.009**	31.9	48.6
7**	37.7	40.6	.650	62.3	59.4
14**	27.5	28.0	.933	72.5	72.0
22**	21.7	34.6	**.034**	78.3	65.4
41**	52.2	65.8	**.027**	47.8	34.2
53**	24.6	32.9	.168	75.4	67.1
72**	49.3	59.0	.126	50.7	41.0
101**	18.8	35.9	**.005**	81.2	64.1
139**	27.5	40.3	**.041**	72.5	59.6
166**	30.4	38.6	.189	69.6	61.4

Note. *True prototypal item. **False (reverse-scored). χ^2 asymptotically significant at *p* < .05 are given in boldface.

0 = "Item does not adhere to the personality disorder."
1 = "Item has an association with the personality disorder, but reflects a general concept."
2 = "Item reflects a distinct aspect of the personality disorder, but is not exclusive to this personality disorder."
3 = "Item describes a very specific characteristic of the personality disorder."

The experts independently judged the item specificity and came to a consensus after discussion. Table 16.6 shows the DSM-IV-TR–MCMI-III-D correspondence and item specificity. Except for items 29 and 97, all true prototypal items were related to DSM-IV-TR criteria according to the experts. Since item 29 also reflected a general concept (specificity = 1) and was already rejected by classical test theory, it would probably be better to omit item 29 from the Compulsive scale. The remaining true prototypal items (with the exception of item 114) were linked by the experts to the same criteria as proposed by Millon. Most DSM-IV-TR criteria were represented (criteria 1, 3, 4, 7, and 8, according to Millon [1997] and the experts; criterion 2, according to Millon). Aspects considered of importance for the presence of obsessive–compulsive personality disorder by the DSM-IV-TR taxonomy, but not integrated into the Compulsive scale, were criteria 5 ("is unable to discard worn-out or worthless objects even when they have no sentimental value") and 6 "is reluctant to delegate tasks or to work with others unless they submit to exactly his or her way of doing things"). Several aspects of the DSM-IV-TR criteria are represented in the

TABLE 16.6. DSM-IV-TR–MCMI-III-D Correspondence and Item Specificity

Item	DSM-IV-TR criterion according to Millon (1997)	DSM-IV-TR criterion proposed by all three experts	Specificity (consensus of experts)
2*	8	8, 4	2
29*	A	—	1
59*	7	7	1
82*	1	1	1
97*	3	—	0
114*	2	1	2
137*	3	3	2
172*	4	4	2
7**	NIA	—	0
14**	NIA	—	0
22**	NIA	8	2
41**	NIA	—	1
53**	NIA	—	1
72**	NIA	—	1
101**	NIA	4	1
139**	NIA	—	0
166**	NIA	8,1	1

Note. *True prototypal item. **False (reverse-scored) item. NIA, no information available.

Compulsive scale, but the correspondence with DSM-IV-TR obsessive–compulsive personality disorder is not complete. Moreover, according to the experts, the content of only 9 items (out of 17) corresponded with DSM-IV-TR criteria. However, of the 8 items that did not correspond with DSM-IV-TR criteria, two items (41 and 139) were endorsed significantly differently and in the expected direction by persons with and without compulsive traits. Therefore, the Compulsive scale captures aspects that differentiate people with compulsive traits from people without such traits, but that are not represented in the *DSM* classification.

Striking is that no single item was rated by the three experts as a very specific characteristic of the disorder. Most items that were rated as distinct aspects were true prototypal items (4 of 5). Many items were considered to have an association with compulsive traits (8 items), but also reflect general concepts. Although most items were related to the personality disorder, the items clearly lacked specificity. Most problematic was that 4 of the 17 scale items were rated as not relevant to the personality disorder. One of these 4 items was a true prototypal item: item 97 ("I believe in the saying, 'Early to bed and early to rise . . .' "). As such, it is no surprise that the Compulsive scale had a higher sensitivity than specificity. A meticulous analysis and adjustment of item content could probably enhance the specificity of the scale.

Based on this information, one could expect that the MCMI-III-D would detect compulsive traits/disorder in the woman with compulsions (the first case study in the next section). For the second case study, the man with posttraumatic stress, one could expect that the Post-Traumatic Stress Disorder scale would be elevated (this scale also had an adequate sensitivity level).

Two Case Studies

A Woman from The Netherlands with Compulsions

A 36-year-old woman sought help for her compulsive behavior. She did everything on a fixed schedule, especially cleaning activities. Her husband came with her during the first consultation, owing to the many difficulties in their relationship. Her husband appeared to be a very impulsive and sensation-seeking person. They had rather different points of view regarding the education of their two young children (ages 2 and almost 1). They assessed themselves as being opposites in character, and felt that this led to numerous quarrels. The patient also complained about her moodiness; she felt irritated much of the time, as well as depressed and anxious. Her sense of self-esteem was "changeable" as well. Her husband wanted to discuss their sexual difficulties, but she resisted talking about the topic.

The family background of the patient was complicated. Her mother was 17 when she was born, having been raped by an African man, whom she did not know. The patient's skin was darker than that of her peers. Living with her single mother also made her the subject of negative judgments and bullying by her primary school peers.

Currently, the patient's mother took care of her children 2 days a week; this proved to be complicated. Her communication with her mother was problematic, as her mother did not talk much and never discussed or expressed her feelings about their troubled past. Despite her college education, the patient had no job, but said that she would like to find one.

This woman was administered both the MCMI-III-D and the MMPI-2, producing a valid MCMI-III-D profile. Anxiety was the high-point scale among the Moderate Clinical Syndrome Scales, achieving a BR score of 87 with the Belgian norms and 84 with the U.S. norms. On the Severe Clinical Syndromes Scales, she scored 92 on Thought Disorder with the Belgian BRs, but 70 with the U.S. BRs. The highest scores in the Clinical Personality Patterns with the Belgian BRs were on the Negativistic (BR = 92, or 77 with the U.S. BRs) and Sadistic (BR = 90, or 68 with the U.S. BRs scales). On the Depressive and Dependent scales, the U.S. and Belgian BRs looked much more alike (mid-80s). The Compulsive score was 83 with the Belgian BRs, but only 59 with the U.S. BRs.

The MCMI-III-D pointed to a more complex picture of clinical syndromes and personality disorders than the patient and her husband had presented during the intake phase. The Belgian BRs appear to have come closer to the clinical impressions than the U.S. BRs. This supports the general idea that for different languages and cultures, there is often a need to separate BRs; in this case, the local BRs appear to have improved validity. Some additional research is still needed to compare the efficiency of the Belgian BRs in Belgium and The Netherlands, although both countries share the same language (see the discussion at the start of this chapter of language variations between Flanders and The Netherlands). The MMPI-2 displayed a profile with passive–aggressive traits (scale 4, Psychopathic Deviate = 71T; scale 5, Masculinity/Femininity = 46T; and scale 6, Paranoia = 62T) in combination with anxiety and mood problems (scale 2, Depression = 81T; scale 7, Psychasthenia = 79T). This patient also presented herself on the MMPI-2 as rather cynical and negativistic (scale 3, Hysteria = 83T), and as showing antisocial behavior (scale 4 = 71T, and the content scale Antisocial Practices = 65T).

During treatment, the complex and deeply rooted character of this woman's problems became manifest. It took about 30 sessions to bring her a measure of relief. Her sense of identity was strengthened by interventions that enabled her and her mother to learn more about the man who probably was her father. She became more comfortable with herself, found appropriate work, and could more easily accept her mother's help with her young children.

A Man from Syria with Posttraumatic Stress Symptoms

A 46-year-old man who was born in Syria, had lived in The Netherlands for 20 years, was married to a Dutch woman, and had a 12-year-old son was referred by his family physician because of posttraumatic stress complaints. He was bothered by nightmares. Old memories popped up in his dreams. In one, he found himself locked into a shower stall with blood on the shower curtains. He also dreamed that he was locked in the Damascus airport with no passport and no identity card. He had begun having such dreams as a young boy in Syria. He was the youngest of five children in a family that had been isolated for many years because of its left-wing political persuasions. When he was 13 years old, his father was imprisoned for political reasons, and he and his mother had barely escaped an exploding car bomb; he had seen parts of dead bodies lying all around him. Despite the political persecution, most of his family continued to live in Damascus.

The patient's son had recently been threatened by peers, and the patient himself had had an altercation with an aggressive neighbor who was from Serbia and had threatened to kill another person from the neighborhood. These recent experiences had stirred up nightmares and reactivated general feelings of tension, concentration problems, irritability, and aggression. He had outbursts of anger at his son, but felt very guilty about these. Reluctant to express aggressive behavior toward family members, he became depressed and fatigued, as well as experiencing several somatic and psychosomatic symptoms. He did not trust medical facilities because he had experienced a wrong diagnosis and treatment some years earlier. Recently the members of his family still living in Syria had asked him to visit, but he feared to go there.

The patient worked as an engineer. Previously he had been employed as an oil-drilling engineer in offshore activities, but in The Netherlands he began his own consulting company. In his earlier clinical contact he had appeared to the evaluator to be obsessive–compulsive, because he engaged in obsessive cleaning, was very perfectionistic, and manifested a strict superego. Because of these earlier clinical impressions, he was administered the MCMI-III- D, the MMPI-2, and the Bar-On Emotional Intelligence Inventory (Derksen, 1999).

On the MCMI-III-D he produced a valid profile, but his Desirability score was 93. With the Belgian BRs, his score on the Post-Traumatic Stress Disorder scale was highest among the Clinical Syndrome Scales (BR = 98); with the U.S. norms, his score on the Anxiety scale was highest (BR = 90). His Clinical Personality Patterns with the Belgian BRs showed the highest scores on the Histrionic (BR = 115), Narcissistic (BR = 100), and Compulsive (BR = 98) scales. With the U.S. BRs, his highest scores were on the Narcissistic (BR = 83) and Histrionic (BR = 73) scales. The U.S. BR score on the Compulsive scale, however, was only 58.

To summarize, though the U.S. and Belgian score configurations were similar, it seemed that the Belgian BRs more fully captured this man's observed clinical picture. In general, the MMPI-2 profile supported the findings of the MCMI-III-D. Some additional information was presented by his so-called "conversion V" score: high on scale 1, Hypochondriasis (79*T*), and scale 3, Hysteria (94*T*), but lower on scale 2, Depression (68*T*). Furthermore, the content scale Health Concerns (71*T*) was elevated, as was the supplementary scale Overcontrolled Hostility (68*T*). His total Bar-On Emotional Intelligence Inventory score was high (120*T*); the mean is 100, and the standard deviation is 15). On specific emotional capabilities, he scored high on Emotional Self-Awareness (127*T*), Assertiveness (130*T*), and Optimism (130*T*), but low on Stress Management (81*T*).

After this assessment, the patient was treated for his posttraumatic stress symptoms, and he felt better after six sessions. The treatment was a combination of cognitive-behavioral and psychodynamic approaches. The childhood memories were explored, and the blocked affect was released. Also, he was helped by means of cognitive restructuring to deal with both his aggressive neighbor and his own irritation with his son. The assessment delivered some evidence for further treatment directed at his personality traits. But the patient was not really interested in working at the vulnerabilities in his personality, and having fewer symptoms also slightly softened his compulsive and histrionic traits. The patient and therapist agreed upon termination, with the suggestion to come back if necessary and pay some more attention to his personality traits then.

References

American Psychiatric Association (APA). (2000). *Diagnostic and statistical manual of mental disorders* (4th ed., text rev.). Washington, DC: Author.

Ben-Porath, Y. S. (1995). *Assessing personality disorders with the MMPI-2.* Paper presented at the Clinical Workshops on the MMPI-2 and MMPI-A and the 30th Annual Symposium on Recent Developments in the Use of the MMPI, MMPI-2, and MMPI-A, St. Petersburg, FL.

Butcher, J. N., Graham, J. R., Ben-Porath, Y. S., Tellegen, A., Dahlstrom, W. G., & Kaemmer, B. (2001). *Minnesota Multiphasic Personality Inventory–2: Manual for administration and scoring* (2nd ed.). Minneapolis: University of Minnesota Press.

Choca, J. P., Peterson, C. A., & Shanley, L. A. (1986). Factor analysis of the Millon Clinical Multiaxial Inventory. *Journal of Consulting and Clinical Psychology, 54,* 253–255.

Choca, J. P., Shanley, L. A., & Van Denburg, E. (1992). *Interpretive guide to the Millon Clinical Multiaxial Inventory.* Washington, DC: American Psychological Association.

Craig, R. J. (2005). Alternative interpretations for the histrionic, narcissistic, and compulsive personality disorder scales of the MCMI-III. In R. J. Craig (Ed.), *New directions in interpreting the Millon Clinical Multiaxial Inventory–III (MCMI-III): Essays on current issues* (pp. 71–93). Hoboken, NJ: Wiley.

Craig, R. J., & Bivens, A. (1998). Factor structure of the MCMI-III. *Journal of Personality Assessment, 70,* 190–196.

Craig, R. J., & Weinberg, D. (1993). MCMI: Review of the literature. In R. J. Craig (Ed.), *The Millon Clinical Multiaxial Inventory: A clinical research information synthesis* (pp. 23–70). Hillsdale, NJ: Erlbaum.

Derksen, J. J. L. (1999). *EQ en IQ in Nederland.* Nijmegen, The Netherlands: PEN Tests.

Derksen, J. J. L., De Mey, H. R. A., Sloore, H., & Hellenbosch, G. (2006). *MMPI-2: Handleiding voor afname, scoring en interpretatie* (herziene editie) [*MMPI-2: Manual for administration, scoring, and interpretation* (rev. ed.)]. Nijmegen, The Netherlands: PEN Tests.

Finn, S. E. (1984). A partial cross-sequential analysis of personality ratings on 400 men (Doctoral dissertation, University of Minnesota, 1984). *Dissertation Abstracts International, 45,* 2865B.

Greenblatt, R. L., Modzierz, G. J., Murphy, T. J., & Trimakas, K. (1986). *Nonmetric multidimensional scaling of the MCMI.* Paper presented at the conference on the Millon Clinical Inventories, Miami, FL.

Haddy, C., Strack, S., & Choca, J. P. (2005). Linking personality disorders and clinical syndromes on the MCMI-III. *Journal of Personality Assessment, 84,* 193–204.

Hambleton, R. (1994). Guidelines for adapting educational and psychological tests: A progress report. *European Journal of Psychological Assessment, 10,* 229–244.

Hsu, L. M. (2002). Diagnostic validity statistics and the MCMI-III. *Psychological Assessment, 14,* 410–422.

International Test Commission (ITC). (2000). *Guidelines on Adapting Tests.* Retrieved from *www.intestcom.org*

Kendell, R. E., & Brockington, I. F. (1980). The identification of disease entities and the relationship between schizophrenia and affective psychoses. *British Journal of Psychiatry, 137,* 324–331.

Lewis, S. J., & Harder, D. W. (1990). Factor structure of the MCMI among personality disordered outpatients and in other populations. *Journal of Clinical Psychology, 46,* 613–617.

McCrae, R. R., & Costa, P. T. (1999). A five-factor theory of personality. In L. A. Pervin & O. P. John (Eds.), *Handbook of personality: Theory and research* (2nd ed., pp. 139–153). New York: Guilford Press.

McNiel, D. E., Lam, J. N., & Binder, R. L. (2000). Relevance of interrater agreement to violence risk assessment. *Journal of Consulting and Clinical Psychology, 68,* 1111–1115.

Mertens, J., Baert, H., & Clara, R. (Eds.). (1991). *Welzijnsgids: Gezondheidszorg, welzijnszorg: Noden en behoeften, organisaties en voorzieningen, aanpak en methodiek, beleid. Sociale kaart van Vlaanderen* [*Welfare guide: Health care, public welfare: Needs and necessities, organizations and services, approach and methodology, policy. Social map of Flanders*]. Deurne, Belgium: Kluwer.

Millon, T. (1982). *Millon Clinical Multiaxial Inventory manual* (2nd ed.). Minneapolis, MN: National Computer Systems.

Millon, T. (with Millon, C., & Davis, R. D.). (1994). *MCMI-III manual.* Minneapolis, MN: National Computer Systems.

Millon, T. (with Millon C., & Davis, R. D.). (1997). *MCMI-III Manual* (2nd ed.). Minneapolis, MN: National Computer Systems.

Millon, T. (with Millon, C., Davis, R. D., & Grossman, S.). (2006). *MCMI-III manual* (3rd ed.). Minneapolis, MN: Pearson Assessments.

Morey, L. C., Waugh, M. H., & Blashfield, R. K. (1985). MMPI scales for DSM-III personality disorders: Their derivation and correlates. *Journal of Personality Assessment, 49,* 245–251.

Nunnally, J. C., & Bernstein, I. H. (1994). *Psychometric theory* (3rd ed.). New York: McGraw-Hill.

Nurnberg, H. G., Martin, G. A., Somoza, E., Coccaro, E. F., Skodol, A. E., Oldham, J. M., et al. (2000). Identifying personality disorders: Towards the development of a clinical screening instrument. *Comprehensive Psychiatry, 41,* 137–146.

Pearson Assessments. (2004). *Microtest Q 5.08A* [Computer software]. Minneapolis, MN: Author.

Piersma, H. L. (1986). The factor structure of the Millon Clinical Multiaxial Inventory (MCMI) for psychiatric inpatients. *Journal of Personality Assessment, 50,* 578–584.

Rossi, G. (2004). *Interpersoonlijk uit balans: Empirische validatie van de MCMI-III en de theorie van Millon met betrekking tot de afhankelijke, narcistische, theatrale en antisociale persoonlijkheid* [*Interpersonally imbalanced: Empirical validation of the MCMI-III and the theory of Millon considering the dependent, narcissistic, histrionic and antisocial personality*]. Unpublished doctoral dissertation, Vrije Universiteit Brussel, Brussels, Belgium.

Rossi, G., Hauben, C., Van den Brande, I., & Sloore, H. (2003). Empirical evaluation of the MCMI-III personality disorder scales. *Psychological Reports, 92,* 627–642.

Rossi, G., & Sloore, H. (2005). International uses of the MCMI: Does interpretation change? In R. J. Craig (Ed.), *New directions in interpreting the Millon Clinical Multiaxial Inventory–III (MCMI-III): Essays on current issues* (pp. 144–161). Hoboken, NJ: Wiley.

Rossi, G., Van den Brande, I., Tobac, A., Sloore, H., & Hauben, C. (2003). Convergent validity of the MCMI-III personality disorder scales and the MMPI-2 scales. *Journal of Personality Disorders, 17,* 330–340.

Rossi, G., van der Ark, L. A., & Sloore, H. (2007). Factor analysis of the Dutch language version of the MCMI-III. *Journal of Personality Assessment, 88,* 144–157.

Sloore, H. V., & Derksen, J. J. L. (1997). Issues and procedures in MCMI translations. In T. Millon (Ed.), *The Millon inventories: Clinical and personality assessment* (pp. 286–302). New York: Guilford Press.

Sloore, H. V., Derksen, J. J. L., & De Mey, H. (1994). *MCMI-III: Dutch research form.* Nijmegen, The Netherlands: PEN Tests.

Sloore, H. V., Derksen, J. J. L., Hellenbosch, G., & de Mey, H. R. A. (1993). *MMPI-2 handleiding bij afname, scoring en interpretatie* [*MMPI-2 manual for administration, scoring and interpretation*]. Nijmegen, The Netherlands: PEN Tests.

Smith, G. T., & McCarthy, D. M. (1995). Methodological considerations in the refinement of clinical assessment instruments. *Psychological Assessment, 7,* 300–308.

Somwaru, D. P. (1994). *Assessment of personality disorders with the MMPI-2.* Unpublished master's thesis, Kent State University.

Spitzer, R. L. (1983). Psychiatric diagnoses: Are clinicians still necessary? *Comprehensive Psychiatry, 24,* 399–411.

Swets, J. A., Dawes, R. M., & Monahan, J. (2000). Psychological science can improve diagnostic decisions. *Psychological Science in the Public Interest, 1,* 1–26.

Ten Berge, J. M. F. (1986). Rotation to perfect congruence and the cross validation of component weights across populations. *Multivariate Behavioral Research, 21,* 41–64.

Van de Brande, I. (2002). *Empirische validering van de theorie van Th. Millon m.b.t. de persoonlijkheidsstoornissen [Empirical validation of Th. Millon's theory concerning personality disorders].* Unpublished doctoral dissertation, Vrije Universiteit Brussel, Brussels, Belgium.

Van de Vijver, F., & Tanzer, N. (1997). Bias and equivalence in cross-cultural assessment: An overview. *European Review of Applied Psychology, 47,* 263–279.

West, S. G., & Finch, J. F. (1997). Personality measurement: Reliability and validity issues. In R. Hogan, J. Johnson, & S. Briggs (Eds.), *Handbook of personality psychology* (pp. 143–164). San Diego: Academic Press.

CHAPTER 17

Experiences in Translating and Validating the MCMI in Denmark

Erik Simonsen
Ask Elklit

Theodore Millon introduced his Millon inventories to Europe for the first time at the International Congress "Clinical Implications of the MMPI," held at the Department of Psychiatry, Nordvang Hospital, University of Copenhagen, in 1983. In adapting Jane Loevinger's (1957) three-stage validation model ("theoretical," "internal," and "external"), he launched a new paradigm for constructing clinical psychiatric and psychological inventories that differed from the Minnesota Multiphasic Personality Inventory (MMPI). Millon also presented pertinent historical literature and elaborated on his fundamental perspectives regarding the interaction of personality and psychopathology.

Impressed and inspired by his innovative, systematic, and timely insights into the varying schools of psychopathology, a group of Danish psychiatrists and psychologists formed a "Millon study group." The members of the group were a strong and creative mixture of psychoanalysts, behaviorists, neuropsychologists, experienced clinicians, and researchers, who gathered regularly and had in common a genuine curiosity about psychopathology. Each one paid respect to others' ideas and experiences in working with psychopathology, and all were inspired to broaden their own views.

By furthering their exploration of Millon's inventories and theories, the group members sought to investigate the impact of understanding a patient's psychopathology on the choice and planning of treatment. Important sources for group discussions and clinical vignettes included Millon's newly released seminal book, *Disorders of Personality: DSM-III, Axis II* (Millon, 1981), select Millon Clinical Multiaxial Inventory–I (MCMI-I) patient profiles, and other available clinical evaluations and psychological tests. As one result of the group's meetings, the members agreed that there was a pressing need for a Danish translation of the MCMI. The MCMI is one of the few self-report tests that focus on both symptoms and personality disorders and their relationship. The MCMI-I was developed in 1977, and it was subsequently revised in 1987 and 1994 (Millon, 1977, 1987, 1994).

Inspired by the success and productivity of the Millon study group, the members, in collaboration with Theodore Millon, organized the First International Congress on the Study of Personality Disorders, held in Copenhagen in 1988. They also joined in forming an organization to enhance the international exchange of ideas and to promote research collaboration: the International Society on the Study of Personality Disorders. Subsequently, the Millon study group evolved into the Institute for Personality Theory and Psychopathology. It is evident to all those involved that such landmark organizations owe their existence in large part to Millon's foresight, ingenuity, and organizational endeavors.

In this chapter, we discuss first how the translation of the MCMI-I into Danish took place, and then describe the efforts to improve and revise a subsequent translation with guidance of empirical research.

International Guidelines for Translation of Psychological Tests

The translation of psychological tests should follow the guidelines adopted by a number of international associations, such as the International Association of Cross-Cultural Psychology, the International Union of Psychological Science, and the International Test Commission (Hambleton, 1994). In translating a test into another language, the test developers must consider the following 10 recommendations:

1. The test developers should present evidence that the wording of the items is appropriate for the target population after translation procedures have taken place.
2. The test developers should make sure that the test procedures (i.e., testing techniques, test conventions) are familiar to the target populations, the test administrators, and the patients.
3. The test developers should make sure to present evidence that the purpose of the test and the content of the items are understood by the patients.
4. The test developers should provide empirical evidence to improve the accuracy of the translation, and should compare such evidence for different language versions.
5. The test developers should use appropriate statistical techniques to establish item equivalence between language versions of the instrument.
6. The test developers should apply statistical techniques to identify problematic components or aspects of the instrument that are inadequate for the intended population.
7. The test developers should provide information about validity in the target population.
8. The test developers should provide statistical evidence of the equivalence of questions in the original and target populations.

9. The test developers should ensure that nonequivalent questions intended for different populations should not be used between versions in preparing a common scale.
10. Translations (both forward into the new language and back into the original one) should be done by translators fluent in both languages.

These recommendations and guidelines may seem rather strict and technical; yet, from a more practical and psychological point of view, one may formulate the ideal conditions for a translation.

Issues in Translation of Personality Scales

A psychological test consists of a set of items, a set of administration procedures, relevant scientific theory, and all empirical data that are relevant for the interpretation of the test. Unfortunately, this complex set of procedures and knowledge is often simplified to the point of reification. An essential part of this simplification is to consider only the test items and to ignore theoretical and empirical knowledge about a test. One of the consequences of this reification is a naïve attitude to the problem of translation: When the words of the test items have been more or less literally translated from the source language into the target language, the same test is assumed to exist in both languages.

Before translating the MCMI-I, we engaged in some general consideration of our intended aim. A personality test may be translated from two different perspectives: The intent is either to observe empirically how a good translation of a test behaves differently in various cultures, or to produce an empirically equivalent test in the target language. The first perspective may be called truly "cross-cultural," because its primary goal is to observe cultural differences; the second perspective may be called "psychometric," because the primary goal is to obtain a measurement instrument with certain characteristics in the target language.

An important difference between these two approaches is that the success of the second approach, at least in principle, can be measured empirically: A translation is successful to the extent that the target version of a test has the same psychometric properties of the translated test. To determine the degree of this success, both studies of the internal structure of the test and studies of correlations between the test and other important psychological variables must be conducted.

In this context, a good translation can be considered only one step in the successful transfer of a test from one culture to another, and it is important to realize that a translation may not be necessary in all areas of psychology. If a psychological theory within an area is developed so that it is possible to specify the characteristics of good test items to a sufficient degree, it may be a better procedure simply to construct new items in the target language.

The purpose of translating a personality inventory is usually to obtain an instrument that measures a specified number of personality constructs or personality traits—the same constructs or traits that the original inventory is supposed to measure in the source culture. This is one of the reasons that empirical validation of a translation may fail to relate to between-culture variance in personality constructs: The psychologically important personality constructs may not be the same in various cultures, and even if they are, there may be both qualitative and quantitative differences in their development.

In producing our translation of the MCMI-I, we compared nonclinical samples from the source population (North American) and the target population (Danish). This gave us an idea not only of the quality of the translation, but also of whether there were any striking differences or similarities between the two populations. Before we discuss this, we first give a short description of the most important methods that may be used in the process of translating and validating an inventory in the target language. These methods are divided into linguistic and psychometric procedures.

Linguistic Procedures for Translation

Three different linguistic procedures should be taken into consideration. Each of the following represents a step forward: (1) individual translation, (2) the committee approach, and (3) back-translation.

Individual Translation

The first kind of translation is, of course, limited by the individual translator's knowledge of the two languages and knowledge of the relevant scientific theories. Ideally, the translator should also possess good knowledge of the two cultures. If there is only one translator, he or she should have a basic linguistic education, as well as basic training in the psychological sciences. In most cases, knowledge of the relevant theory is more important than formal language training. The psychological meaning of the wording must be preserved, to ensure that the purpose of the test is fulfilled. In the case of multiconstruct questionnaires like the MCMI, it should be remembered that knowledge of the subscale(s) in which each item is included could be of great help in the translation process. On the one hand, translators with appropriate theoretical knowledge may be better able to use this kind of information; on the other hand, they may also be quite tempted to change individual items substantially. The purpose of these changes may be to make items easier to read and understand. An example is when translators avoid negations used in the source version of a questionnaire. This may be helpful, but in most cases it can be argued that it is the original test constructor who should have avoided negations.

The Committee Approach

In the committee approach, two or more independent translators each produce a first translation. They then meet to discuss differences between their versions and work out an agreement on the most appropriate translation. It is likely that this approach, in most cases, will reduce any bias that the individual translators may have, and it is certainly an advantage that scientists and members with formal language training may supplement each other in a committee.

Back-Translation

One way to investigate different translations is to have one or more translators make a first translation into the target language and then have one or more independent translators make a translation back into the original language (Brislin, 1970). Comparison of the original source version with the back-translated version is a valuable procedure for checking linguistic accuracy. In most cases, this method can detect items that have been poorly translated from a linguistic point of view, and ideally the complete process should be repeated for these items.

If the two versions are highly similar, the comparison suggests that the target version is equivalent to the source language form. However, it must be remembered that apparent equivalence may be created by factors that have nothing to do with the quality of the translation: Translators may have a shared set of rules for translating certain nonequivalent words and phrases, and some back-translators may be able to make sense out of a poor target language version.

Psychometric Procedures in Translation of the Danish MCMI-I

In the analysis on empirical data of translations, a broad selection of psychometric procedures may be used. The most often used are the following: (1) comparing item endorsement frequencies, and (2) calculating correlations between each item and the total scale score (point biserial correlations). The data may also be collected in different ways. One way is to let bilingual responders answer both the source and the target versions. Another way is to have the same group answer different versions of the target questionnaire, or to have two comparable groups answer different target versions.

In this section, we describe as an example how the translation and empirical evaluation took place for the Danish MCMI-I. The MCMI-I has a 175-item true–false self-report format. Its 20 clinical scales cover a span of 9 clinical symptom syndromes (Anxiety, Somatoform, Hypomania, Dysthymia, Alcohol Abuse, Drug Abuse, Psychotic Thinking, Psychotic Depression, Psychotic Delusion); 3 pathological personality disorders (Schizotypal, Borderline, Paranoid); and 8 basic personality patterns (Schizoid, Avoidant, Dependent, Histrionic, Narcissistic, Antisocial, Compulsive, and Passive–Aggressive). There are also two correctional scales of denial versus complaint. The instrument identifies or calculates whether a patient is or is not a member of a diagnostic entity. The raw scores are transformed into base rate scores, a conversion determined by using known prevalence data and by using cutoff points designed to maximize correct classification. The MCMI-I uses an item overlap keying; the reasons for this are theoretical, practical, and empirical. From Millon's theory of psychopathology, one might expect, for example, that the avoidant and the dependent personalities share some common basic features—a finding gauged by empirical covariations. Using item overlap meant that the number of items included in the 20-scale inventory could be kept to a minimum.

To check for translation problems, we compared two different versions of the Danish translation of the MCMI-I in the field pretest phase (Simonsen & Mortensen, 1990). The two versions were given randomly to subjects in a population survey study. Both versions were then translated back into English. The item endorsement frequencies were compared by chi-square tests for all items. Those items with a group difference significant at $p < .01$ were analyzed further for their impact on scale scores. Point biserial correlations between the item and the total scale score were calculated. Altogether, six items were used in significantly different ways. To illustrate the kind of effects that different but still very close translations can have on scale homogeneity and scale scores, we give three examples.

Table 17.1 shows the back-translations of the two Danish versions of MCMI-I item 10. Neither of the two agrees very well with the original English text, and it is noteworthy that considerably more Danes consider themselves satisfied with being a "rank-and-file member" than being "led by others." Moreover, according to the scoring instructions, the item should correlate positively with four subscales: Schizoid, Dependent, Compulsive, and Schizotypal. Clearly, these results indicate that neither of the two Danish versions performs ideally. None of the point biserial correlations should be negative; obviously, either items with substantial negative item–total correlations should be dropped from the scale, or the scoring should be reversed. Items with point correlations close to zero will introduce noise into the measurement and should also be dropped from the scale. In this particular example, neither of the two versions seems close to the original English version, and therefore the first step might be to try an improved translation. If a new translation does not turn out to work better, the best solution may be to construct a new Danish item from scratch. (This, in fact, was what we actually did with this item.)

Table 17.2 shows the same data for MCMI-I item 14. Here there seems to be a very close agreement between the English original text and both translations (the only difference being between "believe" and "think"). The original text uses "think," and the tables show that this version has the highest correlations for four scales, whereas the first version has the highest correlations for three scales. This example illustrates a special problem with the MCMI-I: The fact that items load on several scales makes it even more difficult to obtain an ideal translation, because one particular translation is not the best for all relevant scales.

Finally, Table 17.3 shows text and point biserial correlations for MCMI-I item 37. Danish version 1 has "always tried to avoid," and version 2, like the original, has

---

TABLE 17.1. Text and Statistics for Item 10 of the MCMI-I

Original version: "I am content to be a follower of others."

Danish version 1: "I am satisfied with being a rank-and-file member of a group."

Danish version 2: "I am satisfied with being the type of person who is led by others."

Item endorsement frequencies: 72% (version 1) and 31% (version 2)

Point biserial correlations between item and total scores:

	Version 1	Version 2
Scale 1: Schizoid	−.04	.15
Scale 3: Dependent	.12	.04
Scale 7: Compulsive	.10	−.20
Scale S: Schizotypal	−.03	.17

TABLE 17.2. Text and Statistics for Item 14 of the MCMI-I

Original version: "I think I am a very sociable and outgoing person"
Danish version 1: "I believe that I am a very sociable and outgoing person"
Danish version 2: "I think that I am a very sociable and outgoing person"

Item endorsement frequencies: 89% (version 1) and 50% (version 2)

Point biserial correlations between item and total scale scores:

	Version 1	Version 2
Scale 1: Schizoid	.32	.19
Scale 2: Avoidant	.24	.23
Scale 3: Histrionic	.10	.33
Scale 5: Narcissistic	.28	.37
Scale S: Schizotypal	.29	.11
Scale N: Hypomania	.22	.44
Scale T: Drug Abuse	.23	.37

"always avoided." The table also shows that the point biserial correlations unambiguously confirm that version 2 is more appropriate, and the item can be considered an example of agreement between linguistic and psychometric procedures. When the translation procedures are ended, the final translation should be examined for how well its scale homogeneity is preserved (see below).

Psychometric Properties of the Danish MCMI-III

The MCMI-I in the United States was changed to the MCMI-II in 1987 with new items, a new scoring system, and so forth. And subsequently the MCMI-II was altered in 1994 to the MCMI-III.

After a pilot test of 245 subjects, the Danish version of the MCMI-III was field-tested in a number of treatment centers, psychiatric wards, and in private practice

TABLE 17.3. Text and Statistics for Item 37 of the MCMI-I

Original version: "I have always avoided getting involved with people socially."
Danish version 1: "I have always tried to avoid getting too involved in other people's affairs."
Danish version 2: "I have always avoided associating much with other people."

Item endorsement frequencies: 53% (version 1) and 25% (version 2)

Point biserial correlations between item and total scale scores:

	Version 1	Version 2
Scale 1: Schizoid	.10	.57
Scale 2: Avoidant	.05	.35
Scale S: Schizotypal	.10	.53
Scale SS: Psychotic Thinking	.01	.48

(Table 17.4) with 2,205 participants. The sample consisted of 1,314 women (59.6%) and 891 men (40.4%). Table 17.5 shows the gender differences in base rate scores. Women had higher scores on the Debasement index, as well as on the Histrionic, Narcissistic, and Compulsive scales. There were no gender differences on the Desirability index or on the Dependent, Sadistic (Aggressive), Masochistic (Self-Defeating), Paranoid, Bipolar: Manic, Post-Traumatic Stress Disorder, or Major Depression scales. On all the other scales, men had higher scores.

The sample was divided into six equal-size age groups (18–23, 24–28, 29–34, 35–39, 40–47, 48–73). For most of the Modifying Indices and the scales, increasing age was associated with steadily declining scores. In three cases, the slope was ascending: the Desirability index and the Histrionic and Compulsive scales. Two scales had a regular U-shape with steep slopes: the Somatoform and Major Depression scales. The Schizoid scale had a U-shape with a soft right slope. The Narcissistic scale had an S-shaped slope with a steep rise from age group 2 to age group 3.

Generally, the age-based differences were between 10 and 20 base rate points. Several interpretations are possible: (1) The younger patients were more disturbed than older patients; (2) the younger patients were more sensitive, less denying, less repressive, and/or more honest than the older patients; (3) the various time periods had an impact on the endorsement of disorders (a cohort effect); (4) a selection bias might have existed, in that relatively more disturbed younger patients were asked to participate; or (5) the younger people asked for help at a later point, when their problems had become relatively large (different thresholds for asking for help).

In any case, it is important to be attentive to age in interpreting an MCMI-III profile. In future revisions of the base rate values, age should be considered, as the variation stemming from age seems to be larger than the variation stemming from gender.

The sample was also analyzed according to the type of treatment each patient was referred to. The general picture was that victims of intimate violence had disorders as severe as, or more severe than, those of psychiatric patients and patients who were dependent on alcohol or drugs. Patients with pain were at the opposite end of the spectrum, with few reported psychological problems, not even somatoform disorders (here we interpret the Narcissistic, Histrionic, and Compulsive scales as signs of resources—at least up to some high possible threshold). Forensic patients scored in

TABLE 17.4. Group of Patients Contributing to the Field Testing of the Danish MCMI-III (N = 2,205)

Patient group	Number	%
Patients with pain	287	13.0
Patients abusing alcohol or drugs	206	9.3
Rehabilitation clients	481	21.8
Forensic patients	222	10.1
Psychiatric patients	491	22.3
Patients with organic brain damage	54	2.4
Clients in private practice	279	12.7
Victims of intimate violence	185	8.4
Total	2,205	100.0

TABLE 17.5. MCMI-III Base Rate Scores for Males and Females (*N* = 2,205)

Scale title		Males			Females			*F*
		Mean	SD	Range	Mean	SD	Range	
X.	Disclosure	64.4	18.9	0–100	62.6	20.3	0–100	4.46*
Y.	Desirability	54.4	22.2	0–100	53.9	21.6	0–100	0.33
Z.	Debasement	63.4	20.6	0–100	66.0	20.7	0–100	8.89**
1.	Schizoid	64.8	22.7	0–108	57.5	23.2	0–103	53.71***
2A.	Avoidant	64.0	26.7	0–114	56.5	30.0	0–114	35.93***
2B.	Depressive	71.0	25.8	0–114	61.5	31.2	0–114	55.33***
3.	Dependent	65.7	23.7	0–115	63.9	26.5	0–107	2.65
4.	Histrionic	38.7	19.5	0–84	52.1	24.9	0–98	180.32***
5.	Narcissistic	48.4	20.0	0–114	51.7	21.6	0–115	13.31***
6A.	Antisocial	55.5	23.8	0–99	48.4	21.7	0–102	53.25***
6B.	Sadistic (Aggressive)	49.9	21.3	0–93	50.0	21.6	0–106	0.01
7.	Compulsive	40.7	15.1	0–83	51.0	20.0	0–91	171.23***
8A.	Negativistic (Passive–Aggressive)	57.6	25.6	0–105	52.9	23.8	0–101	19.65***
8B.	Masochistic (Self-Defeating)	54.3	28.5	0–103	56.0	32.2	0–111	1.69
S.	Schizotypal	53.0	27.2	0–106	48.1	27.8	0–105	15.89***
C.	Borderline	57.1	24.9	0–105	54.3	28.1	0–106	6.08**
P.	Paranoid	51.0	26.2	0–111	53.0	26.6	0–114	2.96
A.	Anxiety	69.0	32.3	0–115	65.4	32.0	0–115	6.48**
H.	Somatoform	58.9	23.9	0–111	53.9	27.5	0–115	19.24***
N.	Bipolar: Manic	53.7	19.9	0–98	53.5	21.5	0–113	0.07
D.	Dysthymia	65.5	28.3	0–113	54.8	30.5	0–115	69.40***
B.	Alcohol Dependence	55.1	27.3	0–112	47.4	24.9	0–109	47.02***
T.	Drug Dependence	52.3	23.3	0–106	45.8	25.3	0–113	37.90***
R.	Post-Traumatic Stress Disorder	53.1	26.7	0–109	52.3	26.9	0–114	0.43
SS.	Thought Disorder	59.2	23.7	0–112	54.4	24.4	0–113	21.50***
CC.	Major Depression	59.0	27.5	0–110	57.2	32.5	0–112	1.87
PP.	Delusional Disorder	40.8	28.5	0–105	38.1	30.6	0–115	4.40*

*p < .05. **p .01.; ***p < .0005.

the high range on the Antisocial, Sadistic (Aggressive), Narcissistic, Alcohol Dependence, and Drug Dependence scales. Patients with organic brain damage appeared to score in the lower to middle range on most scales; they had high scores, though, on the Paranoid, Bipolar: Manic, and Delusional Disorder scales.

A number of linear regression analyses were performed to investigate the relative predictive contributions made to scores on each scale by gender, age, and patient group (data not shown). All the regression models were significant. The mean adjusted R^2 value was .06, which represents a small but significant predictive value. The only remarkable adjusted R^2 value was .17 for the Compulsive scale. By comparing the beta values, we could estimate the relative weight for each factor. For the Compulsive scale, female gender β = −.29) and age (β = .28) contributed equally, whereas patient group had a much smaller impact (β = .10). Male gender contributed most to the Schizoid scale (β = .18), while patient group had less impact (β = .11), and age was an insignificant predictor. The reason why patient group was taken into the analyses as an independent factor was that this factor could be considered a continuous variable (even though the placement varied for each scale).

In summary, age appeared to have a larger impact on personality disorders than did gender, but gender predicted the Axis I disorders better than age. Patient group was also an important contributor to a number of scales, with approximately the same degree of impact as gender and age.

Modifying Indices

Table 17.6 compares the base rate scores on scales X, Y, and Z for the Danish and the U.S. norm samples. The distribution of the samples was quite similar. The largest difference was found on Desirability (scale Y), where the U.S. scores were 42% higher (in the 75–115 range).

Reliability and Item Discrimination

Table 17.7 shows the correlation coefficients (Cronbach's alpha) for all indices and scales except for the Disclosure index, which was not relevant due to its large size. Coefficient alpha depends on the correlation between the items of the scale and the number of items in the scale. Many items that approximately measure the same qualities and have high reciprocal correlations, contribute to a high alpha coefficient. With one exception (the Compulsive scale, where $\alpha = .64$), all other alphas were .72 or higher, with a mean for all personality disorders of .81 and for all Axis I disorders of .83. These are very satisfactory levels.

The mean interitem correlation for each scale is also shown in Table 17.7. Values between .20 and .40 are considered optimal (Briggs & Cheek, 1986), as this range reflects an appropriate variation. Very high mean interitem correlations indicate a narrow variation, whereas very low correlations indicate a lack of coherence between items. All 24 mean scale values were between .10 and .34. Seventeen of them were between .20 and .34. The Narcissistic and Compulsive scales had the lowest means. For all the personality scales, the average interitem correlation mean was .23; the similar average mean for scales covering the Axis I disorders was .27.

Table 17.7 also shows the standard error of measurement (*SEM*) for scale raw scores. *SEM* indicates the potential measurement error of a given score. *SEM* is constructed partly from coefficient alpha and partly from the observed standard deviation. The smaller the *SEM*, the more precise confidence levels exist for a test taker's

TABLE 17.6. The Base Rate (BR) Score Ranges for the Modifying Indices in the Danish (*N* = 2,205) and the Millon (*N* = 998) Normative Samples

BR score range	Scale X		Scale Y		Scale Z	
	Millon	Danish	Millon	Danish	Millon	Danish
0–34	14.1%	8.4%	15.7%	18.8%	15.9%	7.6%
35–74	57.8%	58.4%	58.9%	64.9%	53.6%	55.3%
75–84	16.3%	19.3%	16.5%	11.1%	16.6%	21.5%
85–115	11.8%	13.9%	9.0%	5.2%	13.9%	15.6%

TABLE 17.7. Reliability, Interitem Correlations, and *SEM*s of the MCMI-III for the Danish Sample (*N* = 2,205); Alpha Values Added from Millon Normative Sample (*N* = 998)

Scale title		Number of items	α (Danish)	Interitem correlation	*SEM*	α (Millon)
X.	Disclosure	—	—	—	—	—
Y.	Desirability	21	.83	.19	.69	.86
Z.	Debasement	33	.93	.29	.18	.95
1.	Schizoid	16	.78	.18	.11	.81
2A.	Avoidant	16	.88	.32	.14	.89
2B.	Depressive	15	.88	.33	.14	.89
3.	Dependent	16	.82	.22	.13	.85
4.	Histrionic	17	.82	.21	.12	.81
5.	Narcissistic	24	.73	.10	.10	.67
6A.	Antisocial	17	.79	.18	.11	.77
6B.	Sadistic (Aggressive)	20	.81	.17	.12	.79
7.	Compulsive	17	.63	.12	.10	.66
8A.	Negativistic (Passive–Aggressive)	16	.81	.21	.12	.83
8B.	Masochistic (Self-Defeating)	15	.87	.30	.12	.87
S.	Schizotypal	16	.88	.32	.14	.85
C.	Borderline	16	.83	.24	.13	.85
P.	Paranoid	17	.84	.24	.12	.84
A.	Anxiety	14	.87	.31	.12	.86
H.	Somatoform	12	.82	.28	.10	.86
N.	Bipolar: Manic	13	.72	.16	.08	.71
D.	Dysthymia	14	.88	.33	.13	.88
B.	Alcohol Dependence	15	.76	.19	.08	.82
T.	Drug Dependence	14	.83	.25	.09	.83
R.	Post-Traumatic Stress Disorder	16	.89	.32	.13	.89
SS.	Thought Disorder	17	.88	.30	.13	.87
CC.	Major Depression	17	.89	.32	.14	.90
PP.	Delusional Disorder	13	.77	.20	.06	.79

"true" score, which is the average result occurring after a very high number of repeated tests. The potential measurement errors were very small, which signifies that the confidence intervals were very narrow and that the degree of measurement precision was high.

Internal Associations between Scales

Is the Danish version of the MCMI-III comparable to the original Millon sample (Millon, 1997; N = 998) concerning associations among scales? The answer to this is seen in Table 17.8, where the correlations are placed in pairs. A comparison of the U.S. and the Danish α values showed a very high degree of accordance, as all paired correlations had the same direction and were of the same size. The only scale where there were many (16) differences greater than .10 (.11–.14) was the Schizoid scale, where most of the Danish correlations were .12 lower than the U.S. correlations. The

TABLE 17.8. Correlations between MCMI-III Base Rate Scores for the Danish (N = 2,205) and the Millon (N = 998) Normative Samples

Scale title	X	X_M	Y	Y_M	Z	Z_M	1	1_M	2A	2A_M	2B	2B_M	3	3_M	4	4_M	5	5_M	6A	6A_M	6B	6B_M	7	7_M	8A	8A_M
X. Disclosure																										
Y. Desirability	-.59	.62	—																							
Z. Debasement	.79	.80	-.64	-.67	—																					
1. Schizoid	.50	.62	-.58	-.60	.52	.65	—																			
2A. Avoidant	.65	.67	-.75	-.75	.63	.67	.64	.71	—																	
2B. Depressive	.76	.78	-.69	-.69	.74	.77	.52	.64	.71	.72	—															
3. Dependent	.67	.68	-.58	-.61	.63	.66	.38	.48	.65	.65	.68	.63	—													
4. Histrionic	-.56	-.60	.79	.79	-.55	-.60	-.72	-.75	-.80	-.80	-.62	-.65	-.50	-.52	—											
5. Narcissistic	-.40	-.38	.70	.73	-.50	-.45	-.43	-.43	-.65	-.65	-.51	-.48	-.56	-.55	.70	.70	—									
6A. Antisocial	.52	.56	-.25	-.31	.30	.40	.21	.32	.28	.28	.31	.39	.23	.28	-.16	-.14	.06	ns	—							
6B. Sadistic	.60	.59	-.20	-.26	.40	.54	.19	.32	.27	.28	.36	.42	.22	.24	-.14	-.23	.24	.06	.67	.65	—					
7. Compulsive	-.47	-.55	.56	.62	-.38	-.50	-.24	-.38	-.40	-.40	-.41	-.50	-.32	-.39	.46	.46	.24	.36	-.58	-.61	-.42	-.43	—			
8A. Negativistic	.79	.83	-.54	-.52	.68	.75	.45	.57	.61	.61	.66	.69	.54	.56	-.48	-.51	-.33	-.29	.50	.56	.59	.64	-.49	-.63	—	
8B. Masochistic	.77	.78	-.68	-.64	.71	.70	.54	.59	.73	.70	.76	.74	.68	.71	-.58	-.60	-.48	-.45	.35	.42	.38	.40	-.37	-.40	.68	.69
S. Schizotypal	.74	.73	-.63	-.58	.69	.71	.56	.67	.68	.68	.67	.70	.57	.55	-.60	-.61	-.41	-.38	.38	.39	.38	.40	-.41	-.46	.63	.68
C. Borderline	.80	.81	-.60	-.64	.75	.80	.47	.59	.58	.62	.73	.76	.62	.63	-.50	-.55	-.36	-.38	.55	.61	.55	.57	-.55	-.63	.77	.79
P. Paranoid	.71	.74	.41	-.37	.54	.60	.45	.57	.52	.57	.52	.56	.46	.43	-.44	-.47	-.23	-.18	.34	.36	.45	.44	-.26	-.29	.66	.72
A. Anxiety	.69	.69	-.53	-.51	.77	.77	.43	.55	.60	.55	.69	.66	.63	.61	-.48	-.49	-.41	-.37	.28	.32	.35	.40	-.30	-.39	.58	.61
H. Somatoform	.52	.60	-.45	-.53	.77	.79	.49	.61	.46	.54	.56	.65	.43	.55	-.45	-.48	-.38	-.36	.17	.24	.24	.36	-.26	-.35	.46	.55
N. Bipolar: Manic	.57	.62	-.14	-.22	.41	.48	.12	.26	.19	.28	.37	.45	.31	.38	-.28	-.17	ns	ns	.48	.45	.56	.50	-.34	-.36	.48	.59
D. Dysthymia	.70	.72	-.63	-.67	.84	.85	.56	.68	.63	.66	.74	.79	.60	.63	-.60	-.65	-.52	-.48	.29	.36	.33	.37	-.41	-.51	.64	.66
B. Alcohol Dep.	.54	.53	-.29	-.34	.38	.42	.25	.35	.27	.32	.38	.40	.29	.28	-.25	-.37	-.09	-.15	.72	.70	.55	.54	-.46	-.53	.49	.48
T. Drug Dep.	.50	.50	-.20	-.26	.28	.30	.16	.27	.20	.23	.29	.32	.22	.20	-.14	-.22	ns	ns	.83	.82	.58	.48	-.48	-.47	.43	.43
R. PTSD	.73	.74	-.58	-.56	.77	.77	.49	.61	.60	.57	.75	.75	.57	.57	-.51	-.52	-.40	-.37	.32	.36	.38	.39	-.35	-.43	.64	.65
SS. Thought Disor.	.73	.74	-.58	-.58	.82	.82	.51	.62	.60	.60	.74	.76	.60	.60	-.52	-.54	-.40	-.36	.36	.43	.40	.46	-.41	-.48	.66	.68
CC. Major Depres.	.62	.66	-.57	-.64	.84	.85	.52	.62	.58	.58	.63	.69	.51	.58	-.51	-.53	-.46	-.42	.22	.25	.27	.34	-.33	-.41	.54	.57
PP. Delusional Dis.	.56	.58	-.23	-.24	.39	.46	.29	.41	.35	.35	.32	.38	.26	.31	-.27	-.31	ns	ns	.40	.26	.44	.34	-.29	-.22	.48	.53

Scale title	8B	8B_M	S	S_M	C	C_M	P	P_M	A	A_M	H	H_M	N	N_M	D	D_M	B	B_M	T	T_M	R	R_M	SS	SS_M	CC	CC_M
S. Schizotypal	.69	.70	—																							
C. Borderline	.73	.73	.70	—																						
P. Paranoid	.58	.54	.62	.67	.57	.55	—	—																		
A. Anxiety	.64	.60	.67	.64	.67	.67	.51	.55	—																	
H. Somatoform	.49	.56	.49	.57	.52	.58	.33	.46	.60	.66	—															
N. Bipolar: Manic	.39	.47	.44	.50	.55	.57	.39	.50	.39	.48	.25	.32	—													
D. Dysthymia	.69	.70	.64	.65	.70	.74	.45	.51	.68	.68	.74	.78	.34	.35	—											
B. Alcohol Dep.	.39	.41	.42	.40	.55	.54	.36	.34	.35	.35	.22	.26	.45	.39	.37	.38	—									
T. Drug Dep.	.32	.35	.35	.32	.50	.51	.33	.34	.28	.22	.17	.13	.45	.39	.27	.26	.61	.62	—							
R. PTSD	.68	.64	.70	.69	.74	.74	.56	.56	.83	.81	.57	.64	.42	.48	.72	.73	.40	.38	.32	.29	—	—				
SS. Thought Disor.	.67	.67	.76	.76	.78	.79	.51	.57	.76	.77	.63	.71	.47	.52	.79	.79	.41	.42	.33	.33	.77	.76	—			
CC. Major Depres.	.59	.60	.58	.62	.65	.68	.40	.46	.66	.68	.84	.87	.28	.31	.84	.84	.30	.27	.22	.17	.68	.72	.73	.77	—	
PP. Delusional Dis.	.39	.35	.51	.52	.40	.42	.66	.71	.38	.44	.26	.39	.43	.42	.31	.38	.35	.24	.38	.21	.42	.43	.40	.46	.30	.39

Note. Base rate scores for the Millon sample are indicated by a subscript M (e.g., X_M) on scale abbreviations in column heads. ns, nonsignificant.

table shows that there were only three other correlations with a difference greater than .10: the correlations between the Danish and U.S. Histrionic and Alcohol Dependence scales, the Histrionic and Bipolar: Manic scales, and the Antisocial and Delusional Disorder scales.

The Desirability index and the Histrionic, Narcissistic, and Compulsive scales all had a negative sign in relation to all the other scales. The four scales were all positively associated with each other. The Narcissistic scale had a few nonsignificant correlations with other scales.

Correlation analyses supply us with important information about relationships among indices, personality disorders, and Axis I disorders. For example, these analyses reveal that schizoid personality disorder is characterized by a moderate degree of disclosure, little social facade, and moderate debasement, and that it will often co-exist with avoidant personality disorder (possibly combined with depressive, masochistic, and schizotypal traits). Histrionic, narcissistic, and compulsive traits are very unlikely. Among the Axis I disorders, dysthymia is the most likely disorder.

To give an Axis I example, posttraumatic stress disorder is characterized by a high degree of disclosure, strong debasement, and limited social desirability. The most likely comorbid personality disorders are depressive, negativistic, and self-defeating, together with schizotypal, borderline, and paranoid. There is high comorbidity between posttraumatic stress disorder and anxiety, dysthymia, thought disorder, and major depression. These associations are in agreement with recent studies in the field (Schnurr, 1999).

Factor Analysis of the Danish MCMI-III

A scree test was used to reduce the number of factors (Cattell, 1966). The responses were rotated to a four-factor terminal solution, and a cutoff value of .35 was used. The loadings for each item included on each factor are shown in Table 17.9. Items with a secondary positive loading on one factor were ignored if their primary loading on another factor was negative (items 9, 25, 30, 33, 34, 37). The following scales had high loadings on Factor 1: Depressive, Borderline, Anxiety, Somatoform, Dysthymia, Post-Traumatic Stress Disorder, Thought Disorder, and Major Depression. This scale also correlated positively with the Debasement index. The Antisocial, Sadistic (Aggressive), Alcohol Dependence, Drug Dependence, and Bipolar: Manic scales, and to some extent also the Borderline scale, had high loadings on Factor 2. The Compulsive scale had negative loadings on Factor 2. The Histrionic and Narcissistic scales had high positive loadings on Factor 3, whereas the following scales had negative loadings on Factor 3: Schizoid, Avoidant, Dependent, Depressive, and Masochistic (Self-Defeating). This factor was also correlated positively with the Desirability index. The following scales had positive loadings on Factor 4: Negativistic (Passive–Aggressive), Schizotypal, Paranoid, Bipolar: Manic, and Delusional Disorder. This factor also correlated positively with the Debasement index.

We have labeled the factors as follows:

Factor 1: Emotional Instability (Anxiety/Depression/Vulnerability)
Factor 2: Impulsive Aggression versus Constraint

TABLE 17.9. Principal-Components Analysis of the Danish MCMI-III (N = 2,205)

Scale title	Component 1	2	3	4
X. Disclosure				.421
Y. Social Desirability			.810	
Z. Debasement	.831			
1. Schizoid			−.597	
2A. Avoidant			−.774	
2B. Depressive	.468		−.375	
3. Dependent			−.417	
4. Histrionic			.877	
5. Narcissistic			.822	
6A. Antisocial		.966		
6B. Sadistic (Aggressive)		.631		
7. Compulsive		−.776		
8A. Negativistic (Passive–Aggressive)				.362
8B. Masochistic (Self-Defeating)			−.438	
S. Schizotypal			−.355	.422
C. Borderline	.451	.383		
P. Paranoid				.823
A. Anxiety	.686			
H. Somatoform	1.000			
N. Bipolar: Manic		.361		.374
D. Dysthymia	.791			
B. Alcohol Dependence		.778		
T. Drug Dependence		.862		
R. Posttraumatic Stress Disorder	.632			
SS. Thought Disorder	.721			
CC. Major Depression	.966			
PP. Delusional Disorder				.798

Factor 3: Extraversion versus Introversion
Factor 4: Paranoid/Delusional Thinking

There is substantial evidence suggesting a genetic link among anxiety, depression, and neuroticism (Markon, Krueger, Bouchard, & Gottesman, 2002). Factor 1 seems to be measuring this underlining dimension of internalizing disorders and high negative emotionality. Factor 2, on the other hand, is measuring the externalizing disorders with disruptive behavior and substance abuse (Krueger & Tackett, 2003). Substance abuse and antisocial behavior have also been shown to be genetically linked to an impulsive, aggressive personality style (Jang, Vernon, & Livesley, 2000). Factor 3 is capturing one of the more robust findings in personality research: at one pole, stimulus-seeking, histrionic exhibitionism; at the other pole, the schizoid or avoidant personality style. The MCMI-III has scales for severe clinical syndromes, which explains the fourth factor, the psychotic factor: Paranoid–Delusional Thinking. It had the lowest factor loadings. Harkness, McNulty, and Ben-Porath

(1995) also included a psychotic factor, which refers to cognitive and perceptual aberrations, in their Personality Psychopathology Five inventory; however, this construct is seldom included in instruments that have their primary focus on personality. The Paranoid/Delusional Thinking factor and the Emotional Instability factor are unipolar. Normality is the other end of these dimensions.

Rossi, van der Ark, and Sloore (2007; see also Rossi, Sloore, & Derksen, Chapter 16, this volume) also arrived at a four-factor structure for their Dutch version of the MCMI-III, in a sample of 1,210 patients and inmates of European descent. They labeled the four factors General Maladjustment, Aggression/Social Deviance, Paranoid/Delusional Thinking, and Emotional Instability–Detachment. They had a much higher percentage of inpatients, which explains their finding of a General Maladjustment factor. The other factor loadings are quite similar, but the factors are labeled somewhat differently. The differences between the Dutch and the Danish factor loadings are probably more sample-dependent than dependent on cross-cultural differences, the translations, or the constructs of the tests. We have labeled our second and third factors as if they were bipolar dimensions, in which both ends express pathology.

After reviewing the literature on different proposals for classifying personality disorders, Widiger and Simonsen (2005) suggested an alternative dimensional model of four common higher-order bipolar dimensions: Emotional Dysregulation versus Emotional Stability, Impulsivity versus Constraint, Extraversion versus Introversion, Antagonism versus Compliance. In the Danish MCMI-III sample, Impulsivity versus Constraint and Antagonism versus Compliance seem to blend, becoming one factor. Unconventionality versus Closedness to experience seems not to be relevant for assessing personality pathology, but rather more general aspects of personality functioning. On the contrary, the Paranoid/Delusional Thinking factor in the MCMI-III reflects the approach toward general psychopathology.

Reflections on Cross-Cultural Issues in the Assessment of Personality

The issue of whether a personality trait is maladaptive, or causes functional impairment or subjective distress, is obviously related to the cultural context. Different cultures have tended to emphasize different traits as ideal. The Buddhist priests in Asian countries have values and behavior for which they are highly respected; the essential traits include solitary activities, lack of emotional expression, lack of sexual desire, indifference to praise and criticism, and constricted affect—all traits that fall within the definition of schizoid personality disorder. They would not be regarded as having a personality disorder in their own society, however. Similarly, the shamans in other cultures believe in magical thinking, enhance unusual perceptual experiences, show odd and eccentric behavior, and converse in abstract or otherwise "inappropriate" speech, but are not regarded as having schizotypal personality disorder. Each society has its own values and preferences. In Western societies, fashion models, show girls, and actresses are valued for their histrionic traits; grandiose political leaders and businessmen are admired for their narcissistic traits; and scholars, scientists, and ministers are rewarded for their obsessive–compulsive traits. Dependent traits are valued in Inuit cultures.

These examples illustrate that validation of a diagnostic system or a diagnostic instrument like the MCMI has no international "gold standard" to refer to. If the MCMI is to be valid and reliable in cultures outside the United States, the issue of equivalence has to be considered. Equivalence should be obtained in different ways, but each way also presents possible methodological pitfalls:

1. *Linguistic equivalence*. Do the same content and grammar have similar denotative and connotative meanings across cultures? The wording of feelings, thoughts, and behavior often cannot be translated in accurate ways. Each language has its own origin, and vocabularies vary in numbers and content. One way of checking how well the psychological meaning of the original version is kept in the translation procedure is to ensure that a back-translation is carried out. An important example of the connotative problem is the different way in which depression is described in different cultures. Some cultures refer to somatic sensations, others to a set of psychological terms, and still others to external things.

2. *Conceptual equivalence*. As discussed above regarding diagnostic categories, psychological concepts are understood and valued in very different ways across cultures. To be dependent, undemanding, and self-effacing may be valued in one culture, but in another culture it may be regarded as immaturity.

3. *Scale equivalence*. Members of some cultures are not familiar with the principle of scaling their behavior. For example, they may not be able to differentiate among being sad "sometimes," "often," or "all the time." They can only react to such a question with a "yes" or "no" answer.

4. *Norm equivalence*. Patients should be evaluated against culturally applicable norms.

Each culture has its own standards for normal and abnormal behavior, as noted above. There is no such a thing as a universal set of norms.

Conclusion

The MCMI, originally developed in 1977, is now one of the most popular objective personality tests in the United States and in Europe. An important aspect of international research on the MCMI is to validate the test in different cultures and across different diagnostic groups. The MCMI personality scales were originally validated in North American culture, which teaches and reinforces certain values in social behavior. Genetic factors are involved in the expression of personality traits, and, depending on a society's value for such traits, mating patterns will select for them. A society not only idealizes certain traits, but because of cultural learning factors develops its own unique dimensions and patterns of personality, which will establish unique standards of normality. Consequently, we should expect the prevalence of "abnormal" personality types to differ from society to society. Differences in thresholds for abnormal behavior and prevalence of disorders may be a threat to validity of the MCMI subscales in different cultures.

In our translation and validation of the MCMI-III in Denmark, we found that the differences between the original U.S. Millon sample and the Danish sample were quite small, and the MCMI-III appears to be quite robust and consistent with the original norms when applied in a Danish context. The analyses provided some evidence that the age factor may be as important as the gender factor, which may have implications for future changes in base rate scores. The special position of the three "salutogenic" personality scales (Narcissistic, Histrionic, and Compulsive) also deserves future research attention. Is there an upper threshold where these three scales are associated with psychopathology? If this is not the case, then they should be dramatically changed in, or removed from, a future Danish version of the MCMI.

References

Briggs, R. S., & Cheek, J. M. (1986). The role of factor analysis in the development and evaluation of personality scales. *Journal of Personality, 54,* 106–104.

Brislin, R. W. (1970). Backtranslation for cross-cultural research. *Journal of Cross-Cultural Research, 1,* 185–286.

Cattell, R. B. (1966). The scree test for the number of factors. *Multivariate Behavioral Research, 1,* 245–276.

Hambleton, R. (1994). Guidelines for adapting educational and psychological tests: A progress report. *European Journal of Psychological Assessment, 10,* 229–244.

Harkness, A. R., McNulty, J. L., & Ben-Porath, Y. S. (1995). Personality Psychopathology Five (PSY-5): Constructs and MMPI-2 scales. *Personality Assessment, 7,* 104–114.

Jang, K. L., Vernon, P. A, & Livesley, W. J. (2000). Personality traits, family environment, and alcohol misuse: A multivariate behavioral genetic analysis. *Addiction, 95,* 873–888.

Krueger, R. F., & Tackett, J. L. (2003). Personality and psychopathology: Working towards the bigger picture. *Journal of Personality Disorders, 17,* 109–128.

Loevinger, J. (1957). Objective tests as instruments of psychological theory. *Psychological Reports, 3,* 635–694.

Markon, K. E., Krueger, R. F., Bouchard, T. J., & Gottesman, I. I. (2002). Normal and abnormal personality traits: Evidence for genetic and environmental relationships in the Minnesota study of twins reared apart. *Journal of Personality, 70,* 661–693.

Millon, T. (1977). *Millon Clinical Multiaxial Inventory manual.* Minneapolis, MN: National Computer Systems.

Millon, T. (1981). *Disorders of personality: DSM-III, Axis II.* New York: Wiley.

Millon, T. (1987). *Millon Clinical Multiaxial Inventory–II manual.* Minneapolis, MN: National Computer Systems.

Millon, T., & Davis, R. D. (1996). *Disorders of personality: DSM-IV and beyond.* New York: Wiley.

Millon, T. (with Millon, C., & Davis, R. D.). (1994). *Millon Clinical Multiaxial Inventory–III manual.* Minneapolis, MN: National Computer Systems.

Millon, T. (with Millon, C., & Davis, R. D.). (1997). *Millon Clinical Multiaxial Inventory–III manual* (2nd ed.). Minneapolis, MN: National Computer Systems.

Rossi, G., van der Ark, L. A., & Sloore, H. V. (2007). Factor analysis of the Dutch-language version of the MCMI-III. *Journal of Personality Assessment, 85.*

Schnurr, P. P. (1999). Personality as a Risk Factor for PTSD. In R. Yehuda (Ed.), *Risk factors for posttraumatic stress disorder.* Washington, DC, American Psychiatric Press.

Simonsen, E., & Mortensen, E. L. (1990). Difficulties in translation of personality scales. *Journal of Personality Disorders, 4*(3), 290–296.

Widiger, T. A., & Simonsen, E. (2005). Alternative dimensional models of personality disorders: Finding a common ground. *Journal of Personality Disorders, 19,* 110–130.

CHAPTER 18

On the Dimensional Theory, Empirical Support, and Structural Character of the MCMI-III

Stephen Strack
Theodore Millon

As known by readers of this text, the *Millon Clinical Multiaxial Inventory–III* (MCMI-III; Millon, 1997b, 2006) was created to assist clinicians in understanding the psychiatric problems of greatest concern to their patients and to contextualize the patients' presentation features within a personality framework. A guiding assumption of the inventory is that everyone has a personality that influences the kind and severity of problems experienced, the expression of symptoms, and the types of treatments that are most likely to be effective.

The test measures 14 personality disorders (PDs) and 10 clinical syndromes (CSs) via ordinal scales that quantify how much and how well respondents match or fit the constructs being assessed. With regard to the PD scales, items are divided into two groups: one representing core features of the personality that are unique to that disorder, and one representing features that are more peripheral and likely to be shared with one or more similar PDs. For scoring purposes, the core items (also called "prototype items") are weighted 2, while peripheral, overlapping items are weighted 1. Therefore, the highest raw scores for each PD scale are obtained by respondents who acknowledge more of the attitudes, thoughts, feelings, and behaviors that are central to the definition of that personality.

In line with the *Diagnostic and Statistical Manual of Mental Disorders*, fourth edition, and its text revision (DSM-IV and DSM-IV-TR; American Psychiatric Association, 1994, 2000), MCMI-III Axis II PDs are assessed separately from Axis I CSs. To assist in diagnosing patients according to the DSM-IV(-TR), PD scale items cover major diagnostic criteria, and normative data were obtained from psychiatric patients with known DSM-IV(-TR) diagnoses (Millon, 1997b, 2006). Estimating the prevalence of each disorder within the test's normative sample permitted scale scores to be transformed into "base rate" (BR) scores that help in categorizing patients according to DSM-IV(-TR) criteria. For example, knowing that patients in the normative sample who were diagnosed as having schizoid PD had raw scores on the MCMI-III Schizoid scale above a particular point allowed Millon to establish a BR cutoff score that would alert the test user to a patient who was likely to meet DSM-IV(-TR) criteria for a schizoid PD.

The MCMI-III is one of a family of assessment instruments (Millon, 1997a; Strack, 2008) that operationalize Millon's (e.g., 1969, 1990, 2005; Millon & Davis, 1996; Millon & Grossman, 2006) evolutionary model of personality and psychopathology. As noted in earlier chapters of this text, the model represents an attempt to create a mature clinical science of personology by embodying five key elements:

1. *Universal scientific principles*: Science grounded in the ubiquitous laws of nature.
2. *Subject-oriented theories*: Explanatory and heuristic conceptual schemas of nature's expression in what we call "personology" and "psychopathology."
3. *A taxonomy of personality patterns and clinical syndromes*: A classification and nosology derived logically from a coordinated personality–psychopathology theory.
4. *Integrated clinical and personality assessment instruments*: Tools that are empirically grounded and quantitatively sensitive.
5. *Synergistic therapeutic interventions*: Coordinated strategies and modalities of treatment.

According to Millon (2005; Millon & Grossman, 2006), the coordination of these elements so that they are reciprocally enhancing and mutually reinforcing constitutes the essence of a mature clinical science. Just as each person is an intrinsic unity, each component of a clinical science should not remain a separate element of unconnected parts. Rather, each facet of our clinical work—its principles, theories, taxonomy, instrumentation, and therapy—should be integrated into a gestalt, a coupled and synergistic unity in which the whole will be coordinated, and will become more informative and useful than its individual parts.

The Dimensional Model

Contained within Millon's theoretical model are his (e.g., Millon, 2005, 2006; Millon & Davis, 1996; Millon & Grossman, 2006) specifications for a personality taxonomy (see Figure 18.1). Millon believes that it is best for the DSM to employ diagnostic targets that represent complex personality "prototypes" (e.g., schizoid, avoidant, dependent), as opposed to dimensional traits such as dominance–submissiveness or sociability, which he views as subcomponents of the prototypes.[1] Millon also believes that the fundamental building blocks of the prototypes are continuously distributed "domain traits" (see below), and so personality prototypes can be assessed quantitatively as well as categorically. For him, a personality prototype is a superordinate category that subsumes and integrates psychologically covariant

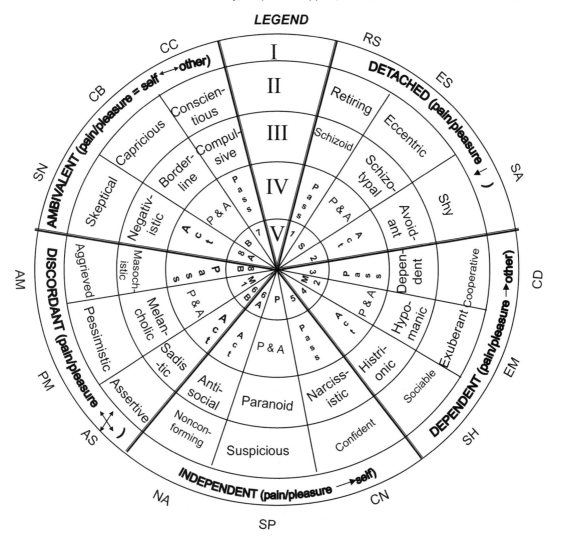

FIGURE 18.1. Personality circulargram I: Normal and abnormal personality patterns. Evolutionary foundations of the normal and abnormal extremes of each personality prototype of the 15 spectra. I, existential orientation; II, normal prototype; III, abnormal prototype; IV, adaptation style; V, MCMI-III scale number/letter. Copyright 2006 by Theodore Millon. Reprinted by permission.

traits, which in turn represent a set of correlated habits that, in their turn, stand for a response displayed in a variety of situations (Millon & Grossman, 2006). In this way, categories and dimensions may be coordinated and are not mutually exclusive.

Millon (see Millon & Davis, 1996) has argued that personality prototypes can be described and differentiated by a set of functional (expressive behaviors, interpersonal conduct, cognitive style, intrapsychic regulatory mechanisms) and structural (self-image, object representations, morphological organization, mood/temperament) domain attributes, which can be optimally assessed using one of four data sources (behavioral, phenomenological, intrapsychic, biophysical). These components, which can be measured quantitatively, are more clinically useful than atheoretically-derived factor traits such as openness (see Figures 18.2 and 18.3, and Table 18.1).

Functional domain attributes represent dynamic processes that occur in the intrapsychic world between the self and psychosocial environment. They represent expressive modes of regulatory action that manage, adjust, transform, coordinate, balance, and otherwise control the give and take of inner and outer life. By contrast, structural attributes represent deeply embedded, relatively enduring templates of imprinted memories, attitudes, needs, fears, and conflicts that guide experience and transform the nature of our ongoing life events. Structural attributes may be conceived as substrates and action dispositions of a quasi-permanent nature that have an orienting and preemptive effect to alter the character of action and the impact of sub-

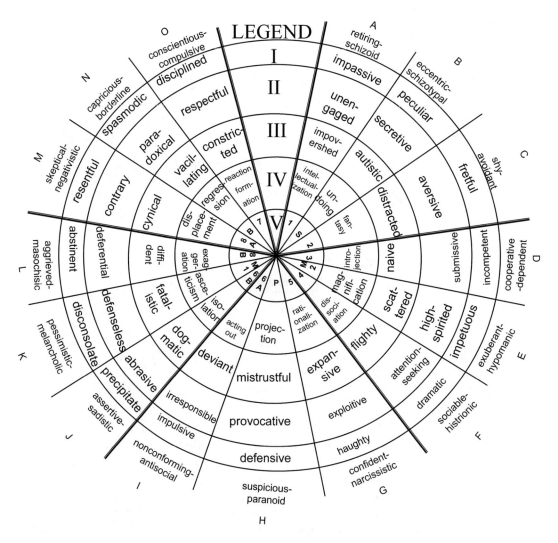

FIGURE 18.2. Personality circulargram IIA: Functional personological domains. I, expressive behaviors; II, interpersonal conduct; III, cognitive style/content; IV, intrapsychic regulatory mechanisms; V, MCMI-III scale. Copyright 2006 by Theodore Millon. Reprinted by permission.

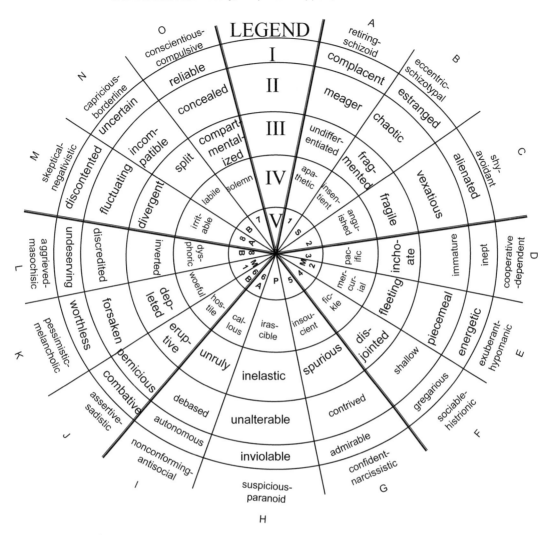

FIGURE 18.3. Personality circulargram IIB: Structural personological domains. I, self-image; II, intrapsychic content; III, intrapsychic structure; IV, mood/temperament; V, MCMI-III scale. Copyright 2006 by Theodore Millon. Reprinted by permission.

sequent experiences in line with the preformed inclinations and expectancies (Millon & Davis, 1996). The rationale for creating the domain traits was that they had to encompass a full range of clinically relevant characteristics (e.g., not just behaviors or cognitions); to provide true distinction among the various prototypes; to parallel or correspond to major therapeutic modalities (e.g., intrapsychic); and to allow for coordination between and among the structural and functional attributes and four levels of data (Millon & Davis, 1996).

Millon (1969; Millon & Davis, 1996) has also specified that the same personality prototypes can be used to describe "normality" and "abnormality." He suggests that normal and abnormal traits lie along a continuum, with no sharp dividing line

TABLE 18.1. Functional and Structural Domains of Personality and Their Optimal Data Sources

Functional domain	Data source	Structural domain
	Behavioral	
Expressive behaviors Interpersonal conduct		
	Phenomenological	
Cognitive style		Object representations Self-image
	Intrapsychic	
Regulatory mechanisms		Morphological organization
	Biophysical	
		Mood/temperament

Note. Although the domains are best measured using the data sources indicated in the table, they can be assessed with some accuracy by using traditional questionnaire and interview methods. Adapted from Millon and Davis (1996, p. 138). Copyright 1996 by John Wiley & Sons, Inc. Adapted by permission.

between the two. Normal and abnormal personality prototypes share similar domain traits, behaviors, and background characteristics. For example, the normally shy personality (see Figures 18.1–18.3) has much in common with the pathological avoidant prototype. The major difference is that the shy person maintains a relatively healthy, flexible adaptation to the environment, whereas the avoidant person lacks the ability to adapt effectively due to rigid and inflexible traits. As such, a diagnostic manual containing Millon's prototypes could be used to assess normal as well as disordered personality.[2]

Furthermore, the model divides personality prototypes into "basic" and "severe" categories. Millon's (1969; Millon & Davis, 1996) group of basic personalities can be found in normal adults as healthy, adaptive styles, or in patients as disorders. The severe personalities—schizotypal, borderline, and paranoid—are viewed as distortions or exaggerations of basic personality types that sometimes have subdiagnostic, almost normal, counterparts (e.g., an eccentric personality is less pathological than a schizotypal style; see Figure 18.1). The logic for differentiating basic and severe personality types comes from the idea that normal personality has evolved over many years to help people survive and adapt, whereas abnormal personality arises from things that go wrong. Finally, the personality prototypes can be usefully combined to describe "subtypes" (e.g., schizoid–narcissistic, avoidant–negativistic, compulsive–dependent). Most people manifest trait characteristics that typify different prototypes in varying degrees.[3] When the domains constituting the several prototypes are measured quantitatively, an overall personality profile can be generated for each person that shows which trait characteristics are most dominant or salient. In this model, the basic personality prototypes (e.g., avoidant, histrionic) are believed to emanate from universal evolutionary processes and are based on semistructured, relatively unchanging characteristics; the subtypes tend to be less fixed, more changeable, and subject to transient environmental influences (Davis & Patterson, 2005; Grossman & del Rio, 2005; Millon & Davis, 1996; Millon & Grossman, 2006).

The MCMI-III PD scales operationalize the standard prototypes of the model directly and quantifiably. Scale scores are continuous, yet enable categorical diagnoses with the use of BRs anchored to the normative sample of DSM-assessed patients. The use of patient norms limits the appropriateness of the scales for assessing normal-range trait characteristics, but respondents can be differentiated as likely to be normal or disordered on the basis of PD scale elevations below and above the clinically significant cutoff of BR = 75. Importantly, a profile of each respondent can be generated to ascertain subtype characteristics, allowing for a rich and complex personality description that has a high probability of matching clinical impressions, especially those based on interpersonal and expressive behaviors (Choca, 2004; Craig, 1999, 2008).

Reliability, Validity, and Factorial Structure

How can the validity of an instrument be assessed in the absence of an objectively defined and consensual criterion? Without an absolute reference point or objective standard, not only does no rigorous feedback loop exist that might directly quantify and therefore guarantee the validity of an instrument, but no such feedback loop *can* exist. Psychological constructs, especially those relating to personality traits, are by definition diverse and largely inferential, and therefore are not anchored to any absolute criterion. This fact requires a different conception of validity from that used with simple and objective observables. Where the constructs are multireferential and hierarchical, validity must be acknowledged as being multireferential and hierarchical as well. Just as any single behavioral act not only will but must fail as an unequivocal measure of the construct of interest, simply because its bandwidth is too narrow to represent the construct in its totality, a single study—conducted as it is in the particularities of time, circumstance, and sample characteristics—must also be viewed as inadequate to establish the construct validity of an instrument.

How, then, is the construction of diagnostic and personality assessment instruments possible at all? Without a construct validity coefficient and the rigorous feedback it would make possible, we have only our expectations concerning what an instrument should do to guide us, both in construction and in evaluation. Two general principles apply.

First, our expectations, whether explicit or not, are really theories about relationships between different gauges of a construct. Accordingly, because all we have with which to evaluate construct validity are our expectations and not some single, external, and absolute criterion, the content of the constructs to be included in the inventory and the relations between them should be specified as precisely as possible. Otherwise, we will be left, despite our time and effort, with something the quality of which can only be determined after the fact—by delineating post hoc what should have been specified from the beginning.

Second, we must distinguish between variables that are internal and external to those of a diagnostic inventory, and specify these internal–external relationships as well. If our inventory is intended to assess personality disorders, we might expect, for example, that those classified as having dependent personalities will also be classified as experiencing depressive episodes more often than will, say, those identified as having antisocial personalities, simply because dependent individuals are likely to feel helpless and hopeless more often than antisocial individuals, who are more likely to take matters into their own hands and change the world around them (albeit in a self-aggrandizing fashion). Together, these internal–internal and internal–external expectations form a set of constraints that our inventory must be constructed to satisfy. The larger this set of constraints, the better, for if the inventory can satisfy many such constraints at the outset, then validity has been built into the instrument from the beginning. In general, the more such constraints the test has been shown to satisfy, the better the instrument, and the greater confidence we can have that it will meet whatever challenges are put to it in the future. Each constraint is an additional point through which the patterns of findings emerging from the instrument are triangulated with reality as it is assumed to exist in theory.

In their thoughtful article more than 50 years ago on the concept of construct validity in psychological tests, Cronbach and Meehl (1955) wrote that the nomological network of relationships among internal concepts and external observables is what provides the basis of an instrument's undergirding theory. The value and interpretability of a test's scores are, in large measure, functions of the comprehensiveness of this network of supporting observables and concepts. No single observable or concept can serve as *the* ultimate criterion, the so-called "gold standard" against which all other parts of the network are to be judged as deficient. The more the instrument is grounded in a range of minicriteria, internal and external, the more likely is it to possess a solid level of generalizable validity and reliability. Such construct validity is, in effect, likely to be more substantial than would any single criterion.

To complicate matters further in test validation, whatever gauge or criterion may be employed must demonstrate a high level of correlation with other established criteria and must be coordinated with the theory's conceptual network. In addition, as Retzlaff (1996) has pointed out, preliminary validation studies of an instrument such as the MCMI-III often prove inadequate to the validation task, owing to methodological deficiencies—for example, the adequacy of the diagnostic criteria employed; the level and frequency of contact between clinical judges and patients; the extent to which clinicians know their patients' traits and difficulties; the diversity in, if not conflicting purposes of, the study; and so on.

We may find it useful to illustrate how detailed knowledge of the characteristics of both specific patients and knowledge of the nomological network of the theory (science?) are necessary to achieve accurate or valid judgments. We use a six-sided die to discuss the pros and cons of this analysis. If we were to roll the die and guess the result, our accuracy level would be approximately 16.67%. However, if we had considerable experience with a particular die and had learned that the number 3 showed up 40% of the time (and the others less than 16%), we would gradually modify our guesses so that the number 3 would be chosen more frequently than any of the others. That is, our BR for guessing would change from some expected chance number in which all possibilities are equally likely to one in which the number 3 would be guessed more frequently, probably until it reached roughly 40% of the time.

We can shift from the preceding example to one in which different die proportions emerge over time. Experience teaches us to approximate what those proportions are. In the case just noted, the number 3 was guessed roughly 40% of the time. In another situation, we might find that the number 5 showed up roughly 50% of the time. In time, the judgments we made for each number would approximate the actual BR for that particular die. Note, however, that the specific individual judgments for each throw in a series might be wrong, although the overall BRs would gradually approximate reality. We would not need to guess any single case correctly for the *overall* BR of our judgments to be quite accurate. Single judgments could remain as erroneous as ever (except that by selecting high BR die numbers, we would make our results more likely to be a little bit better than chance).

This die example approximates what occurs when clinicians make their diagnostic judgments about patients whom they do not know well. Clinicians who work in a particular setting may be very good at estimating that setting's *overall* BRs, but may not be very good at making *specific* diagnostic judgments. How do we improve the accuracy of these judgments? Let us go back to the die. If one has plenty of time to study an individual die (to look at its scratches, chips, etc., so that one can assess its distinctive characteristics), and if one understands enough about the physics of what happens to dice when they are chipped here or marred there, this knowledge should enhance the accuracy of individual judgments—not merely the overall BR proportions. Likewise, if a clinician knows a particular patient very well (and can identify his or her traits, features, history, etc.), *and* if the clinician has studied personality pathology in great detail, he or she then has both general knowledge of the way pathological personality traits interrelate and the distinctive features of the specific patient in question. Consequently, the clinician's judgments should be appreciably better than chance.

Not untypically, most clinical judges in an early MCMI-III validation study saw the subjects only once, and usually without the benefit of clinical interviews or extensive readings of their histories. It was like picking up a die, glancing at it, guessing, and then throwing it. They did not know the subjects well. Nor do we know the level of sophistication the clinicians had concerning PDs. If they had time to study the subjects, and if they had studied the PD literature extensively, then we would have considerable confidence in the accuracy of their individual judgments. Without such background information, their judgments would probably be suitable only for estimating overall BRs. For making individual clinical diagnoses, their lack of familiarity with the subjects and perhaps with the clinical literature on PDs would be likely to result in judgments that were less than satisfactory.

Not all of the innovative ideas developed in the MCMI and its sister inventories have succeeded in fulfilling its aims. Although these instruments can justly be credited with significant areas of success, their notable conceptual goals and validational evaluations have been appraised as lukewarm by some and enthusiastically by others.

Since the introduction of the MCMI in 1977, it has become one of the most frequently used assessment instruments for the examination of PDs and CSs. Only the Rorschach and Minnesota Multiphasic Personality Inventory–2 (MMPI-2) have produced more research during the past 15 years. There are now over 500 empirical studies based on this measure, as well as seven MCMI-related books (Craig, 2008, 2005). A full examination of this literature is beyond our scope, but recent reviews are available (e.g., Choca, 2004; Craig, 1999, 2005; Retzlaff & Dunn, 2003). For our purposes, it will be useful to see whether the MCMI PD scales (1) have been shown to be reliable; (2) yield continuous distributions in patient samples; (3) exhibit concurrent, convergent, and discriminant validity against other PD measures and DSM criteria; (4) yield profile subgroups akin to those proposed by Millon (Davis & Patterson, 2005; Grossman & del Rio, 2005; Millon & Davis, 1996; Millon & Grossman, 2006); and (5) show evidence of continuity in normal populations.

Reliability

The "internal consistency" of test scales refers to how well the items measure the same construct (Nunnally, 1978). High internal consistency (e.g., coefficient alpha ≥ .80) is expected for measures of stable personality characteristics to reflect the cohesiveness of the underlying traits. Lower levels of internal consistency (e.g., coefficient alpha ≥ .70) are acceptable for research instruments and measures of less stable traits in abnormal populations. MCMI PD scales have historically exhibited good levels of internal consistency, although two MCMI-III measures (Compulsive and Narcissistic) exhibited less than desirable values (coefficient alpha = .66 and .67, respectively). As a group, estimates for the scales have ranged from .73 to .95 for the MCMI-I (median = .82; Millon, 1983, p. 47); .86 to .93 for the MCMI-II (median = .90; Millon, 1987, p. 129); and .66 to .89 for the MCMI-III (median = .84; Millon, 2006, p. 58). The lowest internal consistency estimates for the MCMI-III came from two scales assessing a number of normal, healthy attributes that are infrequently found in samples of psychiatric patients (Choca, 2004). The low endorsement frequency of items assessing normal, healthy characteristics in psychiatric samples is not unexpected, since most patients do not advertise their positive features when seeking help.

"Test–retest reliability" indicates how stable test scores are over time (Nunnally, 1978). Personality scales are expected to be reliable over long periods of time among adult respondents, owing to the pervasive and ingrained nature of the underlying traits, attitudes, and behaviors. A variety of studies using different patient populations and test–retest intervals ranging from 5 days to 3 years have shown good stability for MCMI-II and MCMI-III PD scale scores. For the MCMI-I, most studies reported a test–retest interval of about 3 months and yielded a median reliability coefficient for all scales of $r = .71$, with a range of .19 (Passive–Aggressive) to .91 (Histrionic). For the MCMI-II, retest intervals between 21 days and 4 months (average was 2–3 months) yielded a median stability value of $r = .73$ for all scales, with a range of .62 (Borderline) to .78 (Compulsive). For the MCMI-III, retest intervals between 5 days and 4 months have provided a median value across PD scales of $r = .78$, with a range of .58 (Depressive) to .93 (Depressive, Antisocial, Borderline) (Craig, 1999).

Distribution of Scaled Scores

The continuous distribution of a test score is expected when the characteristic being measured is believed to be continuously distributed in the target population (Nunnally, 1978). According to Millon's (e.g., Millon & Davis, 1996) model of personality, the traits underlying PD prototypes, as well as the prototypes themselves, should demonstrate continuity in psychiatric samples. The PD scales of all versions of the MCMI have been shown to have a continuous underlying distribution (Choca, 2004). Owing to the pathological nature of most MCMI test items, the score distributions are not "normal"; rather, they typically show significant positive skew. That is, most respondents have low rates of scale item endorsement, with progressively fewer people showing high endorsement rates. Distributions that approach normality are sometimes found in the MCMI scales measuring more normal characteristics (Histrionic, Narcissistic, Compulsive). For example, in a sample of 2,366 psychiatric patients (see Haddy, Strack, & Choca, 2005, for details), skewness of the MCMI-III weighted raw score PD scales ranged from –.17 to .74, with a median of .25. The Histrionic, Narcissistic, and Compulsive scales exhibited the most (nearly) normal distributions, with skewness coefficients of –.15, .08, and –.17, respectively. Distributions for the least skewed (Narcissistic) and most skewed (Schizotypal) PD scales are given in Figure 18.4.

Empirical Validation Studies

MCMI PD scales have fared well as a group in terms of concurrent, convergent, and discriminant validity when measured against other self-report measures of PDs (Choca, 2004; Craig, 1999; Retzlaff & Dunn, 2003; Rossi, Van den Brande, Tobac, Sloore, & Hauben, 2003). Rossi, Van den Brande, et al. (2003) noted consistent improvements in validity with each new version of the test and found the best concurrent validity between MCMI-III PD scales and the MMPI-2 PD scales developed by Somwaru and Ben-Porath (1995). In their sample of 477 patients and prisoners, who completed a Dutch language version of the MCMI-III, they found that the same PD scales across measures correlated between .56 (Narcissistic) and .75 (Borderline), with the exception of the MCMI-III Compulsive scale, which did not correlate positively with any of the Somwaru and Ben-Porath (1995) or Morey et al. (Colligan, Morey, & Offord, 1994; Morey, Blashfield, Webb, & Jewell, 1988) MMPI-2 PD scales. Their survey of the literature pointed to a pattern of poor concurrent, convergent, and discriminant validity for this scale across all versions of the MCMI, which suggests that Millon's conceptualization of this disorder is different from that of other test developers (see also Choca, 2004, and Craig, 1999).

The MCMI-I (Millon, 1977) was the first multidimensional measure to operationalize Meehl and Rosen's (1955) idea of BRs to assist in clinical diagnosis. All versions of the inventory provide transformations of raw scale scores into BR scores to reflect the distributions of various diagnoses in the normative samples. BR scores increase as a function of the probability that the respondent will meet DSM diagnostic criteria for a particular disorder. A cutoff score of BR $\geq$ 75 is assigned when scale score elevations reach a level where diagnosis is probable, and a cutoff score of BR $\geq$ 85 is assigned when the disorder is likely to be the respondent's most prominent presenting problem. BR cutoff scores allow for categorical diagnosis, as well as the calculation of statistics to estimate how accurate the scales are in identifying "true" cases.

All three versions of the MCMI have been shown to be useful in making DSM diagnoses of PDs in clinical samples, although results vary by scale (Choca, 2004; Millon, 1997b, 2006). As a rule, no self-report measure—including the MCMI—

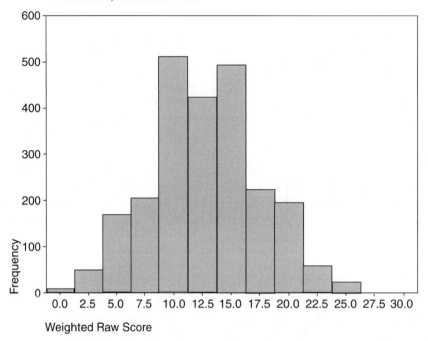

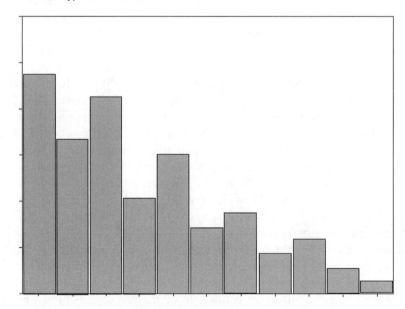

FIGURE 18.4. Distribution of MCMI-III weighted raw scores for the least skewed (top) and most skewed (bottom) PD scales in a sample of 2,366 psychiatric patients. From Strack and Millon (2007, p. 61). Copyright 2007 by Lawrence Erlbaum Associates, Inc. Reprinted by permission of the Taylor & Francis Group.

should be used by itself for making clinical diagnoses (Millon & Davis, 1996; Millon, 1997b, 2006; Rossi, Hauben, Van den Brande, & Sloore, 2003). Nevertheless, research has shown that the MCMI is more diagnostically accurate than clinical interviews, and more accurate than similar self-report measures of personality (e.g., the MMPI-2; Retzlaff & Dunn, 2003), but not more accurate than structured interviews conducted by experienced clinicians (Choca, 2004; Craig, 1999, 2005).[4]

There are several widely used estimates of the diagnostic precision of test scales (Gibertini, Brandenburg, & Retzlaff, 1986; Hsu, 2002). Among them are the following: "Sensitivity" is defined as the percentage of patients identified by clinicians as having a particular diagnosis who were then identified by the scale as having the same disorder. "Positive predictive power" is defined as the percentage of patients identified as having a particular disorder by the scale who were also judged by clinicians as having the same disorder. Conversely, "negative predictive power" is defined as the percentage of patients identified by a test scale as *not* having a particular disorder who were judged by clinicians as also not having the disorder. Each of these estimates provide a different perspective on a test scale's accuracy in making (or not making) a diagnosis. However, they do not fully account for the relationship between test accuracy and the prevalence (BR) rate of various disorders. When the prevalence of a disorder is high (say, 50%), then a test scale will need to accurately diagnose that disorder significantly more than 50% of the time to be useful, because without the test a clinician can accurately make the same diagnosis 50% of the time just based on chance. Alternatively, when the BR of a disorder is quite low (say, 5%), a test scale may make a useful contribution if it correctly diagnoses that disorder 25% of the time, since this signals an increased accuracy of 20% above chance. "Incremental validity" of a positive test diagnosis is an estimate of a scale's accuracy beyond chance, and is calculated by subtracting the BR of a disorder from the scale's positive predictive power (Hsu, 2002).[5]

Table 18.2 provides a summary of the diagnostic efficiency of MCMI-III PD scales. Data were collected from a sample of 322 psychiatric patients and 67 experienced clinicians (for details, see Millon, 1997b, pp. 88–100). The clinicians were asked to select patients from their caseload whom they had seen at least three times (mode = 7), and then to complete a rating scale giving their estimate of each patient's three most prominent PD traits. Clinicians were asked to make their ratings without awareness of the patients' MCMI-III results, but the data collection method did not strictly control for this. As a result, some bias is likely to have accrued, such that the accuracy estimates are probably inflated (Hsu, 2002). In Table 18.2, the "prevalence rate" refers to the percentage of study patients judged as having the particular PD as their primary Axis II diagnosis, while the various statistics were computed based on the patients' highest MCMI-III PD scale elevation. As can be seen in the table, sensitivity ranged from 44% (Negativistic [Passive–Aggressive]) to 92% (Paranoid); positive predictive power ranged from 30% (Masochistic [Self-Defeating]) to 81% (Dependent); negative predictive power was uniformly high at 94% to 100%; and the incremental validity of a positive test diagnosis ranged from a low of 26% (Masochistic) to a high of 75% (Paranoid), with a median of 60%. The scales with the lowest validity estimates (Depressive, Negativistic, and Masochistic) measure PDs that are not included in the current diagnostic manual, which may have been a point of confusion for some raters, and, although the Sadistic (Aggressive) scale measures a PD

TABLE 18.2. Diagnostic Efficiency Estimates for MCMI-III PD Scales

PD scale	Prevalence (%)	Sensitivity (%)	Positive predictive power (%)	Negative predictive power (%)	Incremental validity of a positive test diagnosis (%)
1. Schizoid	6	56	67	97	61
2A. Avoidant	11	65	73	96	62
2B. Depressive	12	57	49	94	37
3. Dependent	13	54	81	94	68
4. Histrionic	7	74	63	98	56
5. Narcissistic	7	59	72	97	65
6A. Antisocial	6	61	50	98	44
6B. Sadistic (Aggressive)	2	71	71	99	69
7. Compulsive	9	73	79	97	70
8A. Negativistic (Passive–Aggressive)	5	44	39	97	34
8B. Masochistic (Self-Defeating)	4	58	30	98	26
S. Schizotypal	3	82	60	99	57
C. Borderline	12	60	71	94	59
P. Paranoid	4	92	79	100	75

Note. Patient *N* = 322; clinician *N* = 67. Data on prevalence, sensitivity, and positive predictive power are from Millon (2006). Data on negative predictive power and incremental validity of a positive test diagnosis are from Hsu (2002). The table itself is adapted from Strack and Millon (2007, p. 63). Copyright 2007 by Lawrence Erlbaum Associates, Inc. Adapted by permission of the Taylor & Francis Group.

that is likewise not included in DSM-IV or DSM-IV-TR (American Psychiatric Association, 1994, 2000), it exhibits good validity. It is possible that the few patients in the sample who demonstrated these personality features were especially salient, and were easily differentiated from antisocial persons who did not exhibit sadistic propensities.

Profile of Personality Scales

Analysis of the profile of MCMI PD scale scores has always been recommended, because most people exhibit a blend of traits from multiple prototype domains (Millon, 1983, 1987, 1997b, 2006). For example, it will be rare for a respondent to obtain an elevation on only the Schizoid scale. Most respondents will show multiple scale elevations identifying the prototype domains that best fit their characteristic way of thinking, feeling, and behaving. Frequently occurring two-point and three-point code types were identified by Millon and others for the MCMI-I and MCMI-II (see Choca, 2004; Millon, 1983, 1987), supporting this element of the model. Millon's experience with these patient groups led him to more formally propose 60 frequently occurring MCMI-III subtypes (Davis & Patterson, 2005; Grossman & del Rio, 2005; Millon & Davis, 1996; Millon & Grossman, 2006). The most recent additions to the test—the Grossman (2004; Grossman & del Rio, 2005; Millon, 2006) Facet Scales—measure subgroups of PD scale items identified by factor analysis (FA) that reflect Millon's structural and functional trait distinctions.

Normal and Abnormal Trait Continuity

All versions of the MCMI were intended for use with patient samples, because their data were based on psychiatric patient norms (Millon, 1983, 1987, 2006). This effectively prohibits direct comparisons between patient and nonpatient samples, and limits the validity studies that can be conducted to evaluate how the test behaves with normal and abnormal persons. Nevertheless, a few studies have been published where the MCMI was given to normal subjects, and their results supported Millon's view that his basic personality prototypes exist in normal form as mild variants of the PDs (Choca, 2004; Retzlaff & Gibertini, 1987; Strack, 1991, 2005a, 2005b). For example, the factor structure of MCMI PD scales is essentially the same in normal and patient samples (Dyce, O'Connor, Parkins, & Janzen, 1997; Retzlaff & Gibertini, 1987; Strack, 1991), and both groups obtained similar personality configurations on the MCMI and other Millon measures that assess normal traits (Craig & Olson, 2001; Strack, 2005a).

Overall, the empirical literature has been supportive of the MCMI PD scales as being reliable and valid measures of continuously distributed prototype trait characteristics that can be useful for diagnosing patients according to DSM criteria. MCMI PD test profiles are useful for identifying subtypes (i.e., personality prototype variants) that follow Millon's (e.g., Millon & Davis, 1996) theoretically and clinically derived formulations. Millon's personality prototypes as measured by the MCMI have also shown consistency across normal and abnormal populations, verifying the hypothesis that the basic PD prototypes are severe forms of the styles found in normal persons.

However, substandard reliability and validity have been noted for a few MCMI PD scales. Problems have cropped up most often at points where Millon's model and the MCMI diverge from the DSM, and from measures that use the DSM for their definitional base (e.g., structured diagnostic interviews). Since the publication of DSM-III (American Psychiatric Association, 1980), Millon's ideas about PDs have strongly shaped the taxonomy of Axis II, but Millon's (1981; Millon & Davis, 1996) model and the DSM's are not the same. As long as there are divergences between the two, the MCMI will remain an imperfect measure of DSM PDs.

Factorial Structure

Over the years a number of debates have arisen about the psychometric properties of the MCMI, its factor structure, and its relationship to Millon's model (Millon & Davis, 1996) of personality and psychopathology. Recent reviews of the MCMI literature (e.g., Choca, 2004; Craig, 1999, 2005) summarize these debates very well, so we limit ourselves here to a discussion of FA as a statistical method for understanding the properties of the instrument, and its relationship to Millon's model.

The MCMI scales were created primarily to operationalize Millon's (Millon & Davis, 1996) taxonomy of PDs, which is polythetic in nature. Personality prototypes are viewed as syntheses of many basic elements and systems that operate within an individual. The prototypes are derived from inherited predispositions, sociocultural influences, and environmental characteristics. Although the prototypes with normal variants evolved over thousands of years, their phenotypic expression varies within and across individuals over time and situations. Personality prototypes are related to one another in a systematic manner, so that some prototypes share basic characteristics, such as a passive or active orientation to shaping the environment and a propensity to seek pleasure and/or avoid pain (Millon & Davis, 1996). MCMI PD scales were created with two groups of items—namely, nonoverlapping prototypal items and overlapping nonprototypal items. The former are viewed as central features of the prototypes, while the latter represent shared characteristics.

As mentioned in numerous publications, Millon (e.g., 1969, 1981; Millon & Davis, 1996) did not create his personality model from the point of view of factorial dimensions. No underlying factor structure has been specified for his taxonomy or for the MCMI. The polythetic nature of the model and the use of overlapping items for scales result in confounded factors, especially when Axis I and II scales are analyzed together (Choca, 2004; Haddy et al., 2005). Nevertheless, the MCMI PD scales can typically be summarized by two or three underlying dimensions that are often labeled Emotionality versus Restraint, Introversion versus Extraversion, and Dominance versus Submissiveness (Craig & Bivens, 1998; Haddy et al., 2005; Millon, 1983, 2006; Retzlaff & Gibertini, 1987; Strack, Choca, & Gurtman, 2001).

Recently, Grossman (2004 and Chapter 6, this volume; Grossman & del Rio, 2005; Millon, 2006) factor-analyzed the items of the MCMI-III's individual PD scales, using the test's normative sample. Employing an alpha factoring technique with oblique rotation, he was able to recover two or three dimensional elements for each personality prototype, which were later refined into subscales by using rational and empirical criteria. Importantly, the prototype subscales were found to measure major structural and functional elements of the personalities, as outlined by Millon (Millon & Davis,1996). A complete listing of the Facet Scales by prototype is given in Table 18.3. The scales can now be calculated for all MCMI-III PD profiles (Millon, 2006).

Owing to Millon's (1969, 1981, 1987, 1997b, 2006) use of the terms "dimension" and "axis" to describe some of the underlying components of his personality prototypes (e.g., active–passive, pleasure–pain, self–other), confusion has occurred as to whether these may be viewed as dimensions that can be recovered in FAs of the MCMI (Piersma, Ohnishi, Lee, & Metcalfe, 2002; Widiger, 1999). The simple answer is "no." The MCMI is based on a theoretical model that uses bipolar axes and dimensions for descriptive and inferential purposes, but these are not to be confused with latent roots identified by FA methods.

At the same time, while the taxonomy as a whole and many of its elements cannot be recovered or adequately tested with FA, some components of the model can be examined in experimental and nonexperimental designs using FA and other statistical techniques that apply to trait characteristics measured on continuous scales. Grossman's (2004; Grossman & del Rio, 2005) work on the MCMI-III PD Facet Scales is an example. He used FA to identify subgroups of PD scale items. Because most MCMI-III items address observable symptoms, feelings, attitudes, and behaviors, it was reasonable to assume that they would cluster together in ways resembling the structural and functional characteristics proposed by Millon and Davis (1996), which are also readily observable or easily inferred (see Table 18.3). Grossman's work showed that some of the trait domains could be recovered, but he noted that there are not enough items on the MCMI-III to adequately represent all of the proposed structural and functional characteristics of each PD. Another example is

TABLE 18.3. Grossman Facet Scales with Alpha Coefficient Reliabilities

Prototype/subscale	Items	Alpha	Prototype/subscale	Items	Alpha
1. Schizoid			6B. Sadistic		
1.1 Temperamentally Apathetic	8	.73	6B.1 Temperamentally Hostile	8	.65
1.2 Interpersonally Unengaged	10	.79	6B.2 Eruptive Organization	8	.59
1.3 Expressively Impassive	8	.60	6B.3 Pernicious Representations	11	.71
2A. Avoidant			7. Compulsive		
2A.1 Interpersonally Aversive	9	.79	7.1 Cognitively Constricted	8	.51
2A.2 Alienated Self-Image	10	.85	7.2 Interpersonally Respectful	6	.48
2A.3 Vexatious Representations	8	.78	7.3 Reliable Self-Image	7	.53
2B. Depressive			8A. Negativistic		
2B.1 Temperamentally Woeful	7	.83	8A.1 Temperamentally Irritable	10	.77
2B.2 Worthless Self-Image	9	.83	8A.2 Expressively Resentful	7	.68
2B.3 Cognitively Fatalistic	8	.82	8A.3 Discontented Self-Image	7	.78
3. Dependent			8B. Masochistic		
3.1 Inept Self-Image	8	.84	8B.1 Discredited Representations	8	.75
3.2 Interpersonally Submissive	8	.64	8B.2 Cognitively Diffident	8	.78
3.3 Immature Representations	6	.71	8B.3 Undeserving Self-Image	10	.85
4. Histrionic			S. Schizotypal		
4.1 Gregarious Self-Image	7	.69	S.1 Estranged Self-Image	11	.85
4.2 Interpersonally Attention-Seeking	8	.61	S.2 Cognitively Autistic	10	.79
4.3 Expressively Dramatic	7	.55	S.3 Chaotic Representations	8	.78
5. Narcissistic			C. Borderline		
5.1 Admirable Self-Image	10	.79	C.1 Temperamentally Labile	10	.81
5.2 Cognitively Expansive	7	.50	C.2 Interpersonally Paradoxical	9	.77
5.3 Interpersonally Exploitive	10	.65	C.3 Uncertain Self-Image	9	.83
6A. Antisocial			P. Paranoid		
6A.1 Expressively Impulsive	9	.56	P.1 Cognitively Mistrustful	8	.74
6A.2 Acting-Out Mechanism	10	.71	P.2 Expressively Defensive	7	.64
6A.3 Interpersonally Irresponsible	8	.61	P.3 Projection Mechanism	9	.64

Note. Reliability coefficients were calculated from the MCMI-III normative cross-validation sample, $N = 398$. Reprinted with permission from Millon (2006). Copyright 2006 by DICANDRIEN, Inc. All rights reserved.

Millon's (Millon & Davis, 1996) hypothesis that a continuum exists between normal and abnormal personality traits. Based on the hypothesis it is reasonable to assume that whatever factor structure exists for the MCMI PD scales, the same structure should obtain in normal and abnormal populations. The preceding section ("Normal and Abnormal Trait Continuity") provides references to a number of studies yielding evidence in support of this particular proposition.[6]

Admittedly, some of the hypothesized biological components, and their developmental influence on personality from infancy to adulthood, are extremely difficult to test at this time because of the limitations of current scientific methods (Strack, 2006). An example is the active–passive polarity, which is hypothesized to underlie the expression of most forms of personality. An individual's orientation to an active or passive lifestyle is more than an algebraic function of energy level (e.g., surgency), sociability, dominance, and intelligence. It refers to a complex coping and survival strategy in which an individual actively shapes surrounding events or waits for circumstances to change in order to bring need gratification. An individual's active or passive tendency is linked to inherited genetic dispositions, which are in turn linked to structural and biochemical elements in the brain that can change during childhood due to environmental factors—such as the availability of food and emotional sustenance, the reinforcements of one's family and social groups, and exposure to traumas (Millon, 1990; Millon & Davis, 1996).[7]

Future validation research on the MCMI will be most helpful when investigators view the instrument in the context of Millon's (Millon & Davis, 1996; Millon & Grossman, 2006) overarching clinical science model and appreciate the limitations that exist in the measure for validating the model and the DSM. As noted earlier, the MCMI-III (Millon, 1997b, 2006) measures 14 PDs, not all of which are present in DSM-IV(-TR) (American Psychiatric Association, 1994, 2000). The MCMI-III is theoretically derived from Millon's model of personality, but it does not measure all of the components of the model. In our view, it is a good measure of Millon's PD prototypes, subtypes, and some of the functional and structural domain traits that the prototypes and subtypes are based on. Validation of the larger model, including its bipolar "axes," will require longitudinal research designs that use multiple measures and data sources (Strack, 2006).

The Role of the MCMI Model in Resolving the Dimensional versus Categorical Debate

The MCMI, and the theory from which it was derived, posit the existence of continuous trait characteristics forming the basis of personality prototypes that can be assessed in categorical form. In our view, the future of personality assessment lies with the development of measures that are linked to a comprehensive clinical science, the features of which have been outlined previously. We believe that the resolution of many of the current dilemmas in personality diagnosis will come with a more sophisticated, theory-driven approach—one that gets beyond the simplicities of traditional categorical and dimensional models. Here we briefly present Millon's (2005; Millon & Davis, 1996; Millon & Grossman, 2006) views on the resolution of categorical versus dimensional models of personality.

The PDs found on Axis II of DSM-IV(-TR) (American Psychiatric Association, 1994, 2000) are diagnosed as categories. If a patient is judged to meet or exceed a minimum number of diagnostic features, that patient may be said to have a particular PD. If the patient falls short of the minimum number of required features, no diagnosis is made. Most psychologists dislike categorical diagnosis, because it goes against a body of evidence showing that personality traits are, for the most part, distributed continuously in the human population (e.g., Strack, 2006). Medically trained psychiatrists have favored categorical diagnosis for all types of disorders, whether physical or mental (e.g., Livesley, 2001). This difference in conceptualizing personality reflects historical differences in the way psychologists and psychiatrists have viewed their subject matter. Psychology's substantive realms have been approached with considerable success by employing methods of dimensional analysis and quantitative differentiation (e.g., intelligence measures, aptitude levels, and trait magnitudes). By contrast, medicine has made its greatest progress by increasing its accuracy in identifying and categorizing discrete disease entities. The issue separating these two historic approaches as it relates to the subject domain of normal and abnormal personality may best be stated in the form of a question: Should personality be conceived and organized as a series of *dimensional* traits that combine to form a unique profile for each individual, or should certain central characteristics be selected to exemplify and *categorize* personality types found commonly in clinical populations?

The view that personality might best be conceived in the form of dimensional traits has only recently begun to be taken seriously as an alternative to the more classic categorical approach by medical practitioners (Livesley, 2001; Widiger & Simonsen, 2005). Certain trait dimensions have been proposed in the past as relevant to these disorders (e.g., dominance–submission, introversion–extraversion), but these have not been translated into the full range of personality pathology seen in clinical practice. Some attributes have been formulated so that one extreme of a dimensional pole differs significantly from the other end in terms of clinical implications. An example would be emotional stability versus emotional instability. Other traits are believed to be abnormal at both ends of the continuum while the middle ground is normal. An example of this would be found in an activity dimension such as listlessness versus restlessness.

Despite their seeming advantages, dimensional systems have not taken strong root in the formal diagnosis of abnormal personality (Livesley, 2001). Numerous complications and limitations have been noted in the literature. First is the fact that there is little agreement among dimensional theorists concerning the number of traits necessary to represent personality. Many years ago, Menninger (1963) contended that a single dimension would suffice; Eysenck (1960) asserted that three are needed; and Cattell (1965) claimed to have identified as many as 33. However, recent models, most notably the five-factor model (Costa & McCrae, 1990; Goldberg, 1990; McCrae, 2006; Norman, 1963), have begun to achieve a modest level of consensus. And some suggest that the traits may mutually be understood in a hierarchical fashion (Markon, Kreuger, & Watson, 2005). Nevertheless, problems are still apparent in the literature in terms of how many and which dimensions are needed to cover normal and abnormal functioning, and how to create a workable hierarchy of higher-order and lower-order dimensions and facets (Livesley, 2001; Markon et al., 2005; Panounen, 1998; Strack, 2006). Although the lexical tradition of using personality terms embedded in common language has been useful in creating a taxonomy of trait dimensions among normal persons, the same approach has not been as fruitful in identifying abnormal dimensional elements (Harkness & McNulty, 1994).

Categorical models appear to have been the preferred schema for representing both CSs and PDs (Livesley, 2001). It should be noted, however, that most contemporary categories neither imply, nor are constructed to be, all-or-none typologies. Although singling out and giving prominence to certain features of behavior, they do not overlook the others, but merely assign them lesser significance. It is the process of assigning centrality or relative dominance to particular characteristics that distinguishes a schema of categories from one composed of trait dimensions. Conceived in this manner, a type simply becomes a *superordinate category* that subsumes and integrates psychologically covariant traits, which in turn represent a set of correlated habits that, in their turn, stand for a response displayed in a variety of situations.

There are, of course, objections to the use of categorical typologies in personality. They contribute to the fallacious belief that syndromes of abnormality are discrete entities, even medical diseases, when in fact they are merely concepts that help focus and coordinate observations (Livesley, 2001). Numerous classifications have been formulated in the past century, and one may question whether any system is worth utilizing if there is so little consensus among categorists themselves.

Is it possible to conclude from this review that categorical or dimensional schemas are potentially the more useful for personality classification? An illuminating answer may have been provided by Cattell, who wrote:

> The description by attributes [traits] and the description by types must be considered face and obverse of the same descriptive system. Any object whatever can be defined either by listing measurements for it on a set of [trait] attributes or by sequestering it to a particular named [type] category. (1970, p. 40)

In effect, Cattell has concluded that the issue of choosing between dimensional traits and categorical types is moot, because they are "two sides of the same coin." The essential distinction to be made between these models is that of comprehensiveness. Types are higher-order syntheses of lower-order traits; they encompass a wider scope of generality. For certain purposes, it may be useful to narrow attention to specific traits; in other circumstances, a more inclusive level of integration may be appropriate (Grove & Tellegen, 1991).

An endeavor to resolve some of these issues was described by Millon (1984, 1986, 1990) and has been summarized earlier. Termed "prototypal trait domains," this approach mixes categorical and dimensional elements in a personological classification. As in the official schema, several criteria are specified for each disorder, but these criteria encompass a large set of clinical domains—for example, mood/temperament and cognitive style (see Grossman, Chapter 6, this volume). The diagnostic criterion is conceived to be prototypal, as is the personality as a whole. Each specific domain is given a standard for each PD. For example, if the clinical attribute "interpersonal conduct" is deemed of value in assessing personality, then a specific prototypal criterion would be identified to represent the characteristic or distinctive manner in which each PD ostensibly conducts its interpersonal life (see Figure 18.2 for an example).

By composing a classification schema that includes all relevant trait domains commonly used by clinicians (e.g., self-image, interpersonal conduct, cognitive style), and that specifies a prototypal feature for each domain and PD, the proposed format would then be fully comprehensive in its scope. It would be useful to experienced and sophisticated clinical assessors, and would also possess directly comparable prototypal features for its parallel categories. A schema of this nature would not only be accepted by practitioners, but would also furnish both detailed substance and symmetry to its assessment taxonomy. The 15 prototypes of Millon's most recent personality model and its associated functional and structural domains have been described earlier (see Figures 18.1–18.3).

To enrich its qualitative categories (the several prototypal features constituting the trait range seen in each domain) with quantitative discriminations (numerical intensity ratings), personologists would not only identify which prototypal features (e.g., "woeful," "hostile," "labile") in a trait domain (e.g., mood/temperament) best characterize a person, but would record a rating or number (e.g., from 1 to 10) to represent the degree of prominence or pervasiveness of the chosen feature(s). Personologists would be encouraged in such a prototypal schema to record and quantify more than one feature per psychological domain (e.g., if suitable, to note both "woeful" and "labile" moods, should their observations lead them to infer the presence of these two prototypal characteristics in that domain). Reference to the descriptive trait domains of all but one personality may be found in Millon and Davis (1996). Information concerning the most recent personality format and details may be found in Millon (2006), Millon and Grossman (2006), and Grossman (Chapter 6, this volume).

The prototypal domain model illustrates that *categorical* (qualitative distinction) and *dimensional* (quantitative distinction) approaches need not be framed in opposition, much less be considered mutually exclusive. Assessments can be formulated, first, to recognize qualitative (categorical) distinctions in what prototypal features best characterize a person, permitting the multiple listing of several such features; and, second, to differentiate these features quantitatively (dimensionally) so as to represent their relative degrees of clinical prominence or pervasiveness. The prototypal domain approach includes the specification and use of categorical attributes in the form of distinct prototypal characteristics, yet allows for a result that permits the diversity and heterogeneity of a dimensional schema of clinically relevant domains.

Acknowledgment

This chapter is adapted from Strack and Millon (2007). Copyright 2007 by Lawrence Erlbaum Associates, Inc. Adapted by permission of the Taylor & Francis Group.

Notes

1. The word "prototype" is commonly used in the English language to mean the model on which something is based or formed. Applied to personality science, the term refers to the most common features or properties of members of a category—in this case, a personality type, style, or disorder. A personality prototype is a theoretical ideal or standard against which real people can be evaluated. All of the prototype's properties are assumed to characterize at least some members of the category, but no one property is necessary or sufficient for membership in the category. It is possible that no actual person would match the theoretical prototype perfectly. Different people approximate it to different degrees, and the closer a person comes to matching all the definitional criteria, the more closely that person typifies the concept (Rosch, 1978). Millon's (2006; Millon & Davis, 1996) taxonomy describes personality in terms of prototypes, but for stylistic purposes we use the terms "type," "style," "disorder," and "prototype" interchangeably in this chapter.
2. Should the American Psychiatric Association adopt a diagnostic system that included normal personality, the MCMI would have to be revised to measure a broader range of normal traits. Current MCMI-III PD scales assess mostly abnormal features.

3. The concept of personality subtypes does not negate the validity or importance of personality prototypes, any more than color blends negate the reality of the primary colors from which they are derived.

4. Although the MCMI-III and other assessment instruments can be summarized as being "accurate" or "inaccurate" for making particular diagnoses within particular parameters, the research literature is still far from complete in terms of assaying all of the variables that affect clinical diagnosis, such as state–trait effects, comorbidity, and neurological factors. As such, readers are cautioned not to overgeneralize the empirical findings presented here and elsewhere regarding the MCMI-III's diagnostic accuracy.

5. "Specificity" is also frequently used as an estimate of a measure's diagnostic accuracy. This is defined as the number of patients who are determined by clinicians as not having a particular disorder who are also shown not to have the disorder by the measure. Research on the MCMI-I demonstrated that the PD scales have high specificity (range = .85 to .95; Gibertini, Brandenburg, & Retzlaff, 1986), and this was confirmed for the MCMI-III (mean for all scales = .97; Hsu, 2002). Specificity is similar to "negative predictive power," which we present in Table 18.2.

6. While Millon (Millon & Davis, 1996) hypothesize that many phenotypically expressed personality characteristics will show continuous distributions in both normal and abnormal samples (e.g., introversion–extraversion), other features important to personality classification (such as active–passive orientation) will not necessarily emerge in dimensional form. Because of this, he believes that FA and dimensionalized traits alone cannot serve as an adequate foundation for a taxonomy of PDs; too many elements would be lost.

7. In this regard, it is unfortunate that the vast majority of published studies on Millon's body of work have focused on his assessment measures rather than his model of personality and psychopathology. We strongly encourage research on his model that is independent of his measures, because assessment instruments like the MCMI are imperfect and limited in how they operationalize many theoretical variables.

References

American Psychiatric Association. (1980). *Diagnostic and statistical manual of mental disorders* (3rd ed.). Washington, DC: Author.

American Psychiatric Association. (1994). *Diagnostic and statistical manual of mental disorders* (4th ed.). Washington, DC: Author.

American Psychiatric Association. (2000). *Diagnostic and statistical manual of mental disorders* (4th ed., text rev.). Washington, DC: Author.

Cattell, R. B. (1965). *The scientific analysis of personality.* Chicago: Aldine.

Cattell, R. B. (1970). The integration of function and psychometric requirements in a quantitative and computerized diagnostic system. In A. R. Mahrer (Ed.), *New approaches to personality classification* (pp. 9–52). New York: Columbia University Press.

Choca, J. P. (2004). *Interpretive guide to the Millon Clinical Multiaxial Inventory* (3rd ed.). Washington, DC: American Psychological Association.

Colligan, R. C., Morey, L. C., & Offord, K. P. (1994). The MMPI/MMPI-2 personality disorder scales: Contemporary norms for adults and adolescents. *Journal of Clinical Psychology, 50,* 168–200.

Costa, P. T., & McCrae, R. R. (1990). Personality disorders and the five-factor model of personality. *Journal of Personality Disorders, 4,* 362–371.

Craig, R. J. (1999). Overview and status of the Millon Clinical Multiaxial Inventory. *Journal of Personality Assessment, 72,* 390–406.

Craig, R. J. (Ed.). (2005). *New directions in interpreting the Millon Clinical Multiaxial Inventory–III (MCMI-III).* Hoboken, NJ: Wiley.

Craig, R. J. (2008). Essentials of MCMI-III assessment. In S. Strack (Ed.), *Essentials of Millon inventories assessment* (3rd ed., pp. 1–55). Hoboken, NJ: Wiley.

Craig, R. J., & Bivens, A. (1998). Factor structure of the MCMI-III. *Journal of Personality Assessment, 70,* 190–196.

Craig, R. J., & Olson, R. E. (2001). Adjectival descriptions of personality disorders: A convergent validity study of the MCMI-III. *Journal of Personality Assessment, 77,* 259–271.

Cronbach, L. J., & Meehl, P. E. (1955). Construct validity in psychological tests. *Psychological Bulletin, 52,* 281–302.

Davis, R. D., & Patterson, M. J. (2005). Diagnosing personality disorder subtypes with the MCMI-III. In R. J. Craig (Ed.), *New directions in interpreting the Millon Clinical Multiaxial Inventory–III (MCMI-III)* (pp. 32–70). Hoboken, NJ: Wiley.

Dyce, J. A., O'Connor, B. P., Parkins, S. Y., & Janzen, H. L. (1997). Correlational structure of the MCMI-III personality disorder scales and comparisons with other data sets. *Journal of Personality Assessment, 69,* 568–582.

Eysenck, H. (1960). *The structure of human personality.* London: Routledge & Kegan Paul.

Gibertini, M., Brandenburg, N. A., & Retzlaff, P. D. (1986). The operating characteristics of the Millon Clinical Multiaxial Inventory. *Journal of Personality Assessment, 50,* 554–567.

Goldberg, L. R. (1990). An alternative "description of personality": The Big-Five factor structure. *Journal of Personality and Social Psychology, 59,* 1216–1229.

Grossman, S. D. (2004). *Facets of personality: A proposal for the development of MCMI-III content scales.* Unpublished doctoral dissertation, Carlos Albizu University, Miami, FL.

Grossman, S. D., & del Rio, C. (2005). The MCMI-III facet subscales. In R. J. Craig (Ed.), *New directions in interpreting the Millon Clinical Multiaxial Inventory–III (MCMI-III)* (pp. 3–31). Hoboken, NJ: Wiley.

Grove, W. M., & Tellegen, A. (1991). Problems with classification of personality disorders. *Journal of Personality Disorders, 5,* 31–41.

Haddy, C., Strack, S., & Choca, J. P. (2005). Linking personality disorders and clinical syndromes on the MCMI-III. *Journal of Personality Assessment, 84,* 193–204.

Harkness, A. R., & McNulty, J. L. (1994). The personality psychopathology five (PSY-5): Issue from the pages of a diagnostic manual instead of a dictionary. In S. Strack & M. Lorr (Eds.), *Differentiating normal and abnormal personality* (pp. 291–315). New York: Springer.

Hsu, L. M. (2002). Diagnostic validity statistics and the MCMI-III. *Psychological Assessment, 14,* 410–422.

Livesley, W. J. (2001). Conceptual and taxonomic issues. In W. J. Livesley (Ed.), *Handbook of personality disorders* (pp. 3–38). New York: Guilford Press.

Markon, K. E., Krueger, R. F., & Watson, D. (2005). Delineating the structure of normal and abnormal personality: An integrative hierarchical appraisal. *Journal of Personality and Social Psychology, 88,* 139–157.

McCrae, R. R. (2006). Psychopathology from the perspective of the five-factor model. In S. Strack (Ed.), *Differentiating normal and abnormal personality* (2nd ed., pp. 51–64). New York: Springer.

Meehl, P. E., & Rosen, A. (1955). Antecedent probability and the efficiency of psychometric signs, patterns, or cutting scores. *Psychological Bulletin, 52,* 194–216.

Menninger, K. (1963). *The vital balance.* New York: Viking.

Millon, T. (1969). *Modern psychopathlogy.* Philadelphia: Saunders.

Millon, T. (1977). *Millon Clinical Multiaxial Inventory manual.* Minneapolis, MN: National Computer Systems.

Millon, T. (1981). *Disorders of personality.* New York: Wiley.

Millon, T. (1983). *Millon Clinical Multiaxial Inventory (MCMI) manual* (3rd ed.). Minneapolis, MN: National Computer Systems.

Millon, T. (1984). On the renaissance of personality assessment and personality theory. *Journal of Personality Assessment, 48,* 450–466.

Millon, T. (1986). Personality prototypes and their diagnostic criteria. In T. Millon & G. L.

Klerman (Eds.), *Contemporary directions in psychopathology: Toward the DSM-IV* (pp. 671–712). New York: Guilford Press.

Millon, T. (1987). *Manual for the MCMI-II* (2nd ed.). Minneapolis, MN: National Computer Systems.

Millon, T. (1990). *Toward a new personology: An evolutionary model.* New York: Wiley-Interscience.

Millon, T. (Ed.). (1997a). *The Millon inventories: Clinical and personality assessment.* New York: Guilford Press.

Millon, T. (2005). Reflections on the future of personology and psychopathology. In S. Strack (Ed.), *Handbook of personology and psychopathology* (pp. 527–546). Hoboken, NJ: Wiley.

Millon, T., & Davis, R. D.. (1996). *Disorders of personality: DSM-IV and beyond.* New York: Wiley.

Millon, T., & Grossman, S. D. (2006). Millon's evolutionary model for unifying the study of normal and abnormal personality. In S. Strack (Ed.), *Differentiating normal and abnormal personality* (2nd ed., pp. 3–49). New York: Springer.

Millon, T. (with Millon, C., & Davis, R. D.). (1997b). *Millon Clinical Multiaxial Inventory–III (MCMI-III) manual* (2nd ed.). Minneapolis, MN: National Computer Systems.

Millon, T. (with Millon, C., Davis, R. D., & Grossman, S. D.). (2006). *Millon Clinical Multiaxial Inventory–III (MCMI-III) manual* (3rd ed.). Minneapolis, MN: Pearson Assessments.

Morey, L. C., Blashfield, R. K., Webb, W. W., & Jewell, J. J. (1988). MMPI scales for DSM-III personality disorders: A preliminary validation study. *Journal of Clinical Psychology, 44,* 47–50.

Norman, W. (1963). Toward an adequate taxonomy of personality attributes: Replicated factor structure in peer nomination personality ratings. *Journal of Abnormal and Social Psychology, 66,* 574–583.

Nunnally, J. (1978). *Psychometric theory* (2nd ed.). New York: McGraw-Hill.

Panounen, S. V. (1998). Hierarchical organization of personality and prediction of behavior. *Journal of Personality and Social Psychology, 74,* 538–556.

Piersma, H. L., Ohnishi, H., Lee, D. J., & Metcalfe, W. E. (2002). An empirical evaluation of Millon's dimensional polarities. *Journal of Psychopathology and Behavioral Assessment, 24,* 151–158.

Retzlaff, P. (1996). MCMI-III validity: Bad test or bad validity study? *Journal of Personality Assessment, 66,* 431–437.

Retzlaff, P. D., & Dunn, T. (2003). The Millon Clinical Multiaxial Inventory–III. In L. E. Beutler & G. Groth-Marnat (Eds.), *Integrative assessment of adult personality* (2nd ed., pp. 192–226). New York: Guilford Press.

Retzlaff, P. D., & Gibertini, M. (1987). Factor structure of the MCMI basic personality scales and common-item artifact. *Journal of Personality Assessment, 51,* 588–594.

Rosch, E. (1978). Principles of categorization. In E. Rosch & B. B. Lloyd (Eds.), *Cognition and categorization* (pp. 27–48). Hillsdale, NJ: Erlbaum.

Rossi, G., Hauben, C., Van den Brande, I., & Sloore, H. (2003). Empirical evaluation of the MCMI-III personality disorder scales. *Psychological Reports, 92,* 627–642.

Rossi, G., Van den Brande, I., Tobac, A., Sloore, H., & Hauben, C. (2003). Convergent validity of the MCMI-III personality disorder scales and the MMPI-2 scales. *Journal of Personality Disorders, 17,* 330–340.

Somwaru, D. P., & Ben-Porath, Y. S. (1995, March). *Development and reliability of MMPI–2 based personality disorder scales.* Paper presented at the 30th Annual Workshop and Symposium on Recent Developments in Use of the MMPI–2 and MMPI–A, St. Petersburg Beach, FL.

Strack, S. (1991). Factor analysis of MCMI-II and PACL basic personality scales in a college sample. *Journal of Personality Assessment, 57,* 345–355.

Strack, S. (2005a). Combined use of the PACL and MCMI-III to assess normal range personality styles. In R. Craig (Ed.), *New directions in interpreting the Millon Clinical Multiaxial Inventory–III (MCMI-III)* (pp. 94–128). Hoboken, NJ: Wiley.

Strack, S. (2005b). Measuring normal personality the Millon way. In S. Strack (Ed.), *Handbook of personology and psychopathology* (pp. 372–389). Hoboken, NJ: Wiley.

Strack, S. (Ed.). (2006). *Differentiating normal and abnormal personality* (2nd ed.). New York: Springer.

Strack, S. (Ed.). (2008). *Essentials of Millon inventories assessment* (3rd ed.). Hoboken, NJ: Wiley.

Strack, S., Choca, J. P., & Gurtman, M. B. (2001). Circular structure of the MCMI-III personality disorder scales. *Journal of Personality Disorders, 15,* 263–274.

Strack, S., & Millon, T. (2007). Contributions to the dimensional assessment of personality disorders using Millon's model and the Millon Clinical Multiaxial Inventory–III (MCMI-III). *Journal of Personality Assessment, 89*(1), 56–69.

Widiger, T. A. (1999). Millon's dimensional polarities. *Journal of Personality Assessment, 72,* 365–389.

Widiger, T. A., & Simonsen, E. (2005). Introduction to the special section: The American Psychiatric Association's research agenda for the DSM-V. *Journal of Personality Disorders, 19,* 103–109.

PART III

A GUIDE TO ASSOCIATED
MILLON CLINICAL INVENTORIES

Using the Millon Behavioral Medicine Diagnostic (MBMD)

Michael H. Antoni
Carrie M. Millon
Theodore Millon

The Role of Psychosocial Factors in Health Preservation and Health Care Delivery

Maintaining our nation's health is one of the most poignant, perplexing, and costly agendas in the United States. Because medical diseases influence millions of American lives and consume billions of American dollars each year, the health care revolution is one of the greatest wars that our country has ever fought. Whereas infectious diseases were the major health challenges for the United States at the beginning of the 20th century, chronic medical diseases—the most expensive kind to treat—are the major health challenges as we move through the first decade of the 21st century. The most prevalent among these diseases remain arthritis, cancer, diabetes mellitus, stroke and cerebrovascular disease, and coronary heart disease (CHD). Other conditions, though lower in prevalence, can exact a heavy financial toll and remain the objects of preventative and treatment research. These include, among others, asthma, human immunodeficiency virus and acquired immune deficiency syndrome (HIV/AIDS), end-stage renal disease (ESRD), liver disease, spinal cord injury, and neurological disease. They also include disturbances in physiological regulation of circulation (e.g., hypertension), digestion (e.g., gastrointestinal disorders), respiration (e.g., chronic obstructive pulmonary disease), energy/arousal (e.g., chronic fatigue syndrome), sensation (e.g., chronic pain), reproduction (e.g., gynecological disorders), metabolism (e.g., thyroid disorders), and inflammation and immune function (e.g., allergies and autoimmune diseases).

Because people often live for several decades with several of these conditions, health care costs for "chronic disease management" are astronomical. At the end of the 1980s, cost figures were surpassing $500 billion annually (Taylor & Aspinwall, 1990). By 1992 the total cost of health care in the United States was $838 billion, accounting for one-seventh of the money spent on all domestic goods and services (U.S. Department of Health and Human Services, 1992), and at the writing of this chapter it is well over $1 trillion annually. In a prior version of this chapter (Antoni, Millon, & Millon, 1997), we asked: "*Were more people getting sicker, were the services getting costlier, or were the providers getting greedier?*" (p. 410, emphasis in original). One alarming trend identified in the 1990s was that huge amounts of health care costs were incurred for unnecessary procedures. This, as well as the significant evidence of abuse in the use of medical interventions, led in part to what is often termed the "managed care revolution" (Regier, 1994). The major mission of this revolution was the long-term reform of our nation's health care system, addressing in particular methods to increase the accessibility, efficacy, and cost-efficiency of procedures and services designed to preserve health and manage disease.

Clinical health psychology gained most of its momentum in parallel with the managed care revolution and the heightened appreciation for the role of psychosocial factors in disease prevention on the one hand and chronic disease management on the other. Sobel (1994) stated that clinical behavioral medicine (e.g., educational, behavioral, and psychosocial) interventions may reduce the frequency of medical utilization by 17% to 56% for such services as total ambulatory care visits, pediatric acute illness visits, acute asthma services, cesarean section and epidural anesthesia during labor and delivery, and major surgery. Sobel's report went on to note that a substantial proportion of health care costs are for treatments for conditions with psychosocial sources; that increasing a person's sense of control and optimism can improve health outcomes and decrease health care costs; and that social-support-building groups are cost-effective ways to deliver interventions to medical patients. Sobel also reported that psychosocial interventions can improve both health outcomes and cost outlays for such conditions as minor and acute illnesses, stress-related disorders, chronic pain, diabetes, asthma, arthritis, surgery, and childbirth. Over the latter part of the 1990s, ongoing research addressed similar questions in the context of other major medical conditions including (but not limited to) CHD, different forms of cancer, and AIDS (Schneiderman, Antoni, Saab, & Ironson, 2001). Most of the gains made in these areas of clinical research and practice were initiated following the observations that patients with similar medical diagnoses and treatments showed wide variability in the physical course and psychological sequelae of the disease being treated, and that much of this variance could be predicted on the basis of the patients' psychosocial characteristics at the time of screening or intake.

The first portion of this chapter identifies many points of intersection between psychosocial processes and the optimization of health maintenance and health care delivery. As in the first edition, we have separated these intersection points into those concerned with health maintenance and those dealing with health care delivery. As regards the health maintenance arena, we focus on psychosocial factors related to (1) health preservation and the primary prevention of disease, and (2) patient responses to disease and secondary/tertiary prevention efforts. Within the context of health care delivery, we focus on the role of psychosocial factors in (1) medical utilization and health care cost containment, as well as (2) treatment success and rehabilitation/ recovery from disease. After summarizing these potential roles for psychosocial factors in these various contexts, we describe some of the methods available for assessing psychosocial characteristics of patients in specific medical environments. We first summarize the empirical support for the use of the Millon Behavioral Health Inventory (MBHI; Millon, Green, & Meagher, 1982) to address both primary and secondary prevention questions in different medical populations. We then review the limitations of the MBHI and present the rationale for the domains targeted by the newest Millon instrument, the Millon Behavioral Medicine Diagnostic (MBMD; Millon, Antoni, Millon, Minor, & Grossman, 2001). After nearly 7 years in development, we completed a series of validation studies with this new instrument, including patients with cardiac disease, transplants, pain, cancer, gastroenterological disorders, infectious disease, and diabetes. The final sections of the chapter focus on the development, validation, and clinical utility of the MBMD to date, and proposed future research and clinical applications for the test in contemporary medical settings.

Psychosocial Factors in Health Maintenance

Health Preservation and Primary Prevention

The type of health maintenance known as "primary prevention" encompasses efforts to preserve a healthy state in specific populations, including activities that reduce the likelihood of developing disease among healthy individuals who are vulnerable to the development of a specific disease. A converging set of psychosocial factors have been associated with several aspects of health maintenance, including frequency of risk behaviors (e.g., substance use, smoking, sun exposure); decisions to utilize diagnostic screening tests (e.g., cholesterol testing, skin cancer screening, mammography, Pap smears, prostate-specific antigen [PSA] testing); the practice of adequate self-care behaviors (e.g., adherence to medications regimens or dietary guidelines); susceptibility to stress-related or trauma-induced symptoms; and resistance to the promotion of preclinical physical and physiological abnormalities and the onset of clinical disease.

Over the past few decades, we have witnessed in the United States an increased public interest and funding base for primary prevention as a means for preventing morbidity and mortality and lowering health care costs due to major disease (Woolf, 1999). There is reason to believe that such efforts have been fruitful, despite the fact that their full potential has not yet been realized. We now know that evidence-based primary prevention methods, such as smoking cessation, exercise, and lowering cholesterol and blood pressure, can prevent significantly more deaths than do assorted tertiary prevention techniques (e.g., use of calcium channel blockers, beta-blockers, aspirin, and warfarin) in patients with cardiovascular disease (Woolf, 1999). Similar results were revealed for primary prevention (e.g., stopping smoking and becoming physically active) versus secondary prevention (e.g., mammography) in lowering the risk of dying from breast cancer (Woolf, 1999). This set of findings emphasizes the importance of making health behavior changes at the earliest possible point in time. Clearly, identifying persons as at risk for any of these diseases (e.g., through family history and related genetic tests) could prevent disease and save medical resources for the portion of the population already suffering from a medical condition. There is growing evidence that several psychosocial factors may be critical to consider as obstacles or facilitators of the use of preventative services. Only recently has there been an appreciation within the medical community that bringing about such preventative behavior changes can be difficult and complex. A huge amount of behavioral research has helped to identify psychosocial variables associated with the adoption and maintenance of specific health activities, including cancer risk behaviors (e.g., smoking, excessive exposure to ultraviolet rays), unprotected sexual behaviors, and obesity and overeating (e.g., Glanz, Lew, Song, & Cook, 1999; Rock et al., 2000). There is also a growing recognition of the importance of studying how certain psychosocial factors (e.g., depression) may interact with a genetic predisposition to engage in these risk behaviors (Lerman, Caporaso, et al., 1998; Lerman, Caporaso, et al., 1999).

PSYCHOSOCIAL FACTORS AND RISK BEHAVIORS

Psychosocial factors associated with engaging in risk behaviors include (but are not limited to) the following characteristics of individuals:

- Appraisals—including their view of self-worth, current health status, and perceived susceptibility to disease; their general outlook toward their future (e.g., optimism–pessimism); their opinions about the health-protective effects of ceasing the risk behaviors; and their personal sense of efficacy for making behavior changes (Becker, Maiman, Kirscht, Haefner, & Drachman, 1977; Rosenstock, 1974; Turk & Meichenbaum, 1989; McCann et al., 1995).
- Repertoire of coping skills or strategies for dealing with internal and external forces that perpetuate the practice of the behaviors.
- Social, economic, familial, and spiritual resources available to them for gaining the tangible and emotional support necessary to make substantial lifestyle changes (Wallston, Alagna, De Vellis, & De Vellis, 1983).
- Context (e.g., external stressors) in which they are attempting to make these changes.

Accordingly, individuals who have a low sense of self-worth, are unconcerned with their health, have a low sense of self-efficacy, maintain a pessimistic outlook, practice maladaptive coping strategies, have few resources for gaining tangible or emotional support, and live in a very stressful environment may be those persons who are most likely to continue engaging in health-compromising risk behaviors. These factors may also act as obstacles to practicing positive self-care behaviors (McCann et al., 1995; Wilson et al., 1986). Moreover, they may work to deter healthy individuals from pursuing diagnostic screenings such as annual physical exams, Pap smears, PSA testing, occult fecal blood testing, skin cancer testing, mammography, and other widely available medical tests that have been shown to dramatically reduce morbidity and mortality as well as health care costs (e.g., Lerman et al., 1993). Most of this work focuses upon psychosocial factors that are associated with the communication of and decisions to undergo these diagnostic tests. Understanding these processes may help to identify disease at its earliest stages, so that biomedical treatments can have maximum effectiveness. Behavioral research has also focused on factors associated with adjustment to positive cancer or cancer risk test results, since personality characteristics and initial reactions to these results may predict whether people make critical follow-up visits after positive Pap smears, mammograms, PSA tests, and colon cancer tests, wherein early interventions may be initiated (Pereira, Antoni, Simon, Efantis-Potter, & O'Sullivan, 2004; Baum & Posluszny, 1999).

As we move into a new era of "personalized" health care and medical treatments, genetic testing is moving to the forefront of research and clinical diagnostics in an effort to identify the groups at greatest risk for the development of future disease. We now know that psychosocial factors can affect decisions to engage in genetic testing that can identify those at elevated risk for specific cancers long before the first signs of cellular (i.e., neoplastic) changes occur (Lerman, Rimer, & Glynn, 1997). These include tests for the risk of breast and ovarian cancer (e.g., BRCA1 and BRCA2 genes) (Lerman, Hughes, et al., 1998; Lerman et al., 1996), and colorectal cancer (hereditary nonpolyposis colon cancer genes, such as msh2, mlh1, pms1, and pms2) (Glanz, Grove, Lerman, Gotay, & Le March, 1999). This work has identified demographic (e.g., socioeconomic status [SES]; Lerman et al., 1996), cognitive (e.g., perceived risk; Glanz, Grove, et al., 1999), and emotional (e.g., depressive symptoms; Lerman, Hughes, et al., 1999) factors that identify those who may be in greatest need of genetic counseling. Psychosocial assessment can potentially be used to determine the best ways to encourage such testing, and then the most effective ways to deliver test information so as to promote appropriate follow-up behaviors (Croyle, Smith, Botkin, Baty, & Nash, 1997; Lerman, 1997).

PSYCHOSOCIAL FACTORS AND HELP SEEKING

Similarly, these factors may contribute to a symptomatic patient's delay in seeking prompt medical attention after the initial onset of physical symptoms, including suspicious skin changes, abnormal bleeding, unexplained weight loss, angina, or even heart attacks (Kolitz, Antoni, & Green, 1985; Cameron, Leventhal, & Leventhal, 1995; Neal, Tilley, & Vernon, 1986). On the other hand, some persons' appraisals, coping strategies, resources, and life context may also cause them to overutilize the health care system when their condition does not warrant such use (Pallak, Cummings, Dorken, & Henke, 1994). Obviously, these aspects of health preservation can have a potentially huge impact on the quality and quantity of patients' lives, as well as on the costs of providing them with health care.

PSYCHOSOCIAL FACTORS AND VULNERABILITY
TO DEVELOPING STRESS-RELATED SYMPTOMS

Psychosocial factors may also contribute to an individual's susceptibility to stress-related symptoms. The experience of stressful life events—ranging from daily hassles and marital discord to more traumatic events, such as sexual and physical abuse, a devastating diagnosis, war, and natural disasters—has been related to the onset or exacerbation of mental and physical symptoms, and underlying physiological changes have been demonstrated in both healthy people (Kiecolt-Glaser & Glaser, 1992; Ironson, Antoni, & Lutgendorf, 1995; Ironson et al., 1997; Cohen, Tyrell, &

Smith, 1991) and those with a preexisting medical condition (Grady et al., 1991; Lutgendorf et al., 1995; Pereira et al., 2003).

Moreover, several psychosocial factors have been shown to be capable of moderating the influence of stressors on physical health changes and physiological regulatory processes. Some of these include an individual's appraisals of self-efficacy (Bandura, Taylor, Williams, Mefford, & Barchas, 1985; O'Leary, 1992; Wiedenfield et al., 1990); an optimistic outlook toward the future (Lutgendorf et al., 1995; Byrnes et al., 1998); adaptive coping strategies, such as acceptance, positive reframing, and active coping (Folkman & Lazarus, 1980; Carver et al., 1993; Taylor, Lichtman, & Wood, 1984; Taylor & Brown, 1988; Antoni, Goldstein, et al., 1995), as well as emotional expressivity (Esterling, Antoni, Kumar, & Schneiderman, 1990; Esterling, Antoni, Fletcher, Marguilles, & Schneiderman, 1994; Pennebaker, Kiecolt-Glaser, & Glaser, 1988); and adequate social support resources (Zuckerman & Antoni, 1995; Cohen & Wills, 1985; Helgeson, Cohen, & Fritz, 1998; Cruess, Antoni, Cruess, et al., 2000).

PSYCHOSOCIAL FACTORS AND THE PROMOTION OF DISEASE PROCESSES

Finally, psychosocial factors may also contribute to an individual's resistance or vulnerability to the promotion of a subclinical pathogenic or pathophysiological process, or to the onset of clinically manifest disease. Some subclinical processes that have been associated with psychosocial factors include the following:

- Coronary artery disease (Schneiderman et al., 2001).
- Hypertension (Dimsdale et al., 1986; Krantz et al., 1987; James, Hartnett, & Kalsbeek, 1984).
- Glucose control (Frenzel, McCaul, Glasgow, & Schafer, 1988; Brand, Johnson, & Johnson, 1986).
- Neoplastic changes in tissue (Antoni, Lutgendorf, et al., 2006).
- Immune system functioning (Kiecolt-Glaser & Glaser, 1992; Antoni, Esterling, Lutgendorf, Fletcher, & Schneiderman, 1995) including the surveillance of acute (Cohen et al., 1991) and chronic (Esterling et al., 1994; Lutgendorf, Antoni, Kumar, & Schneiderman, 1994; McKinnon, Weisse, Reynolds, Bowles, & Baum, 1989; Antoni, Caricco, et al., 2006) viral infections.

Some of the psychosocial factors implicated as contributing to these processes include negative affect and distress states (depressed mood; Herbert & Cohen, 1993), as well as anger and hostility (Dembroski & Costa, 1987); appraisals of self-efficacy or personal control (Cohen & Edwards, 1989; O'Leary, 1992) and optimism (Peterson, Seligman, & Vaillant, 1988; Antoni & Goodkin, 1988; Scheier & Carver, 1985); coping strategies ranging from active coping and engagement to denial, avoidance, and emotional suppression (Holahan & Moos, 1986; Pettingale, Greer, & Tee, 1977; Goodkin, Antoni, & Blaney, 1986; Antoni & Goodkin, 1988); resources, such as social support (House, Landis, & Umberson, 1988; Cohen & Wills, 1985; Cohen, 1988; Zuckerman & Antoni, 1995), religiosity, and spirituality (Levin, 1994); and contextual factors, such as stressful events (Antoni & Goodkin, 1989; Schwartz, Springer, Flaherty, & Kiani, 1986).

Many of these same psychosocial factors may also contribute directly or indirectly to the development of clinical endpoints, such as myocardial infarction (MI) (Booth-Kewley & Friedman, 1987; Friedman & Booth-Kewley, 1987; Kamarck & Jennings, 1991; Frasure-Smith, Lesperance, & Talajic, 1993), different cancers (Fox, 1981; Holland, 1990; Kaplan & Reynolds, 1988; Mulder, van der Pompe, Spiegel, Antoni, & de Vries, 1992; Goodkin, Antoni, Fox, & Sevin, 1993; Goodkin, Antoni, Sevin, & Fox, 1993; Sklar & Anisman, 1981; Antoni, Lutgendorf, et al., 2006), Type II diabetes mellitus (Glasgow, Toobert, Hampson, & Wilson, 1995; Surwit & Feinglos, 1988), gastrointestinal symptoms (Friedman & Booth-Kewley, 1987), rheumatoid arthritis (Anderson, Bradley, Young, McDaniel, & Wise, 1985), and AIDS (Antoni, 2002).

In summary, psychosocial factors have been associated with health-compromising risk behaviors, including decisions to seek diagnostic screening and help seeking following the onset of symptoms; susceptibility to stress-induced health status changes; and the promotion of pathophysiological processes and development of clinical disease. These psychosocial factors do appear to cluster around a finite number of domains, including depression, anxiety, and other psychiatric disorders; cognitive appraisals; coping strategies; economic, social, family, and spiritual resources; and a person's one's life context.

Patient Responses to Diagnosis of Disease and Treatment

A second major domain of health maintenance involves patients' coping resources in response to their initial diagnosis of disease, as well as in their adjustment to chronic disease conditions (i.e., "secondary prevention"). Secondary prevention can refer to the prevention of extreme or maladaptive behavioral or emotional responses to a new diagnosis, a new treatment regimen, or any of the life-changing aspects of a chronic medical condition with which an individual must deal. Although the boundary between secondary and tertiary prevention is not always clear, "tertiary prevention" generally reflects processes that contribute to recovery from, relapse of, or progression of physical disease. In this section, we discuss psychosocial factors that can predict patients' initial reactions to a new diagnosis (e.g., based on positive mammography, Pap smear, or HIV-1 antibody testing); their responses to a stressful or invasive "curative" medical procedure (e.g., surgical mastectomy, hysterectomy, chemotherapy, radiotherapy, cardiac catheterization, or tissue transplantation); and their adjustment to the burdens of a chronic disease (e.g., limitations in physical, mental, vocational, and social activities). These psychosocial factors may also be important in predicting their responses to those regimens concerned with chronic disease management (e.g., renal dialysis, insulin injections, antiviral medications, or lifestyle behavior changes), as well as to the actual physical course of the disease (e.g., recovery, relapse, recurrence, symptom flares, and progressive decline).

PSYCHOSOCIAL FACTORS AND EMOTIONAL RESPONSE TO DIAGNOSIS

There is wide variability in patients' initial psychological reactions to a serious medical diagnosis, with responses often involving either anxiety or depression-related conditions (Taylor & Aspinwall, 1990; Antoni, 1991). Some of the factors that may act to buffer an individual from extreme reactions to serious or life-threatening diagnoses are actually quite similar to those noted in the previous section on health preservation and primary prevention. These include appraisals (interpretation of the meaning of the diagnosis and its ramifications, outlook toward the future, self-efficacy, and treatment efficacy); repertoire of coping strategies (active coping, denial, giving up, cognitive reframing, acceptance); external resources (support of friends and family, spiritual sources of support, economic means); and contextual factors (ongoing life stressors, prior experience with serious disease, functional ability).

There is growing evidence that maintaining an optimistic attitude (Carver et al., 1993) and accepting the reality of and having social or spiritual resources available for dealing with a serious medical diagnosis (Taylor & Aspinwall, 1990; Zuckerman & Antoni, 1995; Woods, Antoni, Ironson, & Kling, 1999a, 1999b; Carver et al., 2005) can be predictive of less distress in the weeks, months, or years after receiving the diagnosis. Conversely, maintaining a pessimistic or hopeless attitude (Carver et al., 1993), using coping strategies such as denial and giving up, and inadequate social support (Zuckerman & Antoni, 1995) or spiritual resources (Woods et al., 1999a, 1999b) may predict greater depression and anxiety reactions after diagnosis of conditions ranging from breast cancer to HIV infection. These initial psychological reactions may abate over the ensuing weeks or months (Jacobson, Perry, & Hirsch, 1990), or may persist and act as obstacles to a patient's future adjustment.

PSYCHOSOCIAL FACTORS AND ADJUSTMENT TO CHRONIC DISEASE

Psychiatric Disturbances. The most widely studied and prevalent psychological problems that come in the period after initial reactions to diagnosis are anxiety and depression (Taylor & Aspinwall, 1990). Anxiety and depression can act as obstacles to a patient's ability to make and adapt to lifestyle changes; to recover from demanding medical procedures; to engage successfully in a rehabilitation program; and in some cases to return to the work force or to premorbid levels of physical, mental, and interpersonal functioning (Bremer, 1995; Taylor & Aspinwall, 1990). Taylor and Aspinwall (1990) note that sources of excessive anxiety in medical patients may include invasive procedures, aversive medication side effects, and fears of disease recurrence, among others. Anxiety reactions may vary considerably across patients as a function of their premorbid personality characteristics and psychiatric history, as well as their specific medical disease, its stage at the time of diagnosis, and the nature of the medical regimen. For instance, uncertainties about the risk that behaviors (e.g., sexual relations) carry for future heart attacks constitute one key source of anxiety among patients with MI (Christman et al., 1988). On the other hand, the greatest concerns and sources of anxiety among women having mastectomies include fears of disease recurrence, loss of femininity, and their partners' reactions to their surgery (Carver et al., 1993; Taylor & Aspinwall, 1990). Other psychosocial (e.g., dependence, self-esteem, pessimism) and sociodemographic (e.g., age, ethnicity, SES) characteristics may delineate which of these potential anxiety sources is most salient for different patient populations.

Depressive reactions to medical diagnosis may have a negative impact on adjustment and health outcomes as well. It has been estimated that up to 25% of medical inpatients suffer from severe depression (Taylor & Aspinwall, 1990). The prevalence of Axis I depressive disorders is known to be substantial among men diagnosed with HIV infection. In fact, the suicide rate in this population has been documented as 36 times higher than that observed in men in the same age group in the general population. Depressive symptoms may last for years after surgery for conditions such as breast cancer (Meyerowitz, 1980). Depressed affect and related symptoms may interfere with adjustment to the lifestyle changes and treatment regimens that accompany a variety of medical diseases. Lustman, Griffith, and Clouse (1988) found that depressed patients with diabetes had significantly greater difficulties with glucose control than did their nondepressed counterparts. Persisting depressed affect in HIV-infected men receiving highly active antiretroviral therapy (HAART) was associated with poorer control over HIV viral load, measured as the concentration of viral RNA in repeated peripheral blood samples collected over a 15-month period (Antoni, Carrico, et al., 2006). It is plausible that identifying psychiatric disorders or mood disturbance early in the medical diagnosis process may increase the efficacy of medical interventions.

Personality and Coping Style. In general, coping strategies characterized by avoidance are associated with increased distress in people dealing with stressors (Holahan & Moos, 1986; Taylor & Aspinwall, 1990). We know that medical patients using denial as a coping strategy after a medical diagnosis of breast cancer (Carver et al., 1993) or HIV infection (Antoni, Goldstein, et al., 1995) have greater levels of distress over the subsequent year. Some have suggested that the effectiveness of denial as a coping strategy in patients with chronic disease may vary as a function of the type as well as the stage of disease (Meyerowitz, 1980). One study found that denial among patients with MI actually predicted fewer days in intensive care and less cardiac dysfunction during hospitalization, but was associated with poorer adaptation to disease in the long term, including poorer adherence to aftercare recommendations and a greater number of days of rehospitalization (Levine et al., 1988). The use of coping strategies such as positive reframing and acceptance tends to predict less distress in the period after diagnosis (e.g., Carver et al., 1993; Lutgendorf et al., 1998). There is also evidence that these associations hold in patients from varying chronic disease groups who are dealing with the longer-term stress of their disease (Taylor & Aspinwall, 1990; Young, 1992). One study found that across patients diagnosed with cancer, hypertension, diabetes, and rheumatoid arthritis—four major chronic disease categories—cognitive restructuring predicted better emotional adjustment, while self-blame and fantasizing, among others, were associated with poorer adjustment (Felton, Revenson, & Hinrichsen, 1984). There is some evidence that those psychosocial characteristics associated with patients' immediate emotional reactions to diagnosis also predict their psychological responses (depressive and anxiety symptoms) to the medical treatment regimens administered in the initial postdiagnosis period. Some work noted that positive active responses to stress, a high locus of control, and greater perceived control over an illness are predictive of better psychological adjustment in patients with different chronic diseases such as cancer (Burgess, Morris, & Pettingale, 1988). One study found that lower levels of helplessness were associated with better psychological functioning and less symptom severity in patients with rheumatoid arthritis (Stein, Wallston, Nicassio, & Castner, 1988). In sum, these studies suggest that medical patients' coping strategies in dealing with the challenges surrounding the initial diagnosis and initial treatment for their disease can have lasting effects on their ability to adjust emotionally.

Social Support and Other Resources. Another psychosocial factor that has been related to patients' ability to adjust to the stressors of their disease is social support. Social support provisions are often grouped into several categories, such as tangible aid, information, and emotional assistance (House, 1981; Schaefer, Coyne, & Lazarus, 1981); others have broken down these categories further into such areas as nurturance, social integration, and sense of belongingness (Cutrona & Russell, 1987). Rewarding personal relationships that provide such things as tangible aid, information, and emotional assistance (House, 1981; Schaefer et al., 1981) in the lives of medical patients have been associated with better psychological adjustment to various conditions, including cancer (Taylor et al., 1984; Helgeson & Cohen, 1996), ESRD (Siegel, Calsyn, & Cuddihee, 1987), HIV/AIDS (Zuckerman & Antoni, 1994), and arthritis (Fitzpatrick, Newman, Lamb, & Shipley, 1988). The literature relating different aspects of social support to emotional adjustment in patients with cancer is substantial. For instance, patients with breast cancer who perceive greater emotional support from family and health care professionals evidence better emotional adjustment after the stress of mastectomy (Jamison, Wellisch, & Pasnau, 1978; Funch & Mettlin, 1982; Northouse, 1988; Helgeson & Cohen, 1996; Alferi, Carver, Antoni, Weiss, & Duran, 2001).

Social support may affect patients' adjustment to a chronic illness via multiple pathways, including ways in which it acts as a stress buffer (Cohen & Wills, 1985; Zich & Temoshok, 1987), facilitates the use of adaptive coping strategies (Dunkel-Schetter, Folkman, & Lazarus, 1987; Leserman, Perkins, & Evans, 1992; Thoits, 1987), and enhances adherence to medication regimens (Wallston et al., 1983; Gonzalez et al., 2004). It is also possible that patients' adverse emotional reactions to the stressors of their disease may act to drive away potential sources of social support (Zuckerman & Antoni, 1995; Wortman & Conway, 1985). Social isolation (Turner, Hays, & Coates, 1993) and social conflict (Leserman et al., 1995) may in turn forestall a person's ability to manage the demands of a chronic disease, resulting in greater distress, depression, and withdrawal, and thereby creating a vicious circle.

Finally, religiosity and spirituality have been associated with a lower prevalence of depression and anxiety in medical patients (Koenig, Pargament, & Nielsen, 1998). One group found that greater use of religion was associated with less depressed mood and anxiety in HIV-infected men (Woods et al., 1999a) and women (Woods et al., 1999b). Another study showed that use of religious coping predicted better adjustment after mastectomy in patients with early-stage breast cancer, though these effects varied as a function of religious orientation (Alferi, Culver, Carver, Arena, & Antoni, 1999).

Contextual Factors. The influence of patients' coping strategies and resources on their psychological adjustment does not act in a vacuum. Rather, it must operate in conjunction with contextual factors such as ongoing major life events and minor hassles; prior skills developed for dealing with illness; and actual functional ability to carry out role-associated responsibilities, vocations, and social activities. The experience of elevated numbers of stressful life events has been associated with depressive symptoms and increased risk of emotional difficulties (Uhlenhuth & Paykel, 1973; Murphy & Brown, 1980; Brown & Siegel, 1988). Ongoing life stress may over-whelm a patient's coping strategies, making it all the more difficult to deal with the challenges of the disease and the associated treatment regimen (Antoni & Emmelkamp, 1995; Antoni et al., 1991). Stressful life events may also interact with negative health behaviors (e.g., alcohol consumption; Morrisey & Schuckitt, 1978; Newcomb & Harlow, 1986), and this interaction can further hamper attempts to cope with new challenges. Patients' perception of their overall quality of life and their ability to carry on premorbid activities can also contribute to their ability to adjust to a demanding medical regimen. Previously, measures such as the Sickness Impact Pro-file (Bergner, Bobbitt, Carter, & Gilson, 1981) and the Index of Daily Activities (Katz, Ford, Moskowitz, Jackson, & Jaffe, 1983) were used to assess functional sta-tus (across psychosocial and physical dimensions) in medical patients, though these measures often do not measure how much the illness has compromised personal or role functioning (Taylor & Aspinwall, 1990). The acute side effects of certain treat-ments (e.g., chemotherapy and radiation) can often have a substantial impact on a patient's perceived quality of life (Lichtman, Taylor, & Wood, 1987), while more subtle chronic side effects of longer-term medication regimens can also greatly com-promise a patient's coping resources (Anderson et al., 1985; Zachariah, 1987).

Psychosocial Interventions. There is also evidence that focused psychosocial interventions (e.g., cognitive-behavioral stress management, or CBSM) that attempt to modify several of the psychosocial factors just noted (e.g., cognitive appraisals, coping strategies, social support) may offset the initial impact of a serious diagnosis (e.g., HIV-1 seropositivity) on distress levels (depressive and anxiety symptoms) and related physiological measures (immune system components) (Antoni, 2003a). There is support for the notion that these sorts of interventions can modify depressed affect and anxiety in medical patients by altering their cognitive appraisals, coping strate-gies, and social resources for managing the disease-specific stressors and challenges emanating from other contextual factors (Antoni, 2003a, 2003b). Many of these interventions feature a social support component, as well as offering patients the opportunity to challenge and change maladaptive cognitive appraisals and coping strategies. Psychosocial interventions have been shown to reduce distress in HIV-infected persons dealing with the stress of diagnosis (Antoni et al., 1991), with the chronic stress of having symptomatic HIV disease (Lutgendorf et al., 1997), the bur-dens of a demanding medication regimen (Antoni, Carrico, et al., 2006), and the stress of partner loss and deaths in their social networks (Chesney & Folkman, 1994; Chesney, Folkman, & Chambers, 1996; Goodkin et al., 1996). Often the effects of these interventions on physiological and health parameters are proportional to reduc-tions in depressed affect (e.g., Antoni, Carrico, et al., 2006); Lutgendorf et al., 1997). Effects of these interventions on negative affect and adjustment appear to be due to a combination of learned stress reduction skills, such as relaxation (Cruess, Antoni, Cruess, et al., 2000); changes in cognitive coping strategies skills, such as positive reframing (Lutgendorf et al., 1998); and improvements in perceived social support (Cruess, Antoni, Cruess, et al., 2000).

Psychosocial interventions have also been used successfully to help patients with cancer deal with the emotional challenges of their disease (Andersen, 1992;

Trijsburg, van Knippenberg, & Rijma, 1992). Many of these interventions feature a social support component and offer patients the opportunity to challenge and change maladaptive cognitive appraisals and coping strategies. Interventions such as group-based CBSM that were developed to help women adapt to the challenges of breast cancer and its treatment (Antoni, 2003b) have been shown to decrease the prevalence of depression (Antoni et al., 2001), to decrease anxiety symptoms and intrusive thoughts about cancer (Antoni, Wimberly, et al., 2006), and to increase positive affect and the sense of finding something positive in the cancer experience (Antoni et al., 2001; Antoni, Kazi, et al., 2006). This intervention was also shown to decrease evening cortisol levels (Cruess, Antoni, McGregor, et al., 2000) and to increase immune (lymphocyte) functioning (McGregor et al., 2004) in these women. Interestingly, the greater the psychological gains reported by these women, the greater the physiological changes. The effects of these interventions seemed to be due to a combination of stress management skills learned (e.g., relaxation) and the emotional processing that women were reporting both in and out of the groups (Antoni, Kazi, et al., 2006). Other work suggests that these forms of psychosocial intervention can reduce stress in tandem with modulating the immune system (Andersen et al., 2004). Many of these effects for CBSM have also been demonstrated in men coping with prostate cancer and its treatment (Penedo et al., 2004, 2006).

Psychosocial interventions have also been shown to facilitate adjustment (1) to other chronic diseases, such as CHD (Oldenberg, Perkins, & Andrews, 1985; Razin, 1982; Gruen, 1975; Williams & Chesney, 1993), arthritis (McCracken, 1991), diabetes mellitus (Glasgow et al., 1995), and melanoma (Fawzy, Cousins, et al., 1990); and (2) to other syndromes, such as chronic pain (Keefe, Dunsmore, & Burnett, 1992) (for a general review, see Schneiderman et al., 2001). The point here is that knowledge of the presence of a psychiatric disturbance or significant emotional distress in a medical patient; information regarding the patient's relative strengths and weaknesses in the domains of cognitive appraisals and coping strategies; support derived from social, familial, or spiritual sources; and an understanding of the ongoing life context can be very useful in determining the way in which the patient will adjust to a new diagnosis and to the demands of a chronic disease. This information can in turn be used to choose appropriate psychosocial services that should be made available to facilitate the adjustment process.

PSYCHOSOCIAL FACTORS AND THE PHYSICAL COURSE OF DISEASE

The psychosocial factors associated with the morbidity and mortality of many chronic diseases are similar to those that predict psychological adjustment to the same maladies. Severity of depressed mood has been shown to be an independent predictor of all-cause mortality in general medical patients (Herrmann et al., 1999); of acute MI and mortality in patients with CHD (Barefoot & Schroll, 1996); and of progression to AIDS in HIV-infected persons (Leserman et al., 1999). Factors such as appraisals, coping styles and different support resources may relate to a better disease course via their ability to moderate the influence of disease-related (and contextual) stressors on emotional adjustment (e.g., depression). Better emotional adjustment may in turn relate to a better disease course through its association with physiological mechanisms that have a protective effect against pathogens (e.g., immune system) or homeostatic dysregulation (e.g., endocrine system) causing the primary disease. Better emotional adjustment may also contribute to better health outcomes by influencing positive health behaviors such as exercise (Blumenthal et al., 1982) and medication adherence (Carney, Freedland, Eisen, et al., 1995).

Personality and Coping Styles. Numerous studies have suggested that patients who use certain coping strategies for dealing with the demands of their disease may actually be able to improve the prognosis for the course of their disease. Although this literature was primarily focused on patients with different types of cancer during the 1960s and 1970s, changes in prevalence patterns of other chronic diseases have broadened this literature to studies of psychosocial characteristics associated with the course of other progressive and usually terminal diseases (e.g., HIV/AIDS), as well as with such chronic but non-life-threatening diseases as arthritis (Grady et al., 1991; Blalock, De Vellis, & Giordino, 1995) and chronic fatigue syndrome (Lutgendorf et al., 1995). The latter are usually tracked in terms of flare-ups. Greater denial coping at the time of a diagnosis of HIV infection predicted greater impairments in immune function 1 year later (Antoni, Goldstein, et al., 1995) and a greater likelihood of progression to full-blown AIDS 2 years later (Ironson et al., 1994). Other studies have related such coping strategies as active confrontation (Mulder, Antoni, Duivenvoorden, Kauffman, & Goodkin, 1995), and realistic acceptance (Reed, Kemeny, Taylor, Wang, & Visseher, 1994) to differences in disease progression for HIV-infected individuals.

Appraisals and Attitudes toward Health and Illness. A large literature suggests that the cognitive appraisals patients use to process life stressors, as well as stressors specific to the burdens of a chronic disease, may be associated with the course of their disease. Reporting efforts to maintain a "fighting spirit" was associated with a slower development of HIV-related symptoms and slower decline in the immune system among HIV-infected men (Solano et al., 1993). Others have found that HIV-infected individuals who show the longest survival time after a diagnosis of AIDS are more likely to maintain an attitude of hope, greater life involvement, and a greater sense of meaningfulness than do those who have shorter survival times (Ironson, Solomon, Cruess, Barroso, & Stivers, 1995; Solomon, Benton, Harker, Bonavida, & Fletcher, 1993). Patients maintaining a fighting spirit in the face of a breast cancer diagnosis have also been shown to have longer survival times than those with a more passive attitude toward the disease (Greer, Morris, Pettingale, & Haybittle, 1990). Women with the combination of a pessimistic attitude and elevated negative life events showed greater promotion of cervical carcinoma (Antoni & Goodkin, 1988, 1989; Goodkin, Antoni, Fox, et al., 1993; Goodkin, Antoni, Sevin, et al., 1993). Among men and women with malignant melanoma, the use of active coping strategies was associated with a greater likelihood of survival up to 6 years later (Fawzy et al., 1993). Other studies have identified associations between attitudinal factors and physiological regulatory indicators that may mediate a faster disease progression. For instance, an external locus of control was associated with poorer diabetes control in both children and adults (Burns, Green, & Chase, 1986). Other work has focused on the personality construct of optimism–pessimism. Lower optimism scores have been related to a lower risk of developing cervical neoplasia (Goodkin, Antoni, Fox, et al.,

1993), and to less likelihood of being rehospitalized after coronary artery bypass graft surgery for such postsurgical complications as wound infections, angina, and MI (Scheier et al., 1999).

Social Support. The resource of social support has been associated with a faster recovery from certain illnesses and may reduce the risk of mortality in some cases (House et al., 1988; Neal et al., 1986). More specifically, adequate levels of social support have been related to faster recovery or rehabilitation from a wide range of diseases, including stroke (Robertson & Suinn, 1968), leukemia (Magni, Silvestro, Tamiello, Zanesco, & Carl, 1988), congestive heart failure (Chambers & Reiser, 1953), and kidney disease (Dimond, 1979). Social support may influence the course of other chronic diseases by improving diabetes control (Marteau, Bloch, & Baum, 1987; Schwartz et al., 1986), by reducing the risk of mortality from MI (Wiklund et al., 1988), by reducing the risk of breast cancer recurrence (Levy, Herberman, Lippman, D'Angelo, & Lee, 1991; Ell, Nishimoto, Mediansky, Mantell, & Hamovitch, 1992), and by slowing down the progressive decline in the immune system (Theorell et al., 1995; Zuckerman & Antoni, 1995) and progression to the clinical manifestations of AIDS (Ironson, Solomon, et al., 1995; Leserman et al., 1999) in those with HIV infection.

Other Resources. There is also a growing appreciation for the importance of other resources. For instance, the ability of patients to use spiritual/religious resources has been related to physiological functions such as blood pressure (Levin & Vanderpool, 1989) and immune function (Woods et al., 1999a). One review of over 100 epidemiological studies noted that religiosity was consistently associated with better physical health (Levin, 1994). One study found that elderly coronary patients who lacked a sense of strength and comfort from religion were more likely to die in the 6 months after open heart surgery than their more religiously comforted counterparts were (Oxman, Freeman, & Manheimer, 1995). Religious involvement or spirituality may influence health in medical patients by multiple pathways, including enhanced social support through the fellowship activities (attending services and praying together), less fear of death, greater practice of health-enhancing behaviors (e.g., adequate sleep and balanced diet), and a decreased likelihood of engaging in health-compromising lifestyle behaviors (e.g., substance use) (Jarvis & Northcott, 1987).

Lifestyle Behaviors. In addition to these psychosocial factors, various lifestyle behavioral factors may play a role in health preservation or adjustment to disease. These include alcohol use (Vaillant, Schnurr, Baron, & Gerber, 1991), illicit drug use (National Institute on Drug Abuse, 1990), overeating patterns (Brownell & Wadden, 1992), caffeine use (Lovallo et al., 1996), tobacco smoking (Epstein & Perkins, 1988), and physical exercise (Dubbert, 1992). Several of these behaviors have also been associated with many of the psychosocial factors mentioned previously, including coping strategies (Marlatt, 1985; Myers, Brown, & Mott, 1993) and social support (Richter, Brown, & Mott, 1991). In addition, there is evidence that contextual factors (e.g., life stressors) may increase the likelihood of such health-compromising behaviors as smoking and drug use (King, Beals, Manson, & Trimble, 1992;

Duberstein, Conwell, & Yeates, 1993), and may decrease the frequency of such health-promoting behaviors as a balanced diet and adequate physical exercise (Epstein & Perkins, 1988; Baum, 1994; Grunberg & Baum, 1985). Moreover, poor emotional adjustment to a chronic disease or to related treatment demands may increase the risk of relapse of smoking, drug, or alcohol use or decrease a patient's ability to maintain a restricted nutritional regimen; and several of these could in turn affect physiological changes in the circulatory system (Krantz, Grunberg, & Baum, 1985) and immune system that are associated with the progression of certain diseases (Levy et al., 1991; Baum, 1994). Identifying chronic disease populations at greatest risk for such negative health behaviors through the use of a comprehensive psychosocial assessment that can integrate information on distress states, stress appraisals and general outlook, coping style, and external resources such as social support and spirituality may be key in providing them with access to psychosocial intervention.

Psychosocial Interventions. Psychosocial interventions capable of modifying several of these psychosocial and behavioral processes may be associated with a decreased rate of disease progression in such conditions as CHD (Ornish et al., 1998; Frasure-Smith & Prince, 1989; Oldenberg et al., 1985; Williams & Chesney, 1993), HIV infection (Ironson et al., 1994; Antoni, 2003a; Antoni, Carrico, et al., 2006), breast cancer (van der Pompe et al., 1994; Spiegel, Kraemer, Bloom, & Gotheil, 1989; Andersen, Kiecolt-Glaser, & Glaser, 1994), and malignant melanoma (Fawzy et al., 1993), to name a few. These studies further emphasize the importance of identifying medical patients who would be most likely to benefit from interventions that modify psychosocial and behavioral factors associated with disease recurrence and survival (Schneiderman et al., 2001).

In sum, the psychosocial factors associated with health preservation (primary prevention) and adjustment to disease (secondary and tertiary prevention) appear to cluster around a number of domains, including cognitive appraisals (self-efficacy, optimism–pessimism, and perceived control); coping strategies (active coping, acceptance and cognitive reframing, avoidance and denial, and emotional suppression); external resources (social, economic, familial, and spiritual); and the individual's life context (stressful events, perceived stress level, and functional ability). The influence of these psychosocial factors on health preservation may be mediated by changes in patients' decisions to engage in risk behaviors, decisions to seek diagnostic screening services, and help-seeking responses after the onset of overt symptoms. The impact of these factors on adjustment to disease and disease course may be mediated by changes in patients' susceptibility to stress-induced emotional (e.g., depressive and anxiety symptoms), physiological (e.g., endocrine, immunological, cardiovascular dysregulation), and physical (e.g., muscle tension, sleep disorders, pain perception) sequelae.

Psychosocial Factors in Health Care Delivery

In addition to the psychosocial factors that may be associated with health maintenance, various psychosocial processes may contribute to optimal health care delivery. The identification of these factors through clinical research and their routine application to medical practice, made possible by comprehensive screening and assessment, may play a pivotal role in containing our nation's accelerating health care cost basis—a liability that has become quite salient in the face of the ongoing managed care revolution. In this section we summarize the effects of this revolution on the delivery of health care in the United States, noting the potentially beneficial effects of efforts directed at cost containment. We then highlight the research providing empirical support for links between specific psychosocial factors and patient medical utilization patterns, and note how these associations in turn can drive up health care costs in the short term. We also point to research relating psychosocial factors to the success rates of certain treatments and to patient recovery and rehabilitation rates from specific illnesses—outcomes that are both instrumental in longer-term cost containment.

The Influence of the Managed Care Revolution on Health Care Delivery

Most managed care systems are designed to manage escalating costs of medical care by providing necessary services to underserved populations, determining the basic criteria for medical need, setting fair prices for services, emphasizing the role of primary care, and monitoring public health (Regier, 1994). We have proposed that addressing these missions could be greatly enhanced with systematic methods for assessing the physical and psychological status of the patients making use of health care services. Improved screening and assessment are relevant for identifying underserved populations who could benefit from enhanced services, determining whether a patient meets criteria for one medical procedure or another, and surveying the utilization of medical services and their relative cost-effectiveness. In addition, one of the most critical ingredients of cost-effective primary care is understanding the factors that predict patients' decisions to utilize early screening and detection services. Another important aspect of primary care involves developing the most reliable and cost-effective techniques for detecting physical and mental disorders in children and adults at the earliest possible stage. Finally, direct and comprehensive assessment of medical patients is a key source of data for predicting and monitoring the effects of medical decisions on recovery and rehabilitation rates, as well as the quality of life of the patients receiving care. In many cases, however, the amount and level of psychosocial/mental health assessment may be grossly disproportionate to the amount of effort and resources spent on high-technology biomedical assessments. In many cases, psychosocial assessment may be totally absent from the screening, intake, and follow-up procedures, despite the remarkably low cost and high payoff potential of these tests.

Even when psychosocial assessments have been incorporated into health care protocols, psychologists have had trouble getting reimbursement from third-party payers for such assessments (Eisen et al., 1998). This has placed at risk the use of psychological assessment for making referrals and decisions about the best level of care and mode of treatment delivery, as well as for preventing early termination from treatment and inadequate adherence to prescriptions and recommendations during convalescence and aftercare (Eisen et al., 1998). Having access to information on personality traits and interpersonal styles is important in making decisions about appropriate psychosocial treatment formats (e.g., group vs. individual-based interventions), which may maximize effectiveness while containing costs (Harkness & Lilienfield, 1997). Moreover, because many health care systems view themselves as acute care providers, they may not appreciate the added value of having a complete patient profile capable of predicting adjustment to treatment and adherence to medication regimens/lifestyle changes—both of which are critical in the management of more costly chronic medical conditions.

Evidence justifying the potential cost savings and quality assurance resulting from integrating adequate mental health benefits into the overall physical health delivery package has been gathered. Epidemiological studies have indicated that 29% of people diagnosed with mental disorders also have substance use disorders (Regier, 1994). This research suggests that people may utilize services for those forms of pathology when they have a comorbid medical condition that can motivate them to seek out health care. Patients with equally serious mental or substance use conditions who are lacking medical comorbidities may fail to seek treatment, or may not seek it as soon or as often as they should. Conversely, many patients with mental or substance use disorders utilize medical services (emergency services, private practice physicians) that are inappropriate for their presenting pathology. The integration of epidemiological and health services research can identify disease comorbidities that account for the highest utilization patterns. Health cost analyses consider the costs of illness and treatment and are important in defining the amounts that should be allocated to benefit packages. Finally, treatment efficacy studies are helpful for developing empirically validated guidelines for primary prevention strategies, as well as recommendations for treatment choices (i.e., triaging) for people already diagnosed with a medical condition. In some cases, triaging decisions may result in a recommendation for a synergistic combination of pharmacological (e.g., antidepressant) and psychosocial (e.g., supportive group therapy or individual counseling) interventions, which can complement the treatment of the primary medical condition (e.g., cancer) by enhancing adherence to a self-care routine/lifestyle change or adjustment to the side effects of the medication. The upshot of these different lines of investigation is that knowledge of patients' psychosocial characteristics and health-relevant behavior patterns could aid in the reduction of the costs of health care delivery across a wide range of medical conditions in affected or at-risk populations.

There are several ways in which researchers have operationalized outcomes for the purpose of studying the influence of psychosocial factors in health maintenance and health care costs. These include indicators of health status, behavior changes, and cost-effectiveness. Health status indicators may be broad categorizations of morbidity and mortality; more disease-specific measures of progression, relapse, or remission; or more functional indices concerning physical and mental capacity or general quality of life. Many of these were used in the studies presented in the previous section. Behavior changes are usually indexed in terms of risk-increasing (e.g., cigarette smoking, fat intake, sun exposure) and risk-decreasing (e.g., exercise, relaxation) activities. Some of these were also included in the studies mentioned previously. Finally, cost-effectiveness can be tracked through actual cash outlay or through hospital admissions, lengths of stay, number of outpatient visits for follow-up, and the use of expensive (e.g., surgery) and less expensive (e.g., medications) procedures. Some of the psychosocial factors associated with health care costs involve those directly related to medical utilization (short-term cost effects), while others relate more directly to treatment success and recovery and rehabilitation rates (longer-term cost effects).

Comprehensive psychological assessments are designed to provide insights about patients' liabilities (e.g., anxiety and depression states, maladaptive coping strategies) as well as assets (e.g., personal and social resources, coping skills, and key targets for psychosocial interventions) (Eisen et al., 1998). The ultimate psychosocial assessment report is a highly synthesized product integrating information about a patient's history, test scores, current medical diagnosis, and comorbidities, to provide predictions about the patient's responses to medical diagnosis and treatment procedures. However, this sort of information gathering and processing can require far more time and effort than that which is reimbursed by current managed care organizations—and this trend is likely to continue or worsen until health insurance companies can see a clear benefit offered by comprehensive psychosocial assessment. What are some of the way in which psychosocial factors can affect health care delivery?

The Influence of Psychosocial Factors on Medical Utilization and Health Care Costs

PSYCHIATRIC DISTURBANCES

There is good evidence that medical patients who display psychiatric disorders, or who are in some way evidencing a poor emotional adjustment to their illness, may generate greater health care costs than do their better adjusted counterparts (Jacobs, Kopans, & Reizes, 1995; Kimmerling, Ouimette, Cronkite, & Moos, 1999; Holland, 1997; Roth et al., 1998). The National Comprehensive Cancer Network (NCCN), made up of 17 comprehensive cancer centers in the United States, has proposed that psychosocial screening begin in the waiting room at the initial visit. Such conditions as dementia, delirium, anxiety disorders, substance abuse, and personality problems would be grounds for a mental health treatment referral. The NCCN report suggests that the benefits of managing distress by providing vulnerable patients with mental health and pastoral counseling may include better patient–physician communication, enhanced compliance with treatment regimens, and lower mood disturbance and stress (Holland, 1997).

These findings are not limited to populations with cancer. For instance, greater state anxiety after gall bladder surgery was associated with longer postoperative hospital stays (Boeke, Stronks, Vehage, & Zwaveling, 1991). Medical patients with depressive disorders may also generate greater costs in the process of obtaining their health care (Greenberg, Stiglin, Finkelstein, & Berndt, 1993; Klerman & Weissman, 1992). Some work has indicated that depressed patients tend to show greater medical utilization (Barsky, Wyshak, & Klerman, 1986; Kimmerling et al., 1999); have longer hospital stays (Jacobs et al., 1995; Narrow, Regier, & Rae, 1993; Cushman, 1986); require more custodial care (e.g., nursing homes; Cushman, 1986); are less able to maintain improvements made during rehabilitation (Thompson, Sobolew-Shubin, Graham, & Janigian, 1989); and may be less able to recapture their premorbid quality of life (Niemi, Laaksonen, Kotila, & Waltimo, 1988), thus increasing the need for further psychological intervention. There is also growing evidence that depressed cardiac patients may be at heightened risk for rehospitalization (Stern, Pascale, &

Ackerman, 1977) and reinfarct (Carney, Freedland, Rich, & Jaffe, 1995; Frasure-Smith, Lesperance, & Talajic, 1993) in the years following their initial MI.

Other work has found that chronically ill patients (drawn from oncology, rheumatology, and gastroenterology services) who showed poor psychosocial adjustment to their illness showed the greatest utilization of medical services (including use of specialist services and number of hospital episodes in the prior 6 months) and generated the highest costs associated with these services (Browne, Arpin, Corey, Fitch, & Gafni, 1990). Another study indicated that patients displaying significant levels of psychopathology had 40% longer hospital stays, incurred 35% greater hospital charges, and also used more procedures; these findings were independent of gender, race, age, and medical diagnosis (Levenson, Hamer, & Rossiter, 1990). Finally, among over 50,000 medical/surgical patients discharged from two major hospitals during 1984, patients with psychiatric comorbidity had nearly double the length of hospital stays of patients without comorbidity (Fulop, Strain, Vita, Lyons, & Hammer, 1987).

PERSONALITY AND COPING STYLE

Stone and Porter (1995) presented a theoretical model for the multiple pathways through which *coping* can affect outcomes in medical patients. They suggested that patients' coping efforts, guided in part by their appraisals of some medical event (e.g., perceiving a physical symptom), can affect their emotional response, their health behaviors, their communications with their health care provider, and their adherence to primary and secondary prevention efforts. These intermediary outcomes may in turn predict the patients' further help seeking, their sense of well-being, and possibly their disease course (Stone & Porter, 1995). Since maladaptive coping strategies lead to poor emotional adjustment, resumption of health risk behaviors, disturbed patient–physician communications, and reduced adherence to recommended treatment regimens, patients using these strategies may require additional medical care with associated escalation in costs.

PSYCHOLOGICAL ISSUES

Other work has found that many of the psychological factors previously associated with emotional adjustment to illness (e.g., social support, life stress) are also associated with medical utilization patterns. One set of psychological characteristics of medical patients that may be related to utilization and health care costs involves such resources as social support. For instance, in a study of social support factors among medical patients attending 43 family practices, those with lower confidante support and lower emotional support showed a significantly greater number of office visits and a greater number of total charges over a 1-year period (Broadhead, Hehlbach, DeGruy, & Kaplan, 1989). Another study found that contextual factors (e.g., elevated life stress) predicted a greater frequency of medical visits, and that this association was strongest among patients whose personality traits included a tendency toward somaticizing (Miranda, Perez-Stable, Munoz, Hargreaves, & Henke, 1991). This study suggested that stress reduction interventions might be particularly cost-effective in reducing overutilization of outpatient medical services, especially among patients who (1) possess this personality characteristic and (2) are undergoing significant life stressors. Thus assessment of key psychological characteristics of medical outpatients within their life context may facilitate triaging into time-limited, focused psychological intervention as a means of substantially containing health care expenditures.

LIFESTYLE BEHAVIORS

The health-compromising behaviors that people engage in may be among the most important factors influencing the cost of their health care. When 2,238 medical records were randomly sampled from over 42,000 discharges from six different hospital populations, such lifestyle behaviors as alcohol use and cigarette smoking were found to be consistently higher among the 13% of patients classified as high-cost utilizers than among the other 87%, the low-cost utilizers (Zook & Moore, 1980). Repeat hospitalizations and unexpected complications during treatment were among the primary causes for the expenditures in the high-cost group. Importantly, these are behaviors that may be modifiable by psychosocial interventions. As noted in prior sections, being able to identify these health behaviors in the context of a patient's mood state, coping strategies, cognitive appraisals and health attitudes, social and external resources, and ongoing life context may enhance the effectiveness of these psychosocial interventions.

PSYCHOSOCIAL INTERVENTIONS

Is there any evidence that psychosocial interventions can significantly reduce health care costs in medical patients? Several reviews addressing the utility of mental health interventions in reducing such costs have been published (e.g., Levenson, 1992). We use the example of behavioral medicine interventions (e.g., educational, behavioral, and psychosocial interventions) to demonstrate the importance of psychosocial factors in cost containment. For instance, one study found that educating patients on self-care reduced doctors' visits for minor illness and related symptoms by 33%, and did so without compromising their health (Vickery, 1983). This program in particular appeared to save $2.50 for every $1 that it cost to implement. Psychological-distress-related physical discomfort (e.g., headaches, gastrointestinal problems, sleep difficulties) is believed to be the most common cause of health care utilization, with up to 60% of all medical visits made by the "worried well" (Cummings & Van den Bos, 1981). Interventions that are directed at the psychosocial sources of these complaints (i.e., stress-reducing techniques) have been estimated to provide a savings of up to $4 for every $1 invested (Schneider, 1987). In one randomized trial, behavioral medicine techniques were found to reduce physical discomfort and to trim off two office visits, on average, in a cohort of patients presenting with stress-related problems (Hellman, 1990). After the costs of the psychosocial intervention were controlled, the health maintenance organization saved thousands of dollars in the first 6 months alone. Pallak et al. (1994) found that a managed mental health treatment intervention reduced medical costs by up to 21% among Medicaid patients, and that these reductions held at 6, 12, and 18 months posttreatment. Another study found that an 11-day psychosocial intervention conducted with inpatients referred for stress-related conditions reduced average numbers of days hospitalized by 68%, with an average cost savings of $3 for each $1 invested (Gonik, 1981).

A large meta-analytic review of this literature revealed that medical utilization was reduced by 10% to 33% and that hospital stays were cut by 1.5 days after brief psychotherapy (Mumford, Schlesinger, Glass, Patrick, & Cuerdon, 1984). Schlesinger, Mumford, Glass, Patrick, and Sharfstein (1983) observed that patients diagnosed with one of four major medical conditions (chronic lung disease, diabetes, ischemic heart disease, and hypertension) showed significantly lower costs for medical services after receiving mental health treatment. Behavioral interventions were also shown to provide relief to patients with chronic pain at a fraction of the cost of medical interventions (Caudill, 1991). This group noted that medical office visits plummeted by 36% in the first year after the program and persisted at this low level over the second year of follow-up, with an average savings achieved by the program of $3.50 for every $1 invested. Jacobs (1987) reviewed the medical cost offsets of different forms of psychosocial intervention in patients presenting with various pain-related disorders. This analysis indicated that biofeedback treatment reduced hospital and clinic utilization by 72% and 63%, respectively; vocational rehabilitation reduced hospital and clinical visits by 89% and 41%, respectively; and a chronic pain program reduced hospital and clinical utilization by 72% and 50%, respectively. On average, these programs were associated with a sustained 47% reduction in hospital utilization and a total of over $7 million in cost savings over a 4-year follow-up period (Jacobs, 1987).

The Influence of Psychosocial Factors on Treatment Success and Recovery from Disease

It is difficult, if not impossible, to separate the contribution of psychosocial interventions to decreased health care utilization from the contribution to treatment success. However, some studies have provided some additional information that may support the role of psychosocial intervention in actually improving the efficacy of a medical intervention regimen. Here we present some examples of behavioral medicine interventions (designed to modify many of the psychosocial factors previously reviewed) for patients with specific diseases or conditions.

DIABETES MELLITUS

One relevant area in this regard is the care of patients diagnosed with diabetes mellitus. One study reviewed nearly 1,000 of such patients' records and found that inadequate self-care contributed to one in every six hospitalizations (Miller, 1981). At least three major studies involving a total of over 20,000 patients showed that psychosocial interventions substantially reduced costs incurred by diabetic patients; some of these studies found a reduction in hospitalization rates of 73% and lengths of stay of 78%, resulting in an estimated savings of over $2,000 per patient participating in the program (Miller & Goldstein, 1972; Miller, 1981). Another found that an outpatient education program reduced the incidence of severe ketoacidosis by 65% and the frequency of lower-extremity amputations by nearly 50%, for a cost savings of over $400,000 per year (Davidson, 1983). Finally, a brief outpatient edu-

cation program reduced the number of hospital days by over 50% in a group of dia-
betics (Assal et al., 1985; Muhlhauser, 1983). Similar forms of interventions conducted with pregnant women with diabetes have also been shown to lower medical
costs for both the mothers' and the infants' care, with savings up to 30.3%, resulting
in over $5 saved for each $1 invested. Beyond these impressive cost savings, the
results of this last study suggest that children's health may be affected to some degree
by diabetic mothers' access to psychosocial intervention.

ASTHMA

Among patients with asthma, psychosocial interventions delivered in small groups
resulted in more symptom-free days, greater physical activity improvements, and
49% fewer office visits for acute attacks than among patients receiving usual care
over a 2-year follow-up period (Wilson et al., 1993). Another study found that
patients with asthma who were offered a brief psychological intervention involving
written disclosure of emotions showed significant improvement in symptoms and
other indicators of clinical status (Smyth, Stone, Hurewitz, & Kaell, 1998).

ARTHRITIS

Among sufferers from chronic rheumatoid arthritis, one health education program
was found to reduce pain reports by 20% and physician visits by 43%. Importantly,
this program also significantly increased patients' perceived self-efficacy—a key characteristic in consistent self-management, adherence to medical regimens, and reducing vulnerability to stressors and mood disturbances. For these patients, the program
saved an estimated $12 over a 4-year period (or $3 annually) for each $1 invested
(Lorig et al., 1993).

SURGERY

There is some evidence that patients may recover from surgery faster with preopera-
tive psychosocial intervention. Studies conducted over the past two decades have
indicated that psychological interventions may speed actual physical recovery rates
from surgery. Such interventions as muscle relaxation have been associated with
improvements in several surgery-related outcome variables, including fewer days in
intensive care, fewer total days in the hospital, and fewer incidents of congestive
heart failure (e.g., Aiken & Henricks, 1971). Among the nearly 200 studies addressing this topic between 1963 and 1989, beneficial effects for various forms of
psychosocial intervention were reported 79% to 84% of the time (Devine, 1992).
Similar to other work with hospital inpatients, length of hospital stay was reduced by
1.5 days on average. Even with a conservative estimate of projected cost savings of
such changes in length of stay, these programs may save up to $10 for each $1
invested. Across 13 other studies, psychosocial intervention reduced hospital days
after MI or surgery by 2 full days (Mumford, Schlesinger, & Glass, 1982). One study
also revealed that conducting an adequate psychological screen and triaging patients
scheduled for surgery to receive psychiatric intervention reduced the average hospital

stay by 2.2 days, for a savings of over $8 for each dollar invested (Strain et al., 1991). Thus greater attention to the role of psychosocial factors is warranted to contain health care costs and to improve success rates of surgeries for a wide range of conditions. There is some indication that psychosocial interventions that reduce stress levels may also affect postsurgical complications by reducing stress hormone output (e.g., urinary cortisol; Doering et al., 2000); improving wound healing (Kiecolt-Glaser, Marucha, Malarkey, Mercado, & Glaser, 1995); or accelerating immune system recovery after surgery, blood transfusions, and anesthesia (van der Pompe, Antoni, & Heijnen, 1998).

DISEASE COMPLICATIONS

Psychosocial interventions may play a significant role in reducing long-term health care costs by reducing the likelihood of such phenomena as diabetic complications, recurrence of heart attacks after MI, and extended rehabilitation costs for spinal injury or stroke due to reinjury. Other long-term effects of psychosocial interventions are currently being explored in terms of reducing the progression rate of conditions such as HIV infection, the recurrence rate of certain cancers (e.g., breast cancer), and life-threatening and costly complications (e.g., kidney failure) of other disease processes.

An intriguing target for future intervention research in patients with cancer involves the proposed link between stress and susceptibility to infectious disease (Bovbjerg & Valdimarsdottir, 1996). It has been suggested that since stress is associated with increased susceptibility to upper respiratory infections (Cohen et al., 1991) and bacterial infections (Bovjberg & Valdimarsdottir, 1996), patients with cancer, especially those who are emotionally distressed and receiving chemotherapy or other immunosuppressive adjuvant therapies, may be quite vulnerable to stress-associated opportunistic infections (Bovbjerg & Valdimarsdottir, 1996). Surprisingly, very little work has examined the effects of stressors or stress management interventions on the incidence of infectious disease in patients receiving adjuvant therapy for cancer, despite the fact that psychosocial intervention participants show increased lymphocyte functioning (McGregor et al., 2004).

Psychosocial-Assessment-Directed Intervention Choices

Despite the impressive cost savings that may be achieved with psychosocial interventions, it is important to note that these are average cost savings and do not reflect individual cases. It is entirely likely that there are subsets of patients who possess certain psychosocial characteristics that make them more or less likely to benefit from psychosocial interventions. The ability to identify these characteristics at the point of screening and intake would further increase cost savings, because all patients in need of such services would be caught, while those not in need of such services would not incur the costs or burden of psychosocial services unnecessarily.

To summarize what we have said up to this point in the chapter, several characteristics are capable of influencing health maintenance on the one hand and health care costs on the other. Together, these factors can be grouped into four major categories as follows:

1. Psychiatric indicators (anxiety, depression, and other Axis I-related disturbances).
2. Personality coping style (behavioral, cognitive, and interpersonal coping style and strategies).
3. Psychosocial issues (appraisals, resources, and contextual factors).
4. Lifestyle behaviors (health-compromising and health-promoting behaviors).

In addition, knowledge of a patient's communication style may be critical for the health care provider to understand the patient's needs and symptoms. At least four components of a patient's communication style may be relevant here: (1) the tendency to be open about sharing personal information; (2) inclination to present him- or herself in a very positive light, even at the expense of concealing symptoms; (3) inclination to present many minor as well as major symptoms, sensations, and experiences; and (4) receptivity to specific details about diagnostic, prognostic, and treatment procedures and outcomes. The ability to identify systematic distortions, biases, and preferences in patients' self-reports to their health care providers can improve the precision of history taking and symptom monitoring. It can also facilitate patient–provider rapport, potentially resulting in improved help seeking upon emergence of new symptoms and better adherence to prescribed and self-care regimens.

Figure 19.1 lists these five sets of psychosocial factors and their relations to various domains of health maintenance (including primary and secondary/tertiary prevention) and health care delivery. Ideally, all of this information can be synthesized to predict a wide range of medical outcomes that are relevant to the management of patients' health care. Some of these treatment prognostics might include the following:

- Patients' compliance with medical regimens.
- Potential difficulties with or misuses of medications.
- Adverse emotional reactions to demanding protocols.
- Managing risks of treatment complications due to the resumption of risk behaviors.
- Patients' potential for positive responses to psychosocial interventions.

Psychosocial Instruments for Assessing Medical Patients

Throughout this chapter, we have referred to various benefits that could be derived from having available a comprehensive psychosocial assessment for medical patients at the earliest possible point of entry into the health care system. This assessment could occur at the point of screening, diagnosis, or initial treatment, or as a person embarks on a chronic disease management regimen. Psychosocial assessment can predict how well patients will maintain their health, as well as how they will interact with health care systems. We have presented the rationale for the development and use of psychosocial assessment in medical patients and those at risk for developing disease. This work has led to the development and validation of a number of psychosocial instruments now in wide use in behavioral medicine research and in the practice of contemporary clinical health psychology. In the remainder of this chapter,

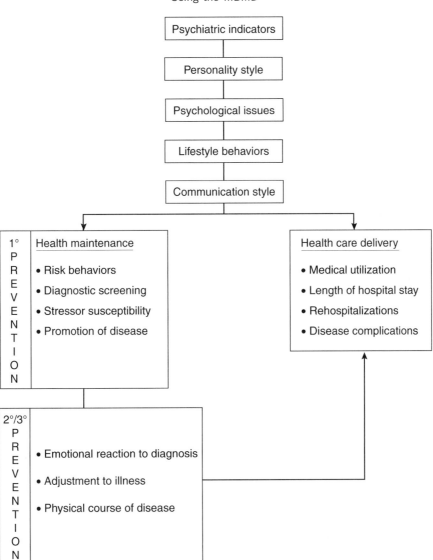

FIGURE 19.1. Five sets of psychosocial characteristics (psychiatric indicators, personality style, psychological issues, lifestyle behaviors, and patient communication style) and their relationship to multiple aspects of health maintenance (primary and secondary/tertiary prevention) and health care delivery.

we highlight two of these instruments: the MBHI (Millon et al., 1982), and a new instrument, the MBMD (Millon et al., 2001). These tools provide integrated information on the psychosocial characteristics of medical patients for the purpose of optimizing health maintenance and health-service-related activities. The extensive body of literature reviewed to this point, in combination with Millon's personality theory, formed the rationale for the choice of the major domains and corresponding scales assessed in these instruments.

The Use of the MBHI with Medical Patients

One objective instrument designed to provide comprehensive information for health psychologists and health care providers in a systematic and explicitly synthesized format is the MBHI (Millon et al., 1982). The MBHI is a 150-item self-report instrument that provides information on patent coping strategies, health-related attitudes (e.g., pessimism and hopelessness), and probable responses to major medical treatments. A good deal of published research has demonstrated the efficacy of the MBHI for evaluating a wide range of medical populations, including patients with cancer (Goodkin et al., 1986; Goldstein & Antoni, 1989), chronic pain (Gatchel et al., 1986; Wilcoxin, Zook, & Zarski, 1988), renal disease (Tracy, Green, & McCleary, 1987), headache (Gatchel et al., 1985), gastrointestinal disorders (Alberts, Lyons, & Anderson, 1988; Richter et al., 1986), and cardiac conditions (Green, Millon, & Meagher, 1983; Katz et al., 1985; Kolitz et al., 1988; Lantinga et al., 1988; Brandwin, Clifford, & Coffman, 1989). These studies have established the utility of the MBHI for predicting the following: help-seeking behaviors after the onset of MI symptoms; the promotion of early neoplastic changes in women at risk for cervical cancer; initial psychological reactions to news of a life-threatening medical diagnosis; psychological adjustment to the burdens of chronic disease; the ability to make lifestyle changes required by certain diseases; appointment keeping and other indices of medical adherence; responses to rehabilitation efforts; decision making concerning treatment choices; the progression of physical disease and related physiological changes (immune system declines); and recovery from and survival after major medical procedures (e.g., heart transplant). Thus the MBHI represented a major contribution by the Millon team, as it provided a research and clinical tool capable of predicting behavioral responses to the onset of new symptoms, reactions to medical diagnosis, adjustment to chronic disease and chronic pain, the efficacy of secondary prevention efforts, and the physical course of disease.

The Use of the MBHI in Health Preservation

The MBHI and Help Seeking in Response to Life-Threatening Symptoms

The MBHI has been used to examine how personality style relates to behavioral and cognitive responses immediately after the onset of acute coronary symptoms in patients experiencing their first MI (Kolitz et al., 1988). Advances in cardio-technology have facilitated the development of life-saving interventions, such as angioplasty and chemical agents capable of removing arterial blockage accompanying MI in as many as 75% of treated cases (Topol et al., 1987). However, these forms of intervention are generally most effective during the first few hours after the onset of acute MI symptoms, after which time the cardiac muscle may be damaged irreparably. Understanding the psychosocial factors (e.g., personality/coping style) that are associated with a patient's decision to pursue help or delay help seeking after the onset of such symptoms may have significant implications for reducing the severity of the MI and its associated costs.

In the first study (Kolitz et al., 1988), 30 patients diagnosed with an MI (23 men and 7 women) completed the MBHI, the Beck Depression Inventory (BDI; Beck, 1978), and a lifestyle behavior interview after they had been transferred from the coronary care unit to the cardiac ward. Using a base rate cutoff score of 70 on the MBHI, the researchers formed three personality code groups and designated these as follows: Angry–Moody (elevations on scales 2, 6, and 8), Dependent–Conforming (elevations on scales 1, 3, and 7), and Confident–Outgoing (elevations on scales 4, 5, and 6). Kolitz et al. found that members of the Angry–Moody group tended to attribute the cause of their MI to external stress, while members of the Dependent–Conforming and Confident–Outgoing groups attributed their heart attacks to their poor lifestyle habits. The Angry–Moody group also reported the longest delay time in seeking medical attention after the onset of their MI symptoms: 81% took longer than 4 hours, and fully 65% took longer than 14 hours to seek help. On the other hand, 91% of the patients in the Confident–Outgoing group and 75% of Dependent–Conforming group members sought medical attention in the first 1 to 4 hours after the onset of MI symptoms. Interestingly, the Angry–Moody group also showed significantly higher BDI scores; higher recent stress; and greater pessimism, hopelessness, and somatic anxiety than did patients in the other two groups. These findings suggested that these subjects were having the most difficulty adjusting emotionally to their MI during their hospital convalescence. A second study by this same group largely replicated these findings in 40 patients with a first-time MI drawn from two different hospitals (Kolitz et al., 1988). These findings, taken together with results of the first study, suggest that personality/coping style, cognitive appraisals (pessimism and hopelessness, as well as attributions for the cause of MI symptoms), and social support resources may act together to play a role in determining patients' decisions to seek help after the onset of life-threatening symptoms.

The MBHI and the Promotion of Subclinical Neoplastic Changes

Another line of investigation has focused on identifying samples of people who possess a genetic, pathophysiological, behavioral, or environmental risk factor for the development of a disease, and then evaluating the incremental proportion of the variance in disease manifestation that can be predicted by knowledge of psychosocial and contextual factors. One application of this paradigm might involve identifying persons who are at risk for the development of CHD because of genetic (family history), pathophysiological (e.g., hypertension, hypercholesterolemia), behavioral (e.g., tobacco smoking and other lifestyle behaviors), and contextual (e.g., high-stress job) risk factors, and examining the incremental predictive power that knowledge of the patients' psychiatric status (e.g., depressive disorder), personality/coping style (e.g., hard-driving, time-urgent, hostile), and psychosocial factors (e.g., low self-esteem, pessimism, social alienation, and lack of resources) provides for predicting the development of overt CHD.

At least four studies have related MBHI-indexed personality coping styles and other psychosocial factors to the subclinical promotion of cervical neoplasia, the cellular changes that precede the development of invasive cervical carcinoma. In one study, 73 women presenting to an obstetrics/gynecology clinic with evidence of repeated abnormal Pap smears completed the MBHI, the Life Experiences Survey (Sarason, Johnson, & Spiegel, 1978), and a lifestyle behavior interview before being colposcopically examined for evidence of neoplastic changes on the surface of the cervix (Goodkin et al., 1986). The women with the highest MBHI Premorbid Pessimism, Future Despair, Social Alienation, and Somatic Anxiety scores showed the strongest association between negative life event stress and level of cervical neoplasia (Goodkin et al., 1986). A second study used a similar paradigm with 75 women undergoing colposcopic examinations for abnormal Pap smears (Antoni & Goodkin, 1988). The researchers found that after they controlled for other risk factors (e.g., Pap smear frequency and cigarette smoking), women with higher scores on the MBHI Respectful style, and Premorbid Pessimism, Future Despair, and Somatic Anxiety scales displayed the greatest level of biopsy-determined cervical neoplasia (Antoni & Goodkin, 1988). A follow-up to this study indicated that the MBHI Respectful style and Psychogenic Attitude scales interacted with recent life event stress in predicting greater levels of cervical neoplasia (Antoni & Goodkin, 1989). These authors proposed that the association between these psychosocial factors and the promotion of cervical neoplasia might be mediated by immune system changes that are associated with stressors and psychosocial factors on the one hand and the surveillance of human papillomavirus (HPV)-induced cervical neoplastic changes on the other (Goodkin, Antoni, Sevin, et al., 1993). A fourth study used the MBHI to pursue this line of reasoning by examining the association between psychosocial factors (personality/coping style, pessimism, contextual factors) and immune system functioning (natural killer cell cytotoxicity, or NKCC) in women at risk for the development of cervical carcinoma due to the presence of multiple risk factors (HPV infection, HIV infection; Byrnes et al., 1998). These researchers found that after they controlled for the presence or absence of two specific types of HPV infection (based on *in situ* hybridization of tissue removed by cervical swabs) and amount of cigarette smoking, higher MBHI Respectful style scores in combination with a greater number of recently experienced negative life events were associated with poorer NKCC. These findings collectively suggest that the MBHI may be useful in identifying psychosocial (personality/coping style, appraisals, resources, and contextual factors) characteristics that combine with lifestyle behavioral risk factors and pathophysiological risk actors to be incrementally predictive of the development of neoplastic disease, as well as changes in underlying surveillance mechanisms that control the growth of the primary pathogenic process.

Another study used the MBHI to examine the association between personality coping styles and immune system functioning in men ultimately diagnosed with HIV infection (Lutgendorf et al., 1996). Healthy, symptom-free, and sexually active gay men enrolled in a study designed to examine the psychological and physiological effects of HIV antibody testing and notification. They completed a battery of psychological tests, including the MBHI, and underwent a blood draw to evaluate the status of their immune systems, approximately 5 weeks before they were tested for and notified of their HIV antibody status. MBHI personality/coping style scores were then correlated with different indices of immune system status within the men who ultimately turned out to be HIV-seropositive (Lutgendorf et al., 1996). As in the case of the cervical neoplasia studies just summarized, the men were unaware of their disease status at the time of psychological testing—thus diminishing the likelihood that test responses were mere reactions to the news of diagnosis, and increasing the likelihood that MBHI responses pertained to long-standing personality/coping styles. As in the case of the cervical neoplasia study, an emotionally nonexpressive coping style was associated with greater impairments in indices of immune system functioning relevant to viral infection surveillance (NKCC and Epstein–Barr virus immunoglobulin G antibody titers) in this cohort of HIV-infected men. Men with greater impairments in immune system surveillance functions at this early, asymptomatic stage of the infection may be at greater risk for a faster progression to full-blown AIDS.

The Use of the MBHI in Assessing Adjustment to Disease and Secondary Prevention

The MBHI and Adjustment to Chronic Disease

We conducted some work testing the utility of the MBHI for identifying associations between personality/coping style and the ways in which HIV-infected people who were already manifesting clinical symptoms adapted to this chronic disease. A number of MBHI coping style scales were found to be associated with several indices of psychosocial and behavioral adjustment in a cohort of symptomatic HIV-infected gay men (Starr et al., 1996). Specifically, elevations of the Inhibited, Forceful, and Sensitive style scales (2, 6, and 8, respectively), as well as higher 2–6–8 composite scores, were associated with higher BDI scores, a lower sense of self-efficacy, less perceived social support, and more frequent use of COPE-indexed (Carver, Scheier, & Weintraub, 1989) denial as a coping strategy for dealing with their infection. On the other hand, higher scores on the MBHI Sociable (scale 4) and Confident (scale 5) style scales were associated with lower BDI depression scores, greater self-efficacy, and less frequent use of denial. Subjects in the highest tercile for the 2–6–8 composite score showed an average BDI score in the clinical range of moderate depression, while the mean of subjects in the remaining two-thirds of the sample had mean BDI scores below the cutoff for mild depression. These results suggested that certain MBHI coping styles may identify HIV-infected persons who are less able to adjust emotionally to their disease.

These psychosocial characteristics may also relate to difficulties in maintaining lifestyle behavior changes. The same study found that higher scores on MBHI scales 6 and 8 were associated with a greater number of sex partners in the past month, and that higher 2–6–8 composite scores were associated with a greater number of different partners and a higher frequency of unprotected sexual episodes (Starr et al., 1996). Transcripts of interviews with these men were rated by independent judges and revealed that men with higher 2–6–8 composites displayed lower self-esteem, poorer problem-solving skills, and less insight as they discussed the ways that they had been dealing with their infection (Starr et al., 1996). Thus HIV-infected individuals (in this study, gay men) with MBHI coping styles characterized according to Millon's theory by active avoidance, active independence, and/or active ambivalence may be less able to adjust emotionally to this life-threatening disease, and may be less able or willing to make the lifestyle changes that are required to maintain their health. Moreover, such individuals appear to maintain a low sense of self-esteem, to utilize maladaptive coping styles (e.g., denial), to display poor problem-solving skills, to have inadequate social support resources, and lack insight into the ways their infection has affected their lives. This work suggests that the MBHI may be useful in identifying HIV-infected persons who could benefit from psychosocial interventions designed to change some of these psychosocial factors.

The MBHI and the Efficacy of Secondary/Tertiary Prevention Efforts

At least two studies have used the MBHI to predict patients' success with interventions designed to help them manage chronic disease. Wilcoxin et al. (1988) found that a composite score based on several MBHI scales (Chronic Tension, Recent Stress, Allergic Inclination, Inhibited style, Respectful style, Pain Treatment Responsivity, Life-Threat Reactivity, and Premorbid Pessimism) successfully predicted gains in time sitting, time standing, number of stairs climbed, time on a treadmill, treadmill speed, and hand grip strength among male and female pain patients completing a 20–day outpatient pain rehabilitation program. A discriminant function analysis revealed that these eight MBHI scales, in combination with demographic information on age, gender, marital status, and educational level, correctly classified 96% (29/30) of patient outcomes.

Another study used the MBHI to relate 42 dialysis patients' psychosocial characteristics to their preferences for types of dialysis and their adjustment to treatment (Weisberg & Page, 1988). All patients completed the MBHI, and a patient questionnaire assessing general emotional factors and current adjustment to dialysis, at the time of their visit to the kidney unit at a large hospital. Patients choosing to receive hospital-based dialysis showed higher scores on the MBHI Chronic Tension, Recent Stress, Premorbid Pessimism, Future Despair, Social Alienation, Somatic Anxiety, Life-Threat Reactivity, and Emotional Vulnerability scales than patients choosing home-based dialysis did. Analysis of personality/coping styles indicated that the patients choosing the hospital-based program had significantly higher MBHI Respectful style scores than did those choosing home-based dialysis. In terms of adjustment to dialysis, higher Recent Stress and Premorbid Pessimism scores were associated with patients' reports of greater difficulty in accepting help from their partners and lower satisfaction with their chosen dialysis modality. Higher scores on Premorbid Pessimism, Future Despair, Social Alienation, Life-Threatening Reactivity, and Emotional Vulnerability were associated with a greater likelihood of the patients' viewing themselves as "sick." Several different MBHI Psychogenic Attitude scales were associated with poorer sexual adjustment and feelings of loss of femininity–masculinity (Weisberg & Page, 1988). Patients scoring higher on MBHI Respectful style were less satisfied with the treatment modality chosen, showed poorer sexual adjustment, and felt less in control of treatment procedures. Higher scores on Forceful style were associated with greater difficulty in asking partners for help, while patients scoring higher on Sociable style were less likely to view themselves as sick and reported greater satisfaction with their treatment. This study demonstrates the usefulness of the MBHI in predicting patients' treatment choices and their ensuing adjustment to the demands of chronic disease. The study may also have implications for health care delivery, as home-based dialysis is associated with substantial cost savings over hospital-based programs. Identifying psychosocial characteristics of patients with kidney disease may help to predict those who are the best candidates for both home- and hospital-based dialysis, and may also direct practitioners to issues that may act as obstacles to successfully implementing either choice.

Development of the MBMD

Despite the impressive results generated by studies using the MBHI to assess psychosocial characteristics relevant to a variety of primary and secondary prevention domains in different patient populations, this instrument did not provide explicit information on several other important psychosocial characteristics. These included (1) psychiatric indicators that may influence patients' adjustment to their medical condition; (2) coping styles reflecting recently derived personality disorders, such as depressive, sadistic, and masochistic personality disorders (Millon & Davis, 1996); (3) other psychosocial factors related to cognitive appraisals (e.g., self-esteem, general efficacy), resources (e.g., spirituality and religion), and contextual factors (e.g., functional abilities); (4) specific lifestyle behaviors (e.g., alcohol and substance abuse, smoking, eating patterns, inactivity and exercise); (5) aspects of patients' communication styles (tendencies toward disclosure, social desirability, devaluation when communicating); and (6) information useful for predicting patient adherence, medication abuses, utilization of medical services, preference for more or less detail when receiving medical information, and emotional responses to stressful medical procedures, which in turn can be useful in informing health care management decision making and mental health treatment triaging. Awareness of the potential usefulness of this information for maximizing health maintenance and minimizing health care costs provided the impetus for the development of a new instrument, the MBMD (Millon et al., 2001), which was designed to address all of these issues in addition to those already tapped by the MBHI.

We developed the MBMD to expand the scope of the MBHI by providing information on those psychosocial characteristics of medical patients that contemporary behavioral medicine research has identified as potentially influencing several domains of health maintenance and health care delivery: (1) Psychiatric Indicators; (2) Coping Style; (3) Stress Moderators; (4) Treatment Prognostics; and (5) Negative Health Habits. Three additional MBMD scales characterize components of the patient's communication style that may affect their test responses as well as the ways in which they interact with health care providers; these scales are Disclosure, Desirability, and Debasement. The Disclosure scale captures patients' tendency to be open about sharing personal information. The Desirability scale characterizes the patients' inclination to present themselves in an overly positive light even at the expense of concealing symptoms. The Debasement scale describes the patients' tendency to present many minor as well as major symptoms, sensations, and experiences in their communications with health care providers. The ability of a health care provider to identify systematic biases and preferences in a patient's self-reports can improve the precision of history taking and symptom monitoring, and can facilitate patient–provider communication. This may ultimately result in improved help seeking upon emergence of new symptoms, as well as better adherence to prescribed pharmacological and self-care regimens.

Empirical Research Using the MBMD in Different Medical Populations

Empirical work supporting the validity of the MBMD in different medical populations includes over 700 patients recruited from comprehensive cancer centers, organ transplant centers, behavioral medicine research centers, diabetes research institutes, and general medical hospitals and clinics (for a fuller description of validation studies, see Millon, Antoni, Millon, Minor, & Grossman, 2006). The studies summarized in this section represent only a sample of the work designed to address specific research questions in real-life medical settings. This research has included studies using the MBMD to predict posttreatment health-related behaviors and medical utilization; outcomes in patients undergoing organ transplant; health behaviors, immune function, and disease activity in persons with HIV infection; and glucose control in persons with diabetes mellitus.

MBMD Validation Studies

In order to establish the predictive validity for an inventory, one must show that it is associated with objective indices of behavior. In the case of the MBMD, we conducted studies to establish correlations between the Treatment Prognostics scales and at least two sets of objective behavioral indicators. In the first set of studies, we related each of these scales to clinical ratings of patients in health care environments representing some of the major patient populations targeted in the validation studies for the instrument: patients with cancers, CHD, or diabetes mellitus. We viewed clinician ratings as another highly valid indicator of health behaviors and predicted responses to treatment to supplement patient self-reports. The six MBMD scales used in this analysis were Interventional Fragility, Medication Abuse, Information Discomfort, Utilization Excess, Problematic Compliance, and a summative score, Adjustment Difficulties, reflecting predictions about overall management risks. In a second set of studies, we related these scales to such objective behaviors as medication adherence in specific medical populations. We now describe the first set of such studies. For this research, 99 patients were rated by clinicians (e.g., nurses, psychologists, social case workers) who were familiar with patients in a variety of settings (diabetes research institutes, comprehensive cancer centers, organ transplant units). The clinicians completed a Staff Rating Scale (SRS) tapping 11 major domains; these domains and their representative items are presented in Table 19.1.

The SRS results indicated that each of the MBMD Treatment Prognostics scales was significantly correlated with the corresponding staff rating for that domain. There was also evidence of discriminant validity, given that the highest MBMD–SRS correlations were for those tapping the same domain. The summative index, Adjustment Difficulties, was associated (as expected) with a number of staff-rated dimensions that would be expected to present management risks. The strongest MBMD correlations here were with SRS Compliance Issues, Pain Experiences, Symptom Fabrication, Medical Complications, Utilization Problems, and Expenditure Excess (r's = .50 to .61, all p's < .001. In addition, scales from other sections of the MBMD were also significantly associated with corresponding SRS domains. For instance, MBMD Pain Sensitivity scores were associated with SRS Pain Experiences ratings (r =-.62, p < .001), and MBMD Negative Health Habits scores such as smoking and eating problems were significantly associated with SRS Lifestyle Difficulties ratings.

When we conceptualized the various scales making up the MBMD, we envisioned that some of these scales might have more salience or be more likely to be elevated in patients with certain types of major diseases. This helped us in determining

TABLE 19.1. Domains and Representative Items from the Staff Rating Scale (SRS) Used in the MBMD Validation Studies

Patient Behavior and Attitudes

Compliance Issues

- Rarely on time for appointment
- Having difficulty following at-home care instructions
- Resists doing what is recommended to improve his/her health
- Not conscientious about taking medications

Medication Problems

- Having difficulty remembering what medications to take or when to take them
- Complaining frequently that he/she is undermedicated
- Taking old prescriptions and/or other people's prescriptions
- Changing prescribed dosages or combining medication without medical consent

Medical Receptivity

- Reluctant to receive important details about his/her test results
- Getting more upset than most when discussing his/her condition
- Resists learning anything about his/her illness
- Seems overwhelmed when given information about his/her medical condition

Lifestyle Difficulties

- Having considerable trouble keeping his/her weight under control
- Overeating to the point that it presents a significant health concern
- Leading a very sedentary life
- Having difficulty with or resists following a regular exercise program
- Unable (or unwilling) to quit smoking
- Having a smoking habit that is a significant health concern

Pain Experiences

- Reporting more pain than others in a similar medical condition
- Reporting pain intense enough to prompt significant life changes
- Constantly asking about what else can be done for pain
- Requesting excessive pain medication

Symptom Fabrication

- Exaggerating symptoms to elicit special medical attention of services
- Seeking procedures and/or medications that are not warranted by his/her diagnosis
- Reporting symptoms that are inconsistent with medical findings
- Likely to be fabricating symptoms

Possible Complications and Outcomes

Medical Complications

- Needing extended at-home care services
- Needing protracted medical treatment
- Needing a prolonged hospital stay
- Having a problematic remedial course
- Failing to respond to standard treatment
- Having numerous side effects or other medical complications

Utilization Problems

- Becoming a doctor shopper
- A hypochondriac
- Seen as demanding of clinical staff
- Becoming impatient with and annoying staff
- Seen as demanding procedures that are not warranted
- Showing up unnecessarily in the ER
- Demanding repeated attention from specialists
- Using up staff time unnecessarily
- Misusing medical services

Expenditure Excess

- A poor risk for a managed care system
- Incurring higher medical expenses
- Requiring numerous medical procedures
- Incurring high inpatient costs
- Requiring repeated hospitalizations or outpatient visits
- Generating inflated or unnecessary expenditures

Therapeutic Outcome Difficulties

- Lacking the qualities of a good support group or psychotherapy candidate
- Too disruptive or hostile for a support group or other psychological intervention
- Too anxious or depressed for a support group or other psychological intervention
- Too self-absorbed or confused for a support group or other psychological intervention

Fragile Reactions

- Overanxious and fearful while awaiting medical procedures
- Needing excessive reassurance while undergoing medical interventions
- Exhibiting bizarre behavior when anticipating stressful medical procedures
- Incoherent or disoriented during medical procedures
- A poor candidate for extended/complicated medical regimens
- A poor candidate for a complex/demanding self-care regimen

which major diseases should be represented in our validation sample. We decided that in addition to sampling from general medical populations, we would oversample from patients in the following major disease groups: cancer, diabetes, HIV/AIDS, and heart disease. We compared mean MBMD scores across patients drawn from these four major disease groups, and analyzed these group differences separately in 105 women and 174 men.

Among women, we found disease group differences on the following scales: Guardedness from the Psychiatric Indicators; Introversive, Inhibited, Nonconforming, Forceful, Respectful, and Oppositional from the Coping Styles; Functional Deficits and Social Isolation from the Stress Moderators; and Medication Abuse, Utilization Excess, Problematic Compliance, Adjustment Difficulties, and Psychological Referral from the Treatment Prognostics and Management Guide sections. Here, patients with HIV/AIDS had the highest scores for Guardedness and for the Introversive, Inhibited, Nonconforming, Forceful, Respectful, and Oppositional coping styles. These group differences were most evident in women, and women also revealed higher prevalence scores than men on nearly all scales. It should be noted, however, that these differences may have been related to factors other than gender, owing to the fact that women within certain disease groups (e.g., HIV/AIDS) were of lower SES than their male counterparts.

From these comparisons, it is apparent that MBMD profiles may vary greatly as a function of gender and disease group, though some of these differences may be brought about by other correlated factors, such as socioeconomic status and education. Nevertheless, these differences by gender justify the use of separate raw prevalence score transformations for men and women. The differences by disease group may reflect inherent differences in personality or demographic characteristics of persons manifesting certain diseases. Caution should be exercised in interpreting these disease group differences as causally related to the development of these diseases. Rather, the differences are likely to reflect demographic factors associated with the nature of the samples used in these validation studies (e.g., most HIV-infected women were inner-city, lower-SES minority women, whereas female patients with cancer were likely to include a greater proportion of middle-aged, middle-SES white women).

Using the MBMD for Predicting Psychological Adjustment in HIV-Infected Persons

The validation studies first associated MBMD scales with well-established indices of mood disturbance, coping strategies, and other stress moderators (e.g., optimism–pessimism, social support, and spirituality) in a group of HIV-infected men and women. Validation studies for the Treatment Prognostics scales pertaining to medication adherence required a different strategy, which we detail in a subsequent section. First, we related MBMD coping style scales with personality measures and indicators of disease-specific coping strategies. Specifically, at the time of the MBMD administration, 40 HIV-positive men and women completed the NEO Personality Inventory—Revised (NEO-PI-R) and the COPE. The COPE measured specific coping strategies used to deal with HIV-related symptoms and stressors.

The pattern of results indicated strong positive correlations between the MBMD Inhibited, Dejected, Oppositional, and Denigrated styles and NEO-PI-R Neuroticism (r's = .58 to .77). In contrast, MBMD Sociable (r = .63) and Confident (r = .46) coping styles were both associated strongly with NEO-PI-R Extraversion. In regard to the use of HIV-specific coping strategies, MBMD Inhibited, Dejected, and Denigrated styles were associated with the use of alcohol and drugs, with denial and behavioral disengagement (giving up), and with less use of more adaptive strategies (such as acceptance and positive reframing) for dealing with HIV infection. The results for analyses of correlates of the MBMD Stress Moderators scales were intuitive. For instance, persons showing elevations in Illness Apprehension might be expected to show greater anxiety levels and to have a more difficult time accepting some of the realities of their illness. Those with elevations in Functional Deficits might be suffering from greater fatigue, confusion, and cognitive deficits, possibly reflecting greater illness-associated compromises in quality of life. This latter MBMD scale comes the closest to representing an overall physical quality-of-life indicator. Persons scoring high in Pain Sensitivity might have more complaints about medication side effects and display more neurotic signs, while having a greater difficulty in using more sophisticated coping strategies (e.g., positive reframing) for dealing with HIV-related challenges. Those with elevations in Social Isolation might be less likely to use seeking support as a coping strategy, and more likely to use a form of disengagement to deal with their illness. Persons showing elevations in Future Pessimism might be more depressed and more prone to disengaging and giving up when faced with the challenges of their illness. Finally, persons scoring higher in Spiritual Absence might be less likely to use spiritual resources or religion in coping with illness and are likely to place less trust in the efficacy of their HIV medications.

Using the MBMD for Predicting Health Behaviors in HIV-Infected Persons

The next set of studies represented an intensive predictive validity investigation of the six MBMD Treatment Prognostics scales' ability to predict actual health behaviors, such as medication adherence (assessed via pill-monitoring forms) and associated improvements in control over disease processes, in HIV-infected men and women who were being treated by complex combination antiretroviral therapy.

Newly emerging antiretroviral medications for HIV/AIDS have been shown to be effective, but require strict adherence in order to achieve success. HIV viral suppression to nondetectable levels, the gold standard for treatment success, is only reached in 40% to 50% of patients (Deeks et al., 1999; Lucas, Chaisson, & Moore, 1999; Valdez et al., 1999). Many suggest that suboptimal levels of adherence to HAART medications can prevent patients from achieving clinically meaningful viral suppression (Bangsberg, Hecht, Charlebois, Chesney, & Moss, 2000; Havlir et al., 2000). Missing as few as 1 or 2 days of medications predicts an increase in viral load and, in some cases, treatment failure (Holzemer, Henry, Portillo, & Miramontes, 1999; Montaner et al., 1998). There is currently great interest in deriving patient factors that may predict optimal medication adherence in HIV-positive persons. This medication regimen requires that patients take up to 18 pills per day. Since compliance of less than 95% can lead to viral mutation and ultimately resistance to the beneficial antiviral effects of these agents (Lewin, 1997), it is quite valuable to be able to forecast compliance levels on the basis of psychosocial assessments.

Behavioral research conducted over the past 20 years has provided clues about individual difference factors underlying medication adherence in other conditions including male patients cardiac rehabilitation (Hershberger, Robertson, & Markert, 1999), patients undergoing renal dialysis (Christensen & Smith, 1995), and patients undergoing heart transplants (Chacko, Harper, Kunik, & Young, 1996). Emerging work has identified psychosocial and behavioral factors related to poorer HAART adherence, including depressive disorders or negative affect states (Gordillo, del Amo, Soriano, & Gonzalez-Lahoz, 1999; Sternhall & Corr, 2002; Weaver et al., 2005), avoidant coping (Weaver et al., 2005), and low social support (Altice, Mostashari, & Friedland, 2001; Singh et al., 1999; Gonzalez et al., 2004). Behavioral factors related to nonadherence to HAART include active drug use (Gordillo et al., 1999) and miscellaneous reasons, such as food restrictions, stressful events, complex schedules, and "forgetting." A study following nearly 1,000 HIV-positive patients up to 5 years found that the primary patient factors related to nonadherence to HAART were depression and lack of support (Carrieri et al., 2006).

We recently conducted a study examining the association of MBMD scores with HAART adherence among 117 HIV-positive individuals on established antiretroviral regimens (Cruess, Meagher, Antoni, & Millon, 2007). The MBMD was administered, and HAART adherence was assessed through patient interview, at a baseline assessment and at 3-month follow-up (at a point after which participants had received medication adherence training from a doctor of pharmacy). As hypothesized, the Medication Abuse scale of the MBMD was uniquely associated with overall adherence at baseline assessment, and also predicted poorer adherence at the 3-month follow-up. Additional MBMD scales (e.g., Depression and Emotional Lability) were also related to overall adherence, as well as to specific adherence behaviors (e.g., missed doses, following specific instructions, and overmedicating). However, the Medication Abuse scale emerged as the most consistent predictor of adherence in the study. These results suggest that the MBMD can be used to predict adherence to HAART medication in a sample of HIV-positive men and women, and may subsequently be used to triage those in need for adherence counseling.

The MBMD and Glucose Control in Patients with Diabetes Mellitus

We also examined associations between MBMD scales and glucose control in patients with diabetes mellitus who were recruited from a diabetes research institute at a large Southeastern medical school. Control of blood glucose levels is a key goal in patients with diabetes, since consistently elevated blood glucose levels may contribute to complications of the disease (Davidson, 1991). We administered the MBMD to patients with diabetes who were receiving regular checkups at the Diabetes Research Institute at the University of Miami Miller School of Medicine. In addition these patients provided blood for tests to determine glycosylated hemoglobin (HBAC1) levels as an indicator of chronic control of blood glucose levels. Elevated HBAC1 levels are indicative of poorer glucose control over the prior 3-month period (Lustman, Frank, & McGill, 1991). Among the 78 patients in this study, higher HBAC1 levels (reflecting poorer glucose control) were associated with higher

MBMD scores for Cognitive Impairment ($r = .22$), Interventional Fragility ($r = .27$), and Medication Abuse ($r = .34$). Higher HBAC1 levels were also marginally associated with the Problematic Compliance score of the MBMD. These findings suggest that the MBMD may be useful in identifying patients with diabetes who are in greatest need of learning skills to manage glucose levels.

An Emerging Application of the MBMD: Bariatric Surgery Consultation

One area where the MBMD is gaining wide use in the clinical community is in the context of presurgical evaluations for patients who are candidates for bariatric surgery. There is great concern about the growing obesity epidemic in the United States (Wadden, Brownell, & Foster, 2002). Over 25% of both the male and female U.S. population is considered to be overweight; some 10% are judged to be "severely overweight," and approximately 2% are considered "morbidly obese." Indeed, obesity may well become to be the leading cause of death in coming years (Flum et al., 2005). Current estimates suggest that approximately 30% of the currently overweight population may be appropriate candidates for a procedure once considered a last resort—that is, bariatric surgery. Bariatric surgery, usually involving some sort of gastric bypass procedure, was employed in just over 13,000 cases in 1998; this number rose to over 100,000 in 2003 and is projected to grow to over 218,000 cases by 2010 if current rates of growth are sustained (Bauchowitz et al., 2005; Santry, Gillen, & Lauderdale, 2005). Patients may have weight loss of up to 60% after gastric bypass surgery and 40% after vertical banded gastroplasty. However, nearly a third of these patients will regain their weight at 2 years postsurgery (Hsu et al., 1998; Delin, Watts, & Bassett, 1995).

Although the effectiveness of bariatric surgery depends on many physical factors, such as age, gender, comorbidities, and surgical volume (Flum et al., 2005), postoperative behaviors are important as well in determining outcomes. Among the most important behavioral predictors of a patient's long-term success is following through with drastic lifestyle changes (Bauchowitz et al., 2005). In other words, maintaining surgical outcomes over the longer term depends in part on the patient's ability to make major lifestyle behavior changes after surgery. These lifestyle changes involve following strict nutritional and exercise guidelines, which may represent marked changes for these individuals (Powers et al., 1997). It is only logical that a lack of success in maintaining lifestyle changes is what has led patients to consider bariatric surgery in the first place (Kalarchian, Wilson, Brolin, & Bradley, 1998). The established link between postoperative behaviors and the ultimate success of bariatric surgery has prompted the National Institutes of Health to recommend psychosocial assessment and counseling before and after such surgery (National Heart, Lung, and Blood Institute, 2000), and guidelines from working groups are in the process of being developed (LeMont, Moorehead, Parish, Reto, & Ritz, 2004).

It is known that numerous psychosocial factors are related to postoperative outcomes for bariatric surgery. Patients with a history of binge eating pose an appreciable risk of reverting to that problematic habit following surgery (Hsu et al., 1998; Green et al., 2004). Similarly significant are a lack of social or familial support, disturbances in body image, and the existence of contradictory or confused motives for undertaking weight loss. Also worthy of note are demographic variables (e.g., ethnicity) and eating style (e.g., cognitive restraint vs. disinhibition), as well as current psychiatric disabilities and general coping or personality styles—all of which will have a bearing on matters of medical compliance, stress tolerance, impulsive acting out, and overutilization of health services (Antoni, 2005).

We now present a case example to illustrate how the MBMD can be used to generate hypotheses in the context of a presurgical consultation for bariatric surgery. This information is elaborated further in a Bariatric Surgery User's Guide for the MBMD, along with a number of other cases (Millon et al., 2007).

The Case of R. C., Female, Age 34

R. C., age 34, was a somewhat anxious, notably obese, yet attractive Native American woman who called the bariatric surgery unit at her local hospital for an exploratory appointment with the unit's intake social worker. Her history was not an unusual one among candidates for this surgical program. She reported that both parents, still living, had always been overweight. She described her own and her younger sister's background of childhood obesity. Although she was currently married, she was experiencing difficulties in her marital relationship following her husband's recent infidelities. Together they had two teenage children: a normally developing 17-year-old boy and a heavy, but not obese, 15-year-old girl.

R. C. had developed Type II diabetes about 8 years prior and was currently on oral medication. The anxiety consequent to her marital difficulties, as well as a series of unsuccessful weight loss programs, prompted R. C. to look into a surgical approach to her problems. Her social life, which included regular activities with several female friends, had mostly been satisfactory. At the time of intake, R. C. worked full-time at a small advertising agency and possessed adequate insurance to cover basic surgical expenses.

She was judged to be an appropriate candidate, following a brief interview with one of the physicians on the surgical staff. Her height was recorded as 5 feet 3 inches, and her weight was 292 pounds. Her goal was to achieve a weight of close to 140 pounds. As part of the standard surgical routine, she was further interviewed by the staff psychologist and was administered the MBMD, the results of which are presented in Figure 19.2.

As can be seen in the profile for this case, there are no marked elevations in Psychiatric Indications, though there is a somewhat elevated score on the Anxiety–Tension scale; this is in line with some of the impressions formed at the interview. The degree to which this level is likely to interfere with her adjustment to surgery or postoperative behaviors is not likely to be significant. Her Coping Styles profile suggests that R. C. is a person who appreciates the company of others and who is diligent in her job and responsive to authority figures. This is a person who is likely to follow medical advice and adhere to treatment guidelines. Among the factors that may insulate this person from stressors and life challenges, her ability to tolerate pain and remain optimistic toward the future (indicated by scores < 35 on the Pain Sensitivity and Future Pessimism scales) may serve her well. The absence of a spiritual source of support for R. C. may be relevant, though her social network may provide the needed external stress buffer, should a need arise to call upon her female friends. The only noteworthy Treatment Prognostics scale is Medication Abuse, suggesting that this woman may have some difficulties following a medication regimen. Given her coping style characterized by respect and trust in authority figures, however, she is likely to respond to clearly structured prescriptions and brief conferences with her physician. There is no indication in the Treatment Prognostics profile that R. C. will have marked difficulty in complying with the requisite postoperative behaviors. The Management Guides section suggests that this patient will experience only moderate adjustment difficulties in the postoperative period.

Norms: Bariatric   Valid Profile
Medical Problem(s):
Code: - // - ** 7 3 * // - *** F * C B A E + // - ** H * I + //

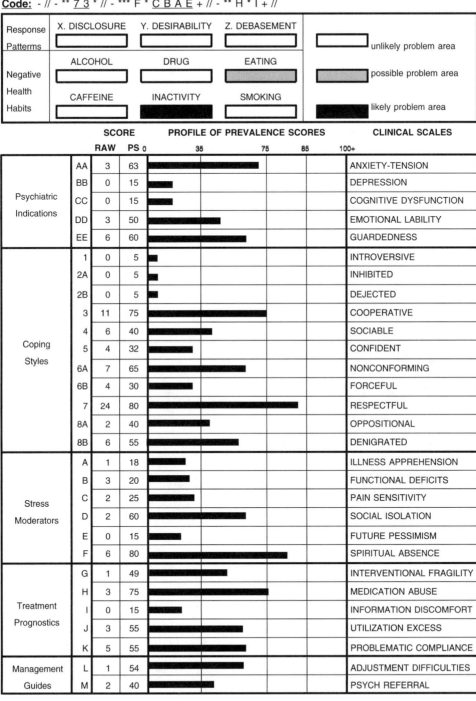

FIGURE 19.2. MBMD Profile and Interpretive Report (Bariatric Norms) for R. C. *(p. 1 of 5)*

BARIATRIC SUMMARY

The following classifications are relevant to patients who are being psychosocially assessed in conjunction with medical plans for gastric surgery. The probabilistic statements below reflect judgments based on clinical experience, the bariatric research literature, and theory-deduced inferences. Nonpsychosocial factors (e.g., BMI, energy metabolism, diabetfc consequences, and hypertension) must also be kept in mind as outcome modifiers.

Studies of 700-plus bariatric surgical patients served as the basis for developing the MBMD's prevalence score (PS) bariatric norms. Further studies to develop probabilistic predictive outcome indices are under way. Data from these studies will be used to further refine plausible hypotheses such as those noted below.

The categorizations in the following tables are based on credible and discriminating probabilistic judgments. As noted, they are not empirically derived, and they should not be considered definitive. They are based on the patient's MBMD bariatric norm scores and profiles, and they are intended to help clinicians make prudent and tentative management decisions for this patient. Inconsistencies between these categorizations and the interpretive statements found in the remainder of this report, while infrequent, may exist. If this occurs, clinicians are encouraged to rely on additional sources of clinical data to gain a better understanding of the patient's condition.

PRESURGICAL INTERVENTION

A. Before the decision to perform surgery is made:	Is considered:
1. An additional psychosocial evaluation	Unnecessary
2. A psychiatric consultation	Unnecessary
3. Supportive psychosocial counseling	Unnecessary
4. A pain management program	Unnecessary

PATIENT BEHAVIOR

B. The likelihood that this patient will:	Is classified as:
1. Be released from the hospital ahead of schedule	Average
2. Change her unhealthy habits	High
3. Refrain from engaging in unhealthy eating behavior	High
4. Follow nutritional advice	Average
5. Comply with a medical regimen	Average
6. Maintain an exercise program	Average
7. Maintain her postsurgical weight loss	High
8. Avoid long-term health complications	High
9. Refrain from taking legal action regarding her surgery	High

POSTSURGICAL OUTLOOK

C. The likelihood that surgery will improve this patient's:	Is classified as:
1. Overall quality of life	Good
2. Psychosocial functioning	Good
3. Body image	Good
4. Physical health	Good
5. Mental outlook	Good
6. Sexual activity	Good
7. Employment/vocational opportunities	Good

POSTSURGICAL CARE

D. The likelihood that this patient will benefit from a:	Is classified as:
1. Physical rehabilitation program	Doubtful
2. Stress and/or sleep management course	Doubtful
3. Bariatric support group	Doubtful
4. Nutritional instruction plan	Doubtful

FIGURE 19.2. *(p. 2 of 5)*

MILLON™ BEHAVIORAL MEDICINE DIAGNOSTIC-INTERPRETIVE REPORT

This report is based on the assumption that the MBMD assessment was completed by a person who is undergoing professional medical evaluation or treatment. MBMD data and analyses do not provide physical diagnoses. Rather; the instrument supplements such diagnoses by identifying and appraising the potential role of psychiatric and psychosomatic factors in a patient's disease and treatment. The statements in this report are derived from cumulative research data and theory. As such, they must be considered probabilistic inferences rather than definitive judgments and should be evaluated in that light by clinicians. The statements contained in the report are of a personal nature and are for confidential professional use only. They should be handled with great discretion and should not be shown to patients or their relatives.

> **Interpretive Considerations**—This section identifies noteworthy response patterns and indicates negative health habits that may be affecting the patient's medical condition.

This patient responded in an open and honest manner with no obvious distortions. Her response style is similar to that of a typical medical patient.

She is probably experiencing problems with maintaining a regular exercise program. Additionally, she may be experiencing problems with overeating.

> **Psychiatric Indications**—This section identifies current psychiatric symptoms or disorders that should be a focus of clinical attention. These symptoms or disorders may affect the patient's response to healthcare treatment and her ability to adjust to or recover from her medical condition.

This patient is not indicating significant psychiatric distress at this time.

> **Coping Styles**—This section characterizes the patient's coping style and/or defenses. These include "normal" parallels of DSM-IV Axis II personality styles that may influence the patient's response to healthcare treatment and her ability to adjust to or recover from her condition.

This patient generally seeks to appear proper, conventional, and socially conforming. Her calm, controlled, and low-key exterior is a superficial veneer, however, that covers a complex of ambivalent feelings that may emerge under stressful circumstances. Nevertheless, she has chosen a lifestyle that reflects a strong sense of commitment to duty and responsibility. She complies with social conventions and has a strict moral sense that rigidly distinguishes right from wrong. This behavioral style is what is seen under most circumstances. It takes a stressful condition, such as an illness, to possibly trigger a display of the underlying layer of ambivalence. The more serious or prolonged the illness, the greater the likelihood that these ambivalent feelings will emerge. At these times, her conventional veneer may give way to blaming others. Shortly after these outbursts, she is likely to express strong feelings of guilt and contrition at having lost control. Psychophysiological ailments are a frequent result of such vacillating and constrained emotions.

This patient's response to a serious physical illness may be initial hesitation in acknowledging that she has a problem. As a consequence, she may find it difficult to share complaint information and her medical history. If sufficient anxiety is present beyond this initial stage, her hesitation and denial may give way to blaming others for some aspect of her discomfort. Although she will be sorry after making critical remarks, reverting to her more conforming behavior, she is likely to be inconsistent and erratic in this regard, periodically switching back and forth from being upset to being conforming and contained.

One of the most helpful approaches to take with this patient is to provide her with specific and concrete written information regarding treatment plans, appointments, and health-promoting regimens. She will not feel fully at ease without structured guidelines such as these. With them, she is likely to be quite cooperative. A formal and professional attitude is most likely to gain her respect and enhance her adherence to a recommended recovery program.

> **Stress Moderators**—This section notes the patient's personal and social assets and liabilities and how they may affect her ability to manage the stressors and burdens of her medical condition and treatment.

Liabilities: Spiritual Absence
Assets: Illness Acceptance, Functional Competence, Pain Tolerance, Future Optimism

FIGURE 19.2. *(p. 3 of 5)*

This patient does not appear to consider her spiritual faith an asset in facilitating recovery from her medical problems. Ifshe is dealing with a serious illness, she may feel unable to carry out self-care responsibilities, especially if she is not in a position to rely on members of her social network. Owing to her passive and conforming nature, it is possible that her failure to access spiritual resources or the support of her church lies in her belief that she has been dealt her fate and must bear the pain and discomfort of it alone. Healthcare providers should inquire into what her premorbid sources of support were and whether she has any religious ties or spiritual beliefs that could help her through this period.

This individual demonstrates appropriate concern about her health and is likely to be an accurate reporter of any changes in her symptoms and functioning. Her conforming style may cause her, at times, to delay acting on changes in her health status. However, her conforming nature can be an advantage because she is likely to closely adhere to a well-structured treatment plan.

This individual demonstrates a strong desire to maintain her independence and daily routines, which are indicators of her ability to function in the world. However, because of her passive and conforming style, she may require explicit assurance from her healthcare provider that she is able to take on her premorbid activities.

This individual appears to handle pain-related symptoms better than other medical patients. If she encounters pain-related problems in the future, her conforming nature may help her adhere to a well-structured treatment plan and derive maximum benefit from any medications prescribed. Allowing her to plan her medication schedule in the context of her daily routines will be helpful for any long-term program of care.

This patient has a good deal of confidence in the likelihood of a speedy recovery from her current condition. Because of her conforming and placid nature, she will probably follow the suggestions of healthcare providers without questioning them. She is likely to place an extraordinary amount of faith in the efficacy of the prescribed treatments. Healthcare providers can make use of this great respect by giving her clear directives for self-care before her discharge, which should lead her to be strongly adherent to the self-care plan.

> **Treatment Prognostics**—This section, which is based on the patient's psychological profile, forecasts her response to medical procedures and medication.

Liabilities: Medication Abuse
Assets: Information Receptivity

This individual may be at heightened risk for having difficulty maintaining a prescribed medication regimen. She may lack the desire to follow through with medication instructions, leading to possible under- or overmedication, She may subconsciously or deliberately abuse her medication as a cry for help. If her distress level is mild, with a moderate risk for apathy toward medication regimens, cognitive therapy may be useful. This may increase her belief in the efficacy of her medications and her own ability to manage the regimen.

This patient is open to receiving information or discussing matters pertaining to her illness. This may help facilitate her adjustment to treatment and may be used by the healthcare team to improve health outcomes.

> **Management Guide**—This section provides recommendations for the general management of this patient based on her psychological profile.

This patient's profile does not suggest extreme difficulty with regard to recovery or elevated expenditures. However, the following issues may be important to monitor or consider when developing a treatment regimen:

| This patient's ability to maintain her prescribed medication regimen may be compromised by her psychological profile.

| This patient does not appear to use spiritual faith as an asset, and she may feel unable to carry out her self-care responsibilities, especially if she is not in a position to rely on members of her social network.

> **Noteworthy Responses**—The patient's endorsement of the following item(s) is particularly worthy of follow-up by the healthcare team.

Panic Susceptibility
   Item # 1   I feel very tense when I think about the day's events.

Adherence Problems
   Item # 116   If I don't get relief from medicine, I may increase the dosage on my own.

FIGURE 19.2. *(p. 4 of 5)*

MILLON BEHAVIORAL MEDICINE DIAGNOSTIC-HEALTHCARE PROVIDER SUMMARY

This patient is a 34-year-old Native American female who is married and is a high school graduate.

PSYCHIATRIC INDICATIONS

This patient is not indicating significant psychiatric distress at this time.

COPING STYLES

This patient is inclined to conform to social expectations and requests, Her stoic front may cover psychic tension and restraint. Denial of her restrained emotions may lead to frequent physical discomfort, which may be further compounded by her efforts to conceal it. Once an Illness is diagnosed, she is likely to want explicit medical instructions, which she will probably carry out faithfully.

CASE MANAGEMENT ISSUES

Stress Moderators

I This patient does not appear to use her spiritual faith to facilitate recovery from her medical problems. The health care provider should ask if she has other sources of support that could help her through this period.

I She is very confident that she will have a speedy recovery. She will probably follow the suggestions of healthcare providers unquestioningly, and she may place an extraordinary amount of faith in the efficacy of the prescribed treatments.

I Her scores indicate that she has other assets in this area. For further information, consult with the attending mental health professional.

Treatment Prognostics

I This individual may be unable or unwililng to follow medication instructlons, which could lead to under- or overmedicating.

I She is open to receiving information or discussing matters pertaining to her illness.

Management Guide

Psychological factors are not likely to contribute to excessive medical complications andlor expenditures for this patient.

FIGURE 19.2. *(p. 5 of 5)*

The Bariatric Summary section of the MBMD is reviewed next. This summary is derived from an algorithm applied to information collected on over 700 bariatric surgery patients completing their treatment in a network of surgery practices who participated in a bariatric-specific normative study (for details, see Millon et al., 2007). Included here are specific guidelines for presurgical interventions; predictions for postsurgical patient behaviors and self-perceptions; and predictions about the need for postsurgical interventions to facilitate longer-term maintenance of treatment gains. Consistent with this patient's MBMD test profile as just reviewed, presurgical interventions (e.g., pain management) and additional psychosocial evaluations are not deemed to be necessary. It is predicted that R. C. will have average to high likelihood of having a positive postsurgical course, that she will be able to adopt and maintain necessary postsurgical health behaviors, and that she will be unlikely to pursue litigation for any aspects of her surgery with which she is unsatisfied. Her postsurgical self-perceptions and outlook toward life are predicted to be positive, and doubt is expressed that she will benefit measurably from postsurgical interventions involving physical rehabilitation, stress/sleep management, nutritional guidance, or support groups.

After the Bariatric Summary, the Interpretive Report goes on to elaborate on the patent's communication style, any potential psychiatric challenges, and the specific nature of her coping style. This information can be of great use in understanding how R. C. conceptualizes her medical condition and can facilitate the ways that the health care team works with this individual. The description of those stress moderators that act as liabilities versus assets provides insight into ways that the physician and staff might help this patient weather the immediate postoperative period and maintain treatment gains thereafter. As can be seen, this patient reports many such assets. The main Interpretive Report concludes with more specific information on treatment prognosticators and management guidelines. The final section of the report, the Healthcare Provider Summary, is a single-page summary that highlights the most salient aspects of the MBMD profile analysis and is designed to be included in the patient's chart for quick reference at future follow-up visits. Overall, this MBMD report consistently indicates an individual who can be considered a good candidate for bariatric surgery, and one who is likely to benefit both physically and psychologically.

Future Research with the MBMD in Bariatric Surgery

The behavioral medicine literature that has accrued in the past three decades and has been reviewed in this chapter provides strong evidence that a comprehensive psychosocial assessment—one that provides information about psychiatric status, coping styles, stress moderators, treatment prognostics, and negative health habits—may play a critical role in maintaining health, optimizing the effects of and recovery from medical treatment, and containing health care costs in a wide variety of medical populations. To return to bariatric surgery as an example, future research should employ prospective designs to test the viability of the MBMD for predicting psychological responses to this surgery, the incidence of success and complications following surgery, costs of medical treatments in surgery candidates with differing psychosocial scale profiles, the likelihood of medication adherence and ability to make lifestyle changes after surgery, and the need for additional clinical services and costs for patients after surgery.

The MBMD may also prove useful in primary care settings for screening patients who are at risk for postsurgical difficulties and for triaging patients for psychosocial services and alternative medical intervention. Some cautionary notes are in order, however. It is plausible that other patient variables may affect the interpretation of information gathered in each of the MBMD domains. These include demographic and medical information. For instance, it will be important to examine the socio-cultural forces that influence the expression of psychiatric indicators and coping styles, as well as the nuances of a patient's communication style. These factors may also affect access to and desire for using various resources (e.g., social vs. spiritual), which in turn may contribute to patients' ability to adjust to their illness, adhere to medication regimens, and make the lifestyle changes that their condition necessitates. It is also critical that specific medical information about diagnosis and treatment, as well as medical and psychiatric comorbidities, be incorporated with other contextual data to enhance the interpretation of each MBMD domain. Establishing the algorithms for how such modifying information can be used to maximize the accuracy of predictions based on the MBMD will require a series of studies using samples that vary systematically in age, gender, ethnicity, and disease type and stage, along with a clear set of psychosocial adjustment and medical outcome variables that are monitored over time.

Summary

The research reviewed in this chapter makes it clear that comprehensive psychosocial assessment can contribute significantly to reducing morbidity and mortality as well as health care costs in different medical populations. We have presented evidence based upon research with the MBHI that information on patients' coping style and attitudes toward health can be important in predicting a variety of health-promoting behaviors, as well as responses to medical treatment. In order both to extend these findings and to address identified limitation in the MBHI, we developed a new instrument, the MBMD, which was designed to embellish the many functions of the MBHI. We first developed a completely new set of items to represent several additional domains, and related scales to address issues that have emerged in contemporary health care. After establishing these new domains and scales, we proceeded to develop a research form of the instrument that could be used to refine items, establish prevalence score transformations, and evaluate the criterion and predictive validity for various scales. We found evidence that several MBMD scales varied as a function of both gender and disease type. This was instrumental in developing prevalence score transformations separately for men and women. Using a validation sample made up of patients with a wide variety of serious medical conditions, we demonstrated that the MBMD Coping Styles scales were correlated with a variety of disease-specific coping strategies and more general personality dimensions in specific medical populations, in a way that supported the underlying theory of the test. We also found evidence that the MBMD Stress Moderators scales were associated with criterion measures as hypothesized. Thus there was widespread evidence for the criterion validity of several MBMD scales drawn from multiple domains.

The continued value of psychosocial evaluations in the medical arena can only be ensured by conducting research demonstrating the ability of such tests as the MBMD to predict quality of life and actual medical outcomes in real-life treatment settings. Specifically, future research should employ prospective designs to test the viability of the MBMD to predict patients' psychological responses to major medical interventions; the incidence of success and medical complications following medical procedures; the costs of different medical treatments and follow-up care; the likelihood of medication abuse; and the ability of patients to participate in needed self-care with newly diagnosed chronic disease. With a solid research base, psychosocial evaluations could ultimately be applied in forecasting utilization and expenditures in large health care systems.

References

Aiken, L., & Henricks, T. (1971). Systematic relaxation as a nursing intervention technique with open heart surgery patients. *Nursing Research, 20*, 212–217.

Alberts, M., Lyons, J., & Anderson, R. (1988). Relations of coping style and illness variables in ulcerative colitis. *Psychological Reports, 62*, 71–79.

Alferi, S., Carver, C. S., Antoni, M. H., Weiss, S., & Duran, R. (2001). An exploratory study of social support, distress, and disruption among low income Hispanic women under treatment for early stage breast cancer. *Health Psychology, 20*, 33–41.

Alferi, S., Culver, J., Carver, C. S., Arena, P., & Antoni, M. H. (1999). Religiosity, religious coping, and distress: A prospective study of Catholic and evangelical Hispanic women in treatment for early-stage breast cancer. *Journal of Health Psychology, 4*, 343–356.

Altice, F. L., Mostashari, F., & Friedland, G. H. (2001). Trust and acceptance of and adherence to antiviral therapy. *Journal of Acquired Immune Deficiency Syndromes, 28*, 47–58.

Andersen, B. L. (1992). Psychological interventions for cancer patients to enhance the quality of life. *Journal of Consulting and Clinical Psychology, 60*, 552–568.

Andersen, B. L., Kiecolt-Glaser, J., & Glaser, R. (1994). A biobehavioral model of cancer stress and disease outcome. *American Psychologist, 49*, 389–404.

Andersen, B. L., Farrar, W. B., Golden-Kreutz, D. M., Glaser, R., Emery, C. F., Crespin, T. R., et al. (2004). Psychological, behavioral, and immune changes after a psychological intervention: A clinical trial. *Journal of Clinical Oncology, 22*, 3570–3580.

Anderson, K. O., Bradley, L. A., Young, L. D., McDaniel, L. K., & Wise, C. M. (1985). Rheumatoid arthritis: Review of psychological factors related to etiology, effects and treatment. *Psychological Bulletin, 98*, 358–387.

Antoni, M. H. (1991). Psychosocial stressors and behavioral interventions in gay men with HIV infection. *International Reviews in Psychiatry, 3*, 383–389.

Antoni, M. H. (2002). Behavioral medicine's role in HIV/AIDS. In A/ Christensen & M. H. Antoni (Eds.), *Chronic medical disorders: Behavioral medicine's perspective.* Oxford: Blackwell.

Antoni, M. H. (2003a). Stress management and psychoneuroimmunology in HIV infection. *CNS Spectrums, 8*, 40–51.

Antoni, M. H. (2003b). *Stress management intervention for women with breast cancer.* Washington, DC: American Psychological Association.

Antoni, M. H. (2005). The study of psychosocial factors influencing medical diseases. In S. Strack (Ed.), *Handbook of personology and psychopathology* (pp. xx–xx). Hoboken, NJ: Wiley.

Antoni, M. H., Baggett, L., Ironson, G., August, S., LaPerriere, A., Klimas, N., et al. (1991). Cognitive–behavioral stress management intervention buffers distress responses and immunologic changes following notification of HIV-1 seropositivity. *Journal of Consulting and Clinical Psychology, 59*(6), 906–915.

Antoni, M. H., Caricco, A., Duran, R., Spitzer, S., Penedo, F., Ironson, G., et al. (2006). Randomized clinical trial of cognitive behavioral stress management on HIV viral load in gay men treated with HAART. *Psychosomatic Medicine, 68*(1), 143–151.

Antoni, M. H., & Emmelkamp, P. (1995). Editorial on special issue on HIV/AIDS. *Clinical Psychology and Psychotherapy, 2*(4), 199–202.

Antoni, M. H., Esterling, B., Lutgendorf, S., Fletcher, M. A., & Schneiderman, N. (1995).

Psychosocial stressors, herpes virus reactivation and HIV-1 infection. In M. Stein & A. Baum (Eds.), *AIDS and oncology: Perspectives in behavioral medicine*. Hillsdale, NJ: Erlbaum.

Antoni, M. H., Goldstein, D., Ironson, G., LaPerriere, A., Fletcher, M. A., & Schneiderman, N. (1995). Coping responses to HIV-1 serostatus notification predict concurrent and prospective immunologic status. *Clinical Psychology and Psychotherapy*, 2(4), 234–248.

Antoni, M. H., & Goodkin, K. (1988). Life stress and moderator variables in the promotion of cervical neoplasia: I. Personality facets. *Journal of Psychosomatic Research*, 32(3), 327–338.

Antoni, M. H., & Goodkin, K. (1989). Life stress and moderator variables in the promotion of cervical neoplasia: II. Life event dimensions. *Journal of Psychosomatic Research*, 33(4), 457–467.

Antoni, M. H., Ironson, G., & Schneiderman, N. (2007). *Stress reduction for HIV-positive adults: A cognitive-behavioral stress management program—therapist guide*. New York: Oxford University Press.

Antoni, M. H., Kazi, A., Lechner, S., Wimberly, S., Gluck, S., & Carver, C. S. (2006). How stress management improves quality of life after treatment for breast cancer. *Journal of Consulting and Clinical Psychology*, 74, 1143–1152.

Antoni, M. H., Lehman, J., Kilbourn, K., Boyers, A., Yount, S., Culver, J., et al. (2001). Cognitive-behavioral stress management intervention decreases the prevalence of depression and enhances benefit finding among women under treatment for early-stage breast cancer. *Health Psychology*, 20, 20–32.

Antoni, M. H., Lutgendorf, S., Cole, S., Dhabhar, F., Sephton, S., McDonald, P., et al. (2006). The influence of biobehavioral factors on tumor biology, pathways and mechanisms. *Nature Reviews Cancer*, 6, 240–248.

Antoni, M. H., Millon, C., & Millon, T. (1997). The role of psychological assessment in health care: The MBHI, MBMC, and beyond. In T. Millon (Ed.), *The Millon inventories: Clinical and personality assessment* (pp. 409–448). New York: Guilford Press.

Antoni, M. H., Wimberly, S., Lechner, S., Kazi, A., Sifre, T., Urcuyo, K., et al. (2006). Stress management intervention reduces cancer-specific thought intrusions and anxiety symptoms among women undergoing treatment for breast cancer. *American Journal of Psychiatry*, 163, 1791–1797.

Assal, J. P., et al. (1985). Patient education as the basis for diabetes care in clinical practice and research. *Diabetologia*, 28, 602–613.

Bandura, A., Taylor, C. B., Williams, S., Mefford, I., & Barchas, J. (1985). Catecholamine secretion as a function of perceived coping self-efficacy. *Journal of Consulting and Clinical Psychology*, 53, 406–414.

Bangsberg, D. R., Hecht, F. M., Charlebois, E. D., Chesney, M., & Moss, A. (2000). Adherence to protease inhibitors, HIV-1 viral load, and development of drug resistance in an indigent population. *AIDS*, 14, 229–234.

Barefoot, J., & Schroll, M. (1996) Symptoms of depression, acute myocardial infarction, and total mortality in a community sample. *Circulation*, 93, 1976–1980.

Barsky, A., Wyshak, G., & Klerman, G. (1986). Medical and psychiatric determinants of outpatient medical utilization. *Medical Care*, 24, 548–560.

Bauchowitz, A. U., Gonder-Frederick, L. A., Olbrisch, M., Azarbad, L., Ryee, M., Woodson, M., et al. (2005). Psychosocial evaluation of bariatric surgery candidates: A survey of present practices. *Psychosomatic Medicine*, 67, 825–832.

Baum, A. (1994). Behavioral, biological, and environmental interactions in disease processes. In S. Blumenthal, K. Matthews, & S. Weiss (Eds.), *New research frontiers in behavioral medicine: Proceedings of the National Conference* (NIH Publication No. 94-3772). Washington, DC: U.S. Government Printing Office.

Baum, A., & Posluszny, D. (1999). Health psychology: Mapping biobehavioral contributions to health and illness. *Annual Review Psychology*, 50, 137–163.

Beck, A. T. (1978). *The Beck Depression Inventory*. Philadelphia: Center for Cognitive Therapy.

Becker, M. H., Maiman, L., Kirscht, J., Haefner, D., & Drachman, R. (1977). The health belief model and dietary compliance: A field experiment. *Journal of Health and Social Behavior, 18,* 348–366.

Bergner, M., Bobbitt, R. A., Carter, W. B., & Gilson, B. S. (1981). The Sickness Impact Profile: Development and final revision of a health status measure. *Medical Care, 19,* 787–805.

Blalock, S., De Vellis, B., & Giordino, K. (1995). The relationship between coping and psychological well-being among people with osteoarthritis: A problem-solving approach. *Annals of Behavioral Medicine, 17,* 107–115.

Blumenthal, J., Williams, R., Wallace, A., et al. (1982). Physiological and psychological variables predict compliance to prescribed exercise therapy in patients recovering from myocardial infarction. *Psychosomatic Medicine, 44,* 519–527.

Boeke, S., Stronks, D., Vehage, F., & Zwaveling, A. (1991). Psychological variables as predictors of the length of post-operative hospitalization. *Journal of Psychosomatic Research, 35,* 281–288.

Booth-Kewley, S., & Friedman, H. S. (1987). Psychological predictors of heart disease: A quantitative review. *Psychological Bulletin, 101,* 343–362.

Bovbjerg, D., & Valdimarsdottir, H. (1996). Stress, immune modulation, and infectious disease during chemotherapy for breast cancer. *Annals of Behavioral Medicine, 18,* S63.

Brand, A. H., Johnson, J. H., & Johnson, S. B. (1986). Life stress and diabetic control in children and adolescents with insulin-dependent diabetes. *Journal of Pediatric Psychology, 11,* 481–495.

Brandwin, M., Clifford, M., & Coffman, K. (1989). The MBHI Life Threat Reactivity Scale as a predictor of mortality in patients awaiting heart transplantation. *Psychosomatic Medicine, 51,* 256.

Bremer, B. (1995). Absence of control over health and the psychological adjustment to end-stage renal disease. *Annals of Behavioral Medicine, 17,* 227–233.

Broadhead, W., Hehlbach, S., DeGruy, F., & Kaplan, B. (1989). Functional versus structural social support and health care utilization in a family medicine outpatient practice. *Medical Care, 27,* 221–233.

Brown, J., & Siegel, J. (1988). Attributions for negative life events and depression: The role of perceived control. *Journal of Personality and Social Psychology, 54,* 316–322.

Browne, G., Arpin, K., Corey, P., Fitch, M., & Gafni, A. (1990). Individual correlates of health service utilization and the cost of poor adjustment to chronic illness. *Medical Care, 28,* 43–58.

Brownell, K. D., & Wadden, T. A. (1992). Etiology and treatment of obesity: Understanding a serious, prevalent, and refractory disorder. *Journal of Consulting and Clinical Psychology, 60,* 505–517.

Burgess, C., Morris, T., & Pettingale, K. W. (1988). Psychological response to cancer diagnosis: II. Evidence for coping styles (coping styles and cancer diagnosis). *Journal of Psychosomatic Research, 32,* 263–272.

Burns, K., Green, P., & Chase, H. (1986). Psychosocial correlates of glycemic control as a function of age in youth with insulin-dependent diabetes. *Journal of Adolescent Health Care, 7,* 311–319.

Byrnes, D., Antoni, M. H., Goodkin, K., Efantis-Potter, J., Simon, T., Munajj, J., et al. (1998). Stressful events, pessimism, natural killer cell cytotoxicity, and cytotoxic/suppressor T-cells in HIV+ black women at risk for cervical cancer. *Psychosomatic Medicine, 60,* 714–722.

Cameron, L., Leventhal, E., & Leventhal, H. (1995). Seeking medical care in response to symptoms and life stress. *Psychosomatic Medicine, 57,* 37–47.

Carney, R., Freedland, K., Eisen, S., et al. (1995). Major depression and medication adherence in elderly patients with coronary heart disease. *Health Psychology, 14,* 88–90.

Carney, R., Freedland, K., Rich, M., & Jaffe, A. (1995). Depression as a risk factor for cardiac events in established coronary heart disease: A review of possible mechanisms. *Annals of Behavioral Medicine, 17,* 142–149.

Carrieri, M. P., Leport, C., Protopopescu, C., Cassuto, J. P., Bouvet, E., Peyramond, D., et al. (2006). Factors associated with nonadherence to highly active antiretroviral therapy: A 5-year follow-up analysis with correction for the bias induced by missing data in the treatment maintenance phase. *Journal of Acquired Immune Deficiency Syndrome, 41,* 477–485.

Carver, C. S., Pozo, C., Harris, S. D., Noriega, V., Scheier, M. F., Robinson, D. S., et al. (1993). How coping mediates the effects of optimism on distress: A study of women with early stage of breast cancer. *Journal of Personality and Social Psychology, 65,* 375–3903.

Carver, C. S., Scheier, M., & Weintraub, J. (1989). Assessing coping strategies: A theoretically-based approach. *Journal of Personality and Social Psychology, 56,* 267–283.

Carver, C. S., Smith, R. G., Antoni, M. H., Petronis, V. M., Weiss, S., & Derhagopian, R. P. (2005). Optimistic personality and psychosocial well-being during treatment predict psychosocial well-being among long-term survivors of breast cancer. *Health Psychology, 24,* 508–516.

Caudill, M. (1991). Decreased clinic use by chronic pain patients: Response to behavioral medicine interventions. *Journal of Clinical Pain, 7*(4), 305–310.

Chacko, R. C., Harper, R. G., Kunik, M., & Young, J. (1996). Relationship of psychiatric morbidity and psychosocial factors in organ transplant candidates. *Psychosomatics, 37,* 100–107.

Chambers, W. N., & Reiser, M. F. (1953). Emotional stress in the precipitation of congestive heart failure. *Medicine, 15,* 38–60.

Chesney, M. A., & Folkman, S. (1994). Psychological impact of HIV disease and implications for intervention. *Psychiatric Clinics of North America, 17,* 163–181.

Chesney, M. A., Folkman, S., & Chambers, D. (1996). The impact of a cognitive–behavioral intervention on coping with HIV disease. *Psychosomatic Medicine, 58,* 86.

Christensen, A. J., & Smith, T. W. (1995). Personality and patient adherence: Correlates of the five-factor model in renal dialysis. *Journal of Behavioral Medicine, 18,* 305–313.

Christman, N. J., McConnell, E. A., Pfeiffer, C., Webster, K. K., Schmitt, M., & Ries, J. (1988). Uncertainty, coping, and distress following myocardial infarction: Transition from hospital to home. *Research in Nursing and Health, 11,* 71–82.

Clark, K. C. (1993). How coping mediates the effect of optimism on distress: A study of women with early stage breast cancer. *Journal of Personality and Social Psychology, 65,* 375–390.

Classen, C., Sephton, E., Diamond, S., & Spiegel, D. (1998). Studies of life-extending psychosocial interventions. In J. C. Holland (Ed.), *Textbook of psycho-oncology* (pp. 730–742). New York: Oxford University Press.

Cohen, S. (1988). Psychosocial models of the role of social support in the etiology of physical disease. *Health Psychology, 7,* 269–297.

Cohen, S., & Edwards, J. R. (1989). Personality characteristics as moderators of the relationship between stress and disorder. In R. W. J. Neufeld (Ed.), *Advances in the investigation of psychological stress.* Hillsdale, NJ: Erlbaum.

Cohen, S., Tyrrell, D. A., & Smith, A. P. (1991). Psychological stress in humans and susceptibility to the common cold. *New England Journal of Medicine, 325,* 606–612.

Cohen, S., & Wills, T. A. (1985). Stress social support, and the buffering hypothesis. *Psychological Bulletin, 98,* 310–357.

Croyle, R., Smith, K., Botkin, J., Baty, B., & Nash, J. (1997). Psychological responses to BRCA1 mutation testing: Preliminary findings. *Health Psychology, 16,* 63–72.

Cruess, D., Meagher, S., Antoni, M. H., & Millon, T. (2007). Utility of the Millon Behavioral Medicine Diagnostic (MBMD) to predict adherence to highly active antiretroviral therapy (HAART) medication regimens among HIV-positive men and women. *Journal of Personality Assessment, 89*(3), 277–290.

Cruess, D. G., Antoni, M. H., McGregor, B. A., Boyers, A., Kumar, M., Kilbourn, K., et al. (2000). Cognitive-behavioral stress management reduces serum cortisol by enhancing positive contributions among women being treated for early stage breast cancer. *Psychosomatic Medicine, 62,* 304–308.

Cruess, S., Antoni, M. H., Cruess, D., Fletcher, M. A., Ironson, G., Kumar, M., et al. (2000). Reductions in HSV-2 antibody titers after cognitive behavioral stress management and relationships with neuroendocrine function, relaxation skills, and social support in HIV+ gay men. *Psychosomatic Medicine, 62,* 828–837.

Cummings, N. A., & Van den Bos, G. R. (1981). The twenty year Kaiser Permanente experience with psychotherapy and medical utilization: Implications for national health policy and national health insurance. *Health Policy Quarterly: Evaluation and Utilization, 1*(2), 159–175.

Cushman, L. A. (1986). Secondary neuropsychiatric complications in stroke: Implications for acute care. *Archives of Physical Medicine Rehabilitation, 69,* 877–879.

Cutrona, C., & Russell, D. (1987). The provision of social relationships and adaptation to stress. In W. H. Jones & D. Perlman (Eds.), *Advances in personal relationships* (Vol. 1). Greenwich, CT: JAI Press.

Davidson, J. K. (1983). The Grady Memorial Hospital Diabetes Programme. In J. I. Mann, K. Pyorala, & A. Teuscher (Eds.), *Diabetes in epidemiological perspective.* Edinburgh: Churchill Livingstone.

Davidson, J. K. (1991). *Clinical diabetes mellitus: A problem-oriented approach* (2nd ed.). New York: Thieme Medical.

Deeks, S. G., Hecht, F. M., Swanson, M., Elbeik, T., Loftus, R., Cohen, P. T., et al. (1999). HIV, RNA, and CD4 cell count response to protease inhibitor therapy in an urban AIDS clinic: Response to both initial and salvage therapy. *AIDS, 13,* 135–143.

Delin, C. R., & Watts, J. M. (1997). A comparison of commonly used indices of weight loss, and a proposed new measure to assess outcomes in research and clinical situations. *Psychology, Health, and Medicine, 2,* 77–86.

Dembroski, T. M., & Costa, P. R., Jr. (1987). Coronary prone behavior: Components of the Type A pattern and hostility. *Journal of Personality, 55,* 211–235.

Devine, E. C. (1992). Effects of psychoeducational care for adult surgical patients: A meta-analysis of 191 studies. *Patient Education and Counseling, 19,* 129–142.

Dimond, M. (1979). Social support and adaptation to chronic illness: The case of maintenance hemodialysis. *Research in Nursing and Health, 2,* 101–108.

Dimsdale, J. E., Pierce, C., Schoenfeld, D., Brown, A., Zusman, R., & Graham, R. (1986). Suppressed anger and blood pressure: The effects of race, sex, social class, obesity, and age. *Psychosomatic Medicine, 48,* 430–436.

Doering, S., Katzlberger, F., Rumpold, G., Roessler, S., Hofstoetter, B., Schatz, D., et al. (2000). Videotape preparation of patients before hip replacement surgery reduces stress. *Psychosomatic Medicine, 62,* 365–373.

Dubbert, P. (1992). Exercise in behavioral medicine. *Journal of Consulting and Clinical Psychology, 60,* 613–618.

Duberstein, P. R., Conwell, Y., & Yeates, E. (1993). Interpersonal stressors, substance abuse, and suicide. *Journal of Nervous and Mental Disease, 181*(2), 80–85.

Dunkel-Schetter, C., Folkman, S., & Lazarus, R. S. (1987). Correlates of social support receipt. *Journal of Personality and Social Psychology, 53,* 71–80.

Eisen, E., Dies, R., Finn, S., Eyde, L., Kay, G., Kubiszyn, T., et al. (1998). *Problems and limitations in the use of psychological assessment in contemporary healthcare delivery: Report of the board of professional affairs, Psychological Assessment Work Group, Part II.* Washington, DC: American Psychological Association.

Ell, K., Nishimoto, R., Mediansky, L., Mantell, J., & Hamovitch, M. (1992). Social relations, social support and survival among patients with cancer. *Journal of Psychosomatic Research, 36,* 531–541.

Epstein, L. H., & Perkins, K. A. (1988). Smoking, stress, and coronary heart disease. *Journal of Consulting and Clinical Psychology, 56,* 342–349.

Esterling, B., Antoni, M. H., Fletcher, M. A., Marguilles, S., & Schneiderman, N. (1994). Emotional disclosure through writing or speaking modulates latent Epstein–Barr virus reactivation. *Journal of Consulting and Clinical Psychology, 62*(1), 130–140.

Esterling, B. A., Antoni, M. H., Kumar, M., & Schneiderman, N. (1990). Emotional repression, stress disclosure responses, and Epstein-Barr viral capsid antigen titers. *Psychosomatic Medicine, 52,* 397–410.

Fawzy, F. I., Cousins, N., Fawzy, N. W., Kemeny, M., Elashoff, R., & Morton, D. (1990). A structured psychiatric intervention for cancer patients: I. Changes over time in methods of coping and affective disturbance. *Archives of General Psychiatry, 47,* 720–725.

Fawzy, F. I., Fawzy, N., Hyun, C., Elashoff, R., Guthrie, D., Fahey, J. L., et al. (1993). Malignant melanoma: Effects of an early structured psychiatric intervention, coping, and affective state on recurrence and survival 6 years later. *Archives of General Psychiatry, 50,* 681–689.

Felton, B. J., Revenson, T. A., & Hinrichsen, G. (1984). Coping and adjustment in chronically ill adults. *Social Science and Medicine, 18,* 889–898.

Fitzpatrick, R., Newman, S., Lamb, R., & Shipley, M. (1988). Social relationships and psychological well-being in rheumatoid arthritis. *Social Science and Medicine, 27,* 399–403.

Flum, D., Salem, L., Broeckel-Elrod, J., Dellinger, E., Cheadle, A., & Chan, L. (2005). Early mortality among medicare beneficiaries undergoing bariatric surgical procedures. *Journal of the American Medical Association, 294,* 1903–1908.

Folkman, S., & Lazarus, R. S. (1980). An analysis of coping in a middle-aged community sample. *Journal of Health and Social Behavior, 21,* 219–239.

Fox, B. H. (1981). Psychosocial factors and the immune system in human cancer. In R. Ader (Ed.), *Psychoneuroimmunology.* New York: Academic Press.

Frasure-Smith, N., Lesperance, F., & Talajic, M. (1993). Depression following myocardial infarction. *Journal of the American Medical Association, 270*(15), 1819–1825.

Frasure-Smith, N., & Prince, R. (1989). Long-term follow-up of the ischemic heart disease life stress monitoring program. *Psychosomatic Medicine, 51,* 485–513.

Frenzel, M. P., McCaul, K. D., Glasgow, R. E., & Schafer, L. C. (1988). The relationship of stress and coping to regimen adherence and glycemic control of diabetes. *Journal of Social and Clinical Psychology, 6,* 77–87.

Friedman, H. S., & Booth-Kewley, S. (1987). The "disease prone" personality: A meta-analytic view of the construct. *American Psychologist, 42,* 539–555.

Fulop, G., Strain, J., Vita, J., Lyons, J., & Hammer, J. (1987). Impact of psychiatric comorbidity on length of hospital stay for medical/surgical patients: A preliminary report. *American Journal of Psychiatry, 144,* 878–882.

Funch, D. P., & Mettlin, C. (1982). The role of support in relation to recovery from breast cancer. *Social Science and Medicine, 16*(1), 91–98.

Gatchel, R., Deckel, A., Weinberg, N., et al. (1985). The utility of the Millon Behavioral Health Inventory in the study of chronic headaches. *Headache, 25,* 49–54.

Gatchel, R., Mayer, T., Capra, P., et al. (1986). Millon Behavioral Health Inventory: Its utility in predicting physical function in patients with low back pain. *Archives of Physical Medicine and Rehabilitation, 67,* 878–882.

Glanz, K., Grove, J., Lerman, C., Gotay, C., & Le Marchand, L. (1999). Correlates of intentions to obtain genetic counseling and colorectal cancer gene testing among at-risk relatives from three ethnic groups. *Cancer Epidemiology, Biomarkers and Prevention, 8,* 329–336.

Glanz, L., Lew, R., Song, V., & Cook, V. (1999). Factors associated with skin cancer prevention practices in a multiethnic population. *Health Education and Behavior, 26,* 344–359.

Glasgow, R., Toobert, D., Hampson, S., & Wilson, W. (1995). Behavioral research on diabetes at the Oregon Research Institute. *Annals of Behavioral Medicine, 17,* 32–40.

Goldstein, D., & Antoni, M. H. (1989). The distribution of repressive coping styles among nonmetastatic and metastatic breast cancer patients as compared to non-cancer patients. *Psychology and Health: An International Journal, 3,* 245–258.

Gonik, U. L. (1981). Cost-effectiveness of behavioral medicine procedures in the treatment of stress-related disorders. *American Journal of Clinical Biofeedback, 4*(1), 16–24.

Gonzalez, J. S., Penedo, F. J., Antoni, M. H., Duran, R. E., Fernandez, M. I., McPherson-Baker, S., et al. (2004). Social support, positive states of mind, and HIV treatment adherence in men and women living with HIV/AIDS. *Health Psychology, 23,* 413–418.

Goodkin, K., Antoni, M. H., & Blaney, P. (1986). Stress and hopelessness in the promotion of cervical intraepithelial neoplasia to invasive squamous cell carcinoma of the cervix. *Journal of Psychosomatic Research, 30,* 67–76.

Goodkin, K., Antoni, M. H., Fox, B. H., & Sevin, B. (1993). A partially testable model of psychosocial factors in the etiology of cervical cancer: II. Psychoneuroimmunological aspects, critique and prospective integration. *Psychooncology, 2*(2), 99–121.

Goodkin, K., Antoni, M. H., Sevin, B., & Fox, B. H. (1993). A partially testable model of psychosocial factors in the etiology of cervical cancer: I. A review of biological, psychological, and social aspects. *Psychooncology, 2*(2), 79–98.

Goodkin, K., Tuttle, R., Blaney, N., Feaster, D., Shapshak, P., Burhalter, J., et al. (1996). A bereavement support group intervention is associated with immunological changes in HIV-1+ and HIV– homosexual men. *Psychosomatic Medicine, 58,* 83.

Gordillo, V., del Amo, J., Soriano, V., & Gonzalez-Lahoz, J. (1999). Sociodemographic and psychological variables influencing adherence to antiretroviral therapy. *AIDS, 13,* 1763–1769.

Grady, K., Reisine, S., Fifield, J., Lee, N., McVay, J., & Kelsey, M. (1991). The impact of Hurricane Hugo and the San Francisco earthquake on a sample of people with rheumatoid arthritis. *Arthritis Care and Research, 2,* 106–110.

Green, A., Dymek-Valentine, M., Pyduk, S., LeGrange, D., & Alverdy, J. (2004). Psychosocial outcome of gastric bypass surgery for patients with and without binge eating. *Obesity Surgery, 14,* 975–985.

Green, C., Millon, T., & Meagher, R. (1983). The MBHI: Its utilization in assessment and management of the coronary bypass surgery patient. *Psychotherapy and Psychosomatics, 39,* 112–121.

Greenberg, P. E., Stiglin, L. E., Finkelstein, S. N., & Berndt, E. R. (1993). The economic burden of depression in 1990. *Journal of Clinical Psychiatry, 54,* 405–417.

Greer, S., Morris, T., Pettingale, K., & Haybittle, J. (1990). Psychological response to breast cancer and 15-year outcome. *Lancet, i,* 49–50.

Gruen, W. (1975). Effects of brief psychotherapy during hospitalization period on the recovery process in heart attacks. *Journal of Consulting and Clinical Psychology, 43,* 232–233.

Grunberg, N., & Baum, A. (1985). Biological commonalities of stress and substance abuse. In S. Schiffman & T. Willis (Eds.), *Coping and substance abuse.* Orlando, FL: Academic Press.

Harkness, A., & Lilienfield, S. (1997). Individual differences science for treatment planning: Personality traits. *Psychological Assessment, 9,* 349–360.

Havlir, D. V., Schrier, R. D., Torriani, F. J., Chervenak, K., Hwang, J. Y., & Boom, W. H. (2000). Effect of potent antiretroviral therapy on immune responses to *Mycobacterium avium* in human immunodeficiency virus-infected subjects. *Journal of Infectious Disease, 182,* 1658–1663.

Helgeson, V., & Cohen, S. (1996). Social support and adjustment to cancer: Reconciling descriptive, correlational, and intervention research. *Health Psychology, 15,* 135–148.

Helgeson, V. S., Cohen, S., & Fritz, H. L. (1998). Social ties and cancer. In J. Holland (Ed.), *Textbook of psycho-oncology.* New York: Oxford University Press.

Hellman, C. J. C. (1990). A study of the effectiveness of two group behavioral medicine interventions for patients with psychosomatic complaints. *Behavioral Medicine, 16,* 165–173.

Herbert, T., & Cohen, S. (1993). Depression and immunity: A meta-analytic review. *Psychological Bulletin, 113,* 472–486.

Herrmann, C., Brand-Driehorst, S., Kaminsky, B., Leibing, E., Staats, H., & Ruger, H. (1998). Diagnostic groups and depressed mood as predictors of 22-month mortality in medical inpatients. *Psychosomatic Medicine, 60,* 570–577.

Hershberger, P. J., Robertson, K. B., & Markert, R. J. (1999). Personality and appointment keeping adherence in cardiac rehabilitation. *Journal of Cardiopulmonary Rehabilitation, 19,* 106–111.

Holahan, C. J., & Moos, R. H. (1986). Personality, coping, and family resources in stress resistance: A longitudinal analysis. *Journal of Personality and Social Psychology, 51,* 389–395.

Holland, J. C. (1990). Behavioral and psychosocial risk factors in cancer: Human studies. In J.

Holland & J. Rowland (Eds.), *Handbook of psychooncology*. New York: Oxford University Press.

Holland, J. C. (1997). Preliminary guidelines for the treatment of distress. *Oncology, 11*, 109–117.

Holzemer, W. L., Henry, S. B., Portillo, C. J., & Miramontes, H. (1999). The client adherence profiling-intervention tailoring (CAP-IT) intervention for enhancing adherence to HIV/AIDS medications: A pilot study. *Journal of Association of Nurses in AIDS Care, 11*, 36–44.

House, J. A. (1981). *Work stress and social support*. Reading, MA: Addison-Wesley.

House, J. S., Landis, K. R., & Umberson, D. (1988). Social relationships and health. *Science, 241*, 540–545.

Hsu, L. K. G., Benotti, P. N., Dwyer, J., Roberts, S. B., Saltzman, E., Shikora, S., et al. (1998). Nonsurgical factors that influence the outcome of bariatric surgery: A review. *Psychosomatic Medicine, 60*, 338–346.

Ironson, G., Antoni, M. H., & Lutgendorf, S. (1995). Can psychological interventions affect immunity and survival?: Present findings and suggested targets with a focus on cancer and human immunodeficiency virus. *Mind/Body Medicine, 1*(2), 85–110.

Ironson, G., Friedman, A., Klimas, N., Antoni, M. H., Fletcher, M. A., LaPerriere, A., et al. (1994). Distress, denial and low adherence to behavioral intervention predict faster disease progression in gay men infected with human immunodeficiency virus. *International Journal of Behavioral Medicine, 1*, 90–105.

Ironson, G., Solomon, G., Cruess, D., Barroso, J., & Stivers, M. (1995). Psychosocial factors related to long-term survival with HIV/AIDS. *Clinical Psychology and Psychotherapy, 2*, 249–266.

Ironson, G., Wynings, C., Schneiderman, N., Baum, A., Rodriguez, M., Greenwood, D., et al. (1997). Post traumatic stress symptoms, intrusive thoughts, and loss of immune function after Hurricane Andrew. *Psychosomatic Medicine, 59*, 128–141.

Jacobs, D. (1987). Cost-effectiveness of specialized psychological programs for reducing hospital stays and outpatient visits. *Journal of Clinical Psychology, 43*, 729–735.

Jacobs, D., Kopans, B., & Reizes, J. M. (1995). Reevaluation of depression: What the general practitioner needs to know. *Mind/Body Medicine, 1*, 17–22.

Jacobson, P., Perry, S., & Hirsch, D. (1990). Behavioral and psychological responses to HIV antibody testing. *Journal of Consulting and Clinical Psychology, 58*, 31–37.

James, S. A., Hartnett, S., & Kalsbeek, W. D. (1984). John Henryism and blood pressure differences among black men. *Journal of Behavioral Medicine, 7*, 259–276.

Jamison, K., Wellisch, D., & Pasnau, R. (1978). Psychosocial aspects of mastectomy: I. The woman's perspective. *American Journal of Psychiatry, 135*, 432–436.

Jarvis, G., & Northcott, H. (1987). Religion and differences in morbidity and mortality. *Social Science and Medicine, 25*, 813–824.

Kalarchian, M., Wilson, G., Brolin, R., & Bradley, L. (1998). Binge eating in bariatric surgery patients. *International Journal of Eating Disorders, 23*, 89–92.

Kamarck, T., & Jennings, J. (1991). Biobehavioral factors in sudden cardiac death. *Psychological Bulletin, 109*, 42–75.

Kaplan, G. A., & Reynolds, P. (1988). Depression and cancer mortality and morbidity: Prospective evidence from the Alameda County study. *Journal of Behavioral Medicine, 11*, 1–13.

Katz, C., Martin, R., Landa, B., et al. (1985). Relationship of psychologic factors to frequent symptomatic ventricular arrhythmia. *American Journal of Medicine, 78*, 589–594.

Katz, S., Ford, A., Moskowitz, R., Jackson, B., & Jaffe, M. (1983). Studies of illness in the aged: The Index of ADL. *Journal of the American Medical Association, 185*, 914–919.

Keefe, F., Dunsmore, J., & Burnett, R. (1992). Behavioral and cognitive-behavioral approaches to chronic pain: Recent advances and future directions. *Journal of Consulting and Clinical Psychology, 60*, 528–536.

Kiecolt-Glaser, J., & Glaser, R. (1992). Psychoneuroimmunology: Can psychological interventions modulate immunity? *Journal of Consulting and Clinical Psychology, 60*(4), 569–575.

Kiecolt-Glaser, J., Marucha, P., Malarkey, W., Mercado, A., & Glaser, R. (1995). Slowing of wound healing by psychological stress. *Lancet, 346,* 1194–1196.

Kimmerling, R., Ouimette, P., Cronkite, R., & Moos, R. (1999). Depression and outpatient medical utilization: A naturalistic 10-year follow-up. *Annals of Behavioral Medicine, 21,* 317–321.

King, J., Beals, J., Manson, S., & Trimble, J. (1992). A structural equation model of factors related to substance use among American Indian adolescents. *Drugs and Society, 6*(3–4), 253–268.

Klerman, G., & Weissman, M. (1992). The course, morbidity, and costs of depression. *Archives of General Psychiatry, 49,* 831–834.

Koenig, H., Pargament, K., & Nielsen, J. (1998). Religious coping and health status in medically ill hospitalized older adults. *Journal of Nervous and Mental Disease, 186,* 513–521.

Kolitz, S., Antoni, M. H., & Green, C. (1988). Personality style and immediate help-seeking responses following the onset of myocardial infarction. *Psychology and Health, 2,* 259–289.

Krantz, D. S., DeQuattro, V., Blackburn, H. W., Eaker, E., Haynes, S., James, S. A., et al. (1987). Task Force 1: Psychosocial factors in hypertension. *Circulation, 76*(Suppl. 1), 184–188.

Krantz, D. S., Grunberg, N. E., & Baum, A. (1985). Health psychology. *Annual Review of Psychology, 36,* 349–383.

Lantinga, L., Sprafkin, R., McCroske, J., et al. (1988). One-year psychosocial follow-up of patients with chest pain and angiographically normal coronary arteries. *American Journal of Cardiology, 62,* 209–213.

LeMont, D., Moorehead, M., Parish, M., Reto, C., & Ritz, S. (2004, October). *Suggestions for the pre-surgical psychological assessment of bariatric surgery candidates.* Gainesville, FL: Allied Health Sciences Section Ad Hoc Behavioral Health Committee. American Society for Metabolic and Bariatric Surgery.

Lerman, C. (1997). Translational behavioral research in cancer genetics. *Preventive Medicine, 26,* S65–S69.

Lerman, C., Caporaso, N., Audrain, J., Main, D., Bowman, E., Lockshin, B., et al. (1999). Evidence suggesting the role of specific genetic factors in cigarette smoking. *Health Psychology, 18,* 14–20.

Lerman, C., Caporaso, N., Main, D., Audrain, J., Boyd, N. R., Bowman, E. D., et al. (1998). Depression and self-medication with nicotine: The modifying influence of the dopamine D4 receptor gene. *Health Psychology, 17,* 56–62.

Lerman, C., Daly, M., Sands, C., Balshem, A., Lustbader, E., Heggan, T., et al. (1993). Mammography adherence and psychological distress among women at risk for breast cancer. *Journal of the National Cancer Institute, 85,* 1074–1080.

Lerman, C., Hughes, C., Lemon, S., Main, D., Snyder, C., Durham, C., et al. (1998). What you don't know can hurt you: Adverse psychologic effects in members of BRCA1-linked and BRCA2-linked families who decline genetic testing. *Journal of Clinical Oncology, 16,* 1650–1654.

Lerman, C., Hughes, C., Trock, B., Myers, R., Main, D., Bonney, A., et al. (1999). Genetic testing in families with hereditary nonpolyposis colon cancer. *Journal of the American Medical Association, 281,* 1618–22.

Lerman, C., Narod, S., Schulman, K., Hughes, C., Gomez-Caminero, A., Bonney, G., et al. (1996). BRCA1 testing in families with hereditary breast–ovarian cancer: A prospective study of patient decision-making and outcomes. *Journal of the American Medical Association, 275,* 1885–1892.

Lerman, C., Rimer, B., & Glynn, T. (1997). Priorities in behavioral research in cancer prevention and control. *Preventive Medicine, 26,* S3—S9.

Leserman, J., DiSantostefano, R., Perkins, D., Murphy, C., Golden, R., & Evans, D. (1995). Longitudinal study of social support and social conflict as predictors of depression and dysphoria among HIV-positive and HIV-negative gay men. *Depression, 2,* 189–199.

Leserman, J., Jackson, E. D., Petitto, J. M., Golden, R. N., Silva, S. G., Perkins, D. O., et al. (1999). Progression to AIDS: The effects of stress, depressive symptoms, and social support. *Psychosomatic Medicine, 61,* 397–406.

Leserman, J., Perkins, D., & Evans, D. (1992). Coping with the threat of AIDS: The role of social support. *American Journal of Psychiatry, 149*, 1514–1520.

Levenson, J. (1992). Psychosocial interventions in chronic medical illness: An overview of outcome research. *General Hospital Psychiatry, 14*(Suppl.), 43–49.

Levenson, J., Hamer, R., & Rossiter, L. (1990). Relation of psychopathology in general medical inpatients to use and cost of services. *American Journal of Psychiatry, 147*, 1498–1503.

Levin, J. (1994). Religion and health: Is there an association, is it valid, and is it causal? *Social Science and Medicine, 38*(11), 9–36.

Levin, J., & Vanderpool, H. (1989). Is religion therapeutically significant for hypertension? *Social Science and Medicine, 29*, 69–78.

Levine, M. N., Guyatt, G. H., Gent, M., DePauw, S., Goodyear, M. D., Hryniuk, W. M., et al. (1988). Quality of life in Stage II breast cancer: An instrument for clinical trials. *Journal of Clinical Oncology, 6*, 1798–1810.

Levy, S., Herberman, R., Lippman, M., D'Angelo, T., & Lee, J. (1991). Immunological and psychosocial predictors of disease recurrence in patients with early-stage breast cancer. *Behavioral Medicine, 17*, 67–75.

Lewin, D. (1997). Protease inhibitors: HIV-1 summons a Darwinian defense. *Journal of the National Institute of Health Research, 8*, 33–35.

Lichtman, R., Taylor, S., & Wood, J. (1987). Responses to treatment and quality of life after radiation therapy for breast cancer. In H. P. Withers & L. Peters (Eds.), *Innovations in radiation oncology research*. New York: Springer-Verlag.

Lorig, K., et al. (1993). Evidence suggesting that health education for self-management in patients with chronic arthritis has sustained health benefits while reducing health care costs. *Arthritis and Rheumatism, 36*, 439–446.

Lovallo, W., d'Absi, M., Pincomb, G., Everson, S., Sung, B., Passey, R., et al. (1996). Caffeine and behavioral stress effects on blood pressure in borderline hypertensive Caucasian men. *Health Psychology, 15*, 11–17.

Lucas, G. M., Chaisson, R. E., & Moore, R. D. (1999). Highly active antiretroviral therapy in a large urban clinic: Risk factors for virologic failure and adverse drug reactions. *Annals of Internal Medicine, 131*, 81–87.

Lustman, P., Frank, B., & McGill, J. (1991). Relationship of personality characteristics to glucose regulation in adults with diabetes. *Psychosomatic Medicine, 53*, 305–312.

Lustman, P. J., Griffith, L. S., & Clouse, R. E. (1988). Depression in adults with diabetes: Results of a 5-year follow-up study. *Diabetes Care, 11*, 605–612.

Lutgendorf, S., Antoni, M. H., Ironson, G., Fletcher, M., Penedo, F., Baum, A., et al. (1995). Physical symptoms of chronic fatigue syndrome are exacerbated by the stress of Hurricane Andrew. *Psychosomatic Medicine, 57*, 310–323.

Lutgendorf, S., Antoni, M. H., Ironson, G., Klimas, N., Starr, K., McCabe, P., et al. (1997). Cognitive behavioral stress management decreases dysphoric mood and herpes simplex virus–type 2 antibody titers in symptomatic HIV-seropositive gay men. *Journal of Consulting and Clinical Psychology, 65*, 31–43.

Lutgendorf, S., Antoni, M. H., Ironson, G., Klimas, N., Starr, K., Schneiderman, N., et al. (1996, March). *Coping and social support predict distress changes in symptomatic HIV-seropositive gay men following a cognitive-behavioral stress management intervention.* Paper presented at the Society of Behavioral Medicine, Washington, DC.

Lutgendorf, S., Antoni, M. H., Ironson, G., Starr, K., Costello, N., Zuckerman, M., et al. (1998). Changes in cognitive coping skills and social support mediate distress outcomes in symptomatic HIV-seropositive gay men during a cognitive behavioral stress management intervention. *Psychosomatic Medicine, 60*, 204–214.

Lutgendorf, S., Antoni, M. H., Kumar, M., & Schneiderman, N. (1994). Changes in cognitive coping strategies predict EBV-antibody titre change following a stressor disclosure induction. *Journal of Psychosomatic Research, 38*(1), 63–78.

Magni, G., Silvestro, A., Tamiello, M., Zanesco, L., & Carl, M. (1988). An integrated approach to the assessment of family adjustment to acute lymphocytic leukemia in children. *Acta Psychiatrica Scandinavica, 78,* 639–642.

Marlatt, G. (1985). Coping and substance abuse: Implications for research, prevention, and treatment. In T. Wills & S. Shiffman (Eds.), *Coping and substance abuse.* Orlando, FL: Academic Press.

Marteau, T. M., Bloch, S., & Baum, J. D. (1987). Family life and diabetic control. *Journal of Child Psychology and Psychiatry, 28,* 823–833.

McCann, B., Bovbjerg, V., Brief, D., Turner, C., Follete, W., Fitzpatrick, V., et al. (1995). Relationship of self-efficacy to cholesterol lowering and dietary change in hyperlipidemia. *Annals of Behavioral Medicine, 17,* 221–226.

McCracken, L. (1991). Cognitive-behavioral treatment of rheumatoid arthritis: A preliminary review of efficacy and methodology. *Annals of Behavioral Medicine, 13,* 57–65.

McGregor, B. A., Antoni, M. H., Boyers, A., Alferi, S., Cruess, D., Kilbourn, K. M., et al. (2004). Cognitive behavioral stress management increases benefit finding and immune function among women with early stage breast cancer. *Journal of Psychosomatic Research, 54,* 1–8.

McKinnon, W., Weisse, C., Reynolds, C., Bowles, C., & Baum, A. (1989). Chronic stress, leukocyte subpopulations, and humoral response to latent viruses. *Health Psychology, 8,* 399–402.

Meyerowitz, B. E. (1980). Psychosocial correlates of breast cancer and its treatments. *Psychological Bulletin, 87,* 108–131.

Miller, L. V. (1981). Assessment of program effectiveness at the Los Angeles County–University of Southern California Medical Center. In G. Stein & P. A. Lawrence (Eds.), *Educating diabetic patients.* New York: Springer.

Miller, L. V., & Goldstein, J. (1972). More efficient care of diabetes in a county hospital setting. *New England Journal of Medicine, 286,* 1388–1391.

Millon, T., Antoni, M. H., Millon, C., Minor, S., & Grossman, S. D. (2001). *Millon Behavioral Medicine Diagnostic (MBMD) manual.* Minneapolis, MN: Pearson Assessments.

Millon, T., Antoni, M. H., Millon, C., Minor, S., & Grossman, S. D. (2006). *Millon Behavioral Medicine Diagnostic (MBMD) manual* (2nd ed.). Minneapolis, MN: Pearson Assessments.

Millon, T., Antoni, M. H., Millon, C., Minor, S., & Grossman, S. (2007). *MBMD manual supplement: Bariatric report.* Minneapolis: Pearson Assessments.

Millon, T., & Davis, R. (1996). *Disorders of personality: DSM-IV and beyond* (2nd ed.). New York: Wiley-Interscience.

Millon, T., Green, C., & Meagher, R. (1982). *The Millon Behavioral Health Inventory manual.* Minneapolis, MN: National Computer Systems.

Miranda, J., Perez-Stable, E., Munoz, R., Hargreaves, W., & Henke, C. (1991). Somatization, psychiatric disorder, and stress in utilization of ambulatory medical services. *Health Psychology, 10,* 46–51.

Montaner, J. S. G., Reiss, P., Cooper, D., Vella, S., Harris, M., Conway, B., et al. (1998). A randomized, double-blind trial comparing combinations of nevirapine, didanosine, and zidovudine for HIV-infected patients. *Journal of the American Medical Association, 279,* 930–937.

Morrissey, E., & Schuckitt, M. (1978). Stressful life events and alcohol problems among women seen at a detoxification center. *Journal of Studies on Alcohol, 39,* 1559.

Muhlhauser, I. (1983). Bicentric evaluation of a teaching and treatment program for Type I (insulin-dependent) diabetic patients: Improvement of metabolic control and other measures of diabetes care for up to 22 months. *Diabetologia, 25,* 470–476.

Mulder, C. L., Antoni, M. H., Duivenvoorden, H. J., Kauffman, R. H., & Goodkin, K. (1995). Active confrontational coping predicts decreased clinical progression over a one year period in HIV-infected homosexual men. *Journal of Psychosomatic Research, 39,* 957–965.

Mulder, C. L., van der Pompe, G., Spiegel, D., Antoni, M. H., & de Vries, M. (1992). Do psychosocial factors influence the course of breast cancer?: A review of recent literature, methodological problems and future directions. *Psychooncology, 1,* 155–167.

Mumford, E., Schlesinger, H. J., & Glass, G. V. (1982). The effects of psychological intervention on recovery from surgery and heart attacks: An analysis of the literature. *American Journal of Public Health, 72*(2), 141–151.

Mumford, E., Schlesinger, H. J., Glass, G. V., Patrick, C., & Cuerdon, T. (1984). A new look at evidence about reduced cost of medical utilization following mental health treatment. *American Journal of Psychiatry, 141*(10), 1145–1158.

Murphy, E., & Brown, G. (1980). Life events, psychiatric disturbances, and physical illness. *British Journal of Psychiatry, 136,* 326–338.

Myers, M. G., Brown, S. A., & Mott, M. (1993). Coping as a predictor of substance abuse treatment outcome. *Journal of Substance Abuse, 5*(1), 15–29.

Narrow, W. E., Regier, D. A., & Rae, D. S. (1993). Use of services by persons with mental and addictive disorders: Findings from the National Institute of Mental Health Epidemiologic Catchment Area Program. *Archives of General Psychiatry, 50,* 95–107.

National Heart, Lung, and Blood Institute. (2000, October). *The practical guide to identification, education and treatment of overweight and obesity in adults* (NIH Publication No. 00-4084). Rockville, MD: U.S. Department of Health and Human Services.

National Institute on Drug Abuse. (1990). *Alcohol and health* (DHHS Publication No. ADM 871519). Rockville, MD: U.S. Department of Health and Human Services.

Neal, A. V., Tilley, B. C., & Vernon, S. W. (1986). Marital status, delay in seeking treatment and survival from breast cancer. *Social Science and Medicine, 23,* 305–312.

Newcomb, M., & Harlow, L. (1986). Life events and substance use among adolescents: Mediating effects of perceived loss of control and meaninglessness in life. *Journal of Personality and Social Psychology, 51,* 564.

Niemi, M. L., Laaksonen, R., Kotila, M., & Waltimo, O. (1988). Quality of life 4 years after stroke. *Stroke, 19,* 1101–1107.

Northouse, A. (1988). Social support in patients' and husbands' adjustment to breast cancer. *Nursing Research, 37,* 91–95.

Oldenberg, B., Perkins, R., & Andrews, G. (1985). Controlled trial of psychological intervention in myocardial infarction. *Journal of Consulting and Clinical Psychology, 53,* 852–859.

O'Leary, A. (1992). Self-efficacy and health: Behavioral and stress–physiological mediation. *Cognitive Therapy and Research, 16,* 229–245.

Ornish, D., Scherwitz, L. W., Billings, J. H., Gould, L., Merritt, T. A., & Sparler, S. (1998). Intensive lifestyle changes for reversal of coronary heart disease. *Journal of the American Medical Association, 280,* 2001–2007.

Oxman, T., Freeman, D., & Manheimer, E. (1995). Lack of social participation or religious strength and comfort as risk factors for death after cardiac surgery in the elderly. *Psychosomatic Medicine, 57,* 5–15.

Pallak, M. S., Cummings, N. A., Dorken, H., & Henke, C. J. (1994). Medical costs, Medicaid, and managed mental health treatment: The Hawaii study. *Managed Care Quarterly, 2,* 64–70.

Penedo, F. J., Dahn, J. R., Molton, I., Gonzalez, J., Roos, B., Schneiderman, N., et al. (2004). Cognitive-behavioral stress management improves quality of life and stress management skill in men treated for localized prostate cancer. *Cancer, 100,* 192–200.

Penedo, F. J., Molton, I., Dahn, J. R., Shen, B. J., Kinsinger, D., Schneiderman, N., et al. (2006). A randomized clinical trial of group-based cognitive-behavioral stress management (CBSM) in localized prostate cancer: Development of stress management skills improves quality of life and benefit finding. *Annals of Behavioral Medicine, 31*(3), 261–270.

Pennebaker, J. W., Kiecolt-Glaser, J. K., & Glaser, R. (1988). Disclosure of traumas and immune function: Health implications for psychotherapy. *Journal of Consulting and Clinical Psychology, 56,* 239–245.

Pereira, D., Antoni, M. H., Simon, T., Efantis-Potter, J., Carver, C. S., Duran, R., et al. (2003). Stress and squamous intraepithelial lesions in women with human papillomavirus and human immunodeficiency virus. *Psychosomatic Medicine, 65,* 427–434.

Pereira, D., Antoni, M. H., Simon, T., Efantis-Potter, J., & O'Sullivan, M. J. (2004). Inhibited interpersonal coping style predicts poor adherence to scheduled clinic visits in HIV infected women at risk for cervical cancer. *Annals of Behavioral Medicine, 28,* 195–202.

Peterson, C., Seligman, M. E. P., & Vaillant, G. E. (1988). Pessimistic explanatory style is a risk factor for physical illness: A thirty-five year longitudinal study. *Journal of Personality and Social Psychology, 55,* 23–27.

Pettingale, K., Greer, S., & Tee, D. (1977). Serum IgA and emotional expression in breast cancer patients. *Journal of Psychosomatic Research, 21,* 395–399.

Powers, P. S., Rosemurgy, A., Boyd, F., & Perez, A. (1997). Outcome of gastric restriction procedures: Weight, psychiatric diagnoses, and satisfaction. *Obesity Surgery, 7,* 471–477.

Razin, A. (1982). Psychosocial intervention in coronary artery disease: A review. *Psychosomatic Medicine, 44,* 363–387.

Reed, G. M., Kemeny, M. E., Taylor, S. E., Wang, H. J., & Visscher, B. R. (1994). Realistic acceptance as a predictor of decreased survival time in gay men with AIDS. *Health Psychology, 13*(4), 299–307.

Regier, D. (1994). Health care reform: Opportunities and challenge. In S. Blumenthal, K. Matthews, & S. Weiss (Eds.), *New research frontiers in behavioral medicine: Proceedings of the National Conference* (NIH Publication No. 94-3772). Washington, DC: U.S. Government Printing Office.

Richter, J., Obrecht, W., Bradley, L., et al. (1986). Psychological comparison of patients with nutcracker esophagus and irritable bowel syndrome. *Digestive Diseases and Sciences, 31,* 131–138.

Richter, S., Brown, S., & Mott, M. (1991). The impact of social support and self-esteem on adolescent substance abuse treatment outcome. *Journal of Substance Abuse, 3*(4), 371–385.

Robertson, E. K., & Suinn, R. M. (1968). The determination of rate of progress of stroke patients through empathy measures of patient and family. *Journal of Psychosomatic Research, 12,* 189–191.

Rock, C., McEligot, A., Flatt, S., Sobo, E., Wilfley, D., Jones, V., et al. (2000). Eating pathology and obesity in women at risk for breast cancer recurrence. *International Journal of Eating Disorders, 27,* 172–179.

Rosenstock, I. M. (1974). The health belief model and preventive health behavior. *Health Education Monographs, 2,* 354–386.

Roth, A. J., Kornblith, A. B., Batel-Copel, L., Peabody, E., Peabody, E., Scher, H. I., et al. (1998). Rapid screening for psychologic distress in men with prostate carcinoma: A pilot study. *Cancer, 82,* 1904–1908.

Santry, H., Gillen, D., & Lauderdale, D. (2005). Trends in bariatric surgical procedures. *Journal of the American Medical Association, 294,* 1909–1917.

Sarason, I., Johnson, J., & Spiegel, J. (1978). Assessing the impact of life changes: Development of the Life Experiences Survey. *Journal of Consulting and Clinical Psychology, 46,* 932–946.

Schaefer, C., Coyne, J. C., & Lazarus, R. S. (1981). The health-related functions of social support. *Journal of Behavioral Medicine, 4,* 381–406.

Scheier, M., Mathews, K., Owens, J., Schultz, R., Bridges, M., Magovern, G., et al. (1999). Optimism and rehospitalization after coronary artery bypass graft surgery. *Archives of Internal Medicine, 159,* 829–835.

Scheier, M. F., & Carver, C. S. (1985). Optimism, coping, and health: Assessment and implication of generalized outcome expectancies. *Health Psychology, 4,* 219–247.

Schlesinger, H. J., Mumford, E., Glass, G. V., Patrick, C., & Sharfstein, S. (1983). Mental health treatment and medical care utilization in a fee-for-service system: Outpatient mental health treatment following the onset of a chronic disease. *American Journal of Public Health, 73*(4), 422–429.

Schneider, C. J. (1987). Cost-effectiveness of biofeedback and behavioral medicine treatments: A review of the literature. *Biofeedback and Self-Regulation, 12*(2), 71–92.

Schneiderman, N., Antoni, M. H., Saab, P., & Ironson, G. (2001). Health psychology: Psychosocial and biobehavioral aspects of chronic disease management. *Annual Reviews in Psychology, 52,* 555–580.

Schwartz, L. S., Springer, J., Flaherty, J. A., & Kiani, R. (1986). The role of recent life events and social support in the control of diabetes mellitus. *General Hospital Psychiatry, 8,* 212–216.

Siegal, B. R., Calsyn, R. J., & Cuddihee, R. M. (1987). The relationship of social support to psychological adjustment in end-stage renal disease patients. *Journal of Chronic Diseases, 40,* 337–344.

Singh, N., Berman, S. M., Swindells, S., Justis, J. C., Mohr, J. A., & Wagener, M. M. (1999). Adherence to immunodeficiency virus-infected patients to antiretroviral therapy. *Clinical Infectious Diseases, 29,* 824–830.

Sklar, L. W., & Anisman, H. (1981). Stress and cancer. *Psychological Bulletin, 89,* 369–406.

Smyth, J., Stone, A., Hurewitz, A., & Kaell, A. (1999). Effects of writing about stressful experiences on symptom reduction in patients with asthma or rheumatoid arthritis: A randomized trial. *Journal of the American Medical Association, 281,* 1304–1309.

Sobel, D. (1994). Mind matters, money matters: The cost-effectiveness of clinical behavioral medicine. In S. Blumenthal, K. Matthews, & S. Weiss (Eds.), *New research frontiers in behavioral medicine: Proceedings of the National Conference* (NIH Publication No. 94-3772). Washington, DC: U.S. Government Printing Office.

Solano, L., Costa, M., Salvati, S., Coda, R., Aiuta, F., Mezzaroma, I., et al. (1993). Psychosocial factors and clinical evolution in HIV-1 infection: A longitudinal study. *Journal of Psychosomatic Research, 37*(1), 39–51.

Solomon, G. F., Benton, D., Harker, J., Bonavida, B., & Fletcher, M. A. (1993). Prolonged asymptomatic states in HIV-seropositive persons with 50 CD4+ T-cells/mm3: Preliminary psychoimmunologic findings. *Journal of Acquired Immunodeficiency Syndromes, 6*(10), 1173.

Spiegel, D., Kraemer, H. C., Bloom, J. R., & Gottheil, E. (1989). Effect of psychosocial treatment on survival of patients with metastatic breast cancer. *Lancet, ii,* 888–891.

Starr, K., Antoni, M. H., Penedo, F., Costello, N., Lutgendorf, S., Ironson, G., et al. (1996, March). *Cognitive and affective correlates of emotional expression in symptomatic HIV-infected gay men.* Paper presented at the annual meeting of the Society of Behavioral Medicine, Washington, DC.

Stein, M. J., Wallston, K. A., Nicassio, P. M., & Castner, N. M. (1988). Correlates of a clinical classification schema for the Arthritis Helplessness subscale. *Arthritis and Rheumatism, 31,* 876–881.

Stern, M. J., Pascale, L., & Ackerman, A. (1977). Life adjustment postmyocardial infarction: Determining predictive variables. *Archives of Internal Medicine, 137,* 1680–1685.

Sternhall, P. S., & Corr, M. J. (2002). Psychiatric morbidity and adherence to antiretroviral medication in patients with HIV/AIDS. *Australian and New Zealand Journal of Psychiatry, 36,* 528–533.

Stone, A., & Porter, L. (1995). Psychological coping: Its importance for treating medical problems. *Mind/Body Medicine, 1,* 46–54.

Strain, J., Lyons, J., Hammer, J., Fahs, M., Lebovitz, A., Paddison, P., et al. (1991). Cost offset from a psychiatric consultation–liaison intervention with elderly hip fracture patients. *American Journal of Psychiatry, 148*(8), 1044–1049.

Surwit, R. S., & Feinglos, M. N. (1988). Stress and autonomic nervous system in Type II diabetes: A hypothesis. *Diabetes Care, 11,* 83–85.

Taylor, S. E., & Aspinwall, L. G. (1990). Psychosocial aspects of chronic illness. In P. Costa & G. van den Bos (Eds.), *Psychological aspects of serious illness: Chronic conditions, fatal diseases, and clinical care.* Washington, DC: American Psychological Association.

Taylor, S. E., Lichtman, R. R., & Wood, J. V. (1984). Attributions, beliefs about control, and adjustment to breast cancer. *Journal of Personality and Social Psychology, 46,* 489–502.

Theorell, T., Blomkvist, V., Jonsson, H., Schulman, S., Berntorp, E., & Stigendal, L. (1995). Social support and the development of immune function in human immunodeficiency virus infection. *Psychosomatic Medicine, 57,* 32–36.

Thoits, P. A. (1987). Gender and marital status differences in control and distress: Common stress versus unique stress explanations. *Journal of Health and Social Behavior, 28,* 7–22.

Thompson, S. C., Sobolew-Shubin, A., Graham, M. A., & Janigian, A. S. (1989). Psychosocial adjustment following a stroke. *Social Science and Medicine, 28,* 239–247.

Topol, E., Califf, R., George, B., Kereiakes, D., Abbotsmith, C., Candela, R., et al. (1987). A randomized trial of immediate versus delayed elective angioplasty after intravenous tissue plasminogen activator in acute myocardial infarction. *New England Journal of Medicine, 317*(10), 581–588.

Tracy, H., Green, C., & McCleary, J. (1987). Noncompliance in hemodialysis patients as measured by the MBHI. *Psychology and Health, 2,* 411–412.

Trijsburg, R. W., van Knippenberg, F. C. E., & Rijma, S. E. (1992). Effects of psychological treatment on cancer patients: A critical review. *Psychosomatic Medicine, 54,* 489–517.

Turk, D., & Meichenbaum, D. (1989). Adherence to self-care regimens: The patient's perspective. In R. H. Rozensky, J. Sweet, & S. Tovian (Eds.), *Handbook of clinical psychology in medical settings.* New York: Plenum Press.

Turner, H. A., Hays, R. B., & Coates, T. J. (1993). Determinants of social support among gay men: The context of AIDS. *Journal of Health and Social Behavior, 34,* 37–53.

Uhlenhuth, E., & Paykel, E. (1973). Symptom intensity and life events. *Archives of General Psychiatry, 28,* 473–477.

U.S. Department of Health and Human Services. (1992). *1992 HCFA Statistics: U.S. Department of Health and Human Services, Health Care Financing Administration, Bureau of Data Management and Strategy* (HCFA Publication No. 03333). Washington, DC: U.S. Government Printing Office.

Vaillant, G. E., Schnurr, P. P., Baron, J. R., & Gerber, P. D. (1991). A prospective study of the effect of smoking and alcohol abuse on mortality. *Journal of General Internal Medicine, 6,* 299–304.

Valdez, L., Lederman, M., Woolley, I., Walker, C. J., Vernon, L. T., Hise, A., et al. (1999). Human immunodeficiency virus 1 protease inhibitors in clinical practice: Predictors of virological outcome. *Archives of Internal Medicine, 159,* 1771–1776.

van der Pompe, G., Antoni, M. H., & Heijnen, C. (1998). The effects of surgical stress and psychological stress on the immune function of operative cancer patients. *Psychology and Health, 13,* 1015–1026.

van der Pompe, G., Antoni, M. H., Mulder, N., Heijnen, C., Goodkin, K., de Graeff, A., et al. (1994). Psychoneuroimmunology and the course of breast cancer, an overview: The impact of psychosocial factors on progression of breast cancer through immune and endocrine mechanisms. *Psychooncology, 3,* 271–288.

Vickery, D. M. (1983). Effect of a self-care education program on medical visits. *Journal of the American Medical Association, 250*(21), 2952–2956.

Wadden, T., Brownell, K., & Foster, G. (2002). Obesity: Responding to the global epidemic. *Journal of Consulting and Clinical Psychology, 70,* 510–525.

Wallston, B. S., Alagna, S. W., De Vellis, B., & De Vellis, R. F. (1983). Social support and physical health. *Health Psychology, 2,* 367–391.

Weaver, K., Llabre, M., Durán, R. E., Antoni, M. H., Ironson, G., Penedo, F., et al. (2005). A stress and coping model of medication adherence and viral load in HIV+ men and women on highly active antiretroviral therapy. *Health Psychology, 24,* 385–392.

Weisberg, M., & Page, S. (1988). Millon Behavioral Health Inventory and perceived efficacy of home and hospital dialysis. *Journal of Social and Clinical Psychology, 6,* 408–422.

Wiedenfield, S., O'Leary, A., Bandura, A., Brown, S., Levine, S., & Raska, K. (1990). Impact of perceived self-efficacy in coping with stressors on components of the immune system. *Journal of Personality and Social Psychology, 59,* 1082–1094.

Wiklund, I., Oden, A., Sanne, H., Ulvenstam, G., Wilhelmsson, C., & Wilhemsen, L. (1988). Prognostic importance of somatic and psychosocial variables after a first myocardial infarction. *American Journal of Epidemiology, 128,* 786–795.

Wilcoxin, M., Zook, A., & Zarski, J. (1988). Predicting behavioral outcomes with two psychological assessment methods in an outpatient pain management program. *Psychology and Health*, 2, 319–333.

Williams, R. B., & Chesney, M. (1993). Psychosocial factors and prognosis in established coronary artery disease: The need for research on interventions. *Journal of the American Medical Association*, 279, 1860–1861.

Wilson, S., Scamagas, P., German, D., Hughes, G., Lulla, S., Coss, S., et al. (1993). A controlled trial of two forms of self-management education for adults with asthma. *American Journal of Medicine*, 94, 564–576.

Wilson, W., Ary, D. V., Biglan, A., Glasgow, R. E., Toobert, D. J., & Campbell, D. R. (1986). Psychosocial predictors of self-care behaviors (compliance) and glycemic control in non-insulin-dependent diabetes mellitus. *Diabetes Care*, 9, 614–622.

Woods, T., Antoni, M. H., Ironson, G., & Kling, D. (1999a). Religiosity is associated with affective and immune status in symptomatic HIV-infected gay men. *Journal of Psychosomatic Research*, 46, 165–176.

Woods, T., Antoni, M. H., Ironson, G., & Kling, D. (1999b). Religiosity is associated with affective status in symptomatic HIV-infected African American women. *Journal of Health Psychology*, 4, 317–326.

Woolf, S. (1999). The need for perspective in evidence-based medicine. *Journal of the American Medical Association*, 282, 2358–2365.

Wortman, C., & Conway, T. (1985). The role of social support in adaptation and recovery from physical illness. In S. Cohen & S. Syme (Eds.), *Social support and health*. New York: Academic Press.

Young, L. (1992). Psychological factors in rheumatoid arthritis. *Journal of Consulting and Clinical Psychology*, 60, 619–627.

Zachariah, P. (1987). Quality of life with antihypertensive medication. *Journal of Hypertension*, 5(Suppl.), 105–110.

Zich, J., & Temoshok, L. (1987). Perceptions of social support in men with AIDS and ARC: Relationships with distress and hardiness. *Journal of Applied Social Psychology*, 17, 193–215.

Zook, C. J., & Moore, F. D. (1980). High cost users of medical care. *New England Journal of Medicine*, 302, 996–1002.

Zuckerman, M., & Antoni, M. H. (1995). Social support and its relationship to psychological physical and immune variables in HIV infection. *Clinical Psychology and Psychotherapy*, 2(4), 210–219.

CHAPTER 20

Using the Millon Adolescent Clinical Inventory (MACI) and Its Facet Scales

Joseph T. McCann

Human development is typically conceptualized as consisting of distinct phases of change and growth, each characterized by unique psychosocial challenges and physical changes. Adolescence is a period marked by many developmental changes and conflicts (Coleman, 1992; Petersen, 1988). Biological forces bring about an increase in hormonal activity, development of secondary sex characteristics, and physical maturation that leads to a more adult-like appearance. Social pressures also define adolescence as a time of conflict. There is the desire to break away from family influences and adopt the norms of one's peer group; yet adolescents also recognize the frequent need for a certain level of emotional and economic dependence on the family. Also, teenagers' continuing individual growth leads to greater autonomy and questions about their identity and direction in life. In short, adolescence is a transitional phase between childhood and adulthood, characterized by change in all aspects of a person's development.

Because of the distinct nature of adolescence, it should be obvious that psychological assessment procedures need to be designed specifically for the measurement of adolescent personality and adjustment. Strangely, however, the early phases of adolescent psychodiagnosis were characterized by the adaptation of instruments originally designed for adults to the assessment of adolescents (Archer & Ball, 1988). An erroneous assumption presumed to underlie this practice was the notion that adolescents were "mini-adults," and that assessment required merely renorming of existing tests and slight alterations in procedures—perhaps through changing instructions and items or modifying scoring procedures—to make the instruments appropriate for adolescent populations.

Over the last two decades, there have been attempts to design objective personality instruments specifically for adolescents. A major psychological test for adolescent populations that has come into widespread use is the Millon Adolescent Clinical Inventory (MACI; Millon, 1993, 2006). The MACI represents a psychodiagnostic instrument constructed not only with the unique challenges of adolescent assessment in mind, but also with ample recognition given to modern test construction and psychometric principles (McCann, 1999; Millon & Davis, 1998). As a test designed especially for adolescents, the MACI measures clinical symptomatology, personality characteristics, and expressed concerns that are both common among and unique to teenagers. Moreover, the MACI is grounded in a comprehensive theory of personality and psychopathology (Millon, 1969, 1981, 1990; Millon & Davis, 1996). With a specific focus on clinical assessment, the MACI is applicable in a wide range of evaluation and treatment settings where the identification of clinical symptomatology is of primary concern. As such, the MACI scales have been designed to correspond to current diagnostic criteria and clinical syndromes outlined in several versions of the *Diagnostic and Statistical Manual of Mental Disorders* (DSM-III-R, American Psychiatric Association, 1987; DSM-IV, American Psychiatric Association, 1994; DSM-IV-TR, American Psychiatric Association, 2000).

Although no diagnostic instrument represents a perfect measure of DSM criteria, the MACI incorporates several innovations and attributes that reflect the diagnostic conceptual model represented in current diagnostic nomenclature, to facilitate its practical use. As such, the MACI incorporates two sets of scales to measure separately the more transient clinical syndromes associated with Axis I of DSM-IV(-TR) and the more stable features of personality on Axis II.

This chapter provides a brief overview of the procedures followed in developing the MACI, as well as various strategies for interpreting the profile. Readers wishing to find a more in-depth discussion of these issues will want to consult the most recent edition of the test manual (Millon, 2006), as well as the interpretive guide (McCann, 1999). The chapter closes with a brief overview of recent trends in MACI research that have emerged in recent years.

Applications and Limitations

The MACI is an objective personality inventory consisting of 160 items that are answered in a true–false format. It was designed to be used in settings where adolescents are likely to come to the attention of mental health professionals, including outpatient clinics, private practice, correctional facilities, inpatient psychiatric hospitals, general hospital units where mental health issues are of concern, residential treatment facilities, and educational counseling settings. The primary focus of the item and scale content on the MACI is on psychological disturbances and concerns that are likely to be encountered in these various settings. Therefore, various problems such as depression, anxiety, eating disorders, substance abuse, acting-out behavior, peer conflict, and feelings of inadequacy are included in the scope of concerns evaluated by the MACI. Similarly, problematic interpersonal behaviors and personality disturbances are also evaluated, including severe introversion, excessive dependency, antisocial and delinquent propensities, egocentricity, and manipulativeness. Because the focus of the MACI is on clinical concerns and its applications are primarily in clinical settings, there are no scales addressing normal or nonclinical issues, such as academic confidence, scholastic achievement, and career goals. In cases where psychopathology is either absent or not suspected, and professionals are seeking information on normal personality traits or academic interests and scholastic aptitude, other psychological assessment instruments should be utilized.

Given that adolescent behavior and development involves unique challenges, psychological testing instruments are not "one-size-fits-all" ventures. If an instrument is to provide clinically useful information in adolescent populations, it must take developmental issues into account. Therefore, several practical applications were implemented during the development of the MACI that would make it widely applicable in settings where adolescents are evaluated. An important consideration was given to the readability of the items. The MACI items assume that an adolescent has at least a sixth-grade reading level (Millon, 2006). However, in some cases—particularly those where an adolescent has a reading disability or cognitive impairment that interferes with reading—the teenager may be unable to read the items adequately. In these cases, the test can be read to the subject either by a nonintrusive, neutral evaluator, or by a standardized tape recording of the MACI that is available from the test publisher (Pearson Assessments).

Another major consideration during development of the MACI that has had an impact on its applications is the normative age range. The test was developed and standardized on a population of adolescents ages 13–19. Therefore, administration of the MACI to individuals below the age of 13 or above the age of 19 is not appropriate. Furthermore, during standardization of the MACI, consideration was given to the fact that various types of psychopathology may manifest themselves differently as a function of either gender or early versus late adolescence. Therefore, the MACI has different norms for younger (i.e., ages 13–15) and older (i.e., ages 16–19) adolescents, and for both males and females.

As any psychometric instrument does, the MACI has both strengths and limitations in terms of its applicability and utility in any particular setting. Among the strengths of the MACI is its brevity. According to Dyer (1985), test length is a critical factor to consider when one is evaluating adolescents, because of a greater prevalence of such barriers to assessment as inattentiveness and resistance to participating in a psychological evaluation. In addition, the MACI is well suited for an integrated approach to assessment that takes into consideration a wide array of concerns and difficulties, and places these problems within the context of the adolescent's personality. Therefore, an adolescent's problems can be understood as having specific meaning when evaluated within the framework of the teenager's behavioral and interpersonal style, cognitive approach to dealing with problems, and basic temperament. Moreover, the MACI's stratified norms across age groups allow clinicians to apply the instrument to both younger and older adolescents, as noted above. Finally, the MACI has excellent psychometric properties, particularly internal consistency reliability and a composition based on modern psychometrics that includes theoretical/substantive, internal/structural, and external/criterion validation considerations (McCann, 1999; Millon, 2006).

Despite the many strengths of the MACI, clinicians may encounter some limitations in its use as well. For instance, more severe forms of psychopathology, such as psychosis, bipolar disorders, and paranoid ideation, are not directly measured by MACI scales. Moreover, some forms of adolescent psychopathology seen in certain settings, such as obsessive–compulsive disorder or attention-deficit/hyperactivity disorder, are likewise not directly measured by MACI scales. Although other assessment techniques and instruments (e.g., clinical interviews, patient history, collateral reports, and issue-specific instruments) are going to be of greatest assistance in answering certain diagnostic questions, the MACI may still be useful as an ancillary tool for providing an overview of an adolescent's psychological adjustment and functioning, regardless of the specific referral question. Any clinician using the MACI must therefore be mindful of not only the advantages in utilizing the test, but also the limitations that dictate conservative interpretation strategies and applications in specific settings and contexts.

Scale Development and Composition

Each scale in the MACI profile was selected according to a number of criteria (Millon, 1993, 2006). Because Millon's (1969, 1981, 1990; Millon & Davis, 1996) integrated theory of personality and psychopathology served as the guiding framework for development of the MACI, individual scales were included to measure each of the theory's basic personality patterns, as well as personality disorders outlined in DSM-III-R and DSM-IV(-TR) (American Psychiatric Association, 1987, 1994, 2000). The 11 basic personality patterns are Introversive, Inhibited, Doleful, Submissive, Dramatizing, Egotistic, Unruly, Forceful, Conforming, Oppositional, and Self-Demeaning. Given the clinical prevalence and professional interest in borderline personality disturbances that often begin to emerge in adolescence, the Borderline Tendency scale was also selected for inclusion in the MACI profile. The selection of scales to measure specific clinical syndromes was based on the relative importance of such syndromes among adolescents; they include eating disorders, delinquency and conduct problems, impulsivity, substance abuse, anxiety, depression, and suicide potential. Several scales were also included in the MACI profile to reflect concerns and difficulties that are common in adolescent populations and are often foci of clinical attention, but that nevertheless may not reflect specific diagnostic entities. These concerns include identity diffusion, peer problems, insensitivity to others, self-devaluation, emerging concerns over sexual feelings and body image, and family problems. Finally, a number of scales were constructed to evaluate the validity of an adolescent's self-reporting on the MACI; these scales allow clinicians to evaluate the consistency and response style of the teenager taking the test.

The resultant strategy of selecting constructs yielded a profile of 31 scales and indices (see Millon, 1993, 2006, for a complete listing). A major distinguishing feature of the MACI is the use of base rate (BR) scores as the standardized measures for converting, plotting, and interpreting raw scores. The BR scores are derived in a manner that reflects the prevalence rates of various disorders, concerns, and syndromes in a clinical setting, in order to enhance the MACI's use as a diagnostic instrument. These scores were derived by first arriving at a set of items that survived repetitive cycling through a three-stage validation process in which the items met strict theoretical/substantive, internal/structural, and external/criterion forms of validity (Millon, 1993, 2006). Once items were written to correspond with the underlying theoretical prototypal personality descriptions, as well as DSM-IV(-TR) criteria for the clinical syndromes and descriptors for the expressed concerns, they were tested to establish endorsement frequencies and internal consistency reliability. Thus the MACI items were designed to discriminate between various diagnostic groups, while also possessing high levels of internal consistency. In addition, the items were further refined to make sure they corresponded to external diagnostic criteria.

Once items for the MACI were selected, the prevalence rates for each diagnostic category measured by scales 9 (Borderline Tendency) through GG (Suicidal Tendency) were established in the normative sample, based on clinician ratings of these categories using external criteria. Next, raw score frequency distributions were constructed for each of these scales, and five anchor points were chosen at arbitrary levels on the BR scale to convert raw scores into the standardized BR scores. The five BR score levels chosen as anchor points were 0, 60, 75, 85, and 115. BR scores of 0 and 115 were selected to represent the minimum and maximum raw score possible on each scale, respectively, and a BR score of 60 was chosen to correspond to the median raw score on each scale. A BR score of 75 was chosen to correspond to the percentile on the raw score distribution reflecting the percentage of adolescents in the normative sample rated as having a personality trait, expressed concern, or clinical syndrome *present*. A BR score of 85 was selected to identify the raw score percentile reflecting the percentage of adolescents in the sample rated as having a trait, concern, or syndrome *prominent*. Finally, algebraic interpolation was used to convert the raw score levels between the anchor points into BR scores. In this manner, four normative BR tables were constructed for 13- to 15-year-old males, 13- to 15-year-old females, 16- to 19-year-old males, and 16- to 19-year-old females.

For scales 1 (Introversive) through 8B (Self-Demeaning), the BR conversions were constructed in a slightly different manner. As outlined in the MACI manuals (Millon, 1993, 2006), these 11 scales were developed in such a manner that a restriction was placed on the BR transformations. That is, a specific scale had to be the highest among the Personality Patterns scales at a rate matching the prevalence for the same characteristic when rated as *prominent* by clinicians making external criterion ratings in the normative sample. The BR score conversions were also designed to have a scale be the second-highest elevation among the personality style scales at a rate matching the prevalence of the characteristic when rated as *present* by the external criterion. Thus linear interpolation was not always calculated uniformly for each of the BR scores for the basic Personality Patterns scales.

With respect to the Modifying Indices (i.e., scales X, Y, and Z), BR scores were based strictly on raw score percentiles. Therefore, on Disclosure (scale X), Desirability (scale Y), and Debasement (scale Z), BR scores above 85 represent the top 10% of adolescents in the normative sample, whereas BR scores between 75 and 84 represent the next 15%; thus BR scores of 75 or above on the MACI Modifying Indices represent the top quartile of the normative sample. The lowest 15% of raw scores on these scales are represented by BR scores below 35, whereas the remainder of the normative sample falls somewhere between BR scores of 35 and 74.

The most recent innovation in development and refinement of the MACI scales is the formal implementation of the Grossman Facet Scales for the Personality Patterns scales, as reported in the second edition of the test manual (Millon, 2006). Based on a factor analysis of individual items on each of the Personality Patterns scales, Davis (1993) identified a number of content domains that were represented in each of the scales. These content scales not only were offered as a means of supporting the validity of the personality scales, but were also considered to be useful in making more specific interpretations when a specific Personality Pattern scale on the MACI profile was elevated (McCann, 1999). The Grossman Facet Scales constitute a refinement of Davis's work, in that three subscales (i.e., Facet Scales) were identified for each of the Personality Patterns scales, and each subscale represents one of the eight structural–functional personality domains outlined in Millon's underlying theory (Millon, 1990; Millon & Davis, 1996): expressive behavior, interpersonal conduct, cognitive style, self-image, object representations, regulatory mechanisms, morphological organization, and mood/temperament. The Grossman Facet Scales were developed through a process of rational/theoretical analysis of item content of the factor-analytic content scales. Since the item and content sampling across the various personality scales varies, different personality domains are represented in the Facet Scales for each personality scale. That is, while each of the MACI Personality Patterns scales has three Grossman Facet Scales, the scales differ from one another in terms of the specific personality domains measured. Those facets that survived scale development were considered to be the domains most prominently represented in each personality style, according to both theory and psychometric analysis of the MACI items (Millon, 2006).

Table 20.1 provides a listing of the Grossman Facet Scales for each of the MACI Personality Patterns scales, along with a brief description of what each facet measures. The Facet Scales represent not only a recent empirical development with the MACI, but also an interpretive innovation. The second edition of the MACI manual (Millon, 2006) states that the Grossman Facet Scales should be utilized to refine interpretations only for those Personality Patterns scales that have BR scores above 65. BR score conversion tables have been developed for the Grossman Facet Scales, and the revised MACI interpretive report provides a complete listing of scores for each of these scales, as well as a graphic depiction of Facet Scales for Personality Patterns scales that are above BRs of 65 on the MACI profile.

Administration and Scoring

The MACI may be scored by either hand or computer. Given the complexity of the psychometric properties (including item weighting and profile adjustments), hand scoring is a useful learning tool for those clinicians who are either beginning users or experienced professionals who prefer to maintain a comprehensive understanding of the various adjustments that have been made to the profile. Nevertheless, the complexity of the scoring procedures and profile adjustment algorithms render the MACI very well suited for computerized scoring for those clinicians who perform a high volume of testing, as computerization secures accuracy and efficiency in test scoring.

Given that the MACI has 160 items, with 31 scales that have anywhere from 16 to 44 items per scale, there is a considerable level of item overlap; this may have an impact on discriminant validity, and spur multiple scale elevations, for a given pro-

TABLE 20.1. The Grossman Facet Scales for the MACI Personality Patterns Scales

Scale/facets	Brief description
1. Introversive	
Expressively Impassive	Lacking energy, robotic, deficient in spontaneity.
Temperamentally Apathetic	Unexcitable, cold, emotions lack depth.
Interpersonally Unengaged	Indifferent, solitary, does not enjoy closeness.
2A. Inhibited	
Expressively Fretful	Uneasy, hesitant, overreacts to criticism.
Interpersonally Aversive	Excessive social anxiety, distrustful, fearful.
Alienated Self-Image	Feels inadequate, inept, justified in being isolated.
2B. Doleful	
Temperamentally Woeful	Gloomy, brooding, chronic dysphoria.
Expressively Disconsolate	Somber, discouraged, chronic hopelessness.
Cognitively Pessimistic	Defeatist, bleak, thinks things will never improve.
3. Submissive	
Interpersonally Docile	Needs constant reassurance, compliant, placid.
Temperamentally Pacific	Warm, tender, noncompetitive, avoids conflict.
Expressively Incompetent	Acts helpless, passive, docile, avoids assertiveness.
4. Dramatizing	
Interpersonally Attention-Seeking	Actively seeks approval, wants to be center of attention.
Gregarious Self-Image	Sees self as sociable, charming, likes to be busy.
Cognitively Flighty	Suggestible, scattered learning and judgment.
5. Egotistic	
Admirable Self-Image	Believes self to be special, deserving of praise.
Cognitively Expansive	Excessive fantasies of success, imagines success.
Interpersonally Exploitive	Entitlement, unempathic, uses others to enhance self.
6A. Unruly	
Expressively Impulsive	Acts without thinking, short-sighted, careless.
Acting-Out Mechanism	Inner conflicts discharged without guilt or remorse.
Interpersonally Irresponsible	Untrustworthy, unreliable, violates rights of others.
6B. Forceful	
Interpersonally Abrasive	Intimidating, coercive, humiliates others.
Expressively Precipitate	Reckless, daring, undeterred by pain or danger.
Isolation Mechanism	Detached and lacks awareness of impact on others.
7. Conforming	
Expressively Disciplined	Highly structured, overly perfectionistic.
Interpersonally Respectful	Too conscientious, excessively polite and formal.
Conscientious Self-Image	Devoted to work, disciplined, rule-bound.
8A. Oppositional	
Discontented Self-Image	Feels misunderstood, unlucky, unappreciated.
Expressively Resentful	Procrastinates, contrary, undermines others.
Interpersonally Contrary	Changeable, conflicted, intolerant, negative.
8B. Self-Demeaning	
Cognitively Diffident	Repeatedly defeatist, unable to see positive side.
Undeserving Self-Image	Puts self down, shamed, deserving of suffering.
Temperamentally Dysphoric	Tormented, unhappy, anxiously apprehensive.
9. Borderline Tendency	
Temperamentally Labile	Changeable to situations, moods change rapidly.
Cognitively Capricious	Vacillating and contradictory reactions, confusing.
Uncertain Self-Image	Immature self, wavering identity, feels empty.

file. Elsewhere (McCann, 1999), I have performed a series of analyses on the effect that item overlap may have on MACI test results. These analyses reveal that common profile configurations are found in various clinical syndromes. However, to reduce the impact of item overlap, the MACI uses a selective item-weighting scheme and a series of profile adjustments. Each item on the MACI was selected for its substantive connection to a particular construct measured by the test and the individual psychometric properties of those items. Moreover, individual items on the MACI tend to tap into more than one of these psychological constructs, so the keying of items is such that items contribute various raw score points to different scales, based on how closely an item represents the particular trait or construct being measured.

Furthermore, once raw scores for the MACI scales have been converted to BR scores, several profile adjustments are implemented to correct for such influences as the overall level of disclosure, acute anxiety and depressive states, social desirability, negative self-evaluation, and personality styles that tend to be associated with a tendency to either complain about or deny personal problems (Millon, 1993, 2006). These adjustments to the MACI profile serve to preserve the elevation frequencies of each individual scale on the test, so that they correspond to the prevalence rates of the Personality Patterns, Expressed Concerns, and Clinical Syndromes in the normative sample. Despite the intuitive sense these profile adjustments make, they also serve the psychometric goal of maintaining correspondence between the frequency of MACI scale elevations and diagnostic prevalence rates in the normative sample.

Interpretation of the MACI

Clinical interpretation of the MACI follows a series of steps (McCann, 1999). First, the clinician must review information from the adolescent's history and clinical examination, to make sure that interpretive hypotheses can be confirmed by case information and that any inconsistencies between the history and test results can be adequately explained. Second, validity of the MACI profile is evaluated by examining the Modifying Indices to determine whether the adolescent engaged in a response style that may have affected on the consistency or accuracy of the test results. Third, each section of the MACI profile should be analyzed to arrive at a proper understanding of an adolescent's basic Personality Patterns, along with the specific Expressed Concerns and Clinical Syndromes that are evident. Finally, results from the different sections of the profile must be integrated. That is, various meanings may be attributed to particular scale elevations, depending on other elevations in the profile. For example, an elevation on Self-Devaluation (scale B) and Depressive Affect (scale FF)—denoting a clinical state of depression associated with feelings of inadequacy and self-doubt—will take on a different meaning if the adolescent's basic personality pattern is introversive–doleful (scales 1 and 2B), as opposed to submissive–oppositional (scales 3 and 8A). Elsewhere (McCann, 1999), I have outlined other complex interpretive strategies involving two-, three-, and four-point code types in various sections of the MACI profile that can be useful in addressing specific referral questions.

In addition to an analysis of individual scales and profile configurations, interpretation of the MACI can also include the analysis of an adolescent's responses to individual items on the test. Among the various diagnostic questions that may require individual analysis are suicide risk, childhood abuse, and substance abuse (McCann, 1999). Although individual item responses are less reliable from a psychometric perspective, interpreting these can be a useful supplement to the formal interpretation of scales on the profile. The MACI Interpretive Report provides a listing of responses to noteworthy items that makes individual item analysis part of the interpretive process.

The following four sections provide a brief descriptive overview of the four types of MACI scales. Although more comprehensive descriptions of the clinical significance of elevations on each scale can be found elsewhere (McCann, 1999; Millon, 2006), this overview will provide readers with the general interpretive significance of each MACI scale. Most of these scales are contained in the formal profile, but a couple consist of recently developed scales that have emerged in the literature. Following this overview, a brief review of more complex interpretive issues is provided, including suggestions for integrating the MACI profile and dealing with interpretive challenges (i.e., profiles that appear to be a "poor fit" with what is known about a particular adolescent, but that yield diagnostic information with potential clinical uses).

Modifying Indices and Response Styles

The scales in the Modifying Indices section of the MACI profile measure response styles and test-taking attitudes, including random or indiscriminate responding, social desirability, exaggeration or overreporting of problems, and denial or minimization.

Scale VV: Reliability

Although the Reliability index is not integrated as a formal scale on the MACI profile, it nevertheless figures prominently in the evaluation of profile validity. The Reliability scale consists of two items (114 and 126) that have very bizarre content and are rarely, if ever, endorsed by even adolescents with severe forms of psychopathology. According to the MACI manual, scores of 0 on this scale indicate that the test results are valid, whereas a score of 1 suggests that the results may be unreliable, and a score of 2 means that the test result are invalid and the profile should not be interpreted (Millon, 2006). When either of the items on this scale have been answered in the affirmative, various possibilities exist as to the adolescent's approach to taking the MACI. Among the various interpretive hypotheses are random responding, extreme oppositionality to taking the test, concentration difficulties, poor reading skills, and marked confusion that impaired the adolescent's ability to complete a self-report psychological test. Given that the endorsement frequency of the items on this scale is so low, I (McCann, 1999) have recommended a more conservative interpretation of this scale (in which a score of 0 is recommended to interpret the resulting profile, while a score of 1 or higher is considered sufficient to invalidate the test).

M-VRIN and M-TRIN

Owing to the fact that no independent research on the MACI Reliability scale has been conducted (aside from that reported in the test manual), and to the limited number of items on scale VV, Pinsoneault (2002) constructed a pair of scales to measure response inconsistency on the MACI. Using a combination of correlational and rational content analyses on pairs of MACI items, Pinsoneault developed Variable Response Inconsistency (M-VRIN) and True Response Inconsistency (M-TRIN) scales for the MACI to evaluate the extent to which adolescents might respond inconsistently on the instrument. The M-VRIN consists of 46 item pairs with similar content, and the M-TRIN consists of 18 item pairs where the keying to each pair is either "true–true" or "false–false." Pinsoneault reported good sensitivity and specificity statistics for the scales in identifying random MACI protocols, although the diagnostic efficiency of the scales varied as a function of the base rate of random profiles. However, Pinsoneault provided detailed tables to help clinicians and researchers establish appropriate diagnostic cutoffs based on the kinds of decisions required. Although M-VRIN and M-TRIN require further study and are not included in the formal MACI profile, they represent promising measures for assisting in the identification of inconsistent or random response tendencies on the MACI.

Scale X: Disclosure

Although listed as a formal scale on the MACI profile, the Disclosure scale actually does not consist of individual items; rather, it is derived from the sum of raw scores from the first 11 Personality Patterns scales (scales 1 through 8B). The Disclosure scale was originally designed to measure an adolescent's willingness to be open and forthcoming about personal concerns and attributes. Although the intent behind the scale's design was to derive a response style scale that would be value-neutral, in that scores were not intended to reflect either negative or positive impression management, scale X correlates highly in the positive direction with scale Z (Debasement; .78) and modestly in the negative direction with scale Y (Desirability; –.44) (Millon, 2006, p. 121). As such, scale X not only measures the degree of openness with which the adolescent approached the MACI, but also reflects response style. A low score (i.e., BR < 35) suggests that the adolescent was defensive and unwilling to reveal personal difficulties. There may be a number of reasons why an adolescent would approach taking the test in this way, including a general suspicion or guardedness around adults, concerns over how the test results will be used, and a need to appear healthy and well adjusted. A high score (i.e., BR > 74) suggests that the adolescent was open and forthright in taking the test, and when results are markedly elevated (i.e., BR > 84), the adolescent may be needing attention and support or may have other needs for secondary gain.

Scale Y: Desirability

The primary purpose of the Desirability scale is to evaluate for the presence of socially desirable responding. High scores generally reflect an adolescent's strong need to be seen as well adjusted by other individuals. In general, teenagers with a high score on Desirability do not readily see their own personal problems, and they tend to minimize or downplay concerns. The items on scale Y overlap with those on some of the Personality Patterns scales, including scales 4 (Dramatizing), 5 (Egotistic), and 7 (Conforming); therefore, it is not uncommon to see elevations on one or more of these scales when Desirability is elevated. Moreover, although elevations on scale Y are not sufficient to invalidate a MACI computer-generated report, I (McCann, 1999) have suggested that when the BR score on Desirability exceeds 90, the adolescent has endorsed most of the items on this scale; in this case, the possibility of a socially desirable response set that clouds much of the diagnostic information in the profile should be considered.

Scale Z: Debasement

The Debasement scale measures the degree to which an adolescent responded to the MACI items in a manner that emphasizes negative self-attributes or magnifies minor symptoms or concerns. High scores generally indicate that the adolescent is exaggerating or overreporting problems and personal attributes in a negative direction. There are many reasons for such a response style, including extreme psychological distress, severe depression, very poor self-image, malingering, a psychological "cry for help," need for attention, and secondary gain. As with Desirability elevations, Debasement elevations will not invalidate the computer-generated report. However, the overall validity of the MACI profile should be questioned when elevations on scale Z exceed 90, and the possibility of extreme levels of distress, malingering, or other forms of negative dissimulation should be investigated (McCann, 1999).

Modifying Indices Configurations

The general configuration of a valid MACI profile on the Modifying Indices is this: Scales X, Y, and Z all fall below a BR of 75, and the raw score value of Disclosure is above 200. On the other hand, the MACI may still be considered valid even if one or more of scales X, Y, or Z exceed a BR of 74. However, socially desirable response sets are identified by scale Y being above 74 and scales X and Z falling below this level. Negative self-report styles are identified by scale Z being above a BR of 74 and scale Y falling below this level. In negative self-report patterns, scale X will often (but not always) be elevated. In unusual cases, both scales Y and Z may be elevated over a BR of 74, reflecting an atypical pattern of both socially desirable and negative self-reports. Possible explanations for this unusual pattern are either inconsistent or indiscriminate self-reporting, or a state of agitated depression in an adolescent with a gregarious, self-centered, and egocentric personality style (McCann, 1999).

Personality Patterns Scales

Some distinguishing features of the MACI Personality Patterns scales differentiate them from similar scales on the adult versions of the Millon inventories. Although the MACI scales are designed to measure stable and enduring characteristics associated with personality disturbances, rather than transient and state-related symptoms, the scale names on the MACI reflect less pathological variants of the DSM-III-R and DSM-IV(-TR) personality disorders. The major reason for this descriptive innovation is that personality styles are still developing in adolescence and may change as teenagers enter into adulthood. Given the dynamic and somewhat changeable nature of personality over long periods of time, the modification in scale names is a means of giving recognition to this developmental phenomenon.

Scale 1: Introversive

The Introversive scale measures features that are associated with schizoid personality disorder as outlined in the DSM-IV(-TR). Elevations on this scale indicate a diminished capacity for experiencing either enjoyment or pain in life. The adolescent's range of emotional expression tends to be markedly restricted, and he or she will appear apathetic, remote, and detached from others. Interpersonal relationships tend to be very limited, as the teenager's preferences tend to be for solitary and isolated activities that do not involve contact or interaction with other people. In the face of challenges or demands by others, the introversive adolescent responds with indifference and does not readily express discomfort, concern, or anxiety. Individuals who score high on the scale tend to avoid looking at problems or environmental situations in a complex manner. Modest elevations on this scale are common in chronically depressed or dysphoric adolescents, though other scales in the profile should be examined to confirm whether depressive symptoms are evident. According to the Grossman Facet Scales, the three most prominent personality features measured by this scale are impassive behavioral expression, an apathetic temperament, and an unengaged interpersonal style.

Scale 2A: Inhibited

The Inhibited scale was designed to measure features associated with avoidant personality disorder in the DSM-IV(-TR). Elevations on this scale reflect extreme sensitivity to rejection and criticism. There is a broad tendency to view life as being filled with unpleasant and painful experiences that interfere with enjoyment in life. Often the adolescent will avoid doing things or initiating projects or social contacts out of fear that things will turn out badly. Interpersonal relationships are avoided because of extreme fears over being rejected or criticized. As such, adolescents with high scores on this scale are often seen by others as shy, ill at ease, and socially awkward. They tend to feel lonely, and lack the confidence and self-assurance that would permit them to excel in various aspects of their lives. When relationships are formed, an inhibited adolescent tends to cling anxiously to others and seek constant reassurance that others are accepting and tolerant. The three dominant features of elevations on the Inhibited scale, according to the Grossman Facet Scales, are fretful behavioral expression, aversive interpersonal style, and an alienated self-image.

Scale 2B: Doleful

The Doleful scale measures characteristics of depressive personality disorder as outlined in Appendix B of DSM-IV(-TR). High scores on this scale are associated with long-standing feelings of dysphoria and depression. Doleful adolescents have great difficulty experiencing joy or pleasure because of their lack of hope about the future. They expect that nothing can be done to change what they see as the sad state of their lives. Moreover, their pessimism carries over into other areas of life and manifests itself in low self-esteem, feelings of worthlessness, and inadequacy over their perceived inability to perform specific activities. In social situations, adolescents with high scores on this scale are seen as lonely and withdrawn, primarily because they do not have a strong interest in interacting with others. High scores on the scale also reflect a propensity to worry excessively and ruminate, often about guilt over past transgressions that are either real or exaggerated. On the Grossman Facet Scales, the three most common personality features measured by the Doleful scale are a woeful/gloomy temperament, disconsolate and somber behavioral expressiveness, and a pessimistic cognitive style.

Scale 3: Submissive

The personality characteristics measured by the Submissive scale are those associated with DSM-IV(-TR) dependent personality disorder. An elevated score on this scale reflects an adolescent who is passive and submissive in interpersonal relationships. Submissive teenagers avoid taking any active leadership role in peer groups, and they are concerned that others may not always be there for them. Adolescents with elevations on this scale tend to have lingering fears that others will leave or abandon them. Moreover, submissive adolescents tend to downplay and minimize their own achievements and abilities, and they prefer to connect with those who can take a more assertive and confident stance in social settings. There are strong needs for attention and affection, as well as strong needs for encouragement and support. Self-confidence is often lacking in many areas, requiring reassurance from others. In relationships, submissive teenagers tend to be overly sentimental and to direct much of their energy toward maintaining connections with others, even when relationships are problematic. The Grossman Facet Scales reveal that the most common personality features associated with this scale are docile interpersonal behavior, a pacific/noncompetitive temperament, and incompetent/helpless behavioral expression.

Scale 4: Dramatizing

The Dramatizing scale is intended to measure characteristics associated with histrionic personality disorder in DSM-IV(-TR). Adolescents who score high on this scale tend to be quite sociable and thrive on having numerous friendships and people in their lives. However, high scores reflect a prominent tendency to display emotions in a dramatic and very changeable manner, and dramatizing teenagers often make decisions that are poorly planned or impulsive. In social settings, these teenagers tend to be very talkative, sensation-seeking, and attention-grabbing. They often become bored very easily, and they require constant stimulation. Moreover, they do not tolerate longer-term relationships very well. Although others may find them interesting at first, dramatizing adolescents' excessive focus on superficial aspects of life situations and their concern for physical appearances often cause friends and acquaintances to become disillusioned and to lose interest. On the Grossman Facet Scales, the three most common personality features measured by the Dramatizing scale are attention-seeking interpersonal behavior, a gregarious self-image, and a flighty/impressionistic cognitive style.

Scale 5: Egotistic

The DSM-IV(-TR) narcissistic personality disorder represents the underlying construct that is measured by the Egotistic scale. High scores reflect an adolescent with a very high level of self-confidence that leads to others' seeing him or her as self-centered, arrogant, and conceited. In relationships, egotistic adolescents require constant admiration, respect, and reinforcement of their self-worth or competence. They expect others to recognize their talents and abilities, and will often become upset or angered if others fail to give them the recognition they believe they deserve. Others tend to see egotistic adolescents as having a strong sense of entitlement and as taking advantage of people to get what they want. Adolescents who score high on this scale are often unable to experience empathy or concern for others. They also tend to spend time fantasizing about having unlimited success or power, leading to periods where they appear aloof or distant. The three most prominent personality features measured by this scale, according to the Grossman Facet Scales, are an admirable/deserving self-image, an expansive cognitive style, and exploitive interpersonal conduct.

Scale 6A: Unruly

The Unruly scale is intended to measure characteristics associated with antisocial personality disorder in DSM-IV(-TR). As such, high scores are found among adolescents who exhibit a range of conduct problems arising from the rejection of social norms and other acceptable standards of behaving. These adolescents are seen as rebellious and reject efforts to have limits placed on their actions. Unruly teenagers are typically uncooperative, although they can engage in cooperative, group-oriented behavior if it involves others who share their antisocial attitudes. Teenagers who score high on this scale value their autonomy, yet they often solve problems in impulsive and irresponsible ways. When these personality propensities are more extreme, illegal activities are often seen, including stealing, truancy, fighting, and other forms of acting out. In social settings, unruly adolescents have little or no regard for the feelings of others, and they may seek revenge for perceived injustices or wrongs that others have committed toward them. They tend not to learn from their mistakes, and therefore a repetitive cycle of acting out and punishment is often observed. On the Grossman Facet Scales, the three most prominent personality features measured by the Unruly scale are impulsive expressive behavior, an acting-out defense mechanism, and irresponsible interpersonal conduct.

Scale 6B: Forceful

Sadistic personality disorder as outlined in the DSM-III-R represents the underlying construct measured by the Forceful scale. Adolescents who score high on this scale are characterized as very strong-willed and tough-minded. They tend to be in constant conflict with authority because of their intolerance for being controlled or having their self-determination limited or restricted. In social situations, forceful teenagers are blunt and hostile, and they are often cruel toward others because they have no empathy or sensitivity for the feelings and rights of others. In some cases, adolescents with high scores on this scale may actually derive pleasure and satisfaction from humiliating, verbally attacking, or in other ways violating the rights of others. When confronted with their behavior, forceful teenagers go on the offensive and become even more hostile and combative. Others tend to see them as controlling, intimidating, and authoritarian. The Grossman Facet Scales reveal that the three most common personality features measured by the Forceful scale are abrasive interpersonal behavior, precipitate/abrupt expressive conduct, and isolation of affect (i.e., they are seen as cold and detached) as a defense mechanism for managing emotions and stress.

Scale 7: Conforming

The Conforming scale is intended to measure obsessive–compulsive personality disorder as outlined in the DSM-IV(-TR). Characteristics of adolescents who score high on this scale are emotional constriction, extreme cognitive rigidity, preoccupation with rules, and a very serious-minded approach to life. In social settings, conforming adolescents keep a tight hold on their feelings and have difficulty accepting others who go against their fixed ideas and beliefs. They tend to be intolerant of those who enjoy being more spontaneous or unpredictable. Thus, while the conforming adolescent sees him- or herself as industrious and hard-working, others tend to see him or her as rigid, stuffy, and too serious. Given that some of the features associated with this scale are seen as desirable (e.g., following rules, working hard), it is not uncommon to see this scale elevated in some teenagers who are not necessarily compulsive in their personalities, but who are exhibiting a socially desirable response set on the MACI. According to the Grossman Facet Scales, the three most prominent personality features measured by the Conforming scale are a disciplined pattern of expressive behavior, respectful interpersonal conduct, and a conscientious self-image.

Scale 8A: Oppositional

Despite the fact that its name might suggest the measurement of features associated with oppositional defiant disorder, the Oppositional scale is actually intended to be a measure of negativistic (passive–aggressive) personality disorder as outlined in Appendix B of the DSM-IV(-TR). Elevations on this scale are associated with teenagers who are resentful over having demands made of them. They tend to be resistant and oppositional toward others when they are asked to do something, and their moods move readily into periods of extreme irritability and anger. In social situations, oppositional adolescents tend to generate considerable confusion in others, since their feelings can fluctuate between sullen withdrawal and irritable acting out. These teenagers are often quick to feel misunderstood and unappreciated by others. They typically spoil the pleasures and enjoyment of others by either engaging in resistant and passive–aggressive behavior, or making indirect hostile comments that are seen as biting. Their stubborn and resistant behavior often results in conflict with teachers, parents, and other authority figures, and oppositional teenagers are very difficult to engage in productive discussion in treatment. On the Oppositional scale, the three major personality features represented on the Grossman Facet Scales are a discontented self-image, resentful expressive conduct, and a contrary/obstructive interpersonal style.

Scale 8B: Self-Demeaning

The Self-Demeaning scale is intended to measure personality features associated with masochistic (self-defeating) personality disorder as outlined in Appendix B of DSM-

III-R. High scores on this scale reflect strong self-effacing and self-punitive beliefs and attitudes. Self-demeaning adolescents often undermine opportunities for personal growth and advancement, because they feel undeserving of success or rewards they experience. They have extremely poor self-esteem and put the needs of others ahead of their own. Those teenagers who score high on this scale deal with conflict by internalizing tension and stress. They blame themselves when problems arise, expect the worst to happen, and frequently complain that they are unable to do anything to change their lives. When offered support, self-demeaning adolescents thwart the efforts of others to help by claiming that they are unworthy. Elevations on this scale are common among chronically depressed teenagers, as well as among some who have been abused or victimized and who have long-standing, unresolved issues over the abuse. On the Grossman Facet Scales, the three prominent personality domains measured by the Self-Demeaning scale are a diffident/self-deprecating cognitive style, an undeserving self-image, and a dysphoric temperament.

Scale 9: Borderline Tendency

Characteristics of borderline personality disorder as outlined in the DSM-IV(-TR) are measured by the Borderline Tendency scale. Adolescents who score high on this scale experience a great deal of emotional turmoil and instability. Their moods change from periods of anxiety to depression, anger, joy, sadness, or restraint. Instability is also found in many areas of the teenagers' lives, including unstable relationships, changing feelings and attitudes toward others, devaluation and idealization of others, and uncertainty about career goals or personal values. Adolescents with borderline tendencies are characteristically lost with respect to personal interests, preferences, and long-term plans. They have a vague, diffuse, or changing sense of identity. Their behavior is often impulsive, self-destructive, and risky, which may be manifested in substance abuse, recurrent suicidal acting out, promiscuous sexual activity, or other forms of recklessness. In relationships, they tend to have intense needs for attention and support that, if left unsatisfied, result in dramatic and extreme attempts to keep others close and involved. The Grossman Facet Scales reveal that the three prominent personality features measured by the Borderline Tendency scale are a labile temperament, a capricious/vacillating cognitive style, and a self-image characterized by uncertainty and confusion.

Expressed Concerns Scales

A major focus of the eight Expressed Concerns scales is the measurement of problems and concerns that adolescents feel are most significant in their lives at the time they are being evaluated. As the name of this section of the MACI profile suggests, these scales are often most useful in beginning a course of treatment, because elevations typically reflect the particular problems or concerns an adolescent is willing to admit. Also, these scales often reflect the adolescent's perception of those issues that are most troublesome (McCann, 1999). That is, when the history or interview suggest a particular problem, but the corresponding Expressed Concerns scale is not elevated, interpretation of the MACI would suggest that the problem is one the adolescent is not willing to admit. On the other hand, a specific elevation or configuration of scales suggests that the problem areas are ones that the adolescent is willing to discuss, and the relative degree of elevation reflects the relative intensity or severity of those particular concerns.

Scale A: Identity Diffusion

Elevations on the Identity Diffusion scale suggest that adolescents have concerns about who they are and what they want out of life. They may have generalized worries about the direction their lives are heading, or specific concerns about a particular issue (e.g., career choice, values, sexual orientation, plans for future education, and life interests). Typically, these teenagers will appear vague and unclear when specific goals or interests are discussed. Individuals who score high on this scale generally have no clear or consistent framework for understanding and thinking about their needs and interests; thus they can often be described as lost, without direction, and unclear about what they want out of life.

Scale B: Self-Devaluation

High scores on the Self-Devaluation scale are associated with feelings of inadequacy, low self-esteem, and unhappiness with oneself. Adolescents with elevations on this scale often feel distress over their lack of accomplishment and are generally discontented with their ability to do things effectively. They fear taking on demands, because they expect to fall short in their attempts to meet goals that either they or others set for them. As a result, they feel weak and inadequate. Research has shown that this scale correlates very strongly in the negative direction with a collateral measure of self-esteem (Pinto & Grilo, 2003).

Scale C: Body Disapproval

Adolescents who obtain elevations on the Body Disapproval scale express marked concerns and high levels of unhappiness with the way in which they feel their physical maturation is occurring. Although adolescence is a time of significant physical changes that are brought about during puberty, this scale is intended to measure the extent to which adolescents are concerned with physical attractiveness and their social appeal. Elevations on the scale tend to reflect a profound tendency to focus on the worst features of one's physical appearance and to compare oneself negatively to peers. Teenagers who view themselves as being deviant physically, having an unusual appearance, or being physically inadequate will show elevations on this scale. In clinical settings, females tend to score higher on this scale, and it is a common elevation among individuals with an eating disorder (Barry & Grilo, 2002).

Scale D: Sexual Discomfort

The Sexual Discomfort scale is intended to measure excessive confusion or discomfort over sexual feelings and impulses that often arise during adolescence. Elevated scores suggest that teenagers are conflicted over various social roles that involve sexual behavior. Moreover, situations that provoke sexual feelings may increase anxiety and worries over sexuality. In addition, this scale sometimes reflects concerns over physical changes that occur with the development of secondary sex characteristics. Some anxieties and worries may be due to a generalized feeling that sexual thoughts and feelings are unwanted and should be avoided.

Scale E: Peer Insecurity

High scores on the Peer Insecurity scale are associated with feelings of unhappiness, discouragement, or anxiety that have been prompted by peer rejection. Sometimes adolescents who score high on this scale shun or avoid relationships because they fear ridicule or teasing; other high scorers may want close relationships, but have found little success in gaining peer acceptance. Overall, the scale is a measure of the extent to which a teenager feels isolated and socially detached, because of either internal feelings of inadequacy, external teasing and ridicule, or both.

Scale F: Social Insensitivity

The characteristics measured by the Social Insensitivity scale include cool indifference to the feelings of others and a lack of empathy. Teenagers who score high on this scale tend to have little regard for the welfare of others and take advantage of other people for personal benefit. I (McCann, 1999) have suggested that this scale can be a useful prognostic indicator in treatment settings, because it reveals the extent to which an adolescent has insight into his or her behavior. When the clinical history reveals that the adolescent has harmed or taken advantage of others, an elevation on this scale reveals that the adolescent has some insight into his or her behavior. On the other hand, if the history reveals insensitivity toward others and the adolescent does not score high on this scale, the interpretation would be a lack of insight that may make treatment and rehabilitation programming more challenging.

Scale G: Family Discord

Elevations on the Family Discord scale reflect conflicted and strained relationships between adolescents and their families. Aside from the specific nature of the family conflict, adolescents who score high on this scale tend to feel that their home lives are tense and full of conflict, and that they are unsupported and cut off from their parents. An examination of other scales in the profile can provide some indication of an adolescent's role or position in the conflict. For example, some adolescents feel overly sensitive to rejection and criticism; others contribute to the conflict through oppositional or rebellious behavior; still others contribute actively to family conflict through emotional volatility and instability.

Scale H: Childhood Abuse

The Childhood Abuse scale is associated with feelings of shame, guilt, or disgust over physical, sexual, or emotional abuse. The items are fairly general and not associated with any particular form of abuse. However, an elevation tends to indicate that a teenager is ruminating about having been abused. Once again, the scale is reflective of the adolescent's perception of his or her experiences and cannot be used to confirm the specifics of a situations involving suspected abuse. Nevertheless, the scale tends to be flexible in representing long-standing perceptions of abuse that occurred in the past, as well as acute exacerbations or recent abuse.

Clinical Syndromes Scales

In most cases, a specific clinical disorder or group of symptoms will be the identifying problem that brings an adolescent to the attention of mental health professionals. The Clinical Syndromes scales measure seven clusters of syndromes that are likely to manifest themselves in the form of a diagnosable condition that will be the focus of treatment. Furthermore, these syndromes often represent extensions of the adolescent's underlying personality style and are best understood within the context of the Personality Patterns scales. Finally, these clinical syndromes are often precipitated by situational stressors or individual concerns and should also be interpreted within the context of the Expressed Concerns scales.

Scale AA: Eating Dysfunctions

Elevations on the Eating Dysfunctions scale reflect difficulties associated with eating problems, such as bulimia, anorexia, and overeating. In addition, high scores may also reflect marked concerns over body image, and thus elevations on scale C (Body Disapproval) may also be present. The adolescent has intense fears about gaining weight or being fat. Some behavioral problems that may be manifested include laxative abuse, binge eating, self-induced vomiting after eating, and compulsive exercising. A factor analysis of MACI items related to eating disorders revealed three dimensions of eating disorder pathology: restrictive behaviors (e.g., starving self, vomiting), body image disturbance, and binge eating (Barry & Grilo, 2002).

Scale BB: Substance Abuse Proneness

The primary clinical concerns reflected in elevations on the Substance Abuse Proneness scale involve excessive use of alcohol and illicit drugs. Common difficulties that are likely to be identified on interview or in the clinical history include excessive time spent trying to obtain drugs and/or alcohol; minimal insight into the adverse effects that substance abuse is having on functioning; and problems in academic, familial, or social settings as a result of substance abuse. In some cases where an adolescent has no history of substance abuse, an elevation on this scale may occur if the teenager has been raised in a family situation where substance abuse is common. Elevations in these cases often reflect attitudes or beliefs (e.g., sensation seeking, risk taking) that are associated with an increased risk of substance abuse. Conversely, some adolescents with a documented history of substance abuse who are in denial or have minimal insight may produce no elevation on this scale.

Scale CC: Delinquent Predisposition

High scores on the Delinquent Predisposition scale represent cognitive attitudes and beliefs that reflect a general disregard for societal norms, rules, and the rights of others. Among the features associated with elevations are a lack of empathy for others. The scale is also associated with features of conduct disorder or delinquent behaviors, which may include hostility, threatening behavior, stealing, frequent fighting, and deception to avoid legal or disciplinary troubles.

Scale DD: Impulsive Propensity

As the scale name implies, high Impulsive Propensity scores are associated with a propensity to act out in an erratic and unstable manner in response to frustration. High scores often indicate a tendency to respond quickly and without considering the adverse consequences of behaviors, usually after a brief or fleeting emotional provocation. The scale is not associated with a specific form of impulsive behavior; it may reflect sexual activity, risk-taking behaviors, angry outbursts, fighting, or similar types of acting out. One study demonstrated that high levels of impulsiveness as measured by scale DD are associated with more frequent marijuana use, less positive sexual attitudes, higher levels of unprotected sexual activity, and a higher perceived risk for susceptibility to HIV infection (Dévieux et al., 2002).

Scale EE: Anxious Feelings

The major features assessed by the Anxious Feelings scale include general feelings of tension, nervousness, and apprehension about the future. Adolescents who score high on this scale often describe feeling anxious about the future and often report a sense of foreboding that something bad is about to happen, although they may sometimes be unable to specify what their concerns are. Some adolescents who score high on this scale feel tense, or are agitated, because they feel that they have had limitations placed on their behavior by parents or the situation in which they find themselves (e.g., hospitalization, incarceration) and do not feel they are free to live their lives as they wish. Other common features of high scores include social anxiety, specific fears or phobias, or physiological signs of tension or worry.

Scale FF: Depressive Affect

The major features associated with elevations on the Depressive Affect scale include depressed mood, a lack of energy, feelings of guilt, and social withdrawal. Features associated with clinical depression are also reflected in high scores, including a loss of confidence or low self-efficacy, feelings of inadequacy, lack of interest in pleasurable activities, and lethargy or a lack of vitality. In addition, other features may include restlessness, rumination, and passive suicidal ideation. Hiatt and Cornell (1999) found moderate support for this scale as a measure of clinical depression, particularly in conjunction with scale 2B (Doleful). Scale FF was strongly correlated with another self-report measure of depression, but Hiatt and Cornell caution that the MACI scales are limited by self-report methodology and should be interpreted in the context of information obtained from the history and clinical interview.

Scale GG: Suicidal Tendency

The Suicidal Tendency scale measures the extent to which an adolescent reports suicidal ideation and planning. Many of the items reflect passive suicidal ideation, such as the belief that others would be better off if the adolescent was dead, generalized feelings of hopelessness, and a lack of purpose in life. Independent research on the scale is limited, but suggests modest correlation with the implementation of suicide precautions in an inpatient setting without specific regard to actual suicidal behavior (Hiatt & Cornell, 1999). I (McCann, 1999) have recommended that elevations on this scale be followed up with an analysis of individual items on the scale to identify specific areas that can be expanded upon in subsequent interviews with the adolescent. When active planning is evident and more direct intervention is required, then consideration should be given to involving family members and collateral supports, or notifying hospital or institutional staff members about relative suicide risk.

Integrating the Profile

Interpretation of the MACI involves not only analysis of single-scale elevations, but also integration of various sections of the profile. A general principle that guides this integrative process is that individual scales (particularly those in the Expressed Concerns and Clinical Syndromes sections) can take on different significance and meaning, depending on the particular personality style of the adolescent. For instance, an elevation on scale FF (Depressive Affect) generally denotes sadness, dysphoria, and pessimism. When this scale is elevated in an adolescent with an unruly and oppositional personality (i.e., scales 6A and 8B), the scale FF elevation will usually occur in situations where the adolescent has been incarcerated, has been punished, or has had severe restrictions placed on his or her freedom. In an inhibited and submissive adolescent (i.e., scales 2A and 3), the scale FF elevation usually occurs in response to severe interpersonal rejection, teasing, or social ostracism.

Another principle that guides integration of the MACI profile is the notion that item overlap can have a major influence on scale elevations, particularly on clusters of scales that share items. Elsewhere (McCann, 1999) I have provided a detailed analysis to assist with identifying these various clusters of scales. For example, scales A (Identity Diffusion) and 9 (Borderline Tendency) share items, as do scales 2B (Doleful), 8B (Self-Demeaning), and FF (Depressive Affect). Common items are found on other scale clusters, such as scales 6A (Unruly), F (Social Insensitivity), and CC (Delinquent Predisposition). Therefore, various Personality Patterns, Expressed Concerns, and Clinical Syndromes scales will show concurrent elevations (although not in every single case), due to common themes that span not only personality style, but also existential concerns and clinical presentation.

Although there are no simple rules or guidelines to follow for integrating the MACI profile, it is best to avoid limiting interpretation of the test to a narrow focus on individual scales. While single-scale elevations are an important part of the interpretive process, clinicians must be also capable of appreciating both the "forest" and the "trees" among MACI elevations. The best tools a clinician has for approaching integrative profile interpretation are sound clinical experience; an understanding of the underlying theory and diagnostic criteria upon which the MACI is based; a clear understanding of the psychometric properties of the test; and a good understanding of the adolescent being evaluated and the context in which the MACI assessment is being undertaken.

Interpretation Challenges: The "Poor-Fit" Profile

In a majority of cases, clinicians will find that the MACI provides an accurate and useful assessment of adolescents' personality and psychological functioning. However, given that the test is a self-report instrument, it is prone to some of the problems that all such instruments have. The impact of response sets, an adolescent's lack of insight or defensiveness, biased self-reports, and other such factors undoubtedly have an adverse influence on psychological test results. Although adjustments are made in the MACI profile to control for such influences, in some cases a clinician will find an MACI profile that is deemed to be reliable and valid based on an analysis of the Modifying Indices, but that does not seem to fit what is known about the teenager's history and clinical presentation.

In these cases, it is tempting to discard the MACI results as inaccurate and useless. However, with careful consideration of the results within the context of the assessment setting, much useful information can often be obtained from these seemingly inaccurate profiles and reports. A good place to begin an analysis of these profiles is by characterizing the nature of the error that is believed to have occurred. Perhaps a scale is not elevated when the history suggests a problem in the particular area. For example, scales D (Sexual Discomfort) and H (Childhood Abuse) may not be elevated when the history reveals that a teenager was sexually abused. Whenever any of the Expressed Concerns scales, for example, are expected to be elevated and they are not, this generally reflects an adolescent's unwillingness or inability to recognize the particular area of difficulty as a concern. Such information can be useful in planning treatment. This same guideline can be utilized for other unexpected results on individual MACI scales.

Another step in analyzing inaccurate profiles is to recognize that personality styles identified on the MACI that do not seem to describe an adolescent may in fact reflect how the adolescent wants to be seen by others. For example, in adolescents with severe conduct disorder who are in correctional settings, or who are undergoing evaluations for legal proceedings, it is common to find elevations on scales 3 (Submissive) and 7 (Conforming). Such adolescents want to be perceived as cooperative and compliant with those who are in a position to evaluate their performance, and who can influence how they are treated within the legal system.

In other instances, some adolescents may report themselves as manifesting certain personality characteristics, clinical symptoms, or other concerns in response to long-term difficulties. Thus adolescents with a chronic mental illness, or those who are severely disabled and have resided for much for their lives in institutional settings, may report excessive submissive or self-demeaning traits because of the perception these teenagers have about themselves as being excessively reliant on others or the system. They may tend to see themselves as inadequate and unable to function independently, which might be an accurate self-evaluation in certain cases.

A basic guideline to follow is to analyze the problematic MACI profile rationally when such profiles occur. It is helpful to ask this question: "Why did *this* adolescent produce *this* profile under *these* circumstances?" Although the MACI will not be accurate 100% of the time, some useful information can generally be gleaned from those profiles that appear to be either slightly or completely inaccurate.

Recent Trends in MACI Research

Although independent research on the MACI was relatively sparse over a period of 5–10 years following the instrument's initial publication in 1993, several studies in recent years show a number of interesting trends. These studies fall into one of three types. In one group of studies, researchers have attempted either to validate specific scales or to use the MACI as a criterion against which to validate another measure of adolescent functioning. Hiatt and Cornell (1999), for example, found that the Doleful and Depressive Affect scales were moderately useful in assessing depression among psychiatrically hospitalized adolescents, while the Suicidal Tendency scale was weakly associated with an external criterion of placement on suicide precautions. Pinto and Grilo (2003) found that the MACI showed good validity for many clinical syndromes, when compared against the criterion of self-report measures of psychopathology and a multidisciplinary team's DSM-IV diagnoses of adolescents. These researchers concluded that the MACI is psychometrically sound and useful as a screen for psychopathology among adolescent psychiatric inpatients. Some researchers have also used the MACI as an external criterion against which to evaluate the validity of other self-report measures, with favorable results (Grisso, Barnum, Fletcher, Cauffman, & Peuschold, 2001).

In another general group of MACI studies, researchers have examined the utility of the instrument among specific clinical groups. For instance, the MACI has been shown to be useful in establishing levels of impulsivity among substance-abusing adolescents with high- and low-risk behaviors for contracting HIV (Dévieux et al., 2002). The MACI has also been used to identify personality-based subtypes or clusters of specific adolescent populations, including sexual abusers (Richardson, Kelly, Graham, & Bhate, 2004) and teenagers in residential treatment (Romm, Bockian, & Harvey, 1999). These studies have demonstrated how the MACI can be used to individualize the assessment of adolescents in programs for the purpose of treatment planning, as has another study on using the MACI to evaluate treatment planning in adolescents with eating disorders (Barry & Grilo, 2002).

The third, and by far most extensive, line of MACI research in recent years has been the use of the instrument to evaluate juvenile offenders and adolescents with psychopathic personality traits. Using the work of Hare (1991, 1996) as a basis, Murrie and Cornell (2000) developed a 20-item MACI scale for the assessment of psychopathy; their findings showed that Substance Abuse Proneness (scale BB) correlated strongly with the Psychopathy Checklist—Revised (Hare, 1991). However, other research has shown that self-report screening measures like the MACI are correlated with external criteria—such as a history of prior violence (Murrie, Cornell, Kaplan, McConville, & Levy-Elkon, 2004)—but that the Psychopathy Checklist: Youth Version has greater utility (Murrie & Cornell, 2002; Stafford & Cornell, 2003) in identifying psychopathic traits. On the other hand, Salekin, Ziegler, Larrea, Anthony, and Bennet (2003) found that the specialized MACI psychopathy scale developed by Murrie and Cornell (2000), as well as a revised scale developed by Salekin and his colleagues, showed adequate validity for predicting general and violent reoffending among adolescent offenders within a 2-year period following discharge from a juvenile court evaluation unit. Also, several studies have shown the MACI to be useful in identifying subtypes of juvenile offenders for the purposes of treatment planning, institutional placement, and disposition planning (Loper, Hoffschmidt, & Ash, 2001; Stefurak, Calhoun, & Glaser, 2004; Taylor, Kemper, Loney, & Kistner, 2006). Overall, these studies support use of the MACI in violence risk assessment, treatment planning for juvenile offenders, and the identification of juvenile offender subtypes.

Conclusion

The purpose of this chapter has been to provide an overview of the composition and clinical uses of the MACI. Strategies for interpretation have also been discussed, as well as approaches to integrating various components and sections of the profile, and confronting unusual test results where the findings may not necessarily fit with other information that is known about the adolescent from the clinical history and presentation. Familiarity with the MACI's composition and psychometric properties, experience in using the instrument in various settings, and a sound understanding of the personality theory underlying the instrument are all hopeful in making maximum use of MACI results in the clinical evaluation of adolescents. Finally, emerging research trends are discussed briefly, in order to provide researchers and clinicians with an overview of how the MACI is being used in various settings.

References

American Psychiatric Association. (1987). *Diagnostic and statistical manual of mental disorders* (3rd ed., revised). Washington, DC: Author.

American Psychiatric Association. (1994). *Diagnostic and statistical manual of mental disorders* (4th ed.). Washington, DC: Author.

American Psychiatric Association. (2000). *Diagnostic and statistical manual of mental disorders* (4th ed., text rev.). Washington, DC: Author.

Archer, R. P., & Ball, J. D. (1988). Issues in the assessment of adolescent psychopathology. In R. L. Greene (Ed.), *The MMPI: Use with specific populations* (pp. 259–277). Philadelphia: Grune & Stratton.

Barry, D. T., & Grilo, C. M. (2002). Eating and body image disturbances in adolescent psychiatric inpatients: Gender and ethnicity patterns. *International Journal of Eating Disorders, 32,* 335–343.

Coleman, J. C. (1992).The nature of adolescence. In J. C. Coleman & C. Warren-Adamson (Eds.), *Youth policy in the 1990s: The way forward* (pp. 8–27). London: Routledge.

Davis, R. D. (1993). *The development of content scales for the Millon Adolescent Clinical Inventory.* Unpublished master's thesis, University of Miami.

Dévieux, J., Malow, R., Stein, J. A., Jennings, T. E., Lucenko, B. A., Averhart, C., et al. (2002). Impulsivity and HIV risk among adjudicated alcohol- and drug-abusing adolescent offenders. *AIDS Education and Prevention, 14*(Suppl. B), 24–35.

Dyer, F. J. (1985). Millon Adolescent Personality Inventory. In D. J. Keyser & R. C. Sweetland (Eds.), *Test critiques* (Vol. 4, pp. 425–433). Kansas City, MO: Test Corporation of America.

Grisso, T., Barnum, R., Fletcher, K. E., Cauffman, E., & Peuschold, D. (2001). Massachusetts Youth Screening Instrument for mental health needs of juvenile justice youths. *Journal of the American Academy of Child and Adolescent Psychiatry, 40,* 541–548.

Hare, R. D. (1991). *The Hare Psychopathy Checklist—Revised.* North Tonawanda, NY: Multi-Health Systems.

Hare, R. D. (1996). Psychopathy: A clinical construct whose time has come. *Criminal Justice and Behavior, 23,* 25–54.

Hiatt, M. D., & Cornell, D. G. (1999). Concurrent validity of the Millon Adolescent Clinical Inventory as a measure of depression in hospitalized adolescents. *Journal of Personality Assessment, 73,* 64–79.

Loper, A. B., Hoffschmidt, S. J., & Ash, E. (2001). Personality features and characteristics of violent events committed by juvenile offenders. *Behavioral Sciences and the Law, 19,* 81–96.

McCann, J. T. (1999). *Assessing adolescents with the MACI: Using the Millon Adolescent Clinical Inventory.* New York: Wiley.

Millon, T. (1969). *Modern psychopathology: A biosocial approach to maladaptive learning and functioning.* Philadelphia: Saunders.

Millon, T. (1981). *Disorders of personality: DSM-III, Axis II.* New York: Wiley.

Millon, T. (1990). *Toward a new personology: An evolutionary model.* New York: Wiley.

Millon, T., & Davis, R. D. (1996). *Disorders of personality: DSM-IV and beyond.* New York: Wiley.

Millon, T., & Davis, R. D. (1998). Millon Adolescent Clinical Inventory (MACI). In G. P. Koocher, J. D. Norcross, & S. S. Hill (Eds.), *Psychologists' desk reference* (pp. 162–168). New York: Oxford University Press.

Millon, T. (with Millon, C., & Davis, R. D.). (1993). *Millon Adolescent Clinical Inventory manual.* Minneapolis, MN: National Computer Systems.

Millon, T. (with Millon, C., Davis, R. D., & Grossman, S. D.). (2006). *Millon Adolescent Clinical Inventory (MACI) manual* (2nd ed.). Minneapolis, MN: Pearson Assessments.

Murrie, D. C., & Cornell, D. G. (2000). The Millon Adolescent Clinical Inventory and psychopathy. *Journal of Personality Assessment, 75,* 110–125.

Murrie, D. C., & Cornell, D. G. (2002). Psychopathy screening of incarcerated juveniles: A comparison of measures. *Psychological Assessment, 14,* 390–396.

Murrie, D. C., Cornell, D. G., Kaplan, S., McConville, D., & Levy-Elkon, A. (2004). Psychopathy scores and violence among juvenile offenders: A multi-measure study. *Behavioral Sciences and the Law, 22,* 49–67.

Petersen, A. C. (1988). Adolescent development. *Annual Review of Psychology, 39,* 583–607.

Pinsoneault, T. B. (2002). A Variable Response Inconsistency scale and a True Response Inconsistency scale for the Millon Adolescent Clinical Inventory. *Psychological Assessment, 14,* 320–330.

Pinto, M., & Grilo, C. M. (2003). Reliability, diagnostic efficiency, and validity of the Millon Adolescent Clinical Inventory: Examination of selected scales in psychiatrically hospitalized adolescents. *Behaviour Research and Therapy, 42,* 1505–1519.

Richardson, G., Kelly, T. P., Graham, F., & Bhate, S. R. (2004). A personality-based taxonomy of sexually abusive adolescents derived from the Millon Adolescent Clinical Inventory (MACI). *British Journal of Clinical Psychology, 43,* 285–298.

Romm, S., Bockian, N., & Harvey, M. (1999). Factor-based prototypes of the Millon Adolescent Clinical Inventory in adolescents referred for residential treatment. *Journal of Personality Assessment, 72,* 125–143.

Salekin, R. T., Ziegler, T. A., Larrea, M. A., Anthony, V. L., & Bennet, A. D. (2003). Predicting dangerousness with two Millon Adolescent Clinical Inventory psychopathy scales: The importance of egocentric and callous traits. *Journal of Personality Assessment, 80,* 154–163.

Stafford, E., & Cornell, D. G. (2003). Psychopathy scores predict adolescent inpatient aggression. *Assessment, 10,* 102–112.

Stefurak, T., Calhoun, G. B., & Glaser, B. A. (2004). Personality typologies of male juvenile offenders using a cluster analysis of the Millon Adolescent Clinical Inventory. *International Journal of Offender Therapy and Comparative Criminology, 48,* 96–110.

Taylor, J. Kemper, T. S., Loney, B. R., & Kistner, J. A. (2006). Classification of severe male juvenile offenders using the MACI clinical and personality scales. *Journal of Clinical Child and Adolescent Psychology, 35,* 90–102.

CHAPTER 21

A Brief Illustrative MACI Case Study

Caryl Bloom

The Millon Adolescent Clinical Inventory (MACI) was designed to be used by mental health professionals as an aid to identifying, predicting, and understanding a wide range of psychological problems that are characteristic of adolescents. In assessing possible strengths as well as weaknesses, the MACI can help the clinician maximize the potential for treatment by building on the full scope of personality attributes rather than focusing on problem areas alone. The following case example illustrates the interplay of biographical facts and MACI scores, and thus should indicate the potential utility of the profile analysis.

Fran is a 16-year-old high school sophomore. Her parents divorced 3 years ago under less than amicable circumstances. This was very disturbing to Fran, who was especially close to her father, an attorney. According to the legal decree, she has an opportunity to spend every other weekend and every Thursday night with her dad. For Fran, this is not sufficient, because she states that she gets along rather poorly with her mother. Fran relies on her dad not only for financial but also for emotional support. Her mother, an executive secretary, is presently dating her boss. This ongoing relationship angers Fran, who blames her mother for initiating the divorce. Fran's two older brothers, who attend out-of-town colleges, appear to have adjusted rather well to the family breakup.

Now that she is 16, Fran contends that she should not have to abide by all of her mother's rules, several of which she judges to be "quite infantile." She defies the curfew set by her mother and refuses to carry out numerous chores assigned to her. There have been tumultuous arguments with her mother about staying out late, not coming home, being sexually active, and failing classes. Her defiance has caused a great deal of anguish for her mother—a consequence that pleases Fran. She had her car taken away after receiving two speeding tickets and being arrested for driving under the influence; her dad was able to void any legal consequences.

Fran feels a measure of fault for her parents' divorce. Her parents' attentions have always been focused on her brothers, and it was when he left for college that the problems between her parents became evident. Fran feels that she has disappointed them both as a daughter and as a student. She believes that this led to her mother's decision to ask for a divorce. By contrast, when she experiences disapproval from her dad, she immediately turns to her studies and spends time with her old friends. Her erratic back-and-forth behaviors have led her parents to think of sending her to finish high school in a distant state. Fran, angry and confused, resists this idea for numerous reasons.

Fran recently began dating a boy who is 3 years her senior and a high school dropout. She likes the excitement of his lifestyle, which includes his selling drugs. Her lifelong earlier friends have largely abandoned her, since she now spends almost all of her time with her new boyfriend and his group. Fran has used drugs such as "crystal meth" and marijuana on occasion, as well as alcohol, especially when she is with her boyfriend and his group. When she does indulge in these behaviors, she says that she suffers problems with sleeping and eating. She is now heavily dependent on her new group of friends, and feels that she wants to become pregnant to keep her intimate relationship permanent. She also says that the baby will give her someone who will always love her.

Fran's parents have decided to have her evaluated by a psychologist before making any further decisions regarding Fran's schooling. The psychologist has requested that Fran take the MACI. Figure 21.1 presents Fran's MACI Profile and Interpretive Report.

PERSONALITY CODE: 8A ** 6B6A*48B2B5//G**F*B//DD**CCBBFF*-//

VALID REPORT   DATE: 03/02/2005

CATEGORY		SCORE		PROFILE OF SR SCORES					DIAGNOSTIC SCALES
		RAW	BR	0	60	75	85	115	
MODIFYING INDICES	X	465	83						DISCLOSURE
	Y	16	95						DESIRABILITY
	Z	8	64						DEBASEMENT
PERSONALITY PATTERNS	1	24	37						INTROVERSIVE
	2A	21	38						INHIBITED
	2B	24	66						DOLEFUL
	3	45	48						SUBMISSIVE
	4	52	73						DRAMATIZING
	5	44	64						EGOTISTIC
	6A	48	76						UNRULY
	6B	27	80						FORCEFUL
	7	37	35						CONFORMING
	8A	45	85						OPPOSITIONAL
	8B	38	68						SELF-DEMEANING
	9	17	47						BORDERLINE TENDENCY
EXPRESSED CONCERNS	A	15	45						IDENTITY DIFFUSION
	B	37	73						SELF-DEVALUATION
	C	15	48						BODY DISAPPROVAL
	D	20	38						SEXUAL DISCOMFORT
	E	4	25						PEER INSECURITY
	F	37	82						SOCIAL INSECURITY
	G	23	90						FAMILY DISCORD
	H	10	37						CHILDHOOD ABUSE
CLINICAL SYNDROMES	AA	26	58						EATING DYSFUNCTIONS
	BB	39	82						SUBSTANCE-ABUSE PRONENESS
	CC	35	83						DELINQUENT PREDISPOSITION
	DD	29	85						IMPULSIVE PROPENSITY
	EE	28	59						ANXIOUS FEELINGS
	FF	19	80						DEPRESSIVE AFFECT
	GG	11	35						SUICIDAL TENDENCY

CONFIDENTIAL INFORMATION FOR PROFESSIONAL USE ONLY

FIGURE 21.1. MACI Profile and Interpretive Report for Fran *(page 1 of 6)*.

The MACI report narratives have been normed on adolescent patients seen in professional treatment settings for either genuine emotional discomforts or social difficulties, and are applicable primarily during the early phases of assessment or psychotherapy. Distortions such as exaggerated severity may occur among respondents who have inappropriately taken the MACI for essentially educational or self-exploratory purposes. Inferential and probabilistic, this report must be viewed as only one aspect of a thorough diagnostic study. Moreover, these inferences should be reevaluated periodically in light of the pattern of attitude change and emotional growth that typifies the adolescent period. For these reasons, it should not be shown to patients or their relatives.

INTERPRETIVE CONSIDERATIONS

In addition to the preceding considerations, the interpretive narrative should be evaluated in light of the following demographic and situational factors. This 16-year-old female is currently in the 10th grade. In the demographic portion of the test, she did not identify any specific problems that are troubling her. Unless this adolescent is a demonstrably well-functioning individual who is currently facing minor life stressors, her responses suggest (1) a need for social approval and commendation, evident in tendencies to present herself in a favorable light; or (2) a marked naivete about psychological matters, including a deficit in self-insight. This interpretive report should be read with these characteristics in mind.

The BR scores reported for this adolescent have been modified to account for the high raw X (Disclosure) scale score, which reflects high self-revealing inclinations and the self-enhancing response tendencies shown by the extreme elevation of scale Y (Desirability) over scale Z (Debasement).

PERSONALITY PATTERNS

This section of the interpretive report pertains to those relatively enduring and pervasive characterological traits that underlie the personal and interpersonal difficulties of this adolescent. Rather than focus on specific complaints and problem areas to be discussed in later paragraphs, this section concentrates on the more habitual, maladaptive methods of relating, behaving, thinking, and feeling.

Most prominent in the MACI profile of this troubled adolescent is the conflict between dependency and self-assertion. She exhibits deep and variable moods, prolonged periods of dejection, and self-deprecation that are intermingled with impulsive and angry outbursts. She anxiously seeks reassurance from her family and peers, and is especially vulnerable to separation fears concerning those who have occasionally provided support. These fears push her to be overly compliant one time, profoundly gloomy the next, and irrationally argumentative and negativistic another. Although she strives to be submissive and self-sacrificing, her behavior has become increasingly unpredictable, irritable, and pessimistic. Repeatedly struggling to express attitudes contrary to her inner feelings, she often exhibits conflicting emotions simultaneously toward others and herself, most notably those of love, rage, and guilt. Also notable are her confusion over her self-image, her highly variable energy levels, her easy fatigability, and her irregular sleep-wake cycle.

Sensitive to external pressure and demands, she vacillates between being sullen, passively aggressive, and contrite. There are irrational and bitter complaints about being victimized, feeling that she deserves to be blamed, being treated unfairly by her peers, a series of behaviors that keep others constantly on edge, never knowing if she will react in a cooperative or sulky manner. Although still making efforts to be obliging, she has learned to anticipate disillusionment and often creates the expected disappointment by provocative questioning and by doubting the interest and support that is shown by others. Self-damaging acts and suicidal gestures may also be employed to gain attention. These irritable testing maneuvers may very well exasperate and alienate those upon

FIGURE 21.1. *(page 2 of 6)*

whom she depends. When threatened by separation and disapproval, she may express guilt, remorse, and self-condemnation in the hope of regaining support, reassurance, and sympathy.

Although she has begun to recognize that others may have grown weary of her erratic behavior, she cannot stop herself from alternating between voicing gloomy self-deprecation and being petulant and bitter. Her struggle between dependent acquiescence and obstructive independence constantly intrudes into most relationships. The inability to regulate her emotional controls, the feeling of being misunderstood, and her erratic moodiness all contribute to innumerable wrangles and conflicts with family and peers, as well as to her persistent tensions, resentment, and depression.

EXPRESSED CONCERNS

The scales in this section pertain to the personal perceptions of this adolescent concerning several issues of psychological development, actualization, and concern. Because experiences at this age are notably subjective, it is important to record how this teenager sees events and reports feelings, not just how others may objectively report them to be. For comparative purposes, her attitudes regarding a wide range of personal, social, and familial matters are contrasted with those expressed by a broad cross-section of teenagers of the same sex and age with psychological problems.

This young woman is not concerned about the welfare of those in need. In fact, she finds their frailties intolerable. She finds it far easier to be rejecting than helpful, and she is willing to override the rights of others in the service of her personal ends.

Serious family problems complicate her other difficulties. Tension and a lack of support appear to be typical. Depending on the personality style described earlier in this report, these problems reflect either persistent parental rejection or, conversely, a sharp break on her part as she asserts her independence from traditional family values.

CLINICAL SYNDROMES

The features and dynamics of the following distinctive clinical syndromes are worthy of description and analysis. They may arise in response to external precipitants, but are likely to reflect and accentuate enduring and pervasive aspects of this young woman's basic personality makeup.

At times, this young woman has periods of unconstrained energy, hyperdistractibility, and flights of ideas in which intense and contrary thoughts and energies are discharged recklessly. She exhibits restlessness and impulsivity in an erratic sequence characterized by both exploitive and hostile facets. One moment she may present a saucy and seductive manner; minutes later, incited by either an inner stimulus or an outer provocation, she may become thoughtlessly enraged and heedlessly belligerent. These quickly discharged impulses intensify her difficulties in an ever-increasing spiral of vicious circles within family and other social settings.

Rebellious acts or social noncompliance or both are indicated in the protocol of this young woman, who is highly erratic, irritable, and negativistic in mood. Her delinquent tendencies are a statement of resentful independence from the constraints of conventional life and a means of disjoining her conflicts and liberating her uncharitable impulses toward others. Likely to be brought to the attention of authorities, her acts of assertive defiance have undertones of self-destruction, and her angry noncompliance is displayed with a careless indifference to its consequences.

Her MACI results suggest that this adolescent may be subject to periods of drug use and alcoholism, probably provoked by frustration and resentment. Generally disposed to vent her brittle

FIGURE 21.1. *(page 3 of 6)*

emotions, she is apt to create stormy scenes with destructive consequences when she is drinking or using drugs heavily. Although her discontent and dissatisfaction may be entwined with moments of guilt and contrition, her anger and reproach rarely subside. They are aired frequently in accusatory statements, irrational jealousy, and recriminations that intimidate members of her family. Added to these denunciations is a self-destructive element that compels her to undermine her good fortune, as well as those she sees as having frustrated and disillusioned her.

Although not disposed to a major depression, this irritable and conflicted young woman appears to be suffering an extended dysthymic disorder that is marked by agitated and erratic qualities. She is likely to exhibit sequential periods of self-deprecation and despair, anxiety and futility, bitter discontent and demanding irritability. Upset by external constraints on her manipulative style and thrown off balance by an upsurge of moods and conflicts that she can neither understand nor control, she periodically turns against herself, voicing anger and self-loathing. Such actions may induce guilt in others, providing her with a measure of retribution for resentments she cannot voice without further jeopardizing her precarious state.

NOTEWORTHY RESPONSES

The client answered the following statements in the direction noted in parentheses. These items suggest specific problem areas that the clinician may wish to investigate.

Acute Distress

  43. Things in my life just go from bad to worse. (True)
  64. I often feel sad and unloved. (True)
109. I get very frightened when I think of being all alone in the world. (True)
133. Lately, I feel jumpy and nervous almost all the time. (True)

Dangerous Ideation

  76. Too many rules get in the way of my doing what I want. (True)
  78. I will sometimes do something cruel to make someone unhappy. (True)
157. I enjoy starting fights. (True)

Emotional Isolation

  20. It is not unusual to feel lonely and unwanted. (True)
158. There are times when nobody at home seems to care about me. (True)

Anorexic Tendency

  48. I always think of dieting, even when people say I'm underweight. (True)
  65. I'm supposed to be thin, but I feel my thighs and backside are much too big. (True)
105. I'm terribly afraid that no matter how thin I get, I will start to gain weight if I eat. (True)
144. I'm willing to starve myself to be even thinner than I am. (True)

Bulimic Tendency

  11. Although I go on eating binges, I hate the weight I gain. (True)
  82. I eat little in front of others; then I stuff myself in private. (True)
124. I go on eating binges a couple of times a week. (True)

FIGURE 21.1. *(page 4 of 6)*

Drug Abuse Inclination

40. I used to get so stoned that I did not know what I was doing. (True)

Alcohol Abuse Inclination

22. Drinking seems to have been a problem for several members of my family. (True)
30. When I have a few drinks I feel more sure of myself. (True)
57. I can hold my beer or liquor better than most of my friends. (True)
90. Drinking really seems to help me when I'm feeling down. (True)
152. When we're having a good time, my friends and I can get pretty drunk. (True)

Childhood Abuse

No items.

DIAGNOSTIC HYPOTHESES

Although the diagnostic criteria used in the MACI differ somewhat from those in the DSM-IV-TR, there are sufficient parallels to recommend consideration of the following assignments. More definitive judgments should draw upon biographical, observational, and interview data in addition to self-report inventories such as the MACI.

Axis II: Personality Disorders, Traits, and Features

Although traits and features of personality disorders are often observable in adolescents, the data from the MACI should not be used to assign diagnostic labels without additional clinical information. Even when assigned, diagnostic labels tend to be less stable for adolescents than for adults. The traits listed below are suggested by the MACI results and may be important adjuncts to the diagnostic process.

> Negativistic and Aggressive/Sadistic Personality Traits
>   with Antisocial and Histrionic Features

Axis I: Clinical Syndromes

The following list contains suggested clinical syndromes and other conditions relating to the DSM-IV-TR that may be a focus of clinical attention.

> 312.9 Disruptive Behavior Disorder NOS

> 312.8 Conduct Disorder
>   Also consider: 313.81 Oppositional Defiant Disorder
>   or V7l.02 Childhood or Adolescent Antisocial Behavior

> 305.90 Other (or Unknown) Substance Abuse

> V6l.20 Parent-Child Relational Problem

PROGNOSTIC AND THERAPEUTIC IMPLICATIONS

The possibility of an acute alcohol- or drug-abuse problem should be carefully considered for this teenager. If verified, appropriate behavioral management or group therapeutic programs should be

FIGURE 21.1. *(page 5 of 6)*

implemented. Once this adolescent has been adequately stabilized, attention may be directed toward the more fundamental goals suggested in the following paragraphs.

Unlikely to be a willing participant in treatment, this adolescent most probably submitted to therapy under the pressure of family, academic, or legal difficulties. Annoyed, sarcastic, and resentful, she will challenge and seek to outwit the therapist by setting up situations to test the therapist's skills, to catch inconsistencies, to arouse ire, and, if possible, to belittle and humiliate the therapist. For the therapist, restraining the impulse to express a condemning attitude will be no easy task. The therapist must expend great effort to check any hostile feelings, keeping in mind that this adolescent's plight is largely of her own making. The patient may actively impede her progress toward conflict resolution and goal attainment. Thus, she may undo what good she has previously achieved in treatment. Driven by contrary feelings, she may retract her kind words to others and replace them with harshness, undermining achievements that she and the therapist have struggled so hard to attain. In short, her ambivalence often robs her of what few steps she has secured toward progress.

This teenager may actively resist exploring her motives. Because she is not a willing participant in therapy, the submissive and help-seeking role is anathema to her. She only submits to therapy under the press of severe family discord or legal problems. For example, she may be in trouble as a consequence of aggressive or abusive behavior or as a result of incessant quarrels or drug involvement. Rarely does she experience guilt or accept blame for the turmoil she causes. To her, a problem can usually be traced to another person's stupidity, laziness, or hostility. Even when she accepts a measure of responsibility for her difficulties, she may resent the therapist for tricking her into admitting it. In this situation, the therapist must restrain any impulse to react with disapproval and criticism. An important step in building rapport with this youth is to see things from her viewpoint. The therapist must convey a sense of trust and a willingness to develop a constructive treatment alliance. A balance of professional authority and tolerance is necessary to diminish the possibility that this teenager will impulsively withdraw from treatment.

Formal behavior modification methods may be fruitfully explored to achieve greater control and responsibility in social behavior. More directive cognitive techniques may be used to confront the patient with the obstructive and self-destructive character of her interpersonal relations. Because of the difficult-to-modify character of these problems and the probability that resistances will impede the effectiveness of other therapeutic procedures, it may be necessary to explore diverse and multipronged therapeutic techniques, A thorough reconstruction of personality may be the best means of altering the pattern. Because family treatment methods focus on the complex network of relationships that often sustain this behavioral style, they may prove to be the most useful techniques to help the patient recognize the source of her own hurt and angry feelings, as well as to appreciate how she provokes hurt and anger in others.

FIGURE 21.1. *(page 6 of 6)*

CHAPTER 22

Development and Validation of the Millon Pre-Adolescent Clinical Inventory (M-PACI)

John Kamp
Robert F. Tringone

The Millon Pre-Adolescent Clinical Inventory (M-PACI; Millon, Tringone, Millon, & Grossman, 2005) is a multidimensional self-report inventory designed for use with 9- to 12-year-olds who are seen in clinical settings. It extends the "family" of Millon clinical inventories from adults (Millon Clinical Multiaxial Inventory–III; MCMI-III) and adolescents (Millon Adolescent Clinical Inventory; MACI) to the preadolescent cohort. The M-PACI consists of 97 true–false items written at a third-grade reading level. The inventory has 14 profile scales that are equally divided into two sets, named Emerging Personality Patterns and Current Clinical Signs. In addition, there are two response validity indicators. The names of all of the M-PACI scales are shown in Table 22.1.

The M-PACI is the outcome of an ambitious project begun in early 2001, the goal of which was to develop a comprehensive yet brief instrument that would provide valuable clinical information from a data source then thought to be suspect—namely, preadolescent self-reports. For example, Loeber, Green, and Lahey (1990) surveyed over 100 mental health professionals who worked with children concerning the usefulness of mothers, teachers, and children themselves as informants in the assessment of behavior problems in 7- to 12-year-olds. Children were viewed as significantly less useful than their mothers as informants in all four general problem areas studied—hyperactivity/inattentiveness, oppositional behaviors, conduct problems, and internalizing problems (e.g., anxiety and depression)—and as significantly less useful than their teachers as informants on hyperactivity/inattentiveness and oppositional behaviors. Overall mean ratings for the four problem domains showed that the surveyed professionals considered information from 7- to 12-year-olds

TABLE 22.1. The M-PACI Scales

Scale set	Scale name
Emerging Personality Patterns	1. Confident
	2. Outgoing
	3. Conforming
	4. Submissive
	5. Inhibited
	6. Unruly
	7. Unstable
Current Clinical Signs	A. Anxiety/Fears
	B. Attention Deficits
	C. Obsessions/Compulsions
	D. Conduct Problems
	E. Disruptive Behaviors
	F. Depressive Moods
	G. Reality Distortions
Response Validity Indicators	IV. Invalidity
	RN. Response Negativity

"slightly useful" in the evaluation of hyperactivity/inattentiveness and oppositional behaviors, and "moderately useful" in the assessment of conduct problems and internalizing problems.

In addition to overall skepticism about the value of preadolescent self-reports, nearly all self-report instruments designed for this age group are single-construct measures that target circumscribed symptom areas (e.g., attention-deficit/hyperactivity disorder [ADHD], anxiety, depression). Instruments intended to provide a comprehensive assessment of personality for the preadolescent age group are virtually nonexistent. Thus one reviewer's evaluation of the landscape at the time when work on the M-PACI began stated, "With regard to the preadolescent age group, the dearth of good general purpose self-report measures has been particularly noticeable" (Merrell, 1999, p. 160). The "MACI Junior" project, as it was first called, set out to develop a new instrument that would meet the need for a multidimensional self-report assessment tool encompassing both personality and clinical symptoms among preadolescents.

This chapter describes the construction and validation of the M-PACI. The inventory's unique features are emphasized, and data supporting its reliability, internal structure, and criterion validity are presented.

Guiding Theoretical System

As it is for the MCMI-III (Millon, 2006a) and the MACI (Millon, 2006b), Millon's personality theory is the underlying and guiding theory for the M-PACI. Initially proposed as a biosocial learning theory (Millon, 1969, 1981), the theory itself has evolved and is now formulated as an evolutionary model (Millon, 1990; Millon & Davis, 1996). At both levels, however, the theory postulates three central polarities that are essential to understanding personality organization: self–other, active–passive, and pleasure–pain. Whereas the biosocial learning model describes these polarities and the personality constructs that are derived from their configurations at clinical levels, the evolutionary model addresses similar processes at more explanatory levels.

According to the biosocial learning theory, personality patterns are learned strategies implemented to secure positive reinforcement and minimize punishment (with these concepts defined in broad terms). The self–other polarity represents the source to which the person turns to enhance his or her life and gain satisfaction, or to avoid psychic pain and discomfort. Those who look to themselves for gratification and/or pain avoidance are termed "independent" on this polarity, while those who look to others are termed "dependent." The term "ambivalent" applies to those individuals who are conflicted regarding whether to look to or to rely on themselves or others in order to meet these needs.

The active–passive polarity represents the nature of the behaviors employed to maximize rewards and minimize pain. Individuals with active personalities typically take the initiative and interact with their environment to achieve gratification and avoid or reduce distress. Those with passive personalities, on the other hand, are much more reserved and maintain a more accommodating stance vis-à-vis their environment. Finally, the pleasure–pain polarity represents the nature of the response elicited from others, which can be positive or negative.

For the MCMI-III, these polarities are combined to derive the 14 scales that correspond to many of the personality disorders recognized by the fourth edition of the *Diagnostic and Statistical Manual of Mental Disorders* (DSM-IV) and its text revision (DSM-IV-TR) (American Psychiatric Association, 1994, 2000). The MACI's 12 Personality Patterns scales have less pathological names and do not represent personality "disorders" per se, because personality disturbances among adolescents may be attributable to their attempts to adjust to and negotiate the numerous internal and external influences, demands, and challenges they face. Adolescent personalities are still developing and are more malleable than adult personalities, which generally consist of more enduring traits.

Among preadolescents, the still-developing and changeable nature of personality is even more pronounced. For that reason, the set of personality scales included in the M-PACI is labeled *Emerging* Personality Patterns. Furthermore, the M-PACI does not assess for, and does not label 9- to 12-year-olds with, personality disorder diagnoses. Finally, a concerted effort was made during the writing of the M-PACI computerized Interpretive Reports to identify an adaptive capacity of each personality pattern in addition to its clinical relevance to the child's problems.

Emerging Personality Patterns Scales

The M-PACI has seven Emerging Personality Patterns scales. Six of these are derived from combinations involving the self–other and active–passive polarities specified by Millon's theory, as shown in Figure 22.1. The seventh scale, Unstable, measures more severe personality problems. As the data presented later in this chapter show, high scores on the Confident, Outgoing, and Conforming scales are generally associated

	Other-Focused (Dependent)	Self-Focused (Independent)	Self–Other Ambivalent	Detached
Passive	Submissive	Confident	Conforming	
Active	Outgoing	Unruly		Inhibited

FIGURE 22.1. Derivation of the Emerging Personality Patterns scales from Millon's theory. From Millon, Tringone, Millon, and Grossman (2005, Figure 2.1). Copyright 2005 by NCS Pearson Inc. Reprinted by permission.

with higher levels of functioning and may represent protective features against stress. The Submissive, Inhibited, Unruly, and Unstable scales reflect troubled personality patterns. The theoretical basis and primary clinical features of each of these personality patterns are described next.

Confident Scale

The Confident scale represents the passive–independent personality style, which involves the development of a superior self-image. Because significant others have continually and often unconditionally showered them with admiration, youngsters with passive–independent personalities have come to believe that they are special, and they have a flourishing appreciation of their self-worth. As a result, they tend to believe that they just need to be themselves in order to feel content and secure. Confident preadolescents who exhibit true talents and abilities often enjoy the attention they receive, and they may attain a high social standing. This is not true of all preadolescents who exhibit this style, however, and an exaggerated or idealized sense of self can sometimes result. Confident preadolescents may also manifest a passive exploitiveness in their relationships, potentially taking others for granted and failing to reciprocate.

Outgoing Scale

The Outgoing scale measures the active–dependent personality style. Outgoing preadolescents are gregarious and sociable. Through their high energy and spirited manner, they develop many friendships and have very active social lives. They often enjoy being the center of attention. In many instances, these children have been showered with approval and have learned to associate receiving rewards (e.g., recognition and praise) with meeting the expectations of others. They may, in turn, learn to implement a behavior set that is designed specifically to elicit attention and affection from others. In extreme instances, they may rely excessively on input from others rather than develop inner guidelines to regulate their efforts, behaviors, and attitudes, and in so doing struggle to establish a stable sense of themselves.

Conforming Scale

Within the Millon model, there are two ambivalent personality patterns. One variant, the passive–ambivalent personality style, is represented on the M-PACI by the

Conforming scale. Conceptually, children with conforming personalities experience an intense intrapsychic conflict between obedience (i.e., being other-oriented and accommodating to others' desires) and defiance (i.e., being self-oriented, expressing their autonomy, and pursuing their own desires). On the surface, these children appear to have resolved the conflict through obedience. They tend to be disciplined and rule-governed, follow directives and meet others' expectations, and pursue achievement-oriented goals. Responsible and conscientious, dependable and reliable, conforming preadolescents are often "model citizens," particularly in school settings. Underneath, however, they may be harboring considerable anger and stress that can occasionally break through their surface calm.

Submissive Scale

The Submissive scale measures the passive–dependent personality pattern. Children with submissive personalities emphasize strong attachments with a few significant others in order to assure themselves of affection, protection, and security. With their tendency to be shy, quiet, and cooperative, they allow and often prefer others to take the lead and make decisions. Submissive children generally avoid taking risks, out of fear that they could get hurt or that an important adult figure might disapprove of their actions. Some may focus on their perceived weaknesses and be visibly lacking in self-confidence. Submissive youngsters are usually quite selective regarding their friends and tend to maintain a small, close-knit social network. They are most comfortable in a safe and protective environment; however, they tend to become anxious when they are encouraged to be more autonomous or in situations requiring assertiveness.

Inhibited Scale

Although the MCMI-III and the MACI each measure three detached personality patterns, the M-PACI measures just one: Inhibited, the active–detached pattern in the Millon schema. Individuals with this style tend to be hypersensitive to anticipated pain and have a limited focus on experiencing pleasure. Inhibited children tend to be apprehensive and socially ill at ease. They have few friends, tend to have trouble fitting in, and often gravitate to the periphery in social situations. Though they wish for acceptance from their peers, their past experiences involving social rejection have taught them to be wary of trusting others and to keep a "low profile" as an effective means of avoiding further rejection or humiliation. They often have low self-esteem and limited coping resources, which make them vulnerable to persistent undercurrents of anxiety, tension, and sadness.

Unruly Scale

The M-PACI Unruly scale represents the active–independent personality pattern. Children with this personality style have often experienced the world as an uncaring, ungiving, or even hostile place (in marked contrast to the nurturing environment experienced by children with the passive–independent confident personality). As a result, unruly preadolescents have learned to mistrust others and to be self-reliant. They are typically proactive in meeting their wants and desires, and will act in hostile and sometimes aggressive ways to do so. They exhibit impulsive tendencies with low frustration tolerance. Their thrill-seeking actions reflect their need for immediate gratification. They will typically have difficulty accepting limits and struggle to take responsibility for their actions. Since they either disregard social rules or fail to heed the possible consequences of their actions, they often present with oppositional and conduct problems. In a distinction common in child psychology, submissive and inhibited personalities are often associated with "internalizing" problems, while unruly personalities are linked with "externalizing" problems.

Unstable Scale

The M-PACI Unstable scale was constructed to assess what appears to be a growing problem in the preadolescent population. Children in this age group who exhibit this pattern are experiencing significant and chronic distress. Unstable preadolescents appear to be facing more family conflicts or disruptions than their peers, and these difficulties are having an adverse effect on their emerging personalities. The impact is evident in their mood lability, their proneness to intense depressive episodes, and their impulsive acting out. Many express suicidal thoughts, and some engage in self-injurious behavior. From the Millon perspective, the unstable personality is conceptualized as a pattern plagued by conflict within all three core polarities. These children experience persistent psychic pain and are vulnerable to both internalizing and externalizing problems, because they are not well integrated in terms of their personality organization. They struggle to cope with life's demands in an effective manner.

Current Clinical Signs Scales

The seven Current Clinical Signs scales assess conditions that present themselves as specific symptom clusters. These conditions are usually the impetus for a referral for evaluation and treatment, since they often affect a child's functioning in home, school, and/or social settings. It is believed that a child's emerging personality provides a critical backdrop for understanding these clinical signs. A clinical syndrome can be seen as an extension of an underlying personality vulnerability or as a potentially biologically driven condition that should be considered within the context of the child's developing personality style.

Anxiety/Fears Scale

Anxiety is a universal emotion that all children experience from time to time. The M-PACI Anxiety/Fears scale assesses problems that tend to be persistent and occur on a frequent basis. The items assess symptoms in the following realms: somatic (e.g., upset stomach), affective (e.g., nervousness), cognitive (e.g., fear of harm to self and family), and behavioral (e.g., missing school due to anxiety).

Attention Deficits Scale

Studies of ADHD indicate that it is a very common presenting problem for preadolescents in clinical settings. Although ADHD is often viewed as a neurologically based condition, inattention and distractibility features may also reflect a child's response to a high level of stress. The Attention Deficits scale items emphasize attention issues and restlessness. When this scale is coelevated with the Disruptive Behaviors scale, which emphasizes impulse control problems, it may be indicative of the symptom triad associated with ADHD, combined type.

Obsessions/Compulsions Scale

Obsessive–compulsive disorder (OCD) is classified in DSM-IV(-TR) as an anxiety disorder. The M-PACI Obsessions/Compulsions scale taps both the cognitive (obsessions) and the ritualistic behavior (compulsions) components of OCD, as well as the anxiety and social discomfort that often accompany the condition. However, it is not clear what percentage of preadolescents present with both components. Some children, for example, may recognize a compulsive behavior or routine, but may not yet have identified the thoughts that may be connected to it or its purpose.

Conduct Problems Scale

There is growing concern over the number of children who engage in hostile, antisocial, and sometimes violent behaviors toward their peers or adults. These behaviors seem more prevalent than ever in our schools and communities. The M-PACI Conduct Problems scale assesses this antisocial behavior pattern. Acts of misconduct often represent the culmination of a protracted pattern of noncompliance, poor frustration tolerance, intermittent aggression, and poor judgment. Underlying anger problems are often present, and peer and family relations often serve in some manner to reinforce the pattern.

Disruptive Behaviors Scale

The M-PACI Disruptive Behaviors scale focuses on impulse control problems. Although many preadolescents will occasionally demonstrate lapses in impulse control, this scale was designed to help identify those with frequent problems in this area. These children's faulty ability to think before they act and to delay a reaction in emotionally charged situations can lead to intense family squabbles and frequent quarrels with their peers. Again, coelevations of this scale with the Attention Deficits scale may signify the presence of ADHD.

Depressive Moods Scale

Depression has become a very common presenting problem in child clinical settings, trailing perhaps only ADHD and concomitant disruptive behavior problems. The M-PACI Depressive Moods scale assesses sad mood, thoughts of death, and feelings of loneliness and despair. Coelevations with the Anxiety/Fears scale may be common, and underlying vulnerabilities appear to be linked to high scores on the Submissive, Inhibited, and Unstable scales.

Reality Distortions Scale

The M-PACI Reality Distortions scale was designed to identify children who may be having cognitive distortions and unusual perceptual experiences. The scale taps reports of auditory and visual hallucinations as well as paranoid ideation. Such experiences often trigger confusion and fear, and a child may begin to think that he or she is "going crazy." Accordingly, the scale also captures a child's subjective distress that would accompany bizarre or frightening perceptions and beliefs.

M-PACI Development and Validation

The development of the M-PACI followed the validation sequence proposed by Loevinger (1957) and Jackson (1970). In her classic monograph, Loevinger delineated three components of construct validity: substantive, structural, and external. Both she and Jackson suggested that these components constituted test construction and validation stages that could be followed sequentially.

As the first step in implementing this test development methodology, 18 initial target constructs were specified for potential inclusion as scales in the final M-PACI inventory. These constructs included the 14 represented by the Emerging Personality Patterns and Current Clinical Signs scales described above, plus 4 in a separate set that was labeled Expressed Concerns. The Expressed Concerns constructs were called Personal Discontent, Peer Insecurity, Family Dysfunction, and School Difficulty.

Substantive Validity

Millon's personality theory (Millon, 1969, 1981, 1990; Millon & Davis, 1996) provides the foundation for the M-PACI's substantive validity, Loevinger's (1957) first level of test validity. The derivation of the seven Emerging Personality Patterns scales from that theory has been described earlier in this chapter. The four Expressed Concerns constructs represented common areas of conscious concern for preadolescents, and the seven Current Clinical Signs constructs captured prevalent presenting problems for this age group in a clinical setting.

Definitions were developed for the 18 initial target constructs to serve as a basis for item writing (as well as for the clinician ratings that are described below). Next, through several rounds of item generation, discussion, and revision, provisional scales were developed for the 18 target constructs. The candidate items for these 18 scales were supplemented with items designed for possible use as indicators of response validity (e.g., paying attention and answering in an honest manner) and assembled with directions into an inventory called the M-PACI Research Form that consisted of 135 true–false items. Because deficits in reading and attention are especially common among 9- to 12-year-olds seen in clinical settings, every effort was made to craft items that were short and simple—and, at the same time, interesting to preadolescents and phrased in the language they use. The intent was to use the research data gathered in the next phase of development to reduce the inventory to fewer than 100 items as an additional way to promote ease of completion for preadolescent clients.

Site Solicitation and Data Collection Materials and Procedures

The collection of research data began with the mailing of a solicitation letter to approximately 350 sites that used the MACI. Sites that returned a postcard indicating willingness to collect data from 9- to 12-year-old clients for this project were mailed a set of data collection materials. These materials included copies of (1) an informed consent form to be signed by a parent or guardian, (2) the M-PACI Research Form, (3) a Clinician's Research Form, and (4) a supplemental self-report test.

The Clinician's Research Form was used to collect clinician ratings, demographic information, and clinical contact data for each research subject. The rating task consisted of choosing the child's most prominent and second most prominent personality patterns, expressed concerns, and clinical signs, using the construct sets and definitions that had been developed for the 18 initial target constructs. Each subject was assigned a clinician rating score of 2, 1, or 0 for each of the 18 variables. If a variable (e.g., the confident personality pattern) was rated most prominent by the subject's clinician, the subject was assigned a score of 2. If the variable was rated second most prominent, a score of 1 was assigned. If the variable was not rated either most prominent or second most prominent, the subject received a score of 0. All correlations involving the clinician ratings were based on these 0/1/2 scores.

To allow the final M-PACI to be validated against other pertinent self-report instruments, three tests that are commonly given to troubled preadolescents were included in the M-PACI development research. These supplemental tests were the multidimensional Behavior Assessment System for Children: Self-Report of Personality Form C (BASC SRP-C; Reynolds & Kamphaus, 1998), and the more narrowly focused Children's Depression Inventory (CDI; Kovacs, 2001) and Revised Children's Manifest Anxiety Scale (RCMAS; Reynolds & Richmond, 2000). Half of the volunteer sites were randomly assigned to administer the BASC SRP-C, one-fourth the CDI, and one-fourth the RCMAS. Copies of the appropriate supplemental test were included in the data collection materials mailed to each site.

Each site was sent a detailed instruction booklet along with the data collection materials described above. The instruction booklet requested that professionals at the site select 9- to 12-year-old clients whose psychological traits and problems they felt they knew reasonably well for potential inclusion in the study. For each client selected, the site was instructed to follow the steps below in sequence:

1. Have the client's parent or guardian read and sign the informed consent form.
2. Have the mental health professional at the site who worked most closely with the child complete the Clinician's Research Form. The instruction booklet emphasized the importance of completing the Clinician's Research Form *before* administering the M-PACI Research Form and the supplemental test,

so that the clinicians' ratings could not be influenced in any way by the subjects' responses to the items on those self-report instruments.

3. Administer the M-PACI Research Form.
4. Administer the supplemental test, either during the same session as the M-PACI Research Form or within the following week. This step was described as optional, but sites were encouraged to administer the supplemental test to as many research subjects as possible.
5. Return the completed materials to the M-PACI research team.

Final Inventory Development

The overall strategy for final inventory development and validation involved dividing the 292 subjects who constituted the total research sample into an inventory development subsample and a cross-validation subsample. Statistics computed with data from the development subsample were used to help select the items and scale composition for the final M-PACI. The reliability and criterion validity of the final scales were then evaluated based on data from the cross-validation subsample, so that those values would not be spuriously inflated by capitalization on chance.

All 292 subjects in the total research sample completed the M-PACI Research Form. However, the M-PACI Research Forms for 6 (2%) of the subjects were judged to be invalid, either because of an excessive number of missing item responses or because of responses to four items that were designed to detect random, careless, or untruthful responding. Of the remaining 286 subjects, 186 were randomly selected for the development subsample and 100 for the cross-validation subsample. Random assignment produced development and cross-validation subsamples that were very similar both demographically and in terms of their psychological characteristics as rated by their clinicians. Chi-square tests for demographic differences between the subsamples were all nonsignificant, as were t tests comparing the mean scores on the 18 clinician rating variables between the two subsamples.

Next, items in the initial pool of 135 were either eliminated or retained and assigned to one or more scales (though item overlap across scales was deliberately limited), based on the following statistics from the development subsample: (1) item endorsement frequencies, (2) correlations of each item with the 18 provisional M-PACI scales, and (3) correlations of each item with the 18 clinician rating scores. This was an iterative process in which scales were formed, evaluated, and revised until no further improvement in their psychometric properties appeared possible. Internal consistency analyses addressed the structural component of test validation cited by Loevinger (1957), and analysis of correlations with the clinician ratings addressed the external component.

During this process, the set of four provisional scales targeting Expressed Concerns was found to be much weaker than the other two scale sets and was dropped. Each of the 14 remaining (and final) M-PACI profile scales includes both "prototype items," which were originally written for that scale and receive a raw score weight of 2, and "subsidiary items," which were originally written for other scales but enhanced the scale's psychometric properties and have content that is conceptually relevant. Subsidiary items receive a raw score weight of 1.

As on the MCMI-III and the MACI, standardized scores on the M-PACI profile scales are reported as base rate (BR) scores, which are scaled to reflect the relative prevalence of the various characteristics measured by the inventory. The M-PACI uses a single set of transformations from raw to BR scores for males and females, and the transformations were determined by using a combined-gender norm group. The final inventory, which consists of 97 items, also includes two Response Validity Indicators called Invalidity and Response Negativity. The M-PACI manual (Millon et al., 2005) provides more detail on the development of the inventory, including the BR scores and Response Validity Indicators.

Structural Validity

Loevinger's (1957) second validation stage, relabeled "internal/structural," pertains to a test's congruence with its underlying theory and is evaluated by examining whether the relationships among items and scales is consistent with the theory's predictions. Within the Millon personality theory, which anticipates shared features or signs between constructs, it is expected that test scales will possess a reasonably high degree of internal consistency and that they will exhibit overlap or correlation with other theoretically related scales.

Reliability

Coefficient alpha internal consistency reliability values for the 14 M-PACI profile scales are shown in Table 22.2. These values were calculated based on the 100 subjects in the cross-validation subsample. The inventory construction goals of keeping the final inventory to fewer than 100 items and permitting only a moderate amount of item overlap among scales resulted in relatively short M-PACI scales, with 7 to 12

TABLE 22.2. Coefficient Alpha Reliability Values for the M-PACI Scales

Scale	No. of items	Alpha
Confident	11	.67
Outgoing	10	.65
Conforming	11	.67
Submissive	12	.66
Inhibited	11	.65
Unruly	12	.84
Unstable	12	.81
Anxiety/Fears	9	.67
Attention Deficits	7	.74
Obsessions/Compulsions	8	.63
Conduct Problems	10	.79
Disruptive Behaviors	9	.79
Depressive Moods	10	.72
Reality Distortions	8	.76

Note. $n = 100$.

items each. Because coefficient alpha is partly a function of scale length, it is not surprising that the alpha values for most of the M-PACI scales are only moderately high. As shown in Table 22.2, these values ranged between .63 (for Obsessions/Compulsions) and .84 (for Unruly), with a mean of .72 and a median of .71 across the 14 scales.

Internal Structure

BR scores on the M-PACI scales were intercorrelated among the 286 subjects in the combined development and cross-validation subsamples. (Because scale intercorrelation data were not used in the development of the final M-PACI, there was no reason not to combine the two subsamples to maximize the sample size for this analysis.) The Confident, Outgoing, and Conforming personality scales correlated positively among themselves. With a few exceptions involving the Conforming scale, these three scales correlated negatively with all of the other scales. The remaining scales—the Submissive, Inhibited, Unruly, and Unstable personality scales, and the seven clinical scales—were all positively intercorrelated except for a handful of very small negative correlations. This pattern suggests that higher scores on the Confident, Outgoing, and Conforming personality scales may in many cases signal positive adjustment. The magnitude of most of the scale intercorrelations was in the low to moderate range, although 8 of the 91 correlations exceeded .60 in magnitude.

In order to explore the intercorrelations among the M-PACI scales more systematically, the correlations were factor-analyzed via principal axis factoring with varimax rotation. The eigenvalues suggested that either a two-factor or a three-factor solution was most appropriate. The two-factor solution proved more interpretable and is shown in Table 22.3.

TABLE 22.3. Factor Loadings for the M-PACI Scales

Scale	Factor I: Externalizing	Factor II: Internalizing
Unruly	.91	−.01
Conduct Problems	.87	−.00
Disruptive Behaviors	.87	.06
Unstable	.68	.41
Conforming	−.67	.08
Attention Deficits	.51	.18
Submissive	−.04	.78
Inhibited	−.11	.78
Depressive Moods	.12	.77
Anxiety/Fears	−.10	.71
Obsessions/Compulsions	.35	.61
Confident	−.23	−.57
Outgoing	−.10	−.42
Reality Distortions	.47	.48
Percent of total variance	28%	26%

Factor I, labeled Externalizing, is characterized by extremely high loadings for the Unruly, Conduct Problems, and Disruptive Behaviors scales. The Unstable, Conforming (with negative sign), and Attention Deficits scales also loaded more highly on this factor. Factor II was labeled Internalizing. The Submissive, Inhibited, Depressive Moods, and Anxiety/Fears scales had high and clear loadings on this factor. The Obsessions/Compulsions scale loaded more highly on Factor II, as did the Confident and Outgoing scales with negative signs. The Reality Distortions scale loaded almost equally on Factors I and II, suggesting that it measures both internalized (i.e., disturbing thoughts) and externalized (i.e., inappropriate behaviors) aspects of reality problems. Apart from Reality Distortions, only two of the M-PACI scales had secondary loadings exceeding .30: The Unstable scale loaded .41 on the Internalizing factor (vs. .68 on the Externalizing factor), and the Obsessions/Compulsions scale loaded .35 on the Externalizing factor (vs. .61 on the Internalizing factor).

External Validity

The third phase of Loevinger's (1957) test validation model, relabeled "external/criterion," involves comparing scores on the test to extratest criterion measures. In the development and validation research reported here, the primary method of external validation of the M-PACI involved correlating BR scores on the 14 profile scales with the clinician ratings of the constructs measured by those scales. To provide secondary validation, M-PACI scores were correlated with scores from the BASC SRP-C, the CDI, and the RCMAS.

Table 22.4 shows the correlation of each M-PACI scale with its clinician rating target in the cross-validation subsample. These convergent validity coefficients were

TABLE 22.4. Correlations between M-PACI Scales and Clinician Ratings of the Same Constructs

Clinician rating variable	Mean	SD	Correlation with corresponding M-PACI scale
Confident	0.33	0.71	.24**
Outgoing	0.36	0.64	.38**
Conforming	0.25	0.59	.33**
Submissive	0.19	0.53	.34**
Inhibited	0.48	0.80	.50**
Unruly	0.76	0.88	.57**
Unstable	0.50	0.73	.46**
Anxiety/Fears	0.51	0.80	.46**
Attention Deficits	0.68	0.88	.41**
Obsessions/Compulsions	0.09	0.38	.19*
Conduct Problems	0.24	0.59	.40**
Disruptive Behaviors	0.78	0.82	.48**
Depressive Moods	0.50	0.73	.37**
Reality Distortions	0.05	0.26	.23*

Note. n = 100.
*p < .05, one-tailed. **p < .01, one-tailed.

quite strong overall, with a mean of .38 and a median of .39 across the 14 M-PACI scales. Eleven of the 14 convergent validity correlations were .33 or greater. The two lowest, .19 for the Obsessions/Compulsions scale and .23 for the Reality Distortions scale, involve clinical syndromes that were attributed to very few research subjects by their clinicians (note the extremely low mean clinician rating scores for these constructs in Table 22.4). The restricted variance of the clinician rating scores for these two clinical signs (reflecting the fact that nearly all subjects received a rating score of 0) would necessarily constrain the ability of any other variable to correlate with them. Thus, on the whole, the M-PACI demonstrated strong convergent validity against the clinician ratings.

Although not shown in Table 22.4, the correlations between the M-PACI scales and the clinician ratings also displayed an impressive convergent–discriminant pattern. There was only one instance in which an M-PACI scale correlated more highly with a clinician rating variable other than its target (the Conduct Problems scale correlated .46 with the clinician ratings of Unruly vs. .40 with the ratings of Conduct Problems). There were only three instances in which a clinician rating variable was predicted better by a scale other than the scale designed to measure that construct (the clinician ratings of Conforming correlated –.40 with the Unruly scale and –.36 with the Conduct Problems scale vs. .33 with the Conforming scale; and the clinician ratings of Obsessions/Compulsions correlated –.22 with the Attention Deficits scale vs. .19 with the Obsessions/Compulsions scale). Thus, of the 182 "off-diagonal" correlations in the full 14 × 14 table of correlations between M-PACI scales and clinician ratings, only 4 exceeded either of their corresponding "on-diagonal" correlations in magnitude. Given the strong conceptual relationships among many of the constructs measured by the M-PACI, this is a remarkable level of discriminant validity.

As noted earlier, half of the data collection sites were asked to optionally administer the BASC SRP-C, one-quarter the CDI, and one-quarter the RCMAS. Of the 160 preadolescents who completed the M-PACI Research Form at "BASC sites," 107 (67%) completed useable BASC SRP-C forms. Of the 63 children who completed the M-PACI Research Form at "CDI sites," 61 (97%) completed the CDI. The RCMAS was completed by 51 (74%) of the 69 children who completed the M-PACI Research Form at "RCMAS sites." Higher completion rates were expected for the 27-item CDI and the 37-item RCMAS than for the 152-item BASC SRP-C. Because scores on these supplemental tests were not used in final M-PACI development, correlations between the M-PACI and each of the other tests were calculated based on all subjects with useable data on each pair of tests.

Table 22.5 presents correlations between the 14 M-PACI profile scales (BR scores) and the 16 BASC SRP-C scales and composites, the Total CDI Score, and RCMAS Total Anxiety. The BASC correlations are based on T-scores using the BASC SRP-C combined-gender general norms (correlations with T-scores using the clinical norms were virtually identical). The CDI and RCMAS correlations are based on raw scores for these two instruments. The exclusion of 6 subjects with invalid M-PACI Research Forms accounts for the slightly smaller sample sizes shown in Table 22.5 compared to those listed in the previous paragraph.

There are many correlations of appreciable magnitude in Table 22.5. The highest of these (i.e., correlations ≥ .60 in magnitude) are all between an M-PACI scale and a BASC, CDI, or RCMAS scale that measures the same construct as the M-PACI scale

TABLE 22.5. Correlations between M-PACI Scales and BASC SRP-C, CDI, and RCMAS Scales

M-PACI scale	B1[a]	B2[a]	B3[a]	B4[a]	B5[a]	B6[a]	B7[a]	B8[a]	B9[a]	B10[a]	B11[a]	B12[a]	B13[a]	B14[a]	B15[a]	B16[a]	CDI[b]	RCMAS[c]
Confident	-.24	-.22	-.33	-.41	-.51	-.54	-.51	-.53	.34	.52	.57	.49	-.26	-.52	.61	-.65	-.58	-.51
Outgoing	-.27	-.14	-.22	-.17	-.35	-.36	-.39	-.39	.15	.51	.32	.49	-.23	-.32	.47	-.48	-.31	-.27
Conforming	-.51	-.45	-.27	-.15	-.19	-.06	-.27	-.37	.44	.21	.33	.48	-.54	-.20	.48	-.29	-.31	-.09
Submissive	.09	.07	.36	.32	.42	.45	.36	.44	-.13	-.27	-.27	-.20	.09	.45	-.27	.44	.49	.55
Inhibited	.14	.05	.34	.37	.45	.49	.45	.38	-.02	-.33	-.26	-.14	.10	.48	-.23	.49	.51	.57
Unruly	.37	.37	.37	.31	.31	.22	.36	.43	-.32	-.28	-.28	-.39	.41	.35	-.41	.38	.18	.38
Unstable	.27	.25	.59	.37	.55	.55	.54	.52	-.34	-.47	-.42	-.39	.29	.60	-.52	.62	.53	.60
Anxiety/Fears	-.04	.00	.34	.26	.43	.51	.27	.34	-.06	-.23	-.35	-.08	-.03	.45	-.22	.44	.33	.54
Attention Deficits	.36	.36	.35	.43	.40	.31	.42	.52	-.23	-.40	-.15	-.37	.41	.43	-.37	.45	.22	.23
Obsessions/Compulsions	.15	.13	.45	.35	.54	.65	.33	.32	-.12	-.33	-.40	-.19	.15	.58	-.32	.53	.57	.75
Conduct Problems	.36	.42	.41	.32	.35	.25	.44	.44	-.44	-.28	-.35	-.36	.44	.39	-.46	.42	.17	.29
Disruptive Behaviors	.35	.35	.40	.32	.37	.28	.36	.42	-.28	-.26	-.28	-.36	.40	.40	-.38	.39	.18	.51
Depressive Moods	.14	.07	.46	.32	.41	.45	.55	.38	-.19	-.38	-.37	-.20	.12	.47	-.36	.52	.65	.50
Reality Distortions	.27	.34	.73	.42	.58	.55	.50	.38	-.34	-.38	-.43	-.27	.35	.67	-.45	.57	.50	.45

Note. B1, BASC Attitude to School; B2, BASC Attitude to Teachers; B3, BASC Atypicality; B4, BASC Locus of Control; B5, BASC Social Stress; B6, BASC Anxiety; B7, BASC Depression; B8, BASC Sense of Inadequacy; B9, BASC Relations with Parents; B10, BASC Interpersonal Relations; B11, BASC Self-Esteem; B12, BASC Self-Reliance; B13, BASC School Maladjustment; B14, BASC Clinical Maladjustment; B15, BASC Personal Adjustment; B16, BASC Emotional Symptoms Index; CDI, Total CDI Score; RCMAS, RCMAS Total Anxiety.

[a] $n = 104$; correlations $\geq .26$ in magnitude are significant at $p < .01$, two-tailed.
[b] $n = 59$; correlations $\geq .34$ in magnitude are significant at $p < .01$, two-tailed.
[c] $n = 50$; correlations $\geq .36$ in magnitude are significant at $p < .01$, two-tailed.

or one with a clear conceptual relationship. Examples include the correlation of .65 between M-PACI Depressive Moods and the Total CDI Score, .75 between M-PACI Obsessions/Compulsions and RCMAS Total Anxiety, .65 between M-PACI Obsessions/Compulsions and BASC Anxiety, .73 between M-PACI Reality Distortions and BASC Atypicality, .60 between M-PACI Unstable and BASC Clinical Maladjustment, and .61 between M-PACI Confident and BASC Personal Adjustment. Thus the correlations with the BASC SRP-C, CDI, and RCMAS provide further evidence for the external/criterion validity of the M-PACI.

Case Example

Working with children in this age group requires considerable time, energy, and effort from many adults. The following case illustrates how to use the M-PACI as an assessment instrument that complements the information and impressions gained from a clinical interview, and as a guide for treatment interventions.

S. P., a 10-year-old male, was seen for psychological assessment and treatment because of depression, debilitating headaches, and obesity. S. P. lived with his parents, had no siblings, and had a small extended family. He had a history of language-based learning disabilities, as well as weaknesses in his gross and fine motor skills. At the time of his first interview, he was placed in a self-contained fourth-grade class and was receiving academic support services. He occasionally played with peers on his block, but had no close friends. He preferred to spend time alone or with his many pets.

S. P.'s parents reported that he was the product of a full-term, unremarkable pregnancy and delivery. They described him as an "easy baby" who was easy to comfort and soothe. Delays, however, were noted in his expressive language skills, and when he began attending nursery school at age 4, he had difficulty making friends. His parents reported that they had to pursue and arrange play dates for their son; otherwise, he would sit at home watching TV or playing video games. Academic struggles were evident early in grammar school, and S. P. received remedial services starting in kindergarten. S. P.'s current teacher described him as shy and quiet in the classroom. He did not disrupt the class in any way, but would participate only when called on. He appeared reluctant to speak out loud on his own, and the teacher believed he might be anxious about making mistakes in front of his peers.

During S. P.'s first interview, he articulated, "I've been feeling depressed. The joy is gone." He endorsed having a depressed mood, diminished interest in and pleasure derived from most activities, hypersomnia with fatigue, psychomotor retardation, and negative self-esteem. S. P. also reported that he experienced frequent headaches, which were often so unbearable that one of his parents would pick him up from school early or he would miss entire school days. Medical consultations were sought, but no medical cause for his headaches was detected. S. P.'s weight was 200+ pounds, with a body mass index of 40. Daily food diaries and exercise logs revealed generally healthy food choices and appropriate portion sizes, but a very sedentary lifestyle.

S. P. was administered the M-PACI test as a part of the assessment process. Figure 22.2 presents S. P.'s M-PACI profile. It is a valid profile, since the Invalidity score is 0 and the Response Negativity percentile score is 50. These scores indicate that S. P. answered the M-PACI test items in an honest way, and that he did not underreport or overreport his clinical problems in comparison to the test's normative sample.

A primary advantage of the M-PACI is that it provides insight into the context within which behavioral or emotional problems are seen. The Emerging Personality Patterns section

MILLON PRE-ADOLESCENT CLINICAL INVENTORY

RESPONSE VALIDITY INDCIATORS
INVALIDITY SCORE: 0
RESPONSE NEGATIVITY RAW SCORE: 17
RESPONSE NEGATIVITY PERCENTILE SCORE: 50

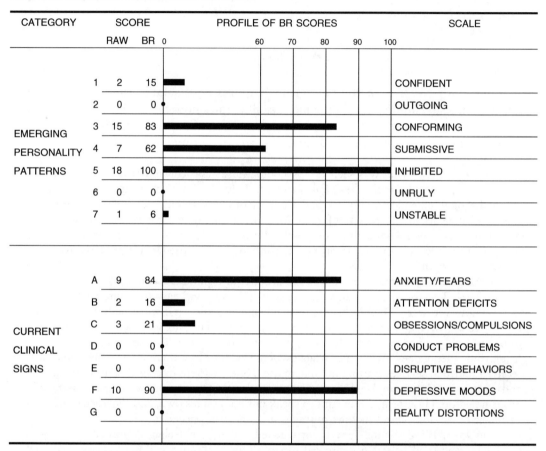

CATEGORY		RAW	BR	PROFILE OF BR SCORES	SCALE
	1	2	15		CONFIDENT
	2	0	0		OUTGOING
EMERGING	3	15	83		CONFORMING
PERSONALITY	4	7	62		SUBMISSIVE
PATTERNS	5	18	100		INHIBITED
	6	0	0		UNRULY
	7	1	6		UNSTABLE
	A	9	84		ANXIETY/FEARS
	B	2	16		ATTENTION DEFICITS
CURRENT	C	3	21		OBSESSIONS/COMPULSIONS
CLINICAL	D	0	0		CONDUCT PROBLEMS
SIGNS	E	0	0		DISRUPTIVE BEHAVIORS
	F	10	90		DEPRESSIVE MOODS
	G	0	0		REALITY DISTORTIONS

CONFIDENTIAL INFORMATION FOR PROFESSIONAL USE ONLY

FIGURE 22.2. M-PACI Profile for S. P., a 10-year-old male.

reveals elevations on the Inhibited and Comforming scales. S. P.'s Inhibited BR score of 100 is the highest obtainable on the test. As noted above, the inhibited personality is conceptualized as the active–detached pattern in the Millon schema. S. P.'s profile reveals how his shyness and apprehensiveness cover underlying needs for acceptance and closeness. He tends to be hypersensitive to anticipated psychic pain and has a limited focus on experiencing pleasure; in the social sphere, these characteristics may be evident in keeping a safe distance emotionally and sometimes physically from others, in spite of his underlying wish to connect with them. It is probable that his previous experiences of rejection, real and perceived, have sensitized him to be wary of trusting others. (These experiences were later verified to have involved peer comments regarding his learning issues, poor motor coordination, and excessive weight.) The short-term adaptive function of protecting himself by keeping to the periphery socially will not prove effective in the long term, because it limits the potentially rewarding experiences he might have otherwise. Furthermore, S. P.'s avoidance of social and emotional involvements with his peers may lead him to drift further toward the periphery. Developmentally, his missing important social interactions at his current age will further inhibit his social skills and ability to cope with social demands later in life. Finally, S. P. possesses limited coping resources, which leave him vulnerable to persistent episodes of anxiety, tension, and sadness.

S. P.'s profile reveals a secondary elevation on the Conforming scale. This scale measures the passive–ambivalent pattern in the Millon schema. Although S. P. may engage in an obedience–defiance conflict, it would appear to be pushed well below the surface, since he respects authority figures, conducts himself in a proper and dependable manner, and is compliant with rules. He takes responsibility for his actions and is quite conscientious. S. P. experiences considerable sadness and anxiety, but suppresses the anger and frustration that he may feel toward others or about his struggles (e.g., with academics, sports). The significant adults in S. P.'s life recognize his attitudes and behaviors, and they are very supportive of him.

Among the Current Clinical Signs scales, S. P.'s endorsements have led to elevated BR scores on the Depressive Moods and Anxiety/Fears scales. These elevations indicate prominent depressive and anxious features. S. P. acknowledges that he is quite sad and distressed. Lacking confidence, he does not believe he can manage the current demands he faces; hence he becomes discouraged and overwhelmed. Internalizing tendencies are apparent in his subjective moods and negative cognitions, which then become manifest in his somatic problems.

The M-PACI also provides guidance regarding treatment interventions. In this case, psychotherapy was recommended, and cognitive-behavioral therapy was noted to be the treatment of choice. S. P. would benefit from identifying and challenging the underlying thoughts that reinforce and perpetuate his sadness and fears. Planning for and engaging in pleasant activities on a regular basis could help reduce his sadness. Social skill building and assertiveness training would be important components for future sessions.

The M-PACI Interpretive Report highlights the role of significant others in a child's life and treatment. For example, discussions should be held regarding the child's core emerging personality features and dynamics, as well as what the parents can do to address them. With S. P., some of the key issues involved his social isolation and lack of trust in others. His parents were enlisted in helping S. P. become more active through their church, which provided group activities and functions for his age; identifying activities he liked and arranging regular opportunities to participate in them; facilitating social contacts; and so forth. The family was also encouraged to address diet and exercise issues. S. P.'s parents were very supportive and involved in his life, and were able to help bolster his self-esteem.

S. P. required other specialists to help him engage in more physical activity. A structured exercise program was necessary in order to address his significant weight problem. Although the M-PACI does not offer diagnostic impressions, at the time of the first interview it was apparent that S. P. met criteria for major depressive disorder. A psychiatric consultation was arranged, and S. P. was started on a selective serotonin reuptake inhibitor (SSRI). He had a positive response to the medication and was eventually weaned from it successfully, without a return of symptoms.

Discussion

A large-scale effort to develop a new multidimensional self-report clinical inventory for use with 9- to 12-year-olds resulted in the 97-item M-PACI. The inventory is scored for seven scales measuring Emerging Personality Patterns and seven measuring

Current Clinical Signs. The inventory's internal consistency reliability, internal structure, and criterion validity against clinician ratings and against other pertinent self-report instruments have been evaluated.

Understandably, the coefficient alpha reliability values for the relatively short M-PACI scales were only moderately high. Very high internal consistency values are considered essential for most tests of ability and achievement, because the constructs measured by those tests are conceptualized as relatively unitary. Lower internal consistency values may be expected for personality or clinical scales measuring constructs that are not as unitary as ability or achievement constructs. For example, some preadolescents may experience obsessions only or compulsions only, which would necessarily lower the internal consistency of a scale measuring both obsessions and compulsions. Thus moderate internal consistency values such as those obtained for the M-PACI scales can be considered acceptable. This is especially true when criterion validity is strong, as the M-PACI results reported here indicate.

M-PACI scale intercorrelations showed that the Confident, Outgoing, and Conforming scales correlated positively among themselves and negatively overall with the remaining scales, which in turn were positively intercorrelated. Factor analysis yielded two readily interpretable factors, labeled Externalizing and Internalizing, that match a commonly applied scheme for classifying psychological problems into two broad categories. The M-PACI scales loaded on these two factors in a way that is consistent with how the scales were conceptualized. In this regard, the factor analysis results support the construct validity of the M-PACI as a whole.

The correlations of the M-PACI scales with the clinician ratings of the constructs measured by those scales showed very strong overall convergent and discriminant validity. Noteworthy from a test validation perspective, these results also seem to counter the skeptical views of the professionals surveyed by Loeber et al. (1990) regarding the value of preadolescents as informants on their own psychological problems. For example, whereas the Loeber et al. survey respondents rated information from preadolescents as only "slightly useful" in the evaluation of hyperactivity/inattentiveness and oppositional behaviors, the M-PACI Attention Deficits scale correlated .41 with the clinician ratings of attention deficits, and the M-PACI Disruptive Behaviors scale correlated .48 with its associated clinician rating variable.

In the Loeber et al. (1990) study, the surveyed professionals rated information from preadolescents as more useful in evaluating problems in the internalizing domain than in the three externalizing domains (hyperactivity/inattentiveness, oppositional behaviors, and conduct problems) about which they were asked. This reflects a widespread and logical view that children's reports of their own affective experiences can contribute unique information to the assessment of affective problems, whereas parent and teacher reports may offer more objectivity than child reports in the assessment of observable behaviors (e.g., see Johnston & Murray, 2003). In the M-PACI validation research, however, correlations with clinician ratings were actually somewhat higher overall for the scales that provided clear markers for the Externalizing factor (.57 for Unruly, .40 for Conduct Problems, .48 for Disruptive Behaviors) than for those loading most clearly on the Internalizing factor (.34 for Submissive, .50 for Inhibited, .37 for Depressive Moods, .46 for Anxiety/Fears). The most important point, however, is that all of these convergent validity correlations were substantial, reflecting both strong criterion validity for the M-PACI scales and the value of the self-reports of preadolescents concerning their own traits and problems.

In addition to the impressive pattern of correlations with the clinician ratings, the M-PACI scales also demonstrated strong correlations with conceptually related scales from the BASC SRP-C, the CDI, and the RCMAS. Overall, the data gathered for the development and initial validation of the M-PACI indicate that the inventory measures a number of important personality patterns and clinical signs with adequate reliability and strong validity. These results suggest that the M-PACI offers a useful addition to the somewhat scanty list of options for the multidimensional self-report assessment of 9- to 12-year-olds being seen in clinical settings.

References

American Psychiatric Association. (1994). *Diagnostic and statistical manual of mental disorders* (4th ed.). Washington, DC: Author.

American Psychiatric Association. (2000). *Diagnostic and statistical manual of mental disorders* (4th ed., text rev.). Washington, DC: Author.

Jackson, D. N. (1970). A sequential system for personality scale development. In C. D. Spielberger (Ed.), *Current topics in clinical and community psychology* (Vol. 2). New York: Academic Press.

Johnston, C., & Murray, C. (2003). Incremental validity in the psychological assessment of children and adolescents. *Psychological Assessment, 15,* 496–507.

Kovacs, M. (2001). *Children's Depression Inventory (CDI) technical manual.* North Tonawanda, NY: Multi-Health Systems.

Loeber, R., Green, S. M., & Lahey, B. B. (1990). Mental health professionals' perception of the utility of children, mothers, and teachers as informants on childhood psychopathology. *Journal of Clinical Child Psychology, 19,* 136–143.

Loevinger, J. (1957). Objective tests as instruments of psychological theory. *Psychological Reports, 3,* 635–694.

Merrell, K. W. (1999). *Behavioral, social, and emotional assessment of children and adolescents.* Mahwah, NJ: Erlbaum.

Millon, T. (1969). *Modern psychopathology.* Philadelphia: Saunders.

Millon, T. (1981). *Disorders of personality: DSM-III, Axis II.* New York: Wiley.

Millon, T. (1990). *Toward a new personology.* New York: Wiley.

Millon, T., & Davis, R. D. (1996). *Disorders of personality: DSM-IV and beyond* (2nd ed.). New York: Wiley.

Millon, T. (with Millon, C., Davis, R. D., & Grossman, S. D.). (2006a). *Millon Clinical Multiaxial Inventory–III (MCMI-III) manual* (3rd ed.). Minneapolis, MN: NCS Pearson.

Millon, T. (with Millon, C., Davis, R. D., & Grossman, S. D.). (2006b). *Millon Adolescent Clinical Inventory (MACI) manual* (2nd ed.). Minneapolis, MN: NCS Pearson.

Millon, T., Tringone, R., Millon, C., & Grossman, S. D. (2005). *Millon Pre-Adolescent Clinical Inventory (M-PACI) manual.* Minneapolis, MN: NCS Pearson.

Reynolds, C. R., & Kamphaus, R. W. (1998). *Behavior Assessment System for Children (BASC) manual.* Circle Pines, MN: American Guidance Service.

Reynolds, C. R., & Richmond, B. O. (2000). *Revised Children's Manifest Anxiety Scale (RCMAS) manual.* Los Angeles: Western Psychological Services.

CHAPTER 23

Using the Millon College Counseling Inventory (MCCI) in Student Services

Stephen Strack

The Millon College Counseling Inventory (MCCI; Millon, 2006c) is a new, multidimensional self-report questionnaire that was designed and normed specifically for today's college counseling population. The measure contains 150 items that are answered with a 5-point Likert format ranging from 1 = "never" to 5 = "always." The MCCI scales (see Table 23.1) include 11 Personality Styles (e.g., Introverted, Sociable, Borderline), 11 Expressed Concerns (e.g., Peer Alienation, Career Confusion), 10 Clinical Signs (e.g., Suicidal Tendencies, Anger Dyscontrol), and 4 Response Tendencies (e.g., Disclosure).

The MCCI provides comprehensive coverage of college students' psychological issues, distinguishing it from the single-construct assessment instruments that are commonly used with college students (Mowbray et al., 2006). Substantive scales cover three distinct but interrelated areas of psychological functioning. First, the Personality Styles scales measure a respondent's characteristic manner of thinking, feeling, and relating to the world. The personality styles measured by the MCCI were derived from Theodore Millon's (e.g., 1969; Millon & Davis, 1996; Strack, 2005) model of personality and psychopathology. Ten scales measure normal, nondisordered styles that are theoretically linked to more severe styles found in psychiatric settings. An 11th (Borderline) scale measures a clinically salient personality that is frequently found in students who exhibit serious difficulties with school adjustment.

TABLE 23.1. MCCI Scale Names and Brief Definitions

Scale group, abbreviation, and name	Brief definition
Personality	
1. Introverted	Nondisordered schizoid personality.
2A. Inhibited	Nondisordered avoidant personality.
2B. Dejected	Nondisordered depressive personality.
3. Needy	Nondisordered dependent personality.
4. Sociable	Nondisordered histrionic personality.
5. Confident	Nondisordered narcissistic personality.
6A Unruly	Nondisordered antisocial personality.
7. Conscientious	Nondisordered compulsive personality.
8A. Oppositional	Nondisordered negativistic personality.
8B. Denigrated	Nondisordered masochistic personality.
9. Borderline	Clinical borderline personality.
Expressed Concerns	
A. Mental Health Upset	Level of general dissatisfaction and unhappiness.
B. Identity Quandaries	Confusion or dissatisfaction with sense of self.
C. Family Disquiet	Problems with family of origin.
D. Peer Alienation	Unable to make friends; feelings of loneliness.
E. Romantic Distress	Problems with current relationship or unable to find a partner.
F. Academic Concerns	Problems with classes, coursework, and homework.
G. Career Confusion	Dissatisfaction with career plans; indecision.
H. Abusive Experiences	Problems with current or past abuse.
I. Living Arrangement Problems	Dissatisfaction with college living situation.
J. Financial Burdens	Difficulty with current finances; trouble managing funds.
K. Spiritual Doubts	Distress over religious or spiritual matters.
Clinical Signs	
AA. Suicidal Tendencies	Thoughts or intentions of self-harm.
BB. Depressive Outlook	Depressive mood and symptoms.
CC. Anxiety/Tension	Symptoms of generalized anxiety.
DD. Post-Traumatic Stress	Symptoms of post-traumatic stress disorder (PTSD).
EE. Eating Disorders	Potentially dangerous eating habits.
FF. Anger Dyscontrol	Trouble controlling or expressing anger.
GG. Attention (Cognitive) Deficits	Problems with concentration and attention.
HH. Obsessions/Compulsions	Unwanted repetitive or obsessive thoughts and behaviors.
II. Alcohol Abuse	Problematic drinking behavior.
JJ. Drug Abuse	Abuse of street drugs or prescription medicine.
Response Tendencies	
V. Validity	Attentiveness to item content and candid responding.
X. Disclosure	Overall level of self-disclosure.
Y. Desirability	Tendency to present self in a favorable light.
Z. Debasement	Tendency to present self in a negative light.

Second, the Expressed Concerns scales assess the kinds of problems that typically cause students to seek help at college counseling centers (e.g., romantic distress, academic concerns). Third, the Clinical Signs scales measure the degree of distress reported by students in clinically relevant content areas, such as suicidal thinking, depression, anxiety, and posttraumatic stress disorder (PTSD).

In this chapter, I provide a comprehensive overview of the MCCI. I describe the rationale for developing the measure; its theoretical derivation from Millon's (e.g., 1969; Millon & Davis, 1996) model; the test's construction and validation; and procedures for administering, scoring, and interpreting the measure. Finally, two case examples are offered that demonstrate how the MCCI can be used for initial assessment and planning treatment in college settings.

Rationale for Test Development

The MCCI was created in response to recent surveys showing that increasing numbers of college students require some kind of mental health assistance, and that the types of presenting concerns are more broad and complex than they were a generation ago (e.g., Benton, Robertson, Tseng, Newton, & Benton, 2003; Cornish, Riva, Henderson, Kominars, & McIntosh, 2000; Erdur-Baker, Aberson, Barrow, & Draper, 2006). Recognizing that available measures did not adequately address the range and severity of problems being brought to college counseling centers in the 21st century (e.g., suicidal behavior, PTSD, eating disorders; Mowbray et al., 2006), the test development team surveyed psychology staff members in several counseling centers in the United States and Canada about the gaps that needed to be filled, and asked them for a "wish list" of what they most wanted in a new assessment instrument. On the basis of these data, we created the MCCI to assess problems frequently seen among college students within the developmental framework offered by Millon (e.g., Millon & Davis, 1996).

Theoretical Derivation

The MCCI is part of a family of assessment instruments (see Millon, 1997; Strack, 2008) that operationalize Millon's (e.g., 1969, 1990, 1999, 2003a; Millon & Davis, 1996) evolutionary model of personality and psychopathology. Developed over a period of nearly 40 years, the model is an attempt to create a mature clinical science of personology that embodies five key elements (Millon, 2003a; Strack, 2005):

1. *Universal scientific principles*: Science grounded in the ubiquitous laws of nature.
2. *Subject-oriented theories*: Explanatory and heuristic conceptual schemas of nature's expression in what we call "personology" and "psychopathology."
3. A *taxonomy of personality patterns and clinical syndromes*: A classification and nosology derived logically from a coordinated personality–psychopathology theory.

4. *Integrated clinical and personality assessment instruments*: Tools that are empirically grounded and quantitatively sensitive.
5. *Synergistic therapeutic interventions*: Coordinated strategies and modalities of treatment.

Basic Personality Model

Millon's (1969) original biosocial learning theory of personality was presented in a graduate textbook titled *Modern Psychopathology*. There he proposed a threefold group of a priori axes, or dimensions, for conceptualizing types of people: active–passive, pleasure–pain, and self–other. The active–passive axis refers to whether an individual takes the initiative in shaping his or her environment to meet personal needs, or is largely reactive to what the environment brings. The pleasure–pain axis refers to how an individual is motivated toward events that are attractive and positively reinforcing, and away from events that are aversive or negatively reinforcing. The self–other axis refers to whether an individual finds primary gratification in the self or is motivated to derive pleasure from external sources. Using this framework, Millon derived personality coping patterns that, for him, characterize the typical operations and behaviors of various persons.

Learned coping patterns can be viewed as complex forms of instrumental behavior—that is, as ways of achieving positive reinforcements and avoiding negative reinforcements. The various strategies that people employ reflect which kinds of reinforcements they have learned to seek or avoid (pleasure–pain), where they look to obtain the reinforcers (self–other), and how they have learned to behave in order to elicit them (active–passive).

In deriving his personality patterns, Millon placed emphasis on whether the primary source of reinforcement is within the self or within others. Five types of people are distinguished in this area. "Dependent" persons have learned to rely on others for pleasure and avoidance of pain. Behaviorally, these persons display a strong need for external support and attention. Deprived of affection and nurturance they experience discomfort or pain. In contrast, "independent" personalities are those for whom dependence on self rather than others leads to maximum pleasure and minimum pain. In both these types of individuals, there tends to be a clear-cut reliance on self or others. However, not all persons demonstrate such strong commitments. "Ambivalent" persons remain uncertain about how to derive the most pleasure. Some vacillate between conformity one moment and independence the next; others display overt dependence and compliance while harboring strong desires to assert independence. A "detached" group is characterized by a diminished capacity to experience pleasure and pain or by a diminished ability to feel pleasurable reinforcers while being noticeably sensitive to pain. Finally, a "discordant" group shows a reversal on the pleasure–pain polarity (i.e., gratification is sought in pain directed toward the self or toward others).

Millon also emphasized the mode in which people instrumentally elicit reinforcements—that is, either actively or passively. Active persons tend to be alert, vigilant, persistent, decisive, and ambitious in goal-directed behavior. Passive persons engage in few overtly manipulative strategies to gain their ends. They often display a lack of ambition and persistence and show a resigned attitude in which they do little to shape events. They typically wait for the circumstances of their environment to take their course.

An Evolutionary Framework

In his 1990 book *Toward a New Personology*, Millon formally explicated the evolutionary foundation of his model. He sought to link the development and shaping of human personality over thousands of generations in reference to survival and reproduction, using concepts he described as "ecological adaptation" and "reproductive strategy." The concept of ecological adaptation is just a broader way of thinking about how people behave, adjust, and cope to achieve their personal goals (active vs. passive), while reproductive strategy is a broader way of thinking about an individual's goals for personal achievement (advancement of self vs. others). These evolutionary principles are demonstrated in four domains or spheres: "existence," "adaptation," "replication," and "abstraction."

> [A]n individual human organism must pass through four "stages" and must fulfill a parallel set of four "tasks" to perform adequately in life. . . . Each stage and task corresponds to one of four evolutionary phases: existence, adaptation, replication, and abstraction. Polarities . . . representing the first three of the phases (pleasure–pain, passive–active, other–self) have been used to construct a theoretically anchored classification of personality styles and disorders. . . .
>
> Within each stage, every individual acquires personologic dispositions representing a balance or predilection toward one of the two polarity inclinations; which inclination emerges as dominant over time results from the inextricable and reciprocal interplay of intraorganismic and extraorganismic factors. (Millon & Davis, 1996, p. 97)

The four evolutionary phases or stages, and tasks, may be described as follows (and are summarized in Table 23.2):

TABLE 23.2. A Developmental Framework for Personality

Evolutionary phase or stage	Polarity	Survival function	Neuropsychological stage	Developmental achievement
Existence	Pleasure–pain	Life enhancement/life preservation	Sensory–attachment	Trust
Adaptation	Active–passive	Ecological modification/ecological accommodation	Sensorimotor–autonomy	Self-confidence
Replication	Other–self	Progeny nurturance/individual propagation	Pubertal–genital identity	Gender identity and sex role
Abstraction	Thinking–feeling	Intellective reasoning/affective resonance	Intracortical integration	Balance of reason and emotion

Note. Adapted from Millon and Davis (1996, p. 110). Copyright 1996 by John Wiley & Sons, Inc. Adapted by permission.

1. *Existence.* A human being's first task is to survive. Evolutionary mechanisms associated with this stage relate to the processes of life enhancement and life preservation. The former processes are concerned with orienting individuals toward improving the quality of life; the latter involve orienting individuals away from actions and environments that decrease the quality of life or jeopardize existence. These superordinate categories may be called "existential aims" and are related to the polarity of pleasure–pain. A person's survival strategy is initially learned during the first year of life—what Millon (Millon & Davis, 1996) calls the "sensory-attachment" phase. Developing a reliable survival strategy is partly a consequence of being able to trust those upon whom one depends, and a willingness to share that trust with others.

2. *Adaptation.* Once survival is assured, human beings learn to adapt to their environment through ecological accommodation and ecological modification—modes of being that are associated with passive–active behavior and coping strategies. These modes of adaptation refer to a person's tendency to move away from conflicts or problems (i.e., to be passive and compliant in response to challenges), versus moving toward them with the goal of confronting and/or changing them. Learning to adapt to one's environment is a complex process that begins roughly in the second year of life—what Millon (Millon & Davis, 1996) calls the "sensorimotor/autonomy" stage—and may extend several years, although many individuals develop effective and often habitual adaptation patterns by the age of 5. Secure self-confidence is an important outcome of healthy adaptation.

3. *Replication.* Successful personal development includes the ability to leave offspring who themselves survive to reproduce. Millon believes that we develop a preference for either a self-propagating or other-nurturing strategy to achieve this aim. Linked to the self–other polarity and Millon's (Millon & Davis, 1996) "pubertal/gender identity" stage of development (roughly 11–15 years of age), these modes of being are exemplified by tendencies toward self-advancement and agency in interpersonal pursuits, versus a preference for communality and nurturance. A secure gender identity and sex role orientation are major consequences of achieving a balance in this realm.

4. *Abstraction.* The first three evolutionary phases are common to other species, but human beings are unique in developing higher cortical functions that permit, among other things, complex language and reasoning. During the ages of 4 to 18—Millon's (Millon & Davis, 1996) "intracortical integration" stage—people develop preferences for intellective reasoning or affective resonance in processing internal and external information. These preferences represent a thinking–feeling polarity exemplified by an inclination toward mental manipulation and abstraction in problem solving, versus a tendency to use emotions and intuition to tackle issues of personal import. Achieving a balance in the use of reasoning and emotion is a sign of success in this developmental arena.

Concepts of Normality and Pathology

An individual's success in achieving a healthy adult personality is due to many factors, including his or her genetic makeup, family environment, and sociocultural influences. In spite of the many vicissitudes that can cause human development to go awry, the vast majority of persons achieve a relatively healthy lifestyle that permits normal adjustment and personal fulfillment. In Millon's (Millon & Davis, 1996) model, the major difference between "normal" and "abnormal" personality is the rigidity and maladaptiveness of the latter. Normal persons are balanced on the three bipolar dimensions; that is, they are capable of both active and passive adaptation, mildly motivated toward pleasure and away from pain, and gratified by both self and others. Pathological persons are unbalanced on the polarities; that is, they are overly passive or active, strongly motivated to avoid pain but not seek pleasure (or to seek pain and avoid pleasure), and overly reliant on self or others. Normal and abnormal personalities lie along a continuum, such that there is no sharp dividing line between the two types.

> When an individual displays an ability to cope with his environment in a flexible and adaptive manner and when his characteristic perceptions and behaviors foster increments in personal gratification, then he may be said to possess a normal and healthy personality pattern. (Millon & Davis, 1996, p. 222)

By contrast, disordered persons tend to exhibit (1) tenuous stability, or a lack of resilience under conditions of stress; (2) an inability to respond flexibly and appropriately to internal and external demands; and (3) a tendency to foster vicious cycles of pathological behavior (Millon, 1969; Millon & Davis, 1996).

Derivation of Personality Prototypes

In *Disorders of Personality: DSM-IV and Beyond* (Millon & Davis, 1996) and the manual for the Millon Clinical Multiaxial Inventory–III (MCMI-III; Millon, 2006b), Millon described how his model allows for the derivation of 11 basic and 3 severe personality patterns, or "prototypes." The 11 basic prototypes are believed to be present in both normal and disordered forms, while the severe styles are believed to be exaggerations and distortions of the basic styles and do not have their roots in normal human development. The entire set of prototypes was created by combining the nature (pleasure–pain) and source (self–other) of reinforcements with the behavioral strategy (active–passive) utilized in obtaining reinforcements; the five coping strategies described earlier (detached, dependent, independent, ambivalent, and discordant); and two evolutionary variables—that is, existential aim (life enhancement vs. life preservation) and replication strategy (reproductive propagation vs. reproductive nurturance).

MCCI Personality Styles

In adult psychiatric settings, it is appropriate to measure each of Millon's (Millon & Davis, 1996) 11 basic and 3 severe personality prototypes, and to focus on disordered trait characteristics (e.g., as in the MCMI-III). For a college counseling population, we followed a strategy used for other Millon measures that were designed for nonpsychiatric populations, such as the Millon Behavioral Medicine Diagnostic (MBMD; Millon, Antoni, Millon, Meagher, & Grossman, 2001) and the Millon Index of Personality Styles *Revised* (MIPS *Revised*; Millon, 2003b). Namely, we

TABLE 23.3. MCCI Personality Styles Scales within Millon's Evolutionary Framework

Coping style →	Existential aim		Replication strategy		
	Life enhancement	Life preservation	Reproductive propagation		Reproductive nurturance
	Detached	Discordant	Dependent	Independent	Ambivalent
Passive adaptation	1. Introverted 2B. Dejected	8B. Denigrated	3. Needy	5. Confident	7. Conscientious
Active adaptation	2A. Inhibited		4. Sociable	6A. Antisocial	8A. Oppositional
Severe pattern		9. Borderline	9. Borderline		9. Borderline

Note. The Borderline personality is included in multiple columns because it is formed from subgroups of traits found in the basic personality styles and may be expressed in different ways, depending on the makeup of the trait subgroup. Adapted from Millon (2006b, p. 16). Copyright 1990, 1994 by DICANDRIEN. Adapted by permission.

assessed primarily normal traits and included measures for only those personality styles that were evident in sufficient numbers to justify separate scales. The MCCI includes scales for 10 basic personality styles and 1 severe style. Our survey of college counseling centers indicated that Millon's aggressive/sadistic, schizotypal, and paranoid prototypes were rarely evident, and so scales for these styles were not included. Table 23.3 presents the MCCI Personality Styles scale numbers and names as they fit into Millon's evolutionary framework.

Relating Personality to Expressed Concerns and Clinical Signs

In Millon's (1990, 2003a; Millon & Davis, 1996) model, personality is an evolution-based, centrally organized (and organizing) system of perceiving, interpreting, and managing internal and external demands of all kinds. It is the executive system by which humans adapt to their environment:

> Persons are the only organically integrated system in the psychological domain, evolved through the millennia and inherently created from birth as natural entities rather than culture-bound and experience-derived gestalts. The intrinsic cohesion of persons is not merely a rhetorical construction but an authentic substantive unity. Personologic features may often be dissonant and may be partitioned conceptually for pragmatic or scientific purposes, but they are segments of an inseparable biopsychosocial entity. (Millon, 2003a, p. 951)

Because of this, personality may be used to grasp and understand the kinds of stressors people will find most difficult to cope with, and the kinds of symptoms they are likely to exhibit when in distress:

> The events a person perceives as threatening or rewarding, and the behaviors and mechanisms he or she employs in response to them, reflect a long history of interwoven biogenic and psychogenic factors that have formed the person's basic personality pattern. (Millon & Davis, 1996, pp. 237–238)

Development of the MCCI Expressed Concerns and Clinical Signs scales was guided by these principles. The Expressed Concerns scales measure problems that are frequently experienced by students who seek help at college counseling centers. Each scale covers a specific content area (e.g., identity, family, peers) and measures the degree of distress expressed by the student in that area. The Clinical Signs scales were designed to measure the kinds of symptoms (e.g., anxiety, depression, anger) experienced by students in response to the problems they are grappling with.

In accordance with Millon's (Millon & Davis, 1996) model, which hypothesizes inherent overlap among the personality prototypes and among personality styles, problems in living, and symptom expression, test items were keyed on multiple scales across the three sets of MCCI measurement domains in a theoretically consistent manner. For example, item 53, which asks whether the respondent feels too upset to function, is included on the Borderline (Personality Styles) scale, the Mental Health Upset (Expressed Concerns) scale, and the Depressive Outlook (Clinical Signs) scale because of a hypothesized link among these constructs.

Taken together, scales from the three MCCI substantive domains give test users theoretically cohesive, multidimensional portraits of college counseling clients in terms of their characteristic manner of thinking, feeling, and behaving in a specific sociocultural milieu (Personality Styles); the kinds of problems they are grappling with at college (Expressed Concerns); and the symptoms they experience in response to the problems (Clinical Signs).

Test Construction and Validation

Definitions for constructs of the MCCI's substantive scales were developed from Millon's (e.g., 1969; Millon & Davis, 1996) model, as well as recommendations from counselors practicing in the field. A pool of items was created to measure each construct, and the pool was later refined to eliminate unclear, overly complex, and redundant stems. A research form was then created with 177 provisional items; this form also included a section asking counselors to rate the problems they felt to be most salient for the student taking the inventory. The research form was distributed to 33 college counseling centers across the United States, and completed test protocols were obtained from 562 students ranging in age from 17 to 45. Data were gathered from a wide variety of clients who took the MCCI either at initial presentation or after entering counseling for a period of time.

Test and counselor rating data were divided into two matched groups. The larger group ($n = 364$) was used for scale construction, while the smaller group ($n = 200$) was used for cross-validation. Substantive scales were developed to maximize internal consistency and expected correlational patterns based on Millon's (e.g., 1969; Millon & Davis, 1996) model and counselor ratings. They were created to contain a set of "primary" or "prototype" items (assessing features that are central to each construct and that do not overlap with other constructs), as well as "secondary" items (measuring characteristics that typically overlap with other constructs). Primary items were given a weight of 2 when endorsed, and secondary items a weight of

1 when endorsed. Number of items for scales ranged from 3 to 9, with a raw score range of 0 to 56.

Raw scores for substantive scales were transformed into "prevalence scores" (PSs), using combined-gender norms of the total sample (N = 562). PSs are different from percentiles and T-scores, which equalize scores across scales and may mask differences in how traits and symptoms are distributed in a given population. PSs on the MCCI reflect the counselor-estimated prevalence of traits and symptoms in the norm sample. Raw test scores were calibrated so that the percentage of clients receiving scores ≥ 75 would reflect the actual numbers estimated in the MCCI normative sample. Three MCCI Response Tendencies scales (X, Y, Z) were transformed into percentile scores rather than PSs, because these do not measure traits or symptoms. The MCCI Validity scale was not transformed and is used as a raw score.

Following scale development, the cross-validation sample was used to verify scale stability, clinical validity, and appropriate relationships with other measures. Internal consistency (coefficient alpha) ranged from .58 to .87 (mean = .77), with 26 of 32 substantive scales having alpha coefficients $\geq .70$. The lowest reliability figure was obtained for Career Confusion, which has only three items. Convergent validity estimates were calculated from correlations of scale scores and counselor ratings for the presence of each trait or symptom cluster. Values ranged from .40 (Sociable and Romantic Distress) to .03 (Unruly), with average correlations being consistent across the three sets of scales: Personality Styles = .23, Expressed Concerns = .21, Clinical Signs = .25. All but four scales attained a significant association with the counselor ratings (i.e., Unruly, Financial Burdens, Spiritual Doubts, and Attention [Cognitive] Deficits). When we examined the ratings for these four constructs, we found that these problems were rare in the normative sample and/or were difficult for counselors to appraise in students who had been seen only briefly.

Correlations with self-report measures were obtained for the Beck Depression Inventory–II (BDI-II; Beck, Steer, & Brown, 1996; n = 88), the State–Trait Anxiety Inventory (STAI; Spielberger, 1983; n = 52), and the Alcohol Use Inventory (AUI; Horn, Wanberg, & Foster, 1990; n = 44). The BDI-II was moderately associated ($r \geq \pm.40$) with 21 of 32 substantive scales, with the highest values obtained for Mental Health Upset and Depressive Outlook (r = .72). The STAI State scale was moderately associated ($r \geq \pm.40$) with 12 MCCI scales, while the Trait scale was moderately linked ($r \geq \pm.40$) to 19 MCCI scales. Mental Health Upset obtained the highest value with the State scale (r = .59), while the Dejected and Denigrated scales obtained the highest values with the Trait scale (r = .74). The AUI General scale was moderately linked ($r \geq \pm.40$) to 5 MCCI scales, with the strongest association found for the Alcohol Abuse scale (r = .65).

The MCCI manual (Millon, 2006c) provides additional information about test development and validation that should be considered by all users of the inventory. Our initial appraisal of the instrument from a psychometric standpoint indicated that the test scales are appropriately linked to Millon's (e.g., 1969; Millon & Davis, 1996) model of personality and psychopathology, and show promising reliability and validity. Research is currently underway to assess the test–retest stability of the scales and to collect additional convergent–discriminant validity data.

Recommendations for Using the MCCI

The MCCI was designed to help counselors identify, predict, and understand a broad range of psychological issues that are common among college students (ages 16 to 40 years) seen primarily in college counseling settings. It is recommended that clinicians working outside college counseling centers administer either the Millon Adolescent Clinical Inventory (Millon, 2006a) or the MCMI-III (Millon, 2006b) to college students. Although the MCCI may be helpful for clinicians who are working with college-age patients, caution should be used in interpreting the results, since the MCCI was normed on students who sought therapy exclusively at college counseling centers (not at a hospital or private practice).

Administration of the MCCI can be beneficial at many points during the assessment and treatment process: as part of the initial psychological assessment, to gauge progress and reevaluate issues during the course of treatment, and as a treatment outcome measure. Because the inventory is quick (20–30 minutes) and easy for most college students to complete, and easy to administer, score, and interpret, it can be useful in a wide variety of clinical circumstances at college counseling centers. Whenever the MCCI is administered, users are cautioned to examine students' responses to critical items before allowing them to leave the testing area, as these may identify dangerous behavior (e.g., suicidal tendencies and substance abuse) and circumstances (e.g., being stalked on campus) that require immediate attention.

Although the MCCI can help identify a student's personality style and clinical signs *at the time of assessment*, it is important for the counselor to keep in mind that even the most well-adjusted college students will question their identities and undergo stress, due to the fact that many are living away from home for the first time and experiencing a lifestyle quite different from what they were used to. For that reason, the MCCI is better viewed as a tool to help *understand* a student's current condition than as an aid to diagnosing him or her.

The MCCI should not be the sole source of information used for problem identification, treatment planning, placement, or other conclusions or decisions about a student. As any evaluation of anyone does, a competent psychological evaluation of a college student requires integrating information from multiple sources. Such sources may include interviews with the student and family members, school records, rating forms, and the results of other psychological tests.

Administration and Scoring

Test Administration

The MCCI was designed for use as part of a clinical assessment for college students who are receiving counseling services at college counseling centers. A student should complete the inventory in a mental state that will allow him or her to concentrate for the 20 to 30 minutes (or less) that are needed. If the student appears to be distracted, highly anxious, confused, fatigued, or under the influence of medication, it is best to postpone MCCI administration until a later time.

Obtaining meaningful MCCI results also depends on a student's willingness to complete the inventory seriously and honestly. Thus it is important to establish rapport with the student concerning the purpose of the inventory. In some cases, establishing rapport with the parents or guardians may also be important to gaining the student's cooperation.

The MCCI was designed to be nonthreatening. It can be presented as a brief inventory that is used to help the counselor better understand the student's thoughts and feelings. Questions about the use of MCCI results should be answered forthrightly.

The MCCI can be administered with a paper-and-pencil booklet or by computer (using Pearson Assessments software). An audio CD is available for students who have visual handicaps or limited reading skills. The paper-and-pencil booklet that is used to administer the MCCI inventory includes an answer sheet. No materials other than the computer software are required for computer administration.

Instructions for completing the MCCI are printed in the booklet or presented on the computer screen and are self-explanatory. However, it is good practice to read the directions aloud while the student follows along and to ask whether the student has any questions. It is usually not necessary for the administrator to monitor the student closely while he or she is completing the inventory. However, the administrator should remain readily available in case the student needs assistance. In some special circumstances, continuous monitoring may be required. There is no time limit for completing the MCCI; however, the student should be encouraged to work quickly without rushing.

If paper-and-pencil administration is used, the administrator should immediately check the completed answer sheet for omitted or multiple-marked responses (i.e., marked a 0 and a 1). If any are found, the student should be encouraged to provide a valid response. In keeping with the directions for the inventory, students should be encouraged to be as honest as they can and try to respond to every statement, even if they are not sure of their choices.

Scoring the MCCI

The inventory can be scored by computer or by hand. Computer scoring of the MCCI offers the highest level of accuracy. Also, computer scoring is required to obtain an Interpretive Report. MCCI users who score the inventory by computer have one report option. The MCCI Interpretive Report includes both the score profile and in-depth interpretive text.

Although hand-scoring the MCCI inventory is straightforward, the human element inevitably increases the possibility of errors. If hand scoring is used, it is recommended that each inventory be scored twice to help ensure accuracy. The materials required for hand scoring include a combined test booklet and answer sheet, the MCCI test manual, a set of plastic overlays (keys) for determining raw scale scores, and a profile form for recording and plotting the scores.

Interpretation of the MCCI

The task of interpreting results from the MCCI is similar to that for other Millon inventories (e.g., the MCMI-III [Millon, 2006b] and the MIPS *Revised* [Millon,

2003b]; see also Strack, 2008). The professional examining the findings goes through a series of steps: a review of available client information; an assessment of MCCI test validity; an appreciation of the respondent's style of responding to the test; an examination of individual scale elevations, critical items, and noteworthy responses (for users of the computer-generated test report); a summary of results that brings together the respondent's personality style, presenting problems, and clinical symptoms; and then integration of findings from the MCCI with results from other assessment measures.

Reviewing Client Information

MCCI test results should not be examined without considering all available information about the student. Prior to assessing the test findings, a counselor should review the respondent's demographic data, background characteristics, and school records; the reason for presentation; and any interview, observation, and test data collected prior to administration of the MCCI.

Assessing Test Validity

The MCCI is not scorable if eight or more items have been left blank or have been marked with multiple answers. To avoid unscorable tests, it is advisable for the administrator to review the student's answer sheet before he or she leaves the testing room, and ask the individual to complete the omitted information or correct the item responses that have multiple marks.

The MCCI Validity (V) scale consists of three items (18, 72, 129). Two of these assess highly improbable events, and the third asks the client whether he or she is deliberately giving inaccurate answers to the inventory. When any of these items is endorsed 2, 3, or 4, one point is added to the V scale score. If V = 0, the inventory is considered valid. If V = 1, the inventory is considered to be of questionable validity. In these cases, the examiner should assess whether the results can be interpreted. Asking the respondent to explain his or her rationale for giving the particular response is usually sufficient. Often the student was uncertain about the meaning of the item, or intended to mark 0 but gave another response. If V = 2 or 3, the MCCI is considered invalid, and no interpretation should be made.

MCCI results are also considered invalid when the client produces a "flat" profile. This rare event occurs when all of the Personality Styles scales have PSs < 60, all of the Expressed Concerns scales have PSs < 65, and all of the Clinical Signs scales have PSs < 65. This would indicate that the student has revealed so little about him- or herself that the test findings may be seriously inaccurate. When this circumstance arises, the examiner can often obtain valid test results by having the client take the MCCI again, with encouragement to answer openly and honestly.

Evaluating the Client's Response Style

An appreciation of the student's style of responding to the MCCI is valuable for interpreting the substantive scales. Because the MCCI was developed and normed for students seeking help at college counseling centers, the typical response styles of counseling center clients are reflected in the PS transformations that are used for test interpretation. In general, we expect that students who come to college counseling centers for help have problems they wish to make known, and that they are motivated to accept treatment. We would expect from these clients a typical response style where they are relatively open in revealing information about themselves, offer details about problem areas, and minimize the presentation of positive features.

The MCCI has three scales to help users understand each client's style of responding: Disclosure (X), Desirability (Y), and Debasement (Z). These were modeled after the Modifying Indices of the MCMI-III (Millon, 2006b). Raw scores for respondents on these scales are converted to *percentile* scores, based on the distribution of scores obtained by members of the MCCI norm group. Percentile scores are different from the PSs used for the substantive scales. Whereas PSs are anchored to the prevalence rates of various personality styles, expressed concerns, and clinical signs, percentile scores reflect a simple, linear transformation of the raw scores that does not change the underlying distribution. Thus, when a student obtains a percentile score of 30 on scale X, Y, or Z, his or her score is higher than that for 29% of the normative sample, and lower than that for 69% of the sample. When a student obtains a percentile score of 70 on one of these same scales, his or her score is higher than that for 69% of the normative sample and lower than that for 29% of the sample. For scales X, Y, and Z, 60% of respondents will obtain percentile scores between 20 and 80. Only 20% will have scores ≤ 20, and only 20% will have scores ≥ 80.

Disclosure (X) Scale

The Disclosure (X) scale is a composite of responses given to seven of the Personality Styles scales. It was intended to be a broad measure of self-disclosure across all content areas of the test. In college counseling settings, most respondents will produce scores on this scale in the percentile range of 20–80, indicating that they disclosed a significant amount of information on the MCCI. In these cases, scores on the substantive scales will accurately reflect the student's personality traits, presenting problems, and clinical symptoms.

A very high score on scale X (percentile ≥ 90) indicates that the client was indiscriminate in reporting on his or her traits, feelings, attitudes, and behaviors. Resulting PS scores on the Personality Styles, Expressed Concerns, and Clinical Signs scales may be *inflated*. Experience with other Millon inventories (e.g., the MCMI-III) suggests that most people who obtain highly elevated X scores (1) were confused about how to respond, (2) tried too hard to self-disclose, or (3) were in significant distress at the time they completed the test and overreported their symptoms. Examination of the Y and Z scale scores may assist in clarifying the student's motivation. In some cases, it may be worthwhile to interview the client and ask him or her to retake the test in order to obtain more reliable results.

A very low score on scale X (percentile ≤ 10) indicates that the respondent was hesitant in revealing information about him- or herself across many areas. Very low scores suggest that the MCCI Personality Styles, Expressed Concerns, and Clinical Signs scale scores will *underestimate* the student's true levels of traits, concerns, and symptoms. Test interpreters should keep this in mind when making conclusions about the respondent, in order to avoid incorrectly deciding that a problem does not exist when, in fact, the client was reticent in disclosing information. When the scale X percentile score is very low, it is advisable to interview the student about his or her approach to the test. Encouraging the client to retake the test in a more open manner may yield more accurate results.

Desirability (Y) Scale

Some individuals are motivated to present themselves in an especially favorable light. Although a positive self-presentation is expected in some social situations (e.g., a job interview), it is unusual among people who are seeking help for personal problems. The MCCI Desirability (Y) scale was designed to detect test protocols that were answered with a favorable bias. The Y scale contains nine items assessing personal virtues. Most college counseling clients will obtain percentile scores on this scale ranging from 20 to 80. Scores in this range indicate that the respondent was able to recognize and report on a modest number of positive personal qualities. Scores in this range are expected and should not affect the PSs on the substantive scales.

A very high Y scale score (percentile ≥ 90) suggests that the respondent was motivated to present him- or herself in an overly positive manner. Experience with the MCMI-III in clinical populations indicates that most people who obtain high scores on this scale do so because they have a compensatory need to exhibit their positive qualities in situations where this is not called for. These clients don't want professionals to miss their positive virtues and have a tendency to exaggerate these in order to make them known. By itself, this is not a problematic response style. It becomes problematic if the client is also unwilling to self-disclose and reveal the nature of his or her problems on the MCCI. An examination of scales X and Z will be useful in making this assessment. A high Y scale score, in the presence of low elevations on scales X and/or Z, indicates that the respondent has biased his or her self-report by underdisclosing. Results are likely to *underestimate* the client's true level of traits, problems, and symptoms.

Y scale scores in the 10–20 range are not uncommon in settings where people are presenting for help, as most of these individuals have focused their efforts on revealing problems. In general, such scores do not indicate low self-esteem or low levels of personal virtue. However, when the Y score is very low (percentile ≤ 10) in the presence of elevated X and/or Z scores, this is further indication that the client disclosed a large amount of information (X) that was primarily negative in nature (Z), and may signal *overreporting* of traits, problems, and symptoms.

Debasement (Z) Scale

Students who present for help with personal problems are expected to endorse a significant number of items with unfavorable or unpleasant content. The Debasement (Z) scale consists of 22 items with generally negative content. Most respondents will obtain Z percentile scores in the range of 20–80, reflecting their admission of personal problems. A very high Z score (percentile ≥ 90) indicates that the respondent may have overreported negative personal features, resulting in inflated PSs on the Personality Styles, Expressed Concerns, and Clinical Signs scales. Experience with the MCMI-III tells us that highly elevated Z scores are produced by clients who are significantly distressed, confused, or motivated to present themselves in an especially negative light (e.g., to obtain disability benefits). Regardless of the reason for the elevated Z score, it is likely that the substantive MCCI scale scores will also be inflated. Interviewing the client will be helpful in determining the reason for the negative bias. Having the student retake the MCCI may yield more accurate results.

As on the X scale, a very low Z score (percentile ≤ 10) indicates that the respondent has underreported his or her personal problems, and signals that most or all of the Personality Styles, Expressed Concerns, and Clinical Signs scores will be artificially low. To avoid errors in making conclusions about the client, when Z is very low we recommend that the student be interviewed about his or her response style—and, if possible, that the student retake the test with encouragement to be more open and honest.

Understanding the Client's Personality Style

In Millon's (Millon & Davis, 1996) model, a full understanding of an individual's problems and symptoms is only possible with a thorough appreciation of his or her characteristic manner of thinking, feeling, and behaving—that is, his or her personality style. Once the client's test-taking approach is evaluated by using scales X, Y, and Z, his or personality style can be assessed by reviewing the Personality Styles scale scores and using the highest two or three scales to create a portrait of the person. The highest scores constitute a framework for understanding a client's self-image, cognitive style, sociability, temperament, mood, interests, and interpersonal style.

Although the Personality Styles scale scores may be interpreted individually, the vast majority of persons will be better served by a portrait that integrates characteristics of the two or three most prominent scales. To interpret individual personality scales, the descriptions given in Table 23.4 may serve as a starting point. These summaries describe Millon's (Millon & Davis, 1996) personality prototypes—that is, personality styles made up of only one cluster of traits. The prototypes allow us to envision how someone might look if he or she exhibited only one set of highly stereotyped characteristics. The prototype descriptions are useful as teaching tools, as they provide easy mnemonics for grasping what idealized personalities (e.g., introverted, inhibited) might be like. They can be used for interpreting MCCI profiles when only one personality scale is prominent (20 PS points above all other such scales).

Most people exhibit a mixture of traits from more than one personality prototype. Clinical experience has shown that for most purposes, a personality portrait based on the highest two or three scales provides enough detail to give reliable and valid information about the respondent. To select the personality scales for interpretation, the evaluator should order the Personality Styles scores from highest to lowest, noting their elevation above the median and in relation to each other. The highest-scoring scale will serve as the base for the overall interpretation, whereas the second highest scale is given secondary importance, and the third highest scale is given tertiary importance.

When deciding on whether to use two or three scales for interpretation, the evaluator should consider whether the third scale is close in elevation to the other two, and whether it adds significantly to the person's portrait. When three scales are close

TABLE 23.4. Interpretation of Elevated MCCI Personality Styles, Expressed Concerns, and Clinical Signs Scales

Personality Styles scales

Scale 1—Introverted

These persons are low-keyed, quiet, and unassuming. They prefer distant or limited involvement with others and have little interest in social activities. Others view them as being easygoing, mild-mannered, and methodical, lacking in spontaneity and resonance, and awkward or timid in group situations. They frequently see themselves as being simple and unsophisticated, and are usually modest in appraising their own skills and abilities. At school these people do well on their own, are typically dependable and reliable, are nondemanding, and are seldom bothered by noise or commotion around them. They are often viewed as level-headed and calm. However, individuals with this personality style do not respond well if asked to assume leadership positions or participate actively in groups.

Scale 2A—Inhibited

Inhibited persons tend to be hesitant with others and are often shy and ill at ease in social situations. They anticipate that others will be critical or rejecting of them, and because of this they frequently seem skittish in unfamiliar surroundings. In this regard, fellow students and acquaintances may see them as being unnecessarily nervous, wary, and fearful. Although inhibited persons tend to get along reasonably well with others, they are often difficult to get to know on a personal level. These individuals usually wish that they could be at ease with others and tend to desire closeness, but they often are just too uncertain of the consequences of closeness and intimacy to let their guard down. As a result, they may experience feelings of loneliness, but be unable or unwilling to do anything about them. Because of their sensitivity to others, inhibited persons are often described as kind, considerate, and empathic by close acquaintances. Inhibited persons often prefer to work alone or in a small group with people they can come to know well. They do best in stable environments where stimulation and commotion are kept at low to moderate levels.

Scale 2B—Dejected

Individuals with this personality style are marked by a pessimistic and gloomy attitude toward themselves and others. They often appear heavy-hearted and frequently have a poor self-image and low self-esteem. They are socially withdrawn and prefer limited involvement with others. Fellow students and family find them to be serious, quiet, passive, deliberate, and slow-paced. They seem to worry and brood over minor concerns, and limit themselves to tasks and circumstances where they can be fairly certain of the outcome. These individuals are sometimes experienced by others as being perfectionistic, because they tend to be fault-finding and are difficult to please. Nevertheless, they have difficulty expressing their feelings openly, even with close friends. They often seek support and reassurance from others, but their tendency to be negative makes it difficult for them to be accepted by others. Like inhibited persons, dejected individuals usually prefer to work alone or in a small group with people they can come to know well. They do best in environments where there are few changes, where tasks are clearly spelled out, and where fellow students and teachers will be appreciative of their sensitive nature.

Scale 3—Needy

Needy persons can be identified by an easygoing personal style and a willingness to live in accord with the desires of others. They adapt their behavior to the standards of others in an effort to obtain attention and approval. Interpersonally, these individuals are often cooperative, reliable, considerate of others, and deferential. They may appear even-tempered, docile, obliging, self-effacing, ingratiating, or naive. Needy individuals often see themselves as being modestly endowed in terms of skills and abilities. They are often pleased when they can rely on others and may feel insecure when left on their own. Especially when faced with difficult or stressful situations, needy persons seek others to provide authority, leadership, and direction. They often prefer group over solitary work environments and will typically excel in them if given support and guidance. Known as team players who thrive in

(continued)

TABLE 23.4. *(continued)*

vigorous social environments, these individuals perform best in supportive work roles under the guidance of strong leaders. These individuals are usually uncomfortable being assertive and often avoid problems, rather than facing them head-on.

Scale 4—Sociable

Sociable individuals are characterized by an outgoing, talkative, and extraverted style of behavior, and tend to be lively, dramatic, and colorful. They are typically viewed by others as spontaneous, clever, enthusiastic, and vigorous. They can be quite sensitive to the needs and wants of people in their immediate environment, at least to those aspects that will help them get the attention they seek. Sociable individuals often have quickly shifting moods, can be fickle in their likes and dislikes, and may come across as shallow and ungenuine. These persons prefer novelty and excitement, and are bored by ordinary or mundane activities. Like needy persons, sociable individuals seem uncomfortable or deflated when left on their own. Not surprisingly, sociable types often excel in group work environments where they can exercise their showy style. They are attentive to their appearance and keep a cheerful optimism, even in difficult circumstances. However, these individuals can be exasperating because of their quickly shifting interests and emotions. They find it difficult to stick with something once they have lost interest, and seldom hesitate to change loyalties if an alternative gives them more of what they want.

Scale 5—Confident

Cool, calm, and self-assured, individuals with this personality style come across as confident and unflappable. They may have a keen sense of their own importance and special talents. Confident individuals enjoy others' attention and may be quite bold socially, although they are seldom garish. They can be self-centered to a fault. They may become so preoccupied with themselves that they lack concern and empathy for others. These persons have a tendency to believe that others share, or should share, their sense of worth. As a result, they may expect others to submit to their wishes and desires, and to cater to them. Ironically, a confident individual's secure appearance may cover feelings of personal inadequacy and sensitivity to criticism and rejection. Unfortunately, they usually do not permit others to see their vulnerable side. When feeling exposed or undermined, these individuals are frequently disdainful, obstructive, or vindictive. In school settings, confident persons like to take charge in an emphatic manner, often doing so in a way that instills confidence in others. Their self-assurance, wit, and charm often win them leadership positions. They do equally well on their own and in social settings, but in groups they have a need to be "one up" and will often resist roles that place them in an equal or deferential position.

Scale 6A—Unruly

Unruly people are characterized by an impulsive, headstrong, and dominant personal style. They view the world as a harsh place where exploitiveness is needed to assure success, and frequently come across to others as blunt and insensitive. They typically place their own needs ahead of others and are not beneath bending or breaking rules to get what they want. In school settings, these persons are often driven to excel. They do well in circumstances where they can take control or work independently. Unruly persons usually have a strong, independent spirit that gives them an edge in situations requiring a steadfast pursuit of goals in difficult circumstances. Although they can tolerate group settings, these persons prefer to be outside the bounds of community rules and regulations. They are self-oriented and do not readily consider the needs of others. They seldom hesitate in stepping on toes, if doing so helps them achieve their ends.

Scale 7—Conscientious

Responsible, industrious, and respectful of authority, these individuals tend to be conforming and work hard to uphold rules and regulations. They have a need for order and are typically conventional in their interests. These individuals can be rule-abiding to a fault, however, and may be

(continued)

TABLE 23.4. *(continued)*

perfectionistic, inflexible, and judgmental. A formal interpersonal style and notable constriction of affect can make some conscientious persons seem cold, aloof, and withholding. Underneath their social propriety, there is often a fear of disapproval and rejection, or a sense of guilt over perceived shortcomings. Indecisiveness and an inability to take charge may be evident in some of these persons due to a fear of being wrong. However, conscientious persons are best known for being well organized, reliable, and diligent. They have a strong sense of duty and loyalty, are cooperative in group efforts, show persistence even in difficult circumstances, and work well under supervision.

Scale 8A—Oppositional

Oppositional persons tend to be unconventional and individualistic in their response to the world. They march to the beat of a different drummer and are frequently unhappy with the status quo. They may be quick to challenge rules or authorities that they deem arbitrary and unjust. They may also harbor resentment without expressing it directly and may revert to passive–aggressive behavior to make their feelings known. Many oppositional people feel as if they don't fit in, and view themselves as lacking in interpersonal skills. In fact, to others they often appear awkward, nervous, or distracted, and seem angry or dissatisfied with themselves and others. They can be indecisive and have fluctuating moods and interests. An air of uncertainty and general dissatisfaction may reflect an underlying dependency and sense of personal inadequacy. With their best side forward, oppositional persons can be spontaneous, creative, and willing to speak out for what they believe in. These qualities make them especially suited to school settings that are not rule-bound, that give them a certain independence from supervision, and that require unusual duties or creative expression.

Scale 8B—Denigrated

Individuals with this personality style often vacillate between selfless devotion to others and a negativistic, self-demeaning pattern of behavior. They tend to be naïvely idealistic and will persist in goal-directed activities that yield few or no positive outcomes. They seek communality and are willing to give 100% of themselves to further group goals. Because of this, others may be impressed by their devotion to serve and their tendency to be kind, considerate, and charitable. Always forgiving, they believe that people should be accepted for who and what they are. Although they put great effort into serving others, they do not like to be singled out. They feel awkward and uncomfortable if the spotlight is directed toward them, reflecting generally poor self-esteem. Denigrated individuals can be submissive to a fault and often ignore their own needs. Beneath their idealistic personae, these individuals are often quite pessimistic. They are frequently moody and irritable. They tend to view themselves as being awkward and lacking in social skills, and often wish they could rely on others for support and reassurance.

Scale 9 (Severe)—Borderline

Borderline persons are characterized by intense emotional displays and vacillation between positive and negative thoughts, feelings, attitudes, and behaviors. They seem to live life on a roller coaster. They seek novelty and excitement and are quickly swept up by the promise of sensational outcomes. They follow their feelings rather than their intellect, and are valued by friends and fellow students for being spontaneous and creative. Socially, these persons are lively and engaging, with an open mind toward experimentation. However, they are also changeable and usually do not stick with something once they have lost interest. Always ready for new opportunities, these persons seem to have a devil-may-care attitude toward the consequences of their behavior. They are characteristically impulsive and even reckless in their headstrong pursuit of what they desire. They often become quickly involved in new activities and relationships, and develop intense attachments that are quickly undone. Borderline persons do best in school environments that are loosely structured and not rule-bound, that give them independence, and that require unusual duties or creative expression.

(continued)

TABLE 23.4. *(continued)*

Expressed Concerns scales

Scale A—Mental Health Upset

Items for this scale measure a student's experience of current dissatisfaction and unhappiness. High scorers feel upset, moody, and confused. They may feel that they can't cope with daily demands, and may experience anxiety and dysphoria. The sense of unhappiness and inability to function adequately manifested by people who score high on this scale is general rather than specific (i.e., not tied to a particular area of concern).

Scale B—Identity Quandaries

Most college students are still developing their personal identity in such areas as personal beliefs, attitudes, religion, and sexuality. General and specific identity-related concerns are identified by this scale, which includes items inquiring about sexuality, self-esteem, feeling lonely and disconnected, and being confused about religious beliefs. High scorers may have trouble in one or more specific areas, so it is important to examine item responses when this scale is elevated.

Scale C—Family Disquiet

Students who obtain high scores on this scale are upset about problems with their family of origin. They may feel unsupported by family members or feel that their family places too many burdens on them. They may express insecurity about the support they receive (or expect to receive) from family members, or feel that things are unpredictable or chaotic at home.

Scale D—Peer Alienation

Many college students struggle to adapt to an unfamiliar social environment with new rules and expectations from peers. This scale assesses feelings of loneliness and alienation. High scorers report being socially isolated and unable to make friends. They may feel different from other students at school, believe that they are not accepted by others, or feel that the people accessible to them are undesirable as potential friends.

Scale E—Romantic Distress

Items for this scale target problems experienced by students in the realm of intimate relationships. High scale elevations are obtained by people who are experiencing emotional upheaval in a romantic relationship, the recent loss of a partner, or an inability to find a satisfactory partner.

Scale F—Academic Concerns

Students who score high on this scale are reporting general problems in managing the demands of their classes and coursework. They may feel too much pressure in balancing their course load and homework, feel overwhelmed by multiple assignments, and be unable to cope as well as they think they should.

Scale G—Career Confusion

Elevations on this scale are obtained by students who report that they are having problems in deciding on a career path. They may express a lack of support in formulating their choice, experience general indecision and confusion, or feel that they are torn between when they want and what their family members want.

Scale H—Abusive Experiences

Items for this scale measure a variety of content areas including current experiences of abuse (being stalked or abused by a partner), recent abuse (date rape), feeling vulnerable to abuse, the experience of traumatic flashbacks, and sleep disturbances due to recurrent memories of abuse. A review of item responses is important to understand the nature of the concerns being reported by the respondent.

(continued)

TABLE 23.4. *(continued)*

Scale I—Living Arrangement Problems

High scores on scale I are obtained by students who are experiencing difficulties with their college living environment and/or the people in it. They report being generally dissatisfied with where they live because of unsatisfactory conditions, too much noise or commotion, or conflicts with roommates.

Scale J—Financial Burdens

Students with elevated scores on this scale report that they are worried about general financial matters. They may fear being unable to pay their tuition and other school expenses, or find that they have to devote too much time to making money to pay debts. Some high scorers report that their schoolwork suffers as a result of their preoccupation and distress.

Scale K—Spiritual Doubts

All of the items in this scale tap general distress about spiritual and religious beliefs. High scorers report being preoccupied by doubts and confusion about their beliefs. They may be experiencing a spiritual crisis or feel turmoil over recent challenges to their belief system.

Clinical Signs scales

Scale AA—Suicidal Tendencies

This scale consists of two groups of items. One set asks about suicidal thoughts and intents, while the other assesses typical emotions for people who are preoccupied with thoughts of self-harm—namely, feeling lonely, unwanted, and worthless. People who score high on this scale are at risk for suicide because of active suicidal ideation or pervasive feelings of dysphoria. To determine level of risk for suicide, test users should carefully interview students who obtain high scale scores about such matters as past attempts, whether they have a clear plan to end their lives, and whether they have access to the means by which they plan to kill themselves.

Scale BB—Depressive Outlook

Students who score high on this scale may show signs of clinical depression. Items ask about mood and physical symptoms of depression. High scorers report that they feel sad, lonely, and dysphoric; lack energy and enthusiasm; get little pleasure from life; and may cry excessively.

Scale CC—Anxiety/Tension

Items for this scale assess generalized feelings of anxiety and tension. People who score high on this scale report being nervous, worried, and preoccupied with various troubles. They may be tense, unable to relax, and panicky. They may have obsessive thoughts and be unable to sleep. They may feel tired and worn out and be ineffective in managing daily demands.

Scale DD—Post-Traumatic Stress

Each item in scale DD taps a specific symptom of PTSD. Items assess nightmares, flashbacks, insomnia, anxiety, panic, and recurrent traumatic memories. High scorers are reporting intense disruptions in their emotional well-being due to anxious arousal, preoccupation with memories of trauma, and an inability to relax or sleep. Some people with elevated scores may be experiencing current traumatic abuse, while others may be reliving past experiences. Therefore, test users are advised to interview students with elevated scores to assess their safety.

Scale EE—Eating Disorders

This scale addresses potentially dangerous eating habits. Items assess bingeing and purging, self-starvation, erratic dieting, and generally poor eating patterns. Also covered are low self-esteem and

(continued)

TABLE 23.4. *(continued)*

worries about health, which often accompany eating disorders. High scores on this scale indicate eating problems of increasing severity, but test users will need to examine item responses to determine the exact nature of the problem identified.

Scale FF—Anger Dyscontrol

Students who score high on this scale report having trouble with expression and control of anger. They may feel irritable and annoyed, and be bossy toward others. They may have an angry attitude and feel that others taunt or bother them. They may express their anger verbally or behaviorally, and may have gotten into trouble recently because of the way they expressed their anger.

Scale GG—Attention (Cognitive) Deficits

Scale GG measures several symptoms found in people who have attention-deficit/hyperactivity disorder (ADHD). Elevations on this scale are obtained by students who are having trouble in school because they are unable to pay attention, concentrate, or sit still. They may be easily distracted and have trouble organizing themselves. They feel inefficient and sense that they are struggling more with their schoolwork than their peers.

Scale HH—Obsessions/Compulsions

This scale assesses cognitive control symptoms of a general obsessive–compulsive nature. High scorers report having repetitive or obsessive thoughts that won't go away. The content of these thoughts may be bothersome or innocuous, and students may feel compelled to act on what they are thinking. Some people may engage in compulsive behavior (e.g., frequent handwashing) or be preoccupied with fear of acting out unpleasant events that go through their minds. Symptoms of this type are experienced as being very disruptive. Students may report being unable to concentrate on their schoolwork, being inefficient because of the time required to act out compulsive behaviors, and being unable to have satisfactory relationships.

Scale II—Alcohol Abuse

Students who score high on this scale report problematic drinking behavior. They may drink excessively to cope with personal problems, drink to the point of drunkenness, use alcohol to calm their nerves in social situations, and/or have trouble controlling an impulse to drink. Some students who obtain high scores may be pressured by friends and family to reduce their drinking, but not all high scorers are ready to admit that they abuse alcohol and need to cut down or become abstinent.

Scale JJ—Drug Abuse

Items for this scale imply the use of illicit drugs (e.g., marijuana), but the problems reported by students may also be caused by misuse of prescription medications. High scorers indicate that drug use is part of their social life and may be causing trouble for them at school or with family. They may express an inability to cut down on their drug use, but, as with the Alcohol Abuse scale, high scorers on this scale may not be ready to admit that they have a substance abuse problem.

in elevation (within 5 PS points), it makes sense to interpret all three. When the third scale is fairly prominent (PS ≥ 75) but not necessarily close in elevation to the highest two scales, the evaluator should consider the prototype descriptions in Table 23.4 to see how the portrait based on the highest two scales would change if descriptors from the third prototype were added. In some cases the third scale will be very useful, and in other cases it will not. Experience in interpreting the MCCI will guide the user in how to make decisions in this realm.

Using two or three scales to develop a personality portrait is basically additive in nature. Characteristics of the most prominent personality style are used as an outline, and features of other prominent styles are brought in to fill in the picture. It is important to remember that with increasing PS elevations above 50, the likelihood that an individual will demonstrate the behaviors and characteristics represented by the prototype also increases. PS ≥ 75 suggests that the client has significantly more traits of the particular personality style than most other people, and that because of this, these traits will be quite salient to other people. In general, high personality scale scores suggest that the person has a strongly defined personal style that will be readily grasped by others. MCCI profiles where the highest personality scale scores are generally low (PS < 60) suggest that the client will exhibit a less well-defined set of trait characteristics. Note also that personality scales with similar elevations (within 5 PS points) should be weighed more equally in the interpretation than scales with quite different elevations.

In Millon's (Millon & Davis, 1996) model, an elevation on the severe personality style scale (i.e., Borderline) warrants special attention. This personality is viewed as more problematic than the basic personality prototypes. People who score high (PS ≥ 75) on the Borderline scale may exhibit features of a personality disorder. They may have low ego strength and be emotionally labile. They may experience significant symptoms of anxiety and dysphoria, and may have significant problems in school and with personal relationships. An examination of Expressed Concerns and Clinical Signs scales, and of noteworthy responses (for users of the computerized Interpretive Report), will help determine whether further scrutiny is warranted.

Identifying Areas of Expressed Concerns

Although for interpretive purposes it is best to examine the student's personality features before moving on to the other scales, the student's Expressed Concerns scores are most likely to explain why he or she is seeking help at this time. The MCCI's 11 Expressed Concerns scales cover problems frequently presented by students who seek help at college counseling centers: mental health concerns, identity issues, family and peer problems, concerns about romantic relationships, academic problems, career confusion, abusive experiences, living arrangement problems, financial hassles, and spiritual doubts. (See Table 23.4.)

All of the scales in this section were normed so that a PS of 50 represents the median for all college counseling clients, while PS ≥ 75 represent a cut-off for clinical significance. As a rule, any Expressed Concerns scale with PS ≥ 75 should be interpreted as representing a significant problem for the respondent. Higher scores indicate greater severity of distress and concern. Users of the computerized Interpretive

Report should consult the "Noteworthy Responses" section to identify specific problems that may not be represented in the scale scores. It is also advisable to review the item responses for elevated scales to ascertain the issues that are most bothersome for the client. For example, the Identity Quandaries and Abusive Experiences scales contain items that measure distinct facets of these problem areas. Only by examining the item responses will the counselor know whether an identity problem involves sexuality, low self-esteem, or religious beliefs, and whether an abusive event being reported involves current or past experiences.

When more than one Expressed Concern scale is elevated (PS ≥ 75), it is useful to rank-order them in the test report so that the scale with the highest elevation is addressed first, followed by scales with lower rank.

Identifying Clinical Symptoms

Whereas the Expressed Concerns scales measure discrete problems reported by students, the 10 MCCI Clinical Signs scales measure clusters of symptoms experienced in response to these problems. Although several of the scales cover symptoms found on Axis I of the *Diagnostic and Statistical Manual of Mental Disorders*, fourth edition, text revision (DSM-IV-TR; American Psychiatric Association, 2000), our intent was not to diagnose clinical disorders, but rather to identify both general and specific areas of symptom expression among students who present for help at college counseling centers. As with the Expressed Concerns scales, all Clinical Signs scales with PS ≥ 75 should be scrutinized and interpreted (see Table 23.4). Item endorsements for elevated scales should be examined to determine which symptoms are most problematic for the client. This is especially important for the Suicidal Tendencies, Eating Disorders, Alcohol Abuse, and Drug Abuse scales, as the client's responses to individual items will alert counselors to active suicidal ideation, potentially life-threatening eating behaviors, and the degree of alcohol and drug abuse reported by the client. For users of the computerized Interpretive Report, the "Noteworthy Responses" section is also important to consider, as these responses may identify problems not measured by the scales themselves.

Summarizing and Integrating the MCCI Profile

By this time, the counselor reviewing the MCCI test results has considered the student's demographic and background information, assessed test validity and response style, created a portrait of the client's personality style, and identified and interpreted significantly elevated Expressed Concerns and Clinical Signs scales. The next step in test interpretation is to integrate data from these areas into a summary of the individual's personality, presenting problems, and symptoms, in order to make coherent treatment recommendations.

Millon's (Millon & Davis, 1996) model is ideal for this task, as it envisions an inherent connection among all of these data sources. The MCCI Interpretive Report available from Pearson Assessments provides this kind of integration for the "Treatment Considerations" section, and is a useful teaching aid for students and novice professionals who are learning about Millon's system of conceptualizing personality and psychopathology. Experience with the MCCI and familiarity with Millon's (e.g., 1969, 1990, 1999, 2003a; Millon & Davis, 1996) writings will help users become more skilled in the integration process.

An initial framework for integration involves a consideration of the respondent's typical personality style in the context of his or her demographic and background characteristics. Grasping these features of the client will make it easier to assess the likely causes of the expressed concerns and their symptomatic impact on the individual. In deductive fashion, this will lead to treatment recommendations that take into consideration the client's unique personal characteristics and personality style.

Integrating MCCI Results with Other Assessment Data

The MCCI is frequently given to clients along with other assessment measures. When this is done, a final step in test interpretation is to bring together findings from these standardized instruments to create an integrated test battery report. The method used for combining results from multiple tests depends on user preferences. Two common methods are often called "test-by-test" and "areas of psychological functioning." The "test-by-test" method involves a discrete section of the report devoted to results from each test administered to the client. Thus there would be a section for the MCCI and a section for each additional measure given. A "Summary and Conclusions" section is often given at the end of the report, where data from the various sources are synthesized, and diagnostic suggestions are offered. A "Treatment Recommendations" section may follow, based on this summary.

The "areas of psychological functioning" test report integrates findings from the various measures as they apply to specific areas of functioning—for example, mood/affect, self-perception, cognitive style, and interpersonal behavior. In this method, results from each test administered to the client to address the specific psychological functioning area are integrated within that section of the report. As with the "test-by-test" method, there are usually "Summary and Conclusions" and "Treatment Recommendations" sections at the end of the report, which fully integrate findings from the various content realms.

Case Examples

Case 1: Emily

Background Information

Emily, a 19-year-old, non-Hispanic white, never-married female, was admitted to her university on an athletic scholarship for her talents as a tennis player. She came to the college counseling center just prior to beginning her second semester. At presentation, she complained of being very anxious and preoccupied about the pressure she felt to keep her weight down to stay competitive in tennis. Although she was able to handle her academic responsibilities during her first semester, she felt unable to balance the demands of her rigorous training schedule and a social life. She stated that she thought about food "constantly," and had gotten into a bad habit of going on fasts to counterbalance the "junk food" she would eat on weekends when socializing with her boyfriend. She felt that she was losing control over her weight, and feared that she might eventually be dismissed from the tennis team or lose her boyfriend.

MCCI Results

Emily's computer-generated MCCI profile is given in Figure 23.1. Examining the top of the profile page, we note that her results are valid and she has exhibited no unusual test-taking biases. With regard to personality, Emily shows a strong Sociable style (PS = 84), with mild elevations on Unruly (PS = 67) and Confident (PS = 64). Her profile indicates that she is a lively, extraverted woman who finds delight in the social world. She probably has very good social skills and knows how to use her warmth, charm, exuberance, and optimism to good effect. She likes to be the center of attention and can be showy and ostentatious toward this end. Not one to let circumstances take their course, Emily actively manipulates others and the environment to obtain what she wants. She can be quite mercurial when frustrated, exhibiting anger and disdain toward those who get in their way. Her social orientation and outward confidence may cover insecurity about her abilities and talents. She may believe that she has to keep up a front in order to please others.

Although none of Emily's Expressed Concerns scales are elevated at a clinically significant level, the highest scores are consistent with her initial complaints of general unhappiness (Mental Health Upset PS = 71) and distress over possibly losing her boyfriend (Romantic Distress PS = 69) and tennis scholarship (Financial Burdens PS = 64).

On the Clinical Signs scales, Emily has admitted to significant problems with her eating habits (Eating Disorders PS = 100), as well as anxiety (Anxiety/Tension PS = 85), dysphoria (Depressive Outlook PS = 77), and possible abuse of alcohol (Alcohol Abuse PS = 75). Examination of endorsed items for these scales indicates that Emily frequently goes on eating binges and then starves herself to lose weight. She often feels "jittery and restless" and gets upset to the point that she feels she could hurt herself. Importantly, she has not endorsed any items indicating active suicidal thinking. Although alcohol abuse was not something she revealed during her initial interview, Emily later admitted to having trouble trying to control an impulse to drink alcohol.

Taken as a whole, Emily's MCCI results tell us that she is an active, outgoing person who places a great deal of value on her social attractiveness. She can be impulsive and moody, and she is having serious difficulty managing her weight appropriately. She is currently feeling very anxious and dysphoric, and may be overusing alcohol.

Treatment Plan

Because bingeing–starving behaviors can have serious health consequences, the counselor made the decision to intervene here first. With Emily's permission, the counselor contacted the sports physician and dietician for campus athletes. The physician and dietician worked out a plan to help Emily manage her weight under medical supervision. With the counselor, Emily explored the sources of her anxiety, dysphoria, and desire to drink alcohol to manage her unhappiness. Recognizing the strengths and limitations of her personality style, the counselor used a direct but supportive therapeutic approach with Emily. The counselor was aware that sociable persons are used to fleeing problem situations rather than facing them, and that because of this they are likely to be deficient in the coping skills that would allow them to manage conflicts effectively and build self-esteem. Cognitive and group therapies are often useful with these persons in building and reinforcing interpersonal problem-solving skills. Accordingly, the counselor developed a treatment plan that helped Emily develop more reasonable expectations for herself by confronting her black-and-white beliefs about the need to be physically perfect in order to stay on the tennis team, counteracting negative self-talk, and helping her to recognize her emotional reactivity. The counselor developed homework assign-

MILLON COLLEGE COUNSELING INVENTORY

VALID REPORT

DISCLOSURE (X): RAW = 163 PERCENTILE = 67
DESIRABILITY (Y): RAW = 17 PERCENTILE = 21
DEBASEMENT (Z): RAW = 33 PERCENTILE = 64

CATEGORY		SCORE		PROFILE OF SR SCORES	DIAGNOSTIC SCALES
		RAW	BR	0 50 75 95 100	
PERSONALITY STYLES	1	12	25		INTROVERTED
	2A	10	31		INHIBITED
	2B	21	56		DEJECTED
	3	18	46		NEEDY
	4	41	94		SOCIABLE
	5	29	64		CONFIDENT
	6A	27	67		UNRULY
	7	26	13		CONSCIENTIOUS
	8A	22	59		OPPOSITIONAL
	8B	18	57		DENIGRATED
SEVERE PERSONALITY TENDENCIES	9	18	50		BORDERLINE
EXPRESSED CONCERNS	A	20	71		MENTAL HEALTH PATIENT
	B	12	42		IDENTITY QUANDRIES
	C	11	45		FAMILY DISQUIET
	D	9	30		PEER ALIENATION
	E	12	69		ROMANTIC DISTRESS
	F	18	62		ACADEMIC CONCERNS
	G	6	45		CAREER CONFUSION
	H	8	56		ABUSIVE EXPERIENCES
	I	6	35		LIVING ARRANGEMENT PROBLEMS
	J	16	64		FINANCIAL BURDENS
	K	0	0		SPIRITUAL DOUBTS
CLINICAL SIGNS	AA	9	52		SUICIDAL TENDENCIES
	BB	18	77		DEPRESSIVE OUTLOOK
	CC	20	85		ANXIETY/TENSION
	DD	20	63		POST-TRAUMATIC STRESS
	EE	36	100		EATING DISORDERS
	FF	22	70		ANGER DYSCONTROL
	GG	26	65		ATTENTION (COGNITIVE) DEFICITS
	HH	20	64		OBSESSIONS/COMPULSIONS
	II	22	75		ALCOHOL ABUSE
	JJ	4	50		DRUG ABUSE

CONFIDENTIAL INFORMATION FOR PROFESSIONAL USE ONLY

FIGURE 23.1. MCCI Profile Report for case 1: Emily.

574

ments for Emily to write down situations where she felt out of control and anxious, and then helped her find ways to reduce her arousal with visualization and relaxation exercises. Finally, Emily participated in a group for women with eating disorders, where she increased her self-esteem and learned new coping skills from the group leader and her fellow students. By the end of the semester, Emily had made good progress in developing healthier eating habits, showed greater flexibility in her thinking about herself and others, and reported normal levels of anxiety and dysphoria.

Case 2: José

Background Information

José, a 21-year-old, never married male of Puerto Rican heritage, was born and raised in a suburb of New York City. He was the fourth of seven children born to his parents, both of whom worked in office jobs throughout his childhood. Growing up, José reported that he got along "okay" with his parents, whom he felt were loving, but he complained that they were "always working" and had little time to spend with him or his younger siblings. He reported that his two older sisters were left in charge of the home when the parents were away, and he experienced them as being "mean" and "uncaring."

Not particularly athletic, José excelled in math and science. He took advantage of after-school programs in his neighborhood that were staffed by students at a local college, where he could receive personalized tutoring and participate in field trips to local museums. In his spare time, José preferred to spend time at the public library, where he read for hours and learned to use computers.

José's hard work paid off when it was time to apply for college. He had an excellent grade point average and high SAT scores, and was offered admission to several good schools. Anxious to try a completely new environment, José settled on a college in Florida that offered him a generous financial aid package.

José came to the college counseling center midway through his sophomore year. He did so at the urging of his dormitory roommate, who noted that José was becoming reclusive and gloomy. During his initial interview, José reported that he felt "completely out of place" in his college and was unable to make "real friends." He had thought that the problem would "take care of itself" by the end of his freshman year, but he still felt alone and isolated as a sophomore. At the beginning of the school year, he became infatuated with one of the women in his biology class. He spent hours by himself thinking of ways to meet and date her, but by the time he got the courage to ask her out, he found that she already had a steady boyfriend. José was crushed by this, and in response he withdrew into himself, becoming steadily more depressed and self-critical. "I'm a loser," he told the intake worker.

MCCI Results

José's computer-generated MCCI profile is given in Figure 23.2. Examining the top of the profile page, we can see that the test is valid and that José, while being somewhat low in self-disclosure (X percentile = 21), has been balanced in presenting positive (Y percentile = 61) and negative (Z percentile = 62) aspects of himself.

José's personality style is dominated by Denigrated traits (PS = 83), with no other scales above PS = 60. People who score high on the Denigrated scale often have deeply rooted pessimistic qualities, including a gloomy outlook toward themselves and the world.

MILLON COLLEGE COUNSELING INVENTORY

VALID REPORT

DISCLOSURE (X): RAW = 137 PERCENTILE = 21
DESIRABILITY (Y): RAW = 22 PERCENTILE = 61
DEBASEMENT (Z): RAW = 32 PERCENTILE = 62

CATEGORY		SCORE RAW	SCORE BR	PROFILE OF SR SCORES	DIAGNOSTIC SCALES
PERSONALITY STYLES	1	20	57		INTROVERTED
	2A	20	60		INHIBITED
	2B	28	83		DEJECTED
	3	19	50		NEEDY
	4	28	50		SOCIABLE
	5	10	8		CONFIDENT
	6A	9	7		UNRULY
	7	37	58		CONSCIENTIOUS
	8A	9	11		OPPOSITIONAL
	8B	16	54		DENIGRATED
SEVERE PERSONALITY TENDENCIES	9	12	37		BORDERLINE
EXPRESSED CONCERNS	A	12	41		MENTAL HEALTH PATIENT
	B	15	53		IDENTITY QUANDRIES
	C	4	12		FAMILY DISQUIET
	D	9	54		PEER ALIENATION
	E	14	75		ROMANTIC DISTRESS
	F	16	56		ACADEMIC CONCERNS
	G	0	0		CAREER CONFUSION
	H	0	0		ABUSIVE EXPERIENCES
	I	2	15		LIVING ARRANGEMENT PROBLEMS
	J	10	54		FINANCIAL BURDENS
	K	0	0		SPIRITUAL DOUBTS
CLINICAL SIGNS	AA	12	57		SUICIDAL TENDENCIES
	BB	22	85		DEPRESSIVE OUTLOOK
	CC	16	90		ANXIETY/TENSION
	DD	4	35		POST-TRAUMATIC STRESS
	EE	20	61		EATING DISORDERS
	FF	0	0		ANGER DYSCONTROL
	GG	4	8		ATTENTION (COGNITIVE) DEFICITS
	HH	8	28		OBSESSIONS/COMPULSIONS
	II	16	62		ALCOHOL ABUSE
	JJ	0	0		DRUG ABUSE

(Profile scale markers: 0, 50, 75, 95, 100)

CONFIDENTIAL INFORMATION FOR PROFESSIONAL USE ONLY

FIGURE 23.2. MCCI Profile Report for case 2: José.

They are sensitive and tend to be loners. They typically view themselves as unattractive and awkward, and they often have difficulty finding pleasurable activities in which to engage. These persons are prone to worry and rumination and may be preoccupied with feelings of guilt and shame over perceived or real failures. José's recent setback with a would-be dating partner is probably just one of many social misfires that have helped to reinforce his beliefs that he is not socially adequate, and that peers are not receptive or sensitive to his needs and desires.

On the Expressed Concerns scales, José has a significant elevation on Romantic Distress (PS = 75), indicating that his current focus is on problems finding a dating partner. Among the Clinical Signs scales, the Depressive Outlook (PS = 85) and Anxiety/Tension (PS = 80) scales are noteworthy. José is reporting symptoms of clinical depression, such as loneliness, sadness, low energy, poor concentration and attention, and trouble meeting daily demands. He is also reporting symptoms of anxiety, such as being tense, restless, ruminative, and unable to sleep. Examination of item responses for the elevated scales reveals that José feels very lonely and worthless and believes he is unable to make friends. He has not endorsed any items suggesting suicidal thoughts or intents.

Together, the Personality Styles, Expressed Concerns, and Clinical Signs scales offer a consistent portrait of an unhappy young man who feels that he is unable to make inroads in connecting with his peers for friendship and romance. Recognizing that José's current difficulties emanate from a personality style that tends to caste a pessimistic light on everything, we are aware that a long-term solution will be unlikely if José's habitual patterns of thinking and behaving are not targeted for intervention, along with his interpersonal skills and acute symptoms of depression and anxiety.

Treatment Plan

After discussing the MCCI results with José, his counselor decided to refer him to the college medical clinic for a psychiatric evaluation to see whether medication would help his acute symptoms. In creating a plan for psychotherapy services, José's counselor was mindful that people who score high on the Denigrated scale typically respond to problems by withdrawing and becoming more distrustful. They are likely to be wary of a counselor's interest and to be fearful of intrusion. It is best to take a direct but nonthreatening approach with such individuals and to take time to build rapport. Because these persons are not likely to be forthcoming about how they feel, counselors will do well regularly to seek their feedback about the relationship and proposed tasks. Even when they appear to be open, they are likely to keep their real feelings to themselves. They can be masters of disguise, appearing to be happy or pleased but actually feeling quite differently.

With these issues in mind, José's counselor first helped him examine his attitudes toward peers, as well as his usual method of initiating relationships. This revealed a number of self-defeating elements, such as José's belief that attractive dating partners would not be interested in him, and his tendency to be self-effacing in initial encounters. The counselor took a practical, problem-solving approach: José was asked to rehearse scenarios for meeting potential dates, asking the person out, and then following through. Negative self-talk was challenged, and alternative ways of seeing himself and others were offered and reinforced through homework assignments. Once José was able to demonstrate success in dating, he was asked to participate in a group for building skills in interpersonal relationships, as a way to consolidate and expand his initial gains. After 6 months of counseling, José completed the MCCI again. Following this he was discharged from the counseling center, having demonstrated successful dating behavior and showing significantly lower scores on the Romantic Distress, Depressive Outlook, and Anxiety/Tension scales.

Summary and Conclusion

The MCCI (Millon, 2006c) is a new, self-report assessment tool for use with college counseling clients ages 16 to 40. It is the first multidimensional measure developed and normed exclusively with this population. Its Personality Styles, Expressed Concerns, and Clinical Signs scales tap the kinds of traits and problems most frequently seen among today's college students, and cover such critical areas as suicidal behavior, PTSD, eating disorders, and substance abuse. The test was created as an operationalization of Theodore Millon's (e.g., 1969; Millon & Davis, 1996) comprehensive model of personality and psychopathology. In that model, the client's personality is considered to be the central system through which daily experiences (including stressors), thoughts, and emotions are perceived, organized, and acted upon. Results from the MCCI Personality Styles scales offer a rich portrait of a client's characteristic manner of thinking, feeling, and behaving, while the Expressed Concerns scales measure the content areas of the student's presenting problems, and the Clinical Signs scales assess the manifestation of these problems in a variety of symptom areas. This fast (20–30 minutes) and easy-to-administer inventory is an ideal assessment tool for intake, treatment planning, and measuring response to treatment.

Acknowledgment

This chapter was prepared with support from the U.S. Department of Veterans Affairs.

References

American Psychiatric Association. (2000). *Diagnostic and statistical manual of mental disorders* (4th ed., text rev.). Washington, DC: Author.

Beck, A. T., Steer, R. A., & Brown, G. K. (1996). *The Beck Depression Inventory–II.* San Antonio, TX: Psychological Corporation.

Benton, S. A., Robertson, J. M., Tseng, W., Newton, F. B., & Benton, S. L. (2003). Changes in counseling center client problems across 13 years. *Professional Psychology: Research and Practice, 34,* 66–72.

Cornish, J. A. E., Riva, M. T., Henderson, M. C., Kominars, K. D., & McIntosh, S. (2000). Perceived distress in university counseling center clients across a six-year period. *Journal of College Student Development, 41,* 104–109.

Erdur-Baker, O., Aberson, C. L., Barrow, J. C., & Draper, M. R. (2006). Nature and severity of college students' psychological concerns: A comparison of clinical and nonclinical national samples. *Professional Psychology: Research and Practice, 37,* 317–323.

Horn, J. L., Wanberg, K. W., & Foster, F. M. (1990). *Guide to the Alcohol Use Inventory.* Minneapolis, MN: National Computer Systems.

Millon, T. (1969). *Modern psychopathology.* Philadelphia: Saunders.

Millon, T. (1990). *Toward a new personology.* New York: Wiley.

Millon, T. (Ed.). (1997). *The Millon inventories: Clinical and personality assessment.* New York: Guilford Press.

Millon, T. (2003a). It's time to rework the blueprints: Building a science for clinical psychology. *American Psychologist, 58,* 949–961.

Millon, T. (2003b). *Millon Index of Personality Styles Revised (MIPS Revised) manual*. Minneapolis, MN: Pearson Assessments.

Millon, T., Antoni, M., Millon, C., Meagher, S., & Grossman, S. (2001). *Millon Behavioral Medicine Diagnostic (MBMD) manual*. Minneapolis, MN: Pearson Assessments.

Millon, T., & Davis, R. D. (1996). *Disorders of personality: DSM-IV and beyond* (2nd ed.). New York: Wiley.

Millon, T. (with Grossman, S., Meagher, S., Millon, C., & Everly, G.). (1999). *Personality-guided therapy*. New York: Wiley.

Millon, T. (with Millon, C., Davis, R., & Grossman, S.). (2006a) *Millon Adolescent Clinical Inventory (MACI) manual* (2nd ed.). Minneapolis, MN: Pearson Assessments.

Millon, T. (with Millon, C., Davis, R., & Grossman, S.). (2006b). *Millon Clinical Multiaxial Inventory–III (MCMI-III) manual* (3rd ed.). Minneapolis, MN: Pearson Assessments.

Millon, T. (with Strack, S., Millon, C., & Grossman, S.). (2006c). *Millon College Counseling Inventory (MCCI) manual*. Minneapolis, MN: Pearson Assessments.

Mowbray, C. T., Megivern, D., Mandiberg, J. M., Strauss, S., Stein, C. H., Collins, K., et al. (2006). Campus mental health services: Recommendations for change. *American Journal of Ortho psychiatry, 76*, 226–237.

Spielberger, C. D. (1983). *Manual for the State–Trait Anxiety Inventory*. Palo Alto, CA: Consulting Psychologists Press.

Strack, S. (Ed.). (2005). *Handbook of personology and psychopathology*. Hoboken, NJ: Wiley.

Strack, S. (Ed.). (2008). *Essentials of Millon inventories assessment* (3rd ed.). Hoboken, NJ: Wiley.

CHAPTER 24

Using the Millon–Grossman Personality Domains Checklist (MG-PDC) to Integrate Diverse Clinical Data

Seth D. Grossman
Robert F. Tringone
Theodore Millon

Consistent with current demands for short-term, focused treatment, with the recent emphasis on more molecular aspects of Millon's evolutionary theory (e.g., the Grossman Facet Scales of the Millon Clinical Multiaxial Inventory–III [MCMI-III] and Millon Adolescent Clinical Inventory [MACI]; Millon, 2006a, 2006b), and with the heightened debate regarding categorical versus dimensional models of personality in the upcoming fifth edition of the *Diagnostic and Statistical Manual of Mental Disorders* (DSM-V) (e.g., Costa & McCrae, 1995; Widiger & Trull, 2007), the call has been made to shift diagnostic emphasis from the neo-Kraepelinian categorical mode of thinking to one that may capture a more quantitative and varied picture of the person, with precision and pragmatism. Unlike popular five-factor models, which address this issue by describing personality traits via everyday language and deriving explanatory models from a purely statistical, inductive process (Davis & Millon, 1993), our current thinking involves returning to well-researched and explored theoretical groundings of Millon's evolutionary model (Millon, 1990; Millon & Davis, 1996) to find clinical utility in functional and structural attributes that, when taken together, provide a rich and detailed glimpse of personological functioning. Furthermore, review of these domains of personological functioning reveals high consistency with dominant models and approaches to therapy (cognitive, pharmacological, behavioral, interpersonal, etc.). Consonant as well with methods of assessment and intervention that have an integrated focus on the personality as a system, there is now a need for treating clinicians to assess the interactive domains of personality efficiently and directly. This chapter serves as a brief treatise of developments, inclusive of historical contributions, that have lead to the most recent endeavor to further illuminate dimensions of personality—the Millon–Grossman Personality Domain Checklist (MG-PDC)—as well as to introduce new therapeutic directions enhanced by this measure.

Historical Perspective

In recent decades, there has been a renewed interest in the area of personology. The most significant catalyst was the development and introduction of a prior DSM, the DSM-III (American Psychiatric Association, 1980)—with its multiaxial format, the placement of the personality disorders (PDs) on a separate axis, and the delineation of specific diagnostic criteria. These changes marked a "paradigmatic shift" in the approach to classification and psychodiagnosis (Klerman, 1986; Millon, 1986a). Whereas DSM-I and DSM-II employed a "classic" perspective to psychodiagnosis, DSM-III utilized a prototypic typology that recognized the diagnostic syndromes' intrinsic heterogeneity, due to the probabilistic nature of their diagnostic features.

Wittgenstein (1953) is credited with first recognizing the inherent ambiguity and multidimensionality involved in categorization. Researchers extrapolated from his notions of the multiplicity of "language games" and applied them to the PDs. The DSM-III (American Psychiatric Association, 1980) represented substantial progress toward this end in its development of a prototypal typology (Frances, 1980; Millon, 1986a, 1987b); however, the advances were not complete (Frances, 1982; Frances & Widiger, 1986). For example, some of the DSM-III Axis II PDs were conceptualized within the prototypal typology, while others required the presence of all their diagnostic criteria within a multiple-choice format. Beyond this, there were yet other PD categories representing DSM-III "holdouts" under the classic monothetic format requiring all diagnostic criteria to be present to meet a diagnosis. In the DSM-III-R (American Psychiatric Association, 1987), the DSM-IV (American Psychiatric Association, 1994), and the DSM-IV TR (American Psychiatric Association, 2000), all Axis II PDs are conceptualized according to the polythetic, prototypal typology.

Debates have raged and continue to abound for the shift from the classic model to a prototypal model, and now to the current consideration of dimensional models (Widiger & Trull, 2007). Historically, psychology and psychiatry have tended to align their views of diagnosis with those of medicine and biology (Garfield, 1986), and the classic approach views categories as possessing clear demarcations indicative of distinct entities. Membership is determined by the presence of distinctive, "necessary and sufficient" characteristics that differentiate persons into homogeneous categories. Advantages of the classic perspective include the ease and convenience with which pertinent information can be communicated. Well-established categories are highlighted by a set of the most salient characteristics, and they provide a standard reference for clinicians (Millon, 1987b). The failure to meet the assumptions of monothetic criteria and homogeneous group membership, however, argues against this position (Cantor, Smith, French, & Mezzich, 1980). Also, no available studies have empirically determined the thresholds or cutoff points that make a clear distinction between the presence and the absence of a PD (Widiger, 1992). In addition, Frances and Widiger (1986) noted that attempts to delineate restrictive diagnostic criteria in an effort to increase the sameness of members in a category have led to an increase in the number of "wastebasket" categories. Ironically, the DSM-III-R Axis II revisions led to dramatic increases in the prevalence rates of the PDs as well as in their comorbidity (Morey, 1988).

The prototypal model allows that instances within categories may display quantitative as well as qualitative differences. The critical contribution of the prototypal model is the assumption of probabilistic features, which demands greater flexibility in determining diagnostic categorization. There is a systematic deemphasis on the presence of "necessary and sufficient" characteristics; hence instances are viewed more along a continuum of similarity to prototypes, or "goodness of fit." Attributes serve as correlated indicators of disorders and carry varying degrees of diagnostic efficiency and validity (Clarkin, Widiger, Frances, Hurt, & Gilmore, 1983; Widiger, Hurt, Frances, Clarkin, & Gilmore, 1984). Within the prototypal model, category members are not likely to meet all inclusive and exclusive criteria of a category. Therefore, one anticipates heterogeneity within a disorder, numerous ambiguous or "atypical" cases, and varying degrees of similarity to the standard of comparison (e.g., a DSM-IV or DSM-IV-TR PD). Other than the issue of within-group heterogeneity, the prototypal model allows for the overlap of categories. Although it has been argued that categories may then no longer be very distinctive, the very nature of personality is one of overlap and covariation between personalities. Research utilizing the Millon Personality Diagnostic Checklist (MPDC), to be reviewed shortly, has provided considerable support for the prototypal model (Millon & Tringone, 1989; Tringone, 1990).

Two variants were proposed within a prototypal typology: summary prototypes and exemplar prototypes (Cantor & Genero, 1986). The most relevant examples of summary prototypes are the DSM-IV(-TR) diagnostic criteria sets, whereas exemplar prototypes emphasize the use of multiple examples for any category. The difference lies in the latter's reliance on known instances or "exemplars" of a category, rather than on the abstract image of a cognitive structure (Cantor & Genero, 1986). Millon's writings on PD subtypes (Millon & Davis, 1996) provide theoretically derived exemplars within each PD category. For example, a person who has a primary narcissistic PD may also possess salient features of histrionic PD (amorous narcissism), antisocial PD (unprincipled narcissism), or the paranoid PD (elitist narcissism).

A common counterargument to the "classic" position states that persons cannot be divided into homogeneous, discrete units (Frances, 1980). In an effort to alleviate the qualitative problems of the "classic" model, numerous dimensional perspectives have recently been proposed and have generated considerable interest. Viewing characteristics and disorders along a continuum of severity from normal to pathological, this model emphasizes quantitative gradations rather than qualitative, all-or-none distinctions (Skinner, 1986; Millon, 1987b). Such latitude allows an individual to possess certain features indicative of various disorders in matters of degree. Though they are perceived to be in opposition, classic and dimensional approaches complement one another (Frances, 1982; Millon, 1987b). Whereas such dimensions account for quantitative differences for criteria, personality constructs can be perceived as qualitative sets of attributes. Dimensional scores can also be translated into categorical diagnoses through the use of cutoff points.

Classification systems that employ dimensions are viewed as more flexible and informative than the classic perspective (Widiger, 1982; Widiger & Trull, 2007). Also, they are better able to classify ambiguous cases than is a "forced-choice" paradigm. Their utility may be lessened, however, when descriptions become too complex and unwieldy (Frances, 1982). Other noted problems involve defining the core dimensions, agreeing on the number of core dimensions needed to represent the personality disorders, and identifying the meaningfulness of increments within the chosen dimensions (Millon, 1987b).

With the shift from the classic perspective to the prototypal view, there has been a dramatic increase in the number of studies investigating the PDs. Although we are progressing in our empirical understanding of these disorders, advances must still be made in our theoretical understanding of their origins, their self-perpetuating tendencies, and the way clinicians must intervene in and treat them (Millon, 1969, 1981, 1990; Millon & Davis, 1996).

The MPDC: Early Explorations of Personality Domains

Prior to introducing the MG-PDC, we must first examine its forerunner, on which much of the current methodology is based. The MPDC (Millon & Tringone, 1989, Tringone, 1990, 1997) was developed initially to assist in the construction and validation of the MCMI-II (Millon, 1987a). This was a time of transitions in terms of psychological diagnosis and categorization. As is understandable, given these complex transitions from classic to prototypal views, no "gold standard" served as a comparison point for the PDs; therefore, clinicians were asked to complete the MPDC and provide up to three PD diagnoses, in their order of salience, while their patients completed the MCMI-II research form. The clinicians' diagnoses helped set the prevalence rates and, in turn, the presence and prominence levels of the MCMI-II personality pattern scales. Concordance rates were then generated between the clinicians' diagnostic impressions and the self-report inventory. As part of this process, the diagnostic efficiency of each MPDC item across all the PDs was then calculated to investigate the MPDC's strength and utility in the diagnostic process, as well as its potential as a stand-alone clinician's checklist (Millon & Tringone, 1989, Tringone, 1990).

As with all Millon inventories, the development of the MPDC has followed the validation sequence proposed by Loevinger (1957) and Jackson (1970). In her classic monograph, Loevinger delineated three components of construct validity: substantive, structural, and external. She suggested that these components are construction and validation stages that can be followed sequentially. Her schema incorporates the thinking of Cronbach and Meehl (1955) on construct validity and of Campbell and Fiske (1959) on convergent and discriminant validity. The intent of following this model was to enhance the MPDC's reliability and validity and to maximize its efficiency in assessing personality characteristics. A brief review of the first stage of development is offered here.

For the first, substantive stage (relabeled "theoretical/substantive"), Millon's (1969, 1981) biosocial learning theory served as the underlying theoretical model for the MPDC's conceptualization of the DSM-III-R and DSM-IV PDs, as the recognized constructs could then be theoretically deduced from Millon's three-polarities model. This model also proposed the relationships of the different constructs to one another. Furthermore, it proposed prototypal features of each PD within common domains. Two steps were involved in compiling and developing items to meet this requirement with the MPDC: (1) creating an initial item pool based on theoretical and empirical grounds, and (2) reducing the initial item pool on empirical and rational grounds. These items, representing the 13 proposed PDs for the DSM-III-R, were ultimately derived from Millon's theory as well as from DSM-III diagnostic criteria, both of which were viewed as having theoretical and empirical support for defining PDs.

Content validity for a classification system is achieved when all of its categories are defined across the full range of clinically relevant domains. The criteria sets for the DSM-III-R and DSM-IV personality disorders were deemed both "noncomprehensive" and "noncomparable" (Millon & Davis, 1996). Some of the constructs' criteria are narrow and restricted to behavior-oriented features, while other constructs' criteria are redundant and reiterate a single theme across multiple criteria. Shea (1992) also noted that the criteria sets vary in the number of underlying dimensions they address and the level of inference required to assess the criteria, with the latter issue amplified in regard to whether or not the underlying motivations of the manifest behaviors have been made explicit. This point is especially important, because similar behaviors can have different determinants, and different behaviors can share similar determinants (Stricker & Gold, 1988).

By the time the MPDC was being developed, Millon (1986b, 1990) had outlined defining features for each PD across eight domain areas. Those features manifested between the person and his or her environment were labeled "functional domains." These domains represented the "behaviors, social conduct, cognitive processes, and unconscious mechanisms which manage, adjust, transform, coordinate, balance, discharge, and control the give and take of inner and outer life" (Millon, 1990, p. 136). Three functional domains were incorporated into the MPDC: Expressive Acts, Interpersonal Conduct, and Cognitive Style. A second group of clinically relevant characteristics were labeled "structural domains," which represent "a deeply embedded and relatively enduring template of imprinted memories, attitudes, needs, fears, conflicts, and so on, which guide experience and transform the nature of ongoing life events" (Millon, 1990, p. 147). The structural domains assessed with the MPDC were Self-Image and Mood/Temperament. These five domains were selected because they were considered to be generally more objective and to require less inference on the part of clinicians than do the three remaining domains: Regulatory Mechanisms, Object Representations, and Morphological Organization.

Further stages of development of the MPDC indicate that the instrument exhibited reasonably strong internal/structural reliability as well as external validity when correlated with Millon's theoretical constructs (Tringone, 1997). It was proven to be of great value in assisting the development of the MCMI-II; it was further thought, owing to the continuity of constructs between the MCMI-II and MCMI-III (Millon, 2006a), that its general structure and content would continue to serve well as a clinician's checklist companion to the more recent MCMI-III. It was with this background—that of providing an additional, coordinated source of data in assessment—that the development of the MG-PDC began.

Development of the MG-PDC

Clinicians and researchers need multiple sources of data for accurate assessments of individuals. These data sources, range from incidental to well-structured observations, casual to highly systematic interviews, and cursory to formal analyses of biographical history; also employed are a variety of laboratory tests, self-report inventories, and performance-based or projective techniques. All of these have proven to be useful grounds for diagnostic study. In this context, several questions arise, including this one: How do we put these diverse data sources together to systematize and quantify the information we have gathered? It is toward the end of organizing and maximizing the clinical utility of our personality findings that the MG-PDC has been developed.

On their own, observations and projective techniques are viewed as excessively subjective. Laboratory procedures (e.g., brain imaging) are not yet sufficiently developed, and biographical data are often too unreliable to depend on. And despite their popularity with many a distinguished psychometrician, the utility of self-report inventories is far from universally accepted.

Whether assessment tools are based on empirical investigations, epidemiological research, mathematical analyses, or theoretical deductions, they often fail to characterize persons in the language and concepts traditionally employed by clinical personologists. Although many instruments have been proven valuable in numerous research studies, such as by demonstrating reasonable intercorrelations or a correspondence with established diagnostic systems (e.g., the DSM), many an astute clinician has questioned whether these tools yield anything beyond the reliability of surface impressions. Some (Westen & Weinberger, 2004) doubt whether self-report instruments, for example, successfully tap into or unravel the diverse, complex, and hidden relationships among difficult-to-fathom processes. Other critics have contended that patient-generated responses may contain *no* clinically relevant information beyond the judgments of nonscientists employing a layperson's lexicon.

Data obtained from patient-based self-judgments may be contrasted with the sophisticated clinical appraisals of mental health professionals. We must ask whether clinical language, concepts, and instruments encoded in the evolving professional language of the past 100 years or so generate information incremental to the naive descriptions of an ordinary person's everyday lexicon. We know that clinical languages differ from laypersons' languages because they serve different and more sophisticated purposes (Livesley, Jackson, & Schroeder, 1989). Indeed, clinical concepts reflect the experienced contributions of numerous historical schools of thought (Millon, 2004). Each of these clinical schools (e.g., psychodynamic, cognitive, interpersonal) have identified a multitude of diverse and complex psychic processes that operate in our mental lives. Surely the concepts of these historical professional lexicons are not reducible to the superficial factors drawn from the everyday vocabulary of nonscientists.

In large part, the accurate representation and integration of the insights and concepts of the several major schools of thought led to the formulation of the MPDC, a domain-based, clinician-rated assessment (Millon, 1969, 1981, 1984, 1986a, 1990; Millon & Davis, 1996; Millon & Tringone, 1989; Tringone, 1990, 1997); they have now led to the development, following numerous empirical and theoretical refinements, of the MG-PDC. In contrast to the five-factor method, popular among research-oriented psychologists, the MG-PDC continues the tradition of basing its primary measures on the contributions of five of the major clinical traditions: the behavioral, the interpersonal, the self-psychological, the cognitive, and the biological. Three optional domains are included in the instrument to reflect the psychoanalytic tradition (the structural, the representational, and the regulatory mechanisms); however, the use of these intrapsychic domains has diminished in recent decades, and they are therefore elective (i.e., not required) components of the instrument.

Several criteria have been used to select and develop the clinical domains included in the checklist:

1. The domains are broad-based and varied in the features they embody; that is, they are not limited to biological temperaments or cognitive processes, but instead encompass a full range of personality characteristics that are based on frequently used clinical terms and concepts.
2. They correspond to the major therapeutic modalities employed by contemporary mental health professionals to treat their patients (e.g., cognitive techniques for altering dysfunctional beliefs, group procedures for modifying interpersonal conduct), and hence are readily employed by practicing therapeutic clinicians.
3. They are coordinated with and reflect the official PD prototypes established by the *International Classification of Diseases* (ICD) and DSM, and thereby can be understood by insurance and other management professionals.
4. A distinctive psychological trait can be identified and operationalized in each of the clinical trait domains for each personality prototype, assuring thereby both scope and comparability among personological criteria.
5. They lend themselves to the appraisal of domain characteristics for both normal and abnormal personalities, and hence promote further advances in the field of normality—one of growing interest in the psychological literature.
6. They can constitute an educational clinical tool to sensitize mental health workers in training (psychologists, psychiatrists, clinical social workers, etc.) to the many distinctions, subtleties, and domain interactions that are worth considering in appraising personality attributes.

The integrative perspective encouraged in the MG-PDC views personality as a multidetermined and multireferential construct. One (albeit problematic) approach taken by some clinical researchers to dealing with the conceptual alternatives that characterize personality study today is to oversimplify the task. That is, they choose to assess each patient in accord with a single conceptual orientation, eliminating thereby the integration of divergent perspectives by an act of regressive dogmatism. A truly effective assessment, however—one that is logically consonant with the modern integrative character of personality, both as a construct and as a reality—requires that the individual be assessed systematically across multiple characterological domains. This approach ensures that the assessment is comprehensive, useful to a broad range of clinicians, and more likely to be valid. In assessing individuals with the MG-PDC, clinicians should refrain, therefore, from regarding each domain as an independent entity and thereby falling into a naive, single-minded approach. Each of the domains is a legitimate but highly contextualized part of a unified or integrated whole, a necessary composite ensuring that the full integrity of the person is represented.

As noted previously, the domains of the instrument can be organized in a manner similar to distinctions drawn in the biological realm; that is, they may be divided into and characterized as "structural" and "functional" attributes. The functional domains of the instrument represent dynamic processes that transpire between the individual and his or her psychosocial environment. These transactions take place through what we have termed the person's "modes of regulatory action"—that is, his or her demeanor, social relations, and thought processes, each of which serve to manage, adjust, transform, coordinate, and control the give and take of inner and outer life. Several functional domains relevant to each personality are included among the major components of the MG-PDC.

In contrast to the functional characteristics, structural domains represent templates of deeply embedded affect dispositions and imprinted memories, attitudes, needs, and conflicts that guide experience and orient ongoing life events. These domains may be conceived of as quasi-permanent substrates for identity and temperament. These residues of the past and relatively enduring affects effectively constrain and even close off innovative learning and limit new possibilities to already established habits and dispositions. Their persistent and preemptive character perpetuates the maladaptive behavior and vicious circles of a patient's extant personality pathology.

Of course, individuals differ with respect to the domains they enact most frequently. People vary not only in the degree to which they approximate each personality prototype, but also in the extent to which each domain dominates their behavior. In conceptualizing personality as a system, we must recognize that different parts of the system will be dominant in different individuals, even when those individuals are patients who share the same prototypal diagnosis. It is the goal of the MG-PDC to differentiate, operationalize, and measure quantitatively those domain features that are primary in contributing to the person's functioning. By identifying these features, the instrument should help the clinical therapist to modify the person's problematic features (e.g., interpersonal conduct, cognitive beliefs), and thereby enable the patient to acquire a greater variety of adaptive behaviors in his or her life circumstances.

The MG-PDC Itself, and Instructions for Its Use

In this section, we introduce the MG-PDC in its entirety (see Figure 24.1), along with procedural steps for completing a basic assessment with the instrument. Following this, we present a case to demonstrate the instrument's operational use. You, our

I. Expressive Behavior Domain

These attributes relate to observables at the *behavioral level* of emotion and are usually recorded by noting how the patient acts. Through inference, observations of overt behavior enable us to deduce what the patient unknowingly reveals about his or her emotions or, often conversely, what he or she wants others to think about him or her. The range and character of expressive actions are wide and diverse and they convey distinctive and worthwhile clinical information, from communicating a sense of personal incompetence to exhibiting emotional defensiveness to demonstrating disciplined self-control, and so on.

1st Best Fit	2nd Best Fit	3rd Best Fit	Characteristic Behavior
1	2	3	**A. Impassive:** Is colorless, sluggish, displaying deficits in activation and emotional expressiveness; appears to be in a persistent state of low energy and lack of vitality (e.g., phlegmatic and lacking in spontaneity).
1	2	3	**B. Peculiar:** Is perceived by others as eccentric, disposed to behave in an unobtrusively aloof, curious, or bizarre manner; exhibits socially gauche habits and aberrant mannerisms (e.g., manifestly odd or eccentric).
1	2	3	**C. Fretful:** Fearfully scans environment for social derogation; overreacts to innocuous events and judges them to signify personal derision and mockery (e.g., anxiously anticipates ridicule/humiliation).
1	2	3	**D. Incompetent:** Ill-equipped to assume mature and independent roles; is passive and lacking functional competencies, avoiding self-assertion and withdrawing from adult responsibilities (e.g., has difficulty doing things on his or her own).
1	2	3	**E. Impetuous:** Is forcefully energetic and driven, emotionally excitable and overzealous; often worked up, unrestrained, rash, and hotheaded (e.g., is restless and socially intrusive).
1	2	3	**F. Dramatic:** Is histrionically overreactive and stimulus-seeking, resulting in unreflected and theatrical responsiveness; describes penchant for sensational situations and short-sighted hedonism (e.g., overly emotional and artificially affected).
1	2	3	**G. Haughty:** Manifests an air of being above conventional rules of shared social living, viewing them as naive or inapplicable to self; reveals an egocentric indifference to the needs of others (e.g., acts arrogantly self assured and confident).
1	2	3	**H. Defensive:** Is vigilantly guarded, hyperalert to ward off anticipated deception and malice; is tenaciously resistant to sources of external influence (e.g., disposed to be wary, envious, and jealous).
1	2	3	**I. Impulsive:** Since adolescence, acts thoughtlessly and irresponsibly in social matters; is shortsighted, heedless, incautious, and imprudent, failing to plan ahead or consider legal consequences (e.g., Conduct Disorder evident before age 15).
1	2	3	**J. Precipitate:** Is stormy and unpredictably abrupt, reckless, thickskinned, and unflinching, seemingly undeterred by pain; is attracted to challenge, as well as undaunted by punishment (e.g., attracted to risk, danger, and harm).
1	2	3	**K. Disconsolate:** Appearance and posture convey an irrelievably forlorn, heavy-hearted, if not grief-stricken quality; markedly dispirited and discouraged (e.g., somberly seeks others to be protective).
1	2	3	**L. Abstinent:** Presents self as nonindulgent, frugal, and chaste, refraining from exhibiting signs of pleasure or attractiveness; acts in an unpresuming and self-effacing manner, placing self in an inferior light (e.g., undermines own good fortune).
1	2	3	**M. Resentful:** Exhibits inefficiency, erratic, contrary, and irksome behaviors; reveals gratification in undermining the pleasures and expectations of others (e.g., uncooperative, contrary, and stubborn).
1	2	3	**N. Spasmodic:** Displays a desultory energy level with sudden, unexpected self-punitive outbursts; endogenous shifts in emotional state; places behavioral equilibrium in constant jeopardy (e.g., does impulsive, self-damaging acts).
1	2	3	**O. Disciplined:** Maintains a regulated, emotionally restrained, and highly organized life; often insists that others adhere to personally established rules and methods (e.g., meticulous and perfectionistic).

FIGURE 24.1. The Millon–Grossman Personality Domains Checklist (MG-PDC). Copyright 2006 by Dicandrien, Inc. Reprinted by permission. All rights reserved *(page 1 of 9).*

II. Interpersonal Conduct Domain

A patient's style of relating to others may be captured in a number of ways, such as how his or her actions affect others, intended or otherwise; the attitudes that underlie, prompt, and give shape to these actions; the methods by which he or she engages others to meet his or her needs; and his or her way of coping with social tensions and conflicts. Extrapolating from these observations, the clinican may construct an image of how the patient functions in relation to others.

1st Best Fit	2nd Best Fit	3rd Best Fit	Characteristic Behavior
1	2	3	**A. Unengaged:** Is indifferent to the actions or feelings of others, possessing minimal "human" interests; ends up with few close relationships and a limited role in work and family settings (e.g., has few desires or interests).
1	2	3	**B. Secretive:** Strives for privacy, with limited personal attachments and obligations; drifts into increasingly remote and clandestine social activities (e.g., is enigmatic and withdrawn).
1	2	3	**C. Aversive:** Reports extensive history of social anxiety and isolation; seeks social acceptance, but maintains careful distance to avoid anticipated humiliation and derogation (e.g., is socially pan-anxious and fearfully guarded).
1	2	3	**D. Submissive:** Subordinates needs to a stronger and nurturing person, without whom will feel alone and anxiously helpless; is compliant, conciliatory, and self-sacrificing (e.g., generally docile, deferential, and placating).
1	2	3	**E. High-Spirited:** Is unremittingly full of life and socially buoyant; attempts to engage others in an animated, vivacious, and lively manner; often seen by others, however, as intrusive and needlessly insistent (e.g., is persistently overbearing).
1	2	3	**F. Attention-Seeking:** Is self-dramatizing, and actively solicits praise in a showy manner to gain desired attention and approval; manipulates others and is emotionally demanding (e.g., seductively flirtatious and exhibitionistic).
1	2	3	**G. Exploitive:** Acts entitled, self-centered, vain, and unempathic; expects special favors without assuming reciprocal responsibilities; shamelessly takes others for granted and uses them to enhance self and indulge desires (e.g., egocentric and socially inconsiderate).
1	2	3	**H. Provocative:** Displays a quarrelsome, fractious, and distrustful attitude; bears serious grudges and precipitates exasperation by a testing of loyalties and a searching preoccupation with hidden motives (e.g., unjustly questions fidelity of spouse/friend).
1	2	3	**I. Irresponsible:** Is socially untrustworthy and unreliable, intentionally or carelessly failing to meet personal obligations of a marital, parental, employment, or financial nature; actively violates established civil codes through duplicitous or illegal behaviors (e.g., shows active disregard for rights of others).
1	2	3	**J. Abrasive:** Reveals satisfaction in competing with, dominating, and humiliating others; regularly expresses verbally abusive and derisive social commentary, as well as exhibiting harsh, if not physically brutal behavior (e.g., intimidates, coerces, and demeans others).
1	2	3	**K. Defenseless:** Feels and acts vulnerable and guilt-ridden; fears emotional abandonment and seeks public assurances of affection and devotion (e.g., needs supportive relationships to bolster hopeless outlook).
1	2	3	**L. Deferential:** Relates to others in a self-sacrificing, servile, and obsequious manner, allowing, if not encouraging others to exploit or take advantage; is self-abasing, accepting undeserved blame and unjust criticism (e.g., courts others to be exploitive and mistreating).
1	2	3	**M. Contrary:** Assumes conflicting roles in social relationships, shifting from dependent acquiescence to assertive independence; is obstructive toward others, behaving either negatively or erratically (e.g., sulky and argumentative in response to requests).
1	2	3	**N. Paradoxical:** Needing extreme attention and affection, but acts unpredictably and manipulatively and is volatile, frequently eliciting rejection rather than support; reacts to fears of separation and isolation in angry, mercurial, and often self-damaging ways (e.g., is emotionally needy, but interpersonally erratic).
1	2	3	**O. Respectful:** Exhibits unusual adherence to social conventions and proprieties; prefers polite, formal, and "correct" personal relationships (e.g., interpersonally proper and dutiful).

FIGURE 24.1. *(p. 2 of 9)*

III. Cognitive Style/Content Domain

How the patient focuses and allocates attention, encodes and processes information, organizes thoughts, makes attributions, and communicates reactions and ideas to others represents key cognitive functions of clinical value. These characteristics are among the most useful indices of the patient's distinctive way of thinking. By synthesizing his or her beliefs and attitudes, it may be possible to identify indications of problematic cognitive functions and assumptions.

1st Best Fit	2nd Best Fit	3rd Best Fit	Characteristic Cognitive Style
1	2	3	**A. Impoverished:** Seems deficient in human spheres of knowledge and evidences vague thought processes about everyday matters that are below intellectual level; social communications are easily derailed or conveyed via a circuitous logic (e.g., lacks awareness of human relations).
1	2	3	**B. Autistic:** Intrudes on social communications with personal irrelevancies; there is notable circumstantial speech, ideas of reference, and metaphorical asides; is ruminative, appears self-absorbed and lost in occasional magical thinking; there is a marked blurring of fantasy and reality (e.g., exhibits peculiar ideas and superstitious beliefs).
1	2	3	**C. Distracted:** Is bothered by disruptive and often distressing inner thoughts; the upsurge from within of irrelevant and digressive ideation upsets thought continuity and interferes with social communications (e.g., withdraws into reveries to fulfill needs).
1	2	3	**D. Naive:** Is easily persuaded, unsuspicious, and gullible; reveals a Pollyanna attitude toward interpersonal difficulties, watering down objective problems and smoothing over troubling events (e.g., childlike thinking and reasoning).
1	2	3	**E. Scattered:** Thoughts are momentary and scrambled in an untidy disarray with minimal focus to them, resulting in a chaotic hodgepodge of miscellaneous and haphazard beliefs expressed randomly with no logic or purpose (e.g., intense and transient emotions disorganize thoughts).
1	2	3	**F. Flighty:** Avoids introspective thought and is overly attentive to trivial and fleeting external events; integrates experiences poorly, resulting in shallow learning and thoughtless judgments (e.g., faddish and responsive to superficialities).
1	2	3	**G. Expansive:** Has an undisciplined imagination and exhibits a preoccupation with illusory fantasies of success, beauty, or love; is minimally constrained by objective reality; takes liberties with facts and seeks to redeem boastful beliefs (e.g., indulges fantasies of repute/power).
1	2	3	**H. Mistrustful:** Is suspicious of the motives of others, construing innocuous events as signifying conspiratorial intent; magnifies tangential or minor social difficulties into proofs of duplicity, malice, and treachery (e.g., wary and distrustful).
1	2	3	**I. Deviant:** Construes ordinary events and personal relationships in accord with socially unorthodox beliefs and morals; is disdainful of traditional ideals and conventional rules (e.g., shows contempt for social ethics and morals).
1	2	3	**J. Dogmatic:** Is strongly opinionated, as well as unbending and obstinate in holding to his or her preconceptions; exhibits a broad social intolerance and prejudice (e.g., closed-minded and bigoted).
1	2	3	**K. Fatalistic:** Sees things in their blackest form and invariably expects the worst; gives the gloomiest interpretation of current events, believing that things will never improve (e.g., conceives life events in persistent pessimistic terms).
1	2	3	**L. Diffident:** Is hesitant to voice his or her views; often expresses attitudes contrary to inner beliefs; experiences contrasting and conflicting thoughts toward self and others (e.g., demeans own convictions and opinions).
1	2	3	**M. Cynical:** Skeptical and untrusting, approaching current events with disbelief and future possibilities with trepidation; has a misanthropic view of life, expressing disdain and caustic comments toward those who experience good fortune (e.g., envious or disdainful of those more fortunate).
1	2	3	**N. Vacillating:** Experiences rapidly changing, fluctuating, and antithetical perceptions or thoughts concerning passing events; contradictory reactions are evoked in others by virtue of his or her behaviors, creating, in turn, conflicting and confusing social feedback (e.g., erratic and contrite over own beliefs and attitudes).
1	2	3	**O. Constricted:** Constructs world in terms of rules, regulations, time schedules, and social hierarchies; is unimaginative, indecisive, and notably upset by unfamiliar or novel ideas and customs (e.g., preoccupied with lists, details, rules, etc.).

FIGURE 24.1. *(p. 3 of 9)*

IV. Self-Image Domain

As the inner world of symbols is mastered through development, one major configuration emerges to impose a measure of sameness on an otherwise fluid environment: the perception of self-as-object, a distinct, ever-present identity. Self-image is significant in that it serves as a guidepost and lends continuity to changing experience. Most patients have an implicit sense of who they are but differ greatly in the clarity, accuracy, and complexity of their introspection of the psychic elements that make up this image.

1st Best Fit	2nd Best Fit	3rd Best Fit	Characteristic Self-Image
1	2	3	**A. Complacent:** Reveals minimal introspection and awareness of self; seems impervious to the emotional and personal implications of his or her role in everyday social life (e.g., minimal interest in own personal life).
1	2	3	**B. Estranged:** Possesses permeable ego boundaries, exhibiting acute social perplexities and illusions as well as experiences of depersonalization, derealization, and dissociation; sees self as "different," with repetitive thoughts of life's confusions and meaninglessness (e.g., self-perceptions are haphazard and fragmented).
1	2	3	**C. Alienated:** Sees self as a socially isolated person, one rejected by others; devalues self-achievements and reports feelings of aloneness and undesirability (e.g., feels injured and unwanted by others).
1	2	3	**D. Inept:** Views self as weak, fragile, and inadequate; exhibits lack of self-confidence by belittling own aptitudes and competencies (e.g., sees self as childlike and/or fragile).
1	2	3	**E. Energetic:** Sees self as full of vim and vigor, a dynamic force, invariably hardy and robust, a tireless and enterprising person whose ever-present energy galvanizes others (e.g., proud to be active and animated).
1	2	3	**F. Gregarious:** Views self as socially stimulating and charming; enjoys the image of attracting acquaintances and pursuing a busy and pleasure-oriented social life (e.g., perceived as appealing and attractive, but shallow).
1	2	3	**G. Admirable:** Confidently exhibits self, acts in a self-assured manner, and publicly displays achievements, despite being seen by others as egotistic, inconsiderate, and arrogant (e.g., has a sense of high self worth).
1	2	3	**H. Inviolable:** Is highly insular, experiencing intense fears of losing identity, status, or powers of self-determination; nevertheless, has persistent ideas of self-reference, asserting as personally derogatory and scurrilous entirely innocuous actions and events (e.g., sees ordinary life events as invariably referring to self).
1	2	3	**I. Autonomous:** Values the sense of being free, unencumbered, and unconfined by persons, places, obligations, or routines; sees self as unfettered by the restrictions of social customs and the restraints of personal loyalties (e.g., values being independent of social responsibilities).
1	2	3	**J. Combative:** Values aspects of self that present tough, domineering, and power-oriented image; is proud to characterize self as unsympathetic and unsentimental (e.g., proud to be stern and feared by others).
1	2	3	**K. Worthless:** Sees self as valueless, of no account, a person who should be overlooked, owing to having no praiseworthy traits or achievements (e.g., sees self as insignificant or inconsequential).
1	2	3	**L. Undeserving:** Focuses on and amplifies the very worst features of self; judges self as worthy of being shamed, humbled, and debased; has failed to live up to the expectations of others and, hence, should be reproached and demeaned (e.g., sees self as deserving to suffer).
1	2	3	**M. Discontented:** Sees self as unjustly misunderstood and unappreciated; recognizes that he or she is characteristically resentful, disgruntled, and disillusioned with life (e.g., sees self as unfairly treated).
1	2	3	**N. Uncertain:** Experiences the marked confusions of a nebulous or wavering sense of identity and self-worth; seeks to redeem erratic actions and changing self-presentations with expressions of contrition and self punitive behaviors (e.g., has persistent identity disturbances).
1	2	3	**O. Reliable:** Sees self as industrious, meticulous, and efficient; fearful of error or misjudgment and, hence, overvalues aspects of self that exhibit discipline, perfection, prudence, and loyalty (e.g., sees self as reliable and conscientious).

FIGURE 24.1. *(p. 4 of 9)*

V. Mood/Affect Domain

Few observables are more clinically relevant than the predominant character of an individual's affect and the intensity and frequency with which he or she expresses it. The meaning of extreme emotions is easy to decode. This is not so with the more subtle moods and feelings that insidiously and repetitively pervade the patient's ongoing relationships and experiences. The expressive features of mood/affect may be revealed, albeit indirectly, in activity level, speech quality, and physical appearance.

1st Best Fit	2nd Best Fit	3rd Best Fit	Characteristic Mood
1	2	3	**A. Apathetic:** Is emotionally impassive, exhibiting an intrinsic unfeeling, cold, and stark quality; reports weak affectionate or erotic needs, rarely displaying warm or intense feelings, and apparently unable also to experience either sadness or anger (e.g., unable to experience pleasure in depth).
1	2	3	**B. Distraught or Insentient:** Reports being *either* apprehensive and ill at ease, particularly in social encounters; anxiously watchful, distrustful of others, and wary of their motives; *or* manifests drab, sluggish, joyless, and spiritless appearance; reveals marked deficiencies in emotional expression and pesonal encounters (e.g., highly agitated and/or affectively flat).
1	2	3	**C. Anguished:** Vacillates between desire for affection, fear of rebuff, and numbness of feeling; describes constant and confusing undercurrents of tension, sadness, and anger (e.g., unusually fearful of new social experiences).
1	2	3	**D. Pacific:** Quietly and passively avoids social tension and interpersonal conflicts; is typically pleasant, warm, tender, and noncompetitive (e.g., characteristically timid and uncompetitive).
1	2	3	**E. Mercurial:** Volatile and quicksilverish, at times unduly ebullient, charged up, and irrepressible; at other times, flighty and erratic emotionally, blowing hot and cold (e.g., has marked penchant for momentary excitements).
1	2	3	**F. Fickle:** Displays short-lived and superficial emotions; is dramatically overreactive and exhibits tendencies to be easily enthused and as easily bored (e.g., impetuously pursues pleasure-oriented social life).
1	2	3	**G. Insouciant:** Manifests a general air of nonchalance and indifference; appears coolly unimpressionable or calmly optimistic, except when self centered confidence is shaken, at which time either rage, shame, or emptiness is briefly displayed (e.g., generally appears imperturbable and composed).
1	2	3	**H. Irascible:** Displays a sullen, churlish, and humorless demeanor; attempts to appear unemotional and objective, but is edgy, touchy, surly, quick to react angrily (e.g., ready to take personal offense).
1	2	3	**I. Callous:** Exhibits a coarse incivility, as well as a ruthless indifference to the welfare of others; is unempathic, as expressed in wide-ranging deficits in social charitableness, human compassion, or personal remorse (e.g., experiences minimal guilt or contrition for socially repugnant actions).
1	2	3	**J. Hostile:** Has an overtly rough and pugnacious temper, which flares periodically into contentious argument and physical belligerence; is fractious, willing to do harm, even persecute others to get own way (e.g., easily embroiled in brawls).
1	2	3	**K. Woeful:** Is typically mournful, tearful, joyless, and morose; characteristically worrisome and brooding; low spirits rarely remit (e.g., frequently feels dejected or guilty).
1	2	3	**L. Dysphoric:** Intentionally displays a plaintive and gloomy appearance, occasionally to induce guilt and discomfort in others (e.g., drawn to relationships in which he or she will suffer).
1	2	3	**M. Irritable:** Is often petulant, reporting being easily annoyed or frustrated by others; typically obstinate and resentful, followed in turn by sulky and grumpy withdrawal (e.g., impatient and easily provoked into oppositional behavior).
1	2	3	**N. Labile:** Fails to accord unstable moods with external reality; has marked shifts from normality to depression to excitement, or has extended periods of dejection and apathy, interspersed with brief spells of anger, anxiety, or euphoria (e.g., mood changes erratically from sadness to bitterness to torpor).
1	2	3	**O. Solemn:** Is unrelaxed, tense, joyless, and grim; restrains overtly warm or covertly antagonistic feelings, keeping most emotions under tight control (e.g., affect is constricted and confined).

FIGURE 24.1. *(p. 5 of 9)*

VI. Intrapsychic Mechanisms Domain

Although mechanisms of self-protection, need gratification, and conflict resolution are consciously recognized at times, they represent data derived primarily at the intrapsychic level. Because the ego or defense mechanisms are internal regulatory processes, they are more difficult to discern and describe than processes that are anchored closer to the observable world. As such, they are not directly amenable to assessment by self-reflective appraisal in their pure form, but only as derivatives that are potentially many levels removed from their core conflicts and their dynamic resolution. Despite the methodological problems they present, the task of identifying which mechanisms are most characteristic of a patient and the extent to which they are employed is extremely useful in a comprehensive clinical assessment.

1st Best Fit	2nd Best Fit	3rd Best Fit	Characteristic Mechanism
1	2	3	**A. Intellectualization:** Describes interpersonal and affective experiences in a matter-of-fact, abstract, impersonal, or mechanical manner; pays primary attention to formal and objective aspects of social and emotional events.
1	2	3	**B. Undoing:** Bizarre mannerisms and idiosyncratic thoughts appear to reflect a retraction or reversal of previous acts or ideas that have stirred feelings of anxiety, conflict, or guilt; ritualistic or "magical" behaviors serve to repent for or nullify assumed misdeeds or "evil" thoughts.
1	2	3	**C. Fantasy:** Depends excessively on imagination to achieve need gratification and conflict resolution; withdraws into reveries as a means of safely discharging affectionate as well as aggressive impulses.
1	2	3	**D. Introjection:** Is firmly devoted to another to strengthen the belief that an inseparable bond exists between them; jettisons any independent views in favor of those of another to preclude conflicts and threats to the relationship.
1	2	3	**E. Magnification:** Engages in hyperbole, overstating and overemphasizing ordinary matters so as to elevate their importance, especially features that enhance not only his or her own virtues but those of others who are valued.
1	2	3	**F. Dissociation:** Regularly alters self-presentations to create a succession of socially attractive but changing facades; engages in self-distracting activities to avoid reflecting on/integrating unpleasant thoughts/emotions.
1	2	3	**G. Rationalization:** Is self-deceptive and facile in devising plausible reasons to justify self-centered and socially inconsiderate behaviors; offers alibis to place self in the best possible light, despite evident shortcomings or failures.
1	2	3	**H. Projection:** Actively disowns undesirable personal traits and motives and attributes them to others; remains blind to own unattractive behaviors and characteristics, yet is overalert to and hypercritical of the defects of others.
1	2	3	**I. Acting Out:** Inner tensions that might accrue by postponing the expression of offensive thoughts and malevolent actions are rarely constrained; socially repugnant impulses are not refashioned in sublimated forms, but are discharged directly in precipitous ways, usually without guilt.
1	2	3	**J. Isolation:** Can be cold-blooded and remarkably detached from an awareness of the impact of his or her destructive acts; views objects of violation impersonally, often as symbols of devalued groups devoid of human sensibilities.
1	2	3	**K. Asceticism:** Engages in acts of self-denial, self-tormenting, and self-punishment, believing that one should exhibit penance and not be rewarded with life's bounties; not only is there a repudiation of pleasures, but there are harsh self-judgments and minor self-destructive acts.
1	2	3	**L. Exaggeration:** Repetitively recalls past injustices and seeks out future disappointments as a means of raising distress to troubled homeostatic levels; misconstrues, if not sabotages, personal good fortunes to enhance or maintain preferred suffering and pain.
1	2	3	**M. Displacement:** Discharges anger and other troublesome emotions either indirectly or by shifting them from their true objective to settings or persons of lesser peril; expresses resentments by substitute or passive means, such as acting inept or perplexed, or behaving in a forgetful or indolent manner.
1	2	3	**N. Regression:** Retreats under stress to developmentally earlier levels of anxiety tolerance, impulse control, and social adaptation; is unable or disinclined to cope with responsible tasks and adult issues, as evident in immature, if not increasingly childlike behaviors.
1	2	3	**O. Reaction Formation:** Repeatedly presents positive thoughts and socially commendable behaviors that are diametrically opposite to his or her deeper, contrary, and forbidden feelings; displays reasonableness and maturity when faced with circumstances that normally evoke anger or dismay in most persons.

FIGURE 24.1. *(p. 6 of 9)*

VII. Intrapsychic Content Domain

Significant experiences from the past leave an inner imprint, a structural residue composed of memories, attitudes, and affects that serve as a substrate of dispositions for perceiving and reacting to life's events. Analogous to the various organ systems in the body, both the character and the substance of these internalized representations of significant figures and relationships from the past can be differentiated and analyzed for clinical purposes. Variations in the nature and content of this inner world, or what are often called *object relations*, can be identified with one or another personality and lead us to employ the following descriptive terms to represent them.

1st Best Fit	2nd Best Fit	3rd Best Fit	Characteristic Content
1	2	3	**A. Meager:** Inner representations are few in number and minimally articulated, largely devoid of the manifold percepts and memories, or the dynamic interplay among drives and conflicts that typify even well-adjusted persons.
1	2	3	**B. Chaotic:** Inner representations consist of a jumble of miscellaneous memories and percepts, random drives and impulses, and uncoordinated channels of regulation that are only fitfully competent for binding tensions, accommodating needs, and mediating conflicts.
1	2	3	**C. Vexatious:** Inner representations are composed of readily reactivated, intense, and anxiety-ridden memories, limited avenues of gratification, and few mechanisms to channel needs, bind impulses, resolve conflicts, or deflect external stressors.
1	2	3	**D. Immature:** Inner representations are composed of unsophisticated ideas and incomplete memories, rudimentary drives and childlike impulses, as well as minimal competencies to manage and resolve stressors.
1	2	3	**E. Piecemeal:** Inner representations are disorganized and dissipated, a jumble of diluted and muddled recollections that are recalled by fits and starts, serving only as momentary guideposts for dealing with everyday tensions and conflicts.
1	2	3	**F. Shallow:** Inner representations are composed largely of superficial yet emotionally intense affects, memories, and conflicts, as well as facile drives and insubstantial mechanisms.
1	2	3	**G. Contrived:** Inner representations are composed far more than usual of illusory ideas and memories, synthetic drives and conflicts, and pretentious, if not simulated, percepts and attitudes, all of which are readily refashioned as the need arises.
1	2	3	**H. Unalterable:** Inner representations are arranged in an unusual configuration of rigidly held attitudes, unyielding percepts, and implacable drives, which are aligned in a semidelusional hierarchy of tenacious memories, immutable cognitions, and irrevocable beliefs.
1	2	3	**I. Debased:** Inner representations are a mix of revengeful attitudes and impulses oriented to subvert established cultural ideals and mores, as well as to debase personal sentiments and conventional societal attainments.
1	2	3	**J. Pernicious:** Inner representations are distinguished by the presence of aggressive energies and malicious attitudes, as well as by a contrasting paucity of sentimental memories, tender affects, internal conflicts, shame, or guilt feelings.
1	2	3	**K. Forsaken:** Inner representations have been depleted or devitalized, either drained of their richness and joyful elements or withdrawn from memory, leaving the person to feel abandoned, bereft, discarded.
1	2	3	**L. Discredited:** Inner representations are composed of disparaged past memories and discredited achievements, of positive feelings and erotic drives transposed onto their least attractive opposites, of internal conflicts intentionally aggravated, of mechanisms of anxiety reduction subverted by processes that intensify discomforts.
1	2	3	**M. Fluctuating:** Inner representations compose a complex of opposing inclinations and incompatible memories that are driven by impulses designed to nullify his or her own achievements and/or the pleasures and expectations of others.
1	2	3	**N. Incompatible:** Rudimentary and expediently devised, but repetitively aborted, inner representations have led to perplexing memories, enigmatic attitudes, contradictory needs, antithetical emotions, erratic impulses, and opposing strategies for conflict reduction.
1	2	3	**O. Concealed:** Only those inner affects, attitudes, and actions that are socially approved are allowed conscious awareness or behavioral expression, resulting in gratification being highly regulated, forbidden impulses sequestered and tightly bound, personal and social conflicts defensively denied, kept from awareness, all maintained under stringent control.

FIGURE 24.1. *(p. 7 of 9)*

VIII. Intrapsychic Structure Domain

The overall architecture that serves as a framework for an individual's psychic interior may display weakness in its structural cohesion; exhibit deficient coordination among its components; and possess few mechanisms to maintain balance and harmony, regulate internal conflicts, or mediate external pressures. The concept of intrapsychic structure refers to a personality's organizational strength, interior congruity, and functional efficacy. Psychoanalytic usage tends to be limited to quantitative degrees of integrative pathology, not to *qualitative variations* in integrative configuration.

1st Best Fit	2nd Best Fit	3rd Best Fit	Characteristic Structure
1	2	3	**A. Undifferentiated:** Given an inner barrenness, a feeble drive to fulfill needs, and minimal pressures to defend against or resolve internal conflicts, or to cope with external demands, internal structures are best characterized by limited coordination and deficient organization.
1	2	3	**B. Fragmented:** Coping and defensive operations are haphazardly organized in a fragile assemblage, leading to spasmodic and desultory actions in which primitive thoughts and affects are directly discharged, with few reality-based sublimations, leading to significant further structural disintegrations.
1	2	3	**C. Fragile:** Tortuous emotions depend almost exclusively on a single modality for their resolution and discharge, that of avoidance, escape, and fantasy; hence, when faced with unanticipated stress, there are few resources available to deploy and few positions to revert to, short of a regressive decompensation.
1	2	3	**D. Inchoate:** Owing to entrusting others with the responsibility to fulfill needs and to cope with adult tasks, there are both a deficit and a lack of diversity in internal structures and controls, leaving a miscellany of relatively undeveloped and immature adaptive abilities and elementary systems for independent functioning.
1	2	3	**E. Fleeting:** Structures are highly transient, existing in momentary forms that are cluttered and disarranged, making effective coping efforts temporary at best. Affect and action are unconstrained owing to the paucity of established controls and purposeful goals.
1	2	3	**F. Disjointed:** A loosely knit structural conglomerate exists in which processes of internal regulation and control are scattered and unintegrated, with few methods for restraining impulses, coordinating defenses, and resolving conflicts, leading to broad and sweeping mechanisms to maintain psychic cohesion and stability and, when employed, only further disarrange thoughts, feelings, and actions.
1	2	3	**G. Spurious:** Coping and defensive strategies are flimsy and transparent; they only appear substantial and dynamically orchestrated—regulating impulses only marginally, channeling needs with minimal restraint, and creating an egocentric inner world in which conflicts are dismissed, failures are quickly redeemed, and self-pride is effortlessly reasserted.
1	2	3	**H. Inelastic:** A markedly constricted and inflexible pattern of coping and defensive methods exists, as well as rigidly fixed channels of conflict mediation and need gratification, creating an overstrung and taut frame that is so uncompromising in its accommodation to changing circumstances that unanticipated stressors are likely to precipitate either explosive outbursts or inner shatterings.
1	2	3	**I. Unruly:** Inner defensive operations are noted by their paucity, as are efforts to curb irresponsible drives and attitudes, leading to easily transgressed social controls, low thresholds for impulse discharge, few subliminatory channels, unfettered self-expression, and a marked intolerance of delay or frustration.
1	2	3	**J. Eruptive:** Despite a generally cohesive structure of routinely modulating controls and expressive channels, surging, powerful, and explosive energies of an aggressive and sexual nature produce precipitous outbursts that periodically overwhelm and overrun otherwise reasonable restraints.
1	2	3	**K. Depleted:** The scaffold for structures is markedly weakened, with coping methods enervated and defensive strategies impoverished and devoid of vigor and focus, resulting in a diminished if not exhausted capacity to initiate action and regulate affect.
1	2	3	**L. Inverted:** Structures have a dual quality, one more or less conventional, the other its obverse— resulting in a repetitive undoing of affect and intention, of a transposing of channels of need gratification with those leading to their frustration, and of actions that produce antithetical, if not self-sabotaging consequences.
1	2	3	**M. Divergent:** There is a clear division in the pattern of internal elements such that coping and defensive maneuvers are often directed toward incompatible goals, leaving major conflicts unresolved and psychic cohesion impossible, as fulfillment of one drive or need inevitably nullifies or reverses another.

FIGURE 24.1. *(p. 8 of 9)*

1st Best Fit	2nd Best Fit	3rd Best Fit	Characteristic Structure
1	2	3	**N. Split:** Inner cohesion constitutes a sharply segmented and conflictful configuration with a marked lack of consistency among elements; levels of consciousness occasionally blur; a rapid shift occurs across boundaries separating unrelated memories/affects, results in schisms upsetting limited extant psychic order.
1	2	3	**O. Compartmentalized:** Psychic structures are rigidly organized in a tightly consolidated system that is clearly partitioned into numerous distinct and segregated constellations of drive, memory, and cognition, with few open channels to permit any interplay among these components.

Spectra That Best Characterize the Person

1st Best Fit	2nd Best Fit	3rd Best Fit	Normal to Abnormal Personality Spectrum
1	2	3	Retiring—Schizoid
1	2	3	Eccentric—Schizotypal
1	2	3	Shy—Avoidant
1	2	3	Needy—Dependent
1	2	3	Exuberant—Hypomanic
1	2	3	Sociable—Histrionic
1	2	3	Confident—Narcissistic
1	2	3	Suspicious—Paranoid
1	2	3	Nonconforming—Antisocial
1	2	3	Assertive—Sadistic
1	2	3	Pessimistic—Melancholic
1	2	3	Aggrieved—Masochistic
1	2	3	Skeptical—Negativistic
1	2	3	Capricious—Borderline
1	2	3	Conscientious—Compulsive

Overall Level of Social and Occupational Functioning

Judgment	Rating Number	Description
Excellent	1	Clearly manifests an effective, if not superior level of functioning in relating to family and social peers, even to helping others in resolving their difficulties, as well as demonstrating high occupational performance and success.
Very Good	2	Exhibits considerable social and occupational skills on a reasonably consistent basis, evidencing few if any major areas of interpersonal stress or occupational difficulty.
Good	3	Displays a higher than average level of social and occupational competence in ordinary matters of everyday life. He or she does experience intermittent difficulties in interpersonal relationships and in efforts to achieve work satisfaction.
Fair	4	Functions about average for a typical patient seen in outpatient clinical work. Although able to meet everyday family, social, and occupational responsibilities adequately, there remain problematic or extended periods of occupational stress and/or interpersonal conflict.
Poor	5	Able to be maintained on an outpatient basis, but often precipitates severe conflicts with others that upset his or her equanimity in either or both interpersonal relationships and occupational settings.
Very Poor	6	There is an inability to function competently in most social and occupational settings. Difficulties are precipitated by the patient, destabilizing job performance and upsetting relationships with significant others. Inpatient hospitalization may be necessary to manage periodic severe psychic disruptions.
Markedly Impaired	7	A chronic and marked disintegration is present across most psychic functions. The loss of physical and behavioral controls necessitate extended stays in residential or hospital settings, requiring both sustained care and self-protection.

FIGURE 24.1. *(p. 9 of 9)*

readers, may wish to review the trait options that constitute the choices for each of the domains. While reading and thinking about the several domain descriptions, and to help guide your choices, feel comfortable in moving freely back and forth within Figure 24.1 as you proceed. For example, while working on reviewing the trait options for the Expressive Behavior domain, do not hesitate to look at the trait descriptions for any of the other domains (e.g., Interpersonal Conduct), if by doing so you may be aided in understanding the characteristics of the Expressive Behavior group of choices.

For each of the domain pages in Figure 24.1, beginning with Expressive Behavior, you will see 15 descriptive trait choices. Locate the descriptive choice that appears to you to be the *best fit* in characterizing a patient you may be thinking about. You will circle that choice in the "1st Best Fit" column. Then, as most people can be characterized by more than one Expressive Behavior trait, locate a second-best-fit descriptive characteristic—one not as applicable to this person as the first best fit you selected, but notable nonetheless. Circle that choice in the "2nd best fit" column. Should there be any other listed descriptive trait features that are applicable to this person, but less so than the one selected as second best, you may encircle up to three choices in the "3rd Best Fit" column. (Note that only one trait description may be marked in each of the first two columns.)

Consider the following points as you proceed. The 15 descriptive traits for each domain were written to characterize patients. Furthermore, each trait is illustrated with several clinical characteristics and examples. Note that the person you are rating need not display precisely the characteristics that are listed; they need only be the best-fitting of the listed group of features. It is important to note also that for rated persons of a nonclinical character (i.e., normal personals who display only minor or mild aspects of the trait characteristic), you should nevertheless fully mark the "Best Fit" columns (even though the descriptor is characterized with a more serious clinical description than suits the person). In short, *do not* leave any of the "Best Fit" columns blank. Circle your choices in best-fit order, even when the features of the trait are only marginally present.

After completing ratings for the Expressive Behavior domain in Figure 24.1, you will proceed to fill in your choices for the next seven domains, one at a time, using the same procedure for first, second, and third ratings you have followed previously. As you, our readers, are not officially completing the MG-PDC, it will be useful for you to know which personality prototype corresponds to the letters that precede each of the descriptors. For example, in the Expressive Behavior domain, note that the letter A precedes the first descriptor, "Impassive." The letter A signifies that this descriptor characterizes the Retiring/Schizoid prototype. Each of the following letters in all eight domains corresponds to the following prototypes:

A. Retiring–Schizoid
B. Eccentric–Schizotypal
C. Shy–Avoidant
D. Needy–Dependent
E. Exuberant–Hypomanic
F. Sociable–Histrionic
G. Confident–Narcissistic

H. Suspicious–Paranoid
I. Nonconforming–Antisocial
J. Assertive–Sadistic
K. Pessimistic–Melancholic (Depressive)
L. Aggrieved–Masochistic
M. Skeptical–Negativistic
N. Capricious–Borderline
O. Conscientious–Compulsive

Once you have made your choices in all eight of the domain categories in Figure 24.1 (or only the first five, if you choose; recall our earlier mention that the final three domains are optional), summarize your judgments by making overall first-, second-, and third-best-fit personality spectrum diagnoses in the "Spectra That Best Characterize the Person" section of Figure 24.1. If you wish, before you proceed, you may want to go back to review your eight (or five) domain best choices and *double-circle* the three that you judge most important to be therapeutically modified.

In the final section of Figure 24.1, use your ratings of this person in the eight (or five) domain categories to assess his or her current overall level of social and occupational functioning. Make your judgment using the 7-point continuum in the "Overall Level of . . . " section of the figure, which ranges from "Excellent" to "Markedly Impaired." Focus your rating on the individual's present mental state and social competencies, overlooking where possible physical impairments or socioeconomic considerations. Circle the number in this section that represents your best judgment.

Domain/Tactical Therapeutic Options

An obvious benefit of an instrument such as the MG-PDC is that it facilitates the coordination of domain-based tactical therapeutic strategies toward an integrative approach focusing on personalized (i.e., personality-guided) treatment (e.g., Millon, 1999; Millon & Grossman, 2007). In concert with strategies and approaches harmonized by the totality of the person that focus on motivating aims/existential polarities (Millon, 1990; Millon & Davis, 1996), leading to sequences and combinations of therapeutic techniques, an instrument focusing on domains assesses and specifies *what* techniques and modalities are likely to be of benefit. Turning to those specific domains of the MG-PDC in which clinical problems exhibit themselves, clinicians can address dysfunctions in the realm of interpersonal conduct by employing interpersonal, family, or group therapeutic methods, for example. Psychodynamic, object relations, and brief dynamic modalities may be especially suited to the realm of object representations; the phenomenological schools subsuming cognitive, existential, and humanistic therapies may be best chosen to modify difficulties of cognitive beliefs and self-esteem.

Therapeutic modalities vary in their degree of specificity and strategic goals; these differences are often merely accidents of history, but can be tied back to assumptions latent in the therapies themselves. However, the progression over time has been toward both greater specificity and clearer goals. The *Zeitgeist* of the modern therapeutic delivery systems demands both of these, and the larger society—with more time restrictions, less luxury in longer-term treatments, and higher volumes of psychotherapy—enforces them. More modern approaches to psychotherapy, such as the cognitive-behavioral approach, put into place highly detailed elements (e.g., agreed-upon goals, termination criteria, and ongoing assessments) in which therapy itself becomes a self-regulating system. Ongoing assessments ensure the existence of a feedback process that is open to inspection and negotiation by both therapist and patient. The mode is one of action rather than talk; the action is more interactive and transactive; and therapy is forward-looking and concentrates on realizing present possibilities as a means of creating or opening up new possibilities. Persons are often changed more through exposure and action than through focusing on and unraveling the problems of the past. Insight may be catalytic, even necessary, but is ultimately limited for its own purposes.

In an early book, Millon (1981) likened personality to an immune system for the psyche, such that stability, constancy, and internal equilibrium become the goals of a personality. These goals, of course, may run directly in opposition to the explicit goal of therapy, which is change. If (or, usually, when) a particular therapy client feels threatened, his or her personality system functions as a form of passive resistance, albeit one that may be experienced as a positive force or trait by the therapist. In fact, the structural grounding of a patient's self-image and object representations are so preemptive and confirmation-seeking that the true meaning of the therapist's comments may never reach the level of conscious processing. Alternatively, even if a patient's equilibrium is initially up-ended by a particular interpretation, his or her defensive mechanisms may kick in to ensure that a therapist's comments are some-how distorted, misunderstood, interpreted in a less threatening manner, or even ignored. The first is a passive form of resistance; the second is an active form. No wonder, then, that effective therapy is often considered anxiety-provoking, for it is in situations where the patient really has no effective response—where the functioning of the psychic immune system is temporarily suppressed—that the scope of his or her response repertoire is most likely to be broadened. Personality goes with what it knows, and it is with the unknown that learning is most possible.

A coordinated schema of strategic goals and tactical modalities for treatment seeks to accomplish change in an effective and efficient psychotherapy (Millon & Grossman, 2007). In coordinating approaches that mirror the synchronized composi-tion of an individual's complex clinical syndrome and personality system, a clinician should make an effort to select domain-focused tactics that will fulfill the strategic goals of treatment. Interventions of an unfocused, rambling, and diffuse nature lead only to minor progressions and passive resistance to change via habitual characteris-tics already intrinsic to the individual's personality system. Ultimately, something must happen that cannot be readily fielded by habitual processes—in other words, something that targets and disrupts the homeostatic domain functions identified by the MG-PDC.

The purpose of this domain or tactical focus—or knowing clearly what to do in therapy and why to do it—is to keep the whole of the therapeutic enterprise from becoming diffused. The person-focused systems model runs counter to the determin-istic universe-as-machine model of the late 19th century, which features slow but incremental gains. In a focused, "punctuated" personalized model, therapeutic advances may clearly be spelled out to have genuine transformational potential—a potential maximized through combinations and/or progressions of domain tactics, such as those we have termed "potentiated pairings" and "catalytic sequences" (see Millon, Boice, & Sinsabaugh, Chapter 2, this volume). Tactical specificity, then, is required in part because the psychic level at which therapy is practiced is fairly explicit. The therapeutic relationship and dialogue are largely dominated by discussions of specific domain behaviors, specific domain feelings, and specific domain cognitions, not by abstract discussions of personality style or clinical syndromes.

For the therapist, operationalizing and redefining such diagnostic entities as domain clusters such as expressive behaviors or cognitive styles can be especially beneficial in selecting tactical modalities. For example, an avoidant individual's social withdrawal can be seen as having enough self-esteem to leave a humiliating situation, while a dependent person's clinging to a significant other can be seen as having the strength to devote time and energy to another's care. Of course, these reframes will not be sufficient in and of themselves to produce change. They do, however, constitute positive attributions and thereby work toward increasing self-esteem, while simultaneously working to disconfirm other beliefs that lower esteem and function to keep the person closed off from trying on new roles and behaviors.

As has been noted previously, there are *strategic goals* of therapy—that is, those that endure across numerous sessions and against which progress is measured—and there are specific *domain modality tactics* by which these goals are pursued. Ideally, strategies and tactics should be integrated, with the tactics chosen to accomplish strategic goals, and the strategies chosen on the basis of what tactics might actually achieve (given other constraints, such as the number of therapy sessions and the nature of the problem). To illustrate, intrapsychic therapies are highly strategic but tactically impoverished; purely behavioral therapies are highly tactical but strategically narrow and inflexible. There are, in fact, many different ways that strategies may be operationalized. Just as diagnostic criteria are neither necessary nor sufficient for membership in a given class, it is likely that no technique is an inevitable consequence of a given clinical strategy. Subtle variations in technique and the ingenuity of individual therapists to invent techniques ad hoc assure an almost infinite number of ways to operationalize or put into action a given clinical strategy.

The following vignette represents a recent case in which such a domain-based, personalized case conceptualization was utilized, and outlines the MG-PDC assessment procedure.

Case Example: Yulya V.

Background Information

Yulya, a 32-year-old woman born in Kiev, Ukraine, to Jewish parents, presented for treatment 8 months after returning from an extended tour of duty in both Afghanistan and Iraq. Her family had emigrated to the United States when she was 7 years old, and, owing to their feelings of persecution and personal limitations at the time of their departure from what was then the Soviet Union, "constantly were overprotective and insistent on keeping me on a short leash." As she recalled, her first years in her new country were marked by shyness and uncertainty, with constant yearning for her parents when they were not immediately present. In her early adolescence, however, she took a very different turn: "I suddenly started resenting the hell out of it, and for a while I did anything and everything I wanted." She reported periods of sexual promiscuity, heavy substance use, and consistently oppositional behaviors. "Basically, if my parents told me to do something, I'd do the opposite. They eventually started to try the opposite—encouraging me to do stupid things—and I'd be a model daughter until they noticed, then I'd go bad. It was when they stopped caring, I didn't know what to do." In her early 20s, Yulya was working as an exotic dancer, and allowed herself to get "picked up" by a club patron who then nearly beat her to death. "Ever since, I've been thankful for that awful experience and everything I do. I've made it a point to ask, 'Is this what's best for me, my family and my world?' "

Hoping to study medicine eventually via subsequent benefits, Yulya enlisted in the U.S. Army as a medical services specialist shortly before the events of 9/11, after which she was deployed to Afghanistan and subsequently to Iraq. "Of course now I question the whole thing, but then I just thought I was acting for a noble cause and would do absolutely anything to support the cause." In the service, she met her future husband, a war contractor, and became pregnant; shortly thereafter, the couple returned to the United States and got married.

Presenting Picture

Approximately 1 year later, Yulya noted that she started experiencing "really scary moments," wherein she felt like she was visualizing and reliving episodes from medical traumas and could not recall any medical training. This sinking, hopeless feeling appeared to lead to her feeling "distanced" from most aspects of her life, and her husband noticed her becoming less engaged, more apathetic, and behaving "like a catatonic zombie." At first Yulya argued that "if you'd been through what I've been through, you'd not want to feel everything either," and "of course, I'm going to remember what I've been through, it's no big deal." However, when her husband noted that he felt she might become a "cold mother" to her newborn son, she decided to address it.

Assessment Procedures

Initial assessment of Yulya via clinical interview and the MCMI-III with the Grossman Facet Scales, as well as other instruments capturing both broad-band and symptom-specific features, indicated an overall personality constellation of primarily skeptical/negativistic and conscientious/compulsive features not meeting full criteria for an Axis II diagnosis, but nevertheless indicating significant patterns that would markedly influence treatment. Also present were some very mild but still influential independent/antisocial characteristics. This pattern was strongly marked by an excessive and troubling conflict between meeting the needs of the self and responding to the expectations of others, as well as difficulties negotiating decisions and actions that would stand to modify her environment versus adjusting her own expectations and sense of self to "fit in" with her given circumstances. Layered on this were mild, agitated depressive symptoms and a fairly clear, moderately severe diagnosis of posttraumatic stress disorder (PTSD).

The clinician also completed the MG-PDC in order to capture more molecular facets of Yulya and her presentation, and to facilitate selection and implementation of specific therapeutic techniques to be coordinated into a tactical treatment plan addressing overt symptomatology and characterological domain traits. The following significant domains were identified:

I. *Expressive Behavioral domain.* Yulya was notably *disciplined* in her overt behavioral tendencies, showing a forthrightness and sense of duty in most all of her actions, although she rarely seemed passionate while performing a task. She did, however, display occasional *resentful* acts, which seemed so more by description than action.

II. *Interpersonal Conduct domain.* In this area, Yulya showed only *respectfulness*, without regard to whom she was interacting with. Once again, there was a sense that this was more a role she was playing than the way she really felt about the interaction. This did not seem to indicate "falseness," but more of an affective "removal."

III. *Cognitive Style domain.* Clearly here, Yulya demonstrated a certain *constriction*, as though to think or act in a manner that would violate established norms would be totally unacceptable. However, she could identify, with some insight, that this was inconsistent with earlier life beliefs that actually fell more in line with an independent/antisocial person's *deviant* stylings.

IV. *Self-Image domain.* Yulya presented herself as both *autonomous* and *reliable*, and this combination typically functioned well when she did not have imperatives from others; however, she frequently did have to answer others' needs, and a certain amount of *discontentment* tended to appear.

V. *Mood/Affect domain.* Clearly, Yulya demonstrated *solemnness* in her affect, keeping tight controls over her expressed emotion. This occasionally appeared to gravitate toward apathy, but it would become clear, with very little engagement on the part of the clinician, that this distancing was more a product of control than of uninterest.

VI. *Intrapsychic Mechanisms domain.* *Displacement* characterized this first, more observable intrapsychic domain, as Yulya would, on specific stressful occasions (and largely out of overall character), "forget" important responsibilities or fail to acknowledge something—blaming her "closet ADD," as she termed it.

VII. *Intrapsychic Content domain.* Intrapsychic objects seemed to be *concealed* with Yulya, as she reported regularly that her feelings regarding important people, events, and relationships would only be recalled or reframed in terms of their positive qualities, and past conflicts or conflictual content had a consistent quality of being "for the best."

VIII. *Intrapsychic Structure domain.* Yulya indicated, through vague inferences, that her inner world often seemed *divergent*, setting up win–lose scenarios in terms of one drive or motivation's effectively nullifying another. At the same time, she cloaked this with a rather rigid, tenuous, *compartmentalized* structure.

When we examine these personological domains, the etiology and presentation of PTSD (the identified catalyst for treatment) appear much more distinctive than in the Axis I symptomatic description. Perhaps in Yulya's case, the intrapsychic turmoil between keeping order and resisting expectation provides a context for the expression of guilt over not feeling able to do what is expected in times of crisis (the content of her symptomatic flashbacks). Perhaps she feels limited by rules and expectations, but her belief system doesn't allow her to express unique ideas. This conflict may have been compounded by her experience, in which she took it upon herself to find less accepted means of survival and ended up nearly dead. A tactical treatment plan, then, may be to begin with acknowledgments, in both the self-image and cognitive domains, of places where Yulya may feel she has "no choice" but to meet expectations, especially *because* she is so capable. This may allow her, then, to become aware of resultant resentfulness that not only percolates beneath the surface of a dutiful front (behavioral realm), but also permeates other domains of her life. Ideally, this will lay the groundwork for Yulya to begin the process of working through her discontentments, and to begin to develop less constricted and more flexible coping measures than those driven only by the expectations of others. This, thematically, should open the doors for a more contextual processing of her "relived experiences."

Conclusion

The MG-PDC is the most recent endeavor in addressing personological domains for purposes of coordinated, tactical treatment planning, such as that found in our recent intervention-oriented writings (e.g., Millon & Grossman, 2007). This method represents a continuation of the MPDC (Tringone, 1990, 1997) methodology, updated to reflect innovations in theory and therapeutic approaches, and modified to be well suited to time-limited assessment and intervention paradigms. The MG-PDC's focus on the domain level of personality description, with its perspective on comprehensiveness and comparability of functional and structural domains, makes it possible to emphasize and operationalize a pragmatic, dimensional approach to personality treatment. Further work is necessary and encouraged in order to better understand psychometric properties of the new instrument, beyond its concordance with an explicated and comprehensive theoretical perspective.

References

American Psychiatric Association. (1980). *Diagnostic and statistical manual of mental disorders* (3rd ed.). Washington, DC: Author.

American Psychiatric Association. (1987). *Diagnostic and statistical manual of mental disorders* (3rd ed., rev.). Washington, DC: Author.

American Psychiatric Association. (1994). *Diagnostic and statistical manual of mental disorders* (4th ed.). Washington, DC: Author.

American Psychiatric Association. (2000). *Diagnostic and statistical manual of mental disorders* (4th ed., text rev.). Washington, DC: Author.

Campbell, D. T., & Fiske, D. W. (1959). Convergent and discriminant validation by the multitrait–multimethod matrix. *Psychological Bulletin, 56*, 81–105.

Cantor, N., & Genero, N. (1986). Psychiatric diagnosis and natural categorization: A close analogy. In T. Millon & G. L. Klerman (Eds.), *Contemporary directions in psychopathology: Toward the DSM-IV* (pp. 233–256). New York: Guilford Press.

Cantor, N., Smith, E. E., French, R., & Mezzich, J. (1980). Psychiatric diagnosis as prototype categorization. *Journal of Abnormal Psychiatry, 89*, 181–193.

Clarkin, J. F., Widiger, T. A., Frances, A., Hurt, S. W., & Gilmore, M. (1983). Prototypic typology and the borderline personality disorder. *Journal of Abnormal Psychology, 92*, 263–275.

Costa, P. T., Jr., & McCrae, R. R. (1992). The five-factor model of personality and its relevance to personality disorders. *Journal of Personality Disorders, 6*, 343–359.

Costa, P. T., Jr., & McCrae, R. R. (1995). Domains and facets: Hierarchical personality assessment using the Revised NEO Personality Inventory. *Journal of Personality Assessment, 64*, 21–50.

Cronbach, L. J., & Meehl, P. E. (1955). Construct validity in psychological tests. *Psychological Bulletin, 52*, 281–302.

Davis, R. D., & Millon, T. (1993). The five-factor model for personality disorders: Apt or misguided? *Psychological Inquiry, 4*, 104–109.

Frances, A. (1980). The DSM-III personality disorders section: A commentary. *American Journal of Psychiatry, 137*, 1050–1054.

Frances, A. (1982). Categorical and dimensional systems of personality diagnosis: A comparison. *Comprehensive Psychiatry, 23*, 516–527.

Frances, A., & Widiger, T. A. (1986). Methodological issues in personality disorder diagnosis. In T. Millon & G. L. Klerman (Eds.), *Contemporary directions in psychopathology: Toward the DSM-IV* (pp. 381–400). New York: Guilford Press.

Garfield, S. (1986). Problems in diagnostic classification. In T. Millon & G. L. Klerman (Eds.),

Contemporary directions in psychopathology: Toward the DSM-IV (pp. 99–114). New York: Guilford Press.

Jackson, D. N. (1970). A sequential system for personality scale development. In C. D. Spielberger (Ed.), *Current topics in clinical and community psychology* (Vol. 2, pp. 61–92). New York: Academic Press.

Klerman, G. L. (1986). Historical perspective on contemporary schools of psychopathology. In T. Millon & G. L. Klerman (Eds.), *Contemporary directions in psychopathology: Toward the DSM-IV* (pp. 3–28). New York: Guilford Press.

Livesley, W. J., Jackson, D. N., & Schroeder, M. L. (1989). A study of the factorial structure of personality pathology. *Journal of Personality Disorders, 3,* 292–306.

Loevinger, J. (1957). Objective tests as instruments of psychological theory. *Psychological Reports, 3,* 635–694.

Millon, T. (1969). *Modern psychopathology: A biosocial approach to maladaptive learning and functioning.* Philadelphia: Saunders.

Millon, T. (1981). *Disorders of personality: DSM-III, Axis II.* New York: Wiley.

Millon, T. (1984). On the renaissance of personality assessment and personality theory. *Journal of Personality Assessment, 48,* 450–466.

Millon, T. (1986a). On the past and future of the DSM-III: Personal recollections and projections. In T. Millon & G. L. Klerman (Eds.), *Contemporary directions in psychopathology: Toward the DSM-IV* (pp. 29–70). New York: Guilford Press.

Millon, T. (1986b). Personality prototypes and their diagnostic criteria. In T. Millon & G. L. Klerman (Eds.), *Contemporary directions in psychopathology: Toward the DSM-IV* (pp. 671–712). New York: Guilford Press.

Millon, T. (1987a). *Millon Clinical Multiaxial Inventory–II manual.* Minneapolis, MN: National Computer Systems.

Millon, T. (1987b). On the nature of taxonomy in psychopathology. In M. Hersen & C. Last (Eds.), *Issues in diagnostic research* (pp. 3–85). New York: Plenum Press.

Millon, T. (1990). *Toward an integrated personology: Providing an evolutionary and ecological foundation for Murray's scaffolding.* New York: Wiley.

Millon, T., & Davis, R. D. (1996). *Disorders of personality: DSM-IV and beyond* (2nd ed.). New York: Wiley.

Millon, T., & Grossman, S. (2007). *Overcoming difficult clinical syndromes: A personalized psychotherapy approach.* New York: Wiley.

Millon, T. (with Grossman, S., & Meagher, S.). (2004). *Masters of the mind.* Hoboken, NJ: Wiley.

Millon, T. (with Grossman, S., Meagher, S., Millon, C., & Everly, G.). (1999). *Personality-guided therapy.* New York: Wiley.

Millon, T. (with Millon, C., Davis, R., & Grossman, S.). (2006a). *The Millon Clinical Multiaxial Inventory-III (MCMI-III) manual* (3rd ed.). Minneapolis, MN: Pearson Assessments.

Millon, T. (with Millon, C., Davis, R., & Grossman, S.). (2006b). *The Millon Adolescent Clinical Inventory (MACI) manual* (2nd ed.). Minneapolis, MN: Pearson Assessments.

Millon, T., & Tringone, R. (1989). [Co-occurrence and diagnostic efficiency statistics]. Unpublished raw data.

Morey, L. C. (1988). Personality disorders in DSM-III and DSM-III-R: Convergence, coverage, and internal consistency. *American Journal of Psychiatry, 145,* 573–577.

Shea, M. T. (1992). Some characteristics of the Axis II criteria sets and their implications for assessment of personality disorders. *Journal of Personality Disorders, 6,* 377–381.

Skinner, H. A. (1986). Construct validation approach to psychiatric classification. In T. Millon & G. L. Klerman (Eds.), *Contemporary directions in psychopathology: Toward the DSM-IV* (pp. 307–330). New York: Guilford Press.

Stricker, G., & Gold, J. R. (1988). A psychodynamic approach to the personality disorders. *Journal of Personality Disorders, 2,* 350–359.

Tringone, R. (1990). *Construction of the Millon Personality Diagnostic Checklist–III—R and per-*

sonality prototypes. Unpublished doctoral dissertation, University of Miami, Coral Gables, FL.

Tringone, R. (1997). The MPDC: Composition and clinical applications. In T. Millon (Ed.), *The Millon inventories* (pp. 449–474). New York: Guilford Press.

Westen, D., & Weinberger, J. (2004). When clinical description becomes statistical prediction. *American Psychologist, 59,* 595–613.

Widiger, T. A. (1982). Prototypic typology and borderline diagnoses. *Clinical Psychology Review, 2,* 115–135.

Widiger, T. A. (1992). Categorical versus dimensional classification. *Journal of Personality Disorders, 6,* 287–300.

Widiger, T. A., Hurt, S. W., Frances, A., Clarkin, J. F., & Gilmore, M. (1984). Diagnostic efficiency and DSM-III. *Archives of General Psychiatry, 41,* 1005–1012.

Widiger, T. A., & Trull, T. J. (2007). Plate tectonics in the classification of personality disorder: Shifting to a dimensional model. *American Psychologist, 62,* 71–83.

Wittgenstein, L. (1953). *Philosophical investigations.* Oxford: Blackwell.

PART IV

A GUIDE TO ASSOCIATED MILLON PERSONALITY INVENTORIES

Using the Personality Adjective Check List (PACL) to Gauge Normal Personality Styles

Stephen Strack

The Personality Adjective Check List (PACL) is a 153-item self-report and observer rating measure of Theodore Millon's (1969) eight basic personality patterns for use with normal adults, counseling clients, and psychiatric patients with nondisordered traits. It features a Problem Indicator (PI) scale that measures aspects of Millon's three severe (schizoid, cycloid, and paranoid) styles, and may be used as a gauge of personality disturbance. PACL personality scales measure theoretically derived, *normal* versions of the character types frequently seen in clinical settings. Test results yield rich descriptions of respondents in a language that closely resembles that found in the *Diagnostic and Statistical Manual of Mental Disorders*, fourth edition, text revision (DSM-IV-TR; American Psychiatric Association, 2000). The measure is frequently used by clinicians who work with relatively high-functioning individuals and who want to understand the *strengths* of their clients as well as their weaknesses. The PACL has been used in numerous research studies that have tested various propositions of Millon's theory and addressed the interface between normal and abnormal personality (e.g., Strack, 1991c, 1993, 2005a, 2005b; Millon & Grossman, 2006).

In this chapter, I present the PACL from the ground up. I begin with its theoretical foundation in Millon's (1969) biopsychosocial model of personality and psychopathology, and describe its development according to Loevinger's (1957) three-stage model of test construction. Next, I present clinical and research findings from a variety of studies, and descriptions of persons who obtain high scale scores. Clinical and research uses of the test are then outlined, and I finish with case examples that demonstrate how to apply the PACL with counseling and employee assistance clients.

Theoretical Foundation of the PACL

The PACL originated at the University of Miami in the early 1980s in a research group led by Theodore Millon, Catherine Green, and the late Robert Meagher, Jr. This was an exciting time. DSM-III (American Psychiatric Association, 1980) had just been published, and the new multiaxial diagnostic system incorporated much of Millon's (1969, 1981) theory into its taxonomy of personality disorders. The original Millon Clinical Multiaxial Inventory (MCMI-I; Millon, 1977) had recently been published, and the Millon Adolescent Personality Inventory (MAPI; Millon, Green, & Meagher, 1982a) and Millon Behavioral Health Inventory (MBHI; Millon, Green, & Meagher, 1982b) were just being launched. At that time very little empirical work had been accomplished using Millon's model, and we sought ways of changing this. Many theses and dissertations were spawned in the research group, including my second-year project, *Development of the Personality Adjective Check List and Preliminary Validation in a Normal College Population* (Strack, 1981). The purpose of creating the PACL was to open the door for research on normal subjects. Although Millon's model posits a direct link between normal and abnormal personalities, the MCMI-I, MAPI, and MBHI were designed for clinical populations. By developing a measure of Millon's personalities for normal individuals, we hoped to capitalize on the large pool of nonclinical research subjects available to investigators in college and business settings. By using an adjective check list method of assessment, we hoped to create a measure that was quick and easy to administer that would allow for observer ratings as well as self reports. Our long-term goals included building an analogue model of personality disorders among normal individuals and demonstrating the inherent continuity between the normal and abnormal domains of personality functioning.

Linking Normality and Pathology

An attractive feature of Millon's (1969, 1981, 1986a, 1986b, 1990, 2006; Millon & Davis, 1996) model, and one that makes the PACL possible, is its assumption that normal and abnormal personalities lie along a continuum, with disordered character representing an exaggeration or distortion of normal traits. Normal and abnormal persons are viewed as sharing the same basic styles. Disordered individuals are depicted as a small subset of the pool of all persons who, for various biological, psychological, environmental, and social reasons, have developed rigid and maladaptive traits.

In deriving his personalities, Millon (1981, 1986a, 1986b, 1990, 2006; Millon & Davis, 1996) distinguished four points along the normal–abnormal continuum— that is, normal character, and styles exhibiting mild, moderate, and severe pathology. Eight personality types were posited to exist in normal form and/or in mild or moderate pathological form: namely, asocial, avoidant, submissive (dependent), gregarious (histrionic), narcissistic, aggressive, conforming (compulsive), and negativistic. Three severe styles—schizoid (schizotypal), cycloid (borderline), and paranoid—were thought to be variants of the mildly and moderately pathological personalities that do not have direct counterparts in the normal domain.

Two sets of concepts were outlined by Millon to distinguish his personalities at the various continuum points. One set of concepts defines the relative position of normal and pathological individuals on his three evolutionary polarities—that is, active–passive, pleasure–pain, and self–other (Millon, 1990). Normal individuals are thought to be balanced in each of these areas (e.g., to possess both moderate self-esteem and empathic regard for others). Mild or moderate pathology is apparent among persons showing excesses or deficits in self- or other-regard, active or passive coping, and/or pleasure–pain orientation. Severe pathology is marked by extremes or distortions on these polarities.

A second set of ideas used by Millon (1969, 1986a) to distinguish normal and abnormal personalities focuses on interpersonal functioning—specifically, an individual's level of flexibility, stability, and tendency to foster vicious cycles. Healthy persons are viewed as interpersonally flexible; adaptive in coping; ego-resilient; and able to avoid, escape from, or move beyond pathogenic attitudes, behaviors, or situations. In contrast, mildly and moderately pathological persons exhibit rigidity in interpersonal relations, nonadaptive coping, low ego strength, and a tendency to become mired in dysfunctional schemas or transactions with others and the environment. More severely disturbed individuals are viewed as strongly rigid and inflexible; lacking in adaptive coping skills; possessing extreme ego deficits; and unable to avoid, escape, or move through pathological thought processes and relationships.

When he expanded his model in the early 1990s (Millon, 1994; Millon & Davis, 1994), Millon described a number of new dimensions that he believes underlie the manifest forms of normal personalities. His pathological personality styles, and their normal variants measured by the PACL, were conceived on the basis of three *motivating* aims: active–passive, pleasure–pain, and self–other. To encompass a wider array of normal personality forms, Millon (1994, 2006) introduced four new axes differentiating various *cognitive* styles and five axes delineating *interpersonal* styles. Interested readers may consult Weiss (Chapter 26, this volume) for a complete description of these theoretical principles.

Development of the PACL

The PACL was developed according to a method outlined by Loevinger (1957), which was used by Millon and his colleagues for creating his clinical measures. In this method, test construction is theory-driven and follows a step-by-step process, with development and validation occurring together.

In the first stage of development and validation, 405 theory-derived adjectives were selected to measure normal versions of Millon's (1969) eight basic and three severe personality styles. Items were drawn from numerous sources, including *Modern Psychopathology*, and were selected based on rater judgments that each item had a clear best fit for one style (for details, see Strack, 1987, 1991c).

The second phase of test construction, structural validity, involves creating scales that match the underlying theory. Toward this end, the 405-item experimental check list was given to 207 men and 252 women from colleges in Ohio and Florida. Preliminary scales were created from items that were endorsed by at least 5% and no more than 80% of subjects; had minimum item–scale correlations of .25; and maximum within-scale item–item correlations of .49 (to prevent redundancy; Strack, 1987, p. 577). With these criteria, measures were created for each of Millon's eight basic styles that had satisfactory internal consistency and temporal reliability. Alpha coefficients ranged from .76 to .89 (new sample median = .83; Strack, 1987, p. 578), while test–retest correlations over a 3-month period ranged from .60 to .85 (median = .72 across sexes; Strack, 1987, p. 578). Additional data showed the scales to be relatively free from social desirability bias (Strack, 1987, p. 581).

Unfortunately, measures could not be developed for the three severe (schizoid, cycloid, and paranoid) personalities because of extremely low endorsement rates (< 5%) for most keyed items. Rather than throw away the handful of good items that remained for these measures, I combined them into an experimental Problem Indicator (PI) scale, which seemed potentially useful in identifying persons with personality disorders.

In addition to the personality and experimental scales, I developed three response bias indices to aid in the detection of faked protocols (Strack, 1991c)—namely, Random (R), Favorable (F), and Unfavorable (UF). Separate groups of college students were asked to complete the PACL randomly, or with intent to give an overly favorable or overly unfavorable self-report. Discriminant function analyses were used to distinguish the faked tests from PACLs completed under the normal instructional set. Equations were derived from these analyses (separately for men and women) and were cross-validated with independent samples. The equations were able to correctly identify a large majority of faked (75% to 91%) and normal tests (60% to 94%).

In accordance with the third stage of test development, extensive external (convergent–discriminant) validity data were collected for the PACL in the form of correlations with tests of personality, mood, and dispositional variables, and reports from subjects about current and past behavior (Strack, 1987, 1991b, 1991c, 1994; Strack & Guevara, 1999; Strack & Lorr, 1990; Strack, Lorr, & Campbell, 1989). This research demonstrated that each PACL scale is in line with theoretical expectations and measures milder versions of Millon's (1969) pathological styles. For example, the scale measuring avoidant personality (Inhibited) was positively associated with measures of shyness, submissiveness, and social anxiety, and negatively associated with measures of sociability, dominance, and emotional well-being (Strack, 1991c). The scale measuring aggressive traits (Forceful) was positively linked to measures of arrogance, dominance, assertiveness, and autonomy, and negatively linked to measures of deference, submissiveness, and conscientiousness (Strack, 1991c). In a study comparing the PI scores of psychiatric patients ($n = 124$) and normal adults ($n = 140$) who completed the PACL using standard instructions, I (Strack, 1991a) found that 84% of the PI T-scores ≥ 60 were obtained by patients (only 16% of the normal adults had T-scores over 59).

PACL Research Findings

Since the late 1980s, several other investigators have reported expected relationships between PACL scales and a variety of measures in correlational and quasi-experimental studies using self-reports and personality ratings.

Wiggins and Pincus (1989; Pincus & Wiggins, 1990) examined the PACL in the context of Minnesota Multiphasic Personality Inventory (MMPI) personality disorder scales (Morey, Waugh, & Blashfield, 1985), the Big Five Interpersonal Adjective Scales (IAS-B5; Trapnell & Wiggins, 1990), the NEO Personality Inventory (NEO-PI; Costa & McCrae, 1985), and a circumplex version of the Inventory of Interpersonal Problems (Alden, Wiggins, & Pincus, 1990). PACL scales exhibited anticipated relationships with each of the tests in correlational, canonical, and factor analyses. For example, PACL Introversive and Sociable were loaded (in opposite directions) on a factor that included the MMPI Schizoid and Histrionic scales, NEO-PI Extraversion, and IAS-B5 Dominance. PACL Forceful was correlated .59 with interpersonal problems associated with dominance behavior, while PACL Cooperative was correlated .48 with problems involving exploitation by others.

Horton and Retzlaff (1991) correlated the PACL with the Moos (1974) Family Environment Scale in a sample of 65 undergraduates. They found that family cohesion and expressiveness were strongly associated with cooperative and sociable personality styles, whereas conflict was most prevalent in the families of sensitive and forceful persons. High scores on the Respectful scale were linked to family environments in which cohesion, organization, and religiosity were salient features. Gontag and Erickson (1996) examined the relationship between undergraduates' ($N = 140$) personality traits and their perceptions of their families of origin, using the PACL and the Self-Report Family Inventory (Beavers & Hampson, 1990). They found that students with elevated scores on the PACL Inhibited, Sensitive, and PI scales rated their families as being low in emotional health and competence, whereas high scores on the PACL Respectful scale were associated with perceptions of families as being emotionally healthy and competent. Family cohesiveness was positively and significantly associated with PACL Respectful scores and negatively associated with PACL Sensitive scores.

Byravan and Ramanaiah (2002) examined the amount of shared variance between PACL scales and the five-factor model (FFM) personality dimensions (Extraversion, Agreeableness, Conscientiousness, Neuroticism, Openness) as assessed by the NEO-PI-R (Costa & McCrae, 1992) among a sample of 258 college students. They used PACL nonoverlapping scale scores with a 9-point Likert response format. By force-entering scores for the FFM global factors into multiple-regression equations that predicted individual PACL scales, they found that the amount of overlapping variance ranged from 48% for Cooperative (Submissive) to 71% for Inhibited (Avoidant). Using similar methodology, Trobst, Ayearst, and Salekin (2004) force-entered FFM scores as measured by the revised IAS-B5 (Trapnell & Wiggins, 1990) into regression equations that predicted seven of nine PACL personality scales (all but Sensitive and PI) in a sample of 617 college students. The strongest significant correlations for each scale were as follows: Introversive (Schizoid) with Extraversion (−.36), Inhibited (Avoidant) with Neuroticism (.49), Cooperative (Dependent) with Agreeableness (.28) and Extraversion (.24), Sociable (Histrionic) with Extraversion (.55), Confident (Narcissistic) with Agreeableness (−.40), Forceful (Antisocial) with Agreeableness (−.52) and Extraversion (.27), and Respectful (Obsessive–Compulsive) with Conscientiousness (.53).

The PACL was correlated and factor-analyzed with MMPI-2 scales in independent samples of psychiatric patients ($n = 196$) and normal adults ($n = 124$) (Strack &

Guevara, 1999). Consistent with previous research, PACL scales measuring Millon's neurotic, introverted styles (Introversive, Inhibited, Sensitive, PI) were positively associated with MMPI-2 scales measuring introversion (Si), affective states (D, Pt), and disturbed thinking (Sc), whereas PACL scales measuring extraverted, socially dominant Millon styles (Sociable, Confident, Forceful) were negatively associated with the same MMPI-2 scales. PACL and MMPI-2 scales were reliably associated along two bipolar dimensions measuring Neuroticism/Introversion versus Extraversion and Emotional Distress versus Emotional Stability, which together accounted for 45% of the variance. A third General Distress factor loaded only MMPI-2 scales. Congruency coefficients indicated that the factors for patients and normal adults were very similar. Results highlighted the consistency of the links among MMPI-2 basic scales, the PACL, and other Millon instruments, as well as the utility of the PACL as a measure of Millon's personality styles in a mental health population.

McHoskey, Worzel, and Szyarto (1998) studied the PACL Forceful and Cooperative scales in the context of Machiavellianism and psychopathy. Their sample consisted of 125 college undergraduates. They found that high Forceful scores were significantly associated with higher scores on measures of Machiavellianism, psychopathy, and self-reported antisocial acts, and negatively associated with self-reported prosocial acts. By contrast, high Cooperative scores were negatively associated with Machiavellianism, psychopathy, and self-reported antisocial acts, while the correlation for self-reported prosocial acts was positive but nonsignificant.

Two published studies used the PACL as a rating instrument. Plante and Boccaccini (1997) had 102 college students complete the PACL so to describe their impression of a "typical Roman Catholic priest." The investigators compared the ratings, which were scored using PACL norms, with self-reports on the check list by 12 "successful applicants to the priesthood." Analysis of variance of the ratings and self reports showed that the students viewed a typical Roman Catholic priest as less inhibited and cooperative, and more confident, forceful, and respectful, than the priest candidates viewed themselves. Analysis of Catholic ($n = 55$) and non-Catholic ($n = 47$) student subgroups showed that the Catholic students viewed a typical priest as more sociable, forceful, respectful, and sensitive than did non-Catholic students. Gould and Hyer (2004) had the caregivers of 68 elderly patients with dementia complete the PACL so as to describe each patient according to "the kind of person he was throughout most of his past life." They correlated factors derived from the personality scales with several measures of cognitive functioning and behavioral disturbance. They found that increased withdrawal and irritability after dementia onset were significantly associated with high Inhibited scores in the premorbid personality trait ratings, while premorbid trait ratings of independence (Confident and Forceful) were linked with less interpersonal withdrawal after onset of dementia.

Finally, in a quasi-experimental study of older combat veterans, Hyer and Boyd (1996) compared the PACL personality scores of 40 veterans diagnosed with post-traumatic stress disorder (PTSD) to a matched group of 80 veterans without PTSD. The group with PTSD had significantly higher Inhibited and Sensitive scores than did the patients without PTSD. The investigators also created a multiple-regression equation designed to predict each patient's PTSD score on the Clinician-Administered PTSD Scale (CAPS; Blake et al., 1990). They first entered eight demographic and psychological variables into the equation before allowing entry of scores for the PACL Inhibited and Sensitive scales. PACL Inhibited, but not Sensitive, scores added significantly to prediction of the patients' PTSD scores after entry of the other variables. Independently, the Inhibited scale was found to be correlated .54 with the total PTSD score of the CAPS.

PACL Norms

In keeping with the emphasis on normality, PACL scales were normed as *T*-scores rather than BR scores. Normative data (Strack, 1991c) were obtained from 2,507 normal adults between the ages of 16 and 72. Men constituted 47.4% of the sample, and women 52.6%. Ethnic makeup was 65.2% non-Hispanic white, 17.3% Hispanic, 9.1% black, 7.6% Asian, and 0.8% Native American Indian or Eskimo.

Available Test Products

The PACL is available as a paper-and-pencil measure that can be hand-scored or entered into a computer file via optical scanner. Full-color, computerized versions of the PACL for Windows (WinPACL; Robbins, 1998) are available that permit computer administration of the test, scoring, and printing of profile plots of scores as well as narrative interpretations. The narrative interpretations were written for use in counseling and personnel settings, and were based on Millon's writings, empirical information obtained during test construction and validation, and clinical experience with the test. These programs allow for unlimited uses on a single computer and, as an aid to researchers, can produce exportable files containing test data for multiple subjects.

Now that clinicians, researchers, and their clients have access to the World Wide Web, the PACL can also be securely administered and scored via the Internet, using PACLOnline and IPACL. The website of the PACL's publisher (*www.21stcenturyassessment.com*) provides information about these services.

Comparison with the MCMI

The PACL was designed exclusively on the basis of Millon's (1969) original model of personality and measures normal trait characteristics. This is in contrast to the three editions of the MCMI, which were designed to match DSM Axis II criteria for personality disorders. In addition, Millon's original model differs somewhat from that found in his more recent writings (Millon, 1986a, 1986b, 1990, 1994, 1997, 2003; Millon & Davis, 1996).

In accordance with Millon's (1969, 1987, 1994, 1997, 2006; Millon & Davis, 1996) model and akin to the MCMI, PACL personality scales contain varying numbers of overlapping items, ranging from one for the Respectful scale to nine for the Sensitive scale. The percentage of overlapping items on PACL scales is substantially lower than that for MCMI scales, and ranges from 5% to 35%. As a result, scale intercorrelations for the PACL are somewhat lower than those for the MCMI (median r = |.35| across sexes; Strack, 1987, p. 579). Also as a result, PACL scales containing only nonoverlapping items have been found to be quite reliable on their own, and to yield essentially the same factors as the overlapping scales (Pincus & Wiggins, 1990; Wiggins & Pincus, 1989; Strack, 1991c).

Table 25.1 lists corresponding personality measures for the PACL, MCMI-I, MCMI-II, and MCMI-III. Two MCMI scales each are listed for the PACL Inhibited, Forceful, and Sensitive scales. This is because Millon (1986a, 1986b, 1994, 2003) divided his original avoidant (inhibited) personality into avoidant and depressive types; his original aggressive (forceful) style into antisocial and aggressive/sadistic; and his original negativistic (sensitive) style into passive–aggressive/negativistic and self-defeating/masochistic. An examination of items for these scales suggests that the MCMI Avoidant, Aggressive, and Passive–Aggressive/Negativistic scales may be closer to the PACL Inhibited, Forceful, and Sensitive scales, respectively, than the MCMI Depressive, Antisocial, and Self-Defeating/Masochistic scales are, although research is needed to verify this impression.

In practice, correspondence between the PACL and various versions of the MCMI is reduced by the dissimilar test formats (adjectives vs. statements), models used, and focus on normality versus pathology. In spite of these differences, I (Strack, 1991b) found the 8 PACL and 10 MCMI-II basic personality scales to be correlated between .39 and .67 (median = .52, using MCMI-II weighted raw scores) in a sample of 65 male and 75 female college students. The lowest values were found for PACL Sensitive/MCMI-II Self-Defeating (.39) and PACL Forceful/MCMI-II Antisocial (.41), suggesting that these MCMI-II scales are not strongly aligned with Millon's original (1969) model. By comparison, the MCMI-II Aggressive scale was correlated

TABLE 25.1. Corresponding Scales for the PACL, MCMI-I, MCMI-II, and MCMI-III

PACL		MCMI-I		MCMI-II		MCMI-III	
1.	Introversive	1.	Schizoid	1.	Schizoid	1.	Schizoid
2.	Inhibited	2.	Avoidant	2.	Avoidant	2A.	Avoidant
						2B.	Depressive
3.	Cooperative	3.	Dependent	3.	Dependent	3.	Dependent
4.	Sociable	4.	Histrionic	4.	Histrionic	4.	Histrionic
5.	Confident	5.	Narcissistic	5.	Narcissistic	5.	Narcissistic
6.	Forceful	6.	Antisocial	6A.	Antisocial	6A.	Antisocial
				6B.	Aggressive	6B.	Sadistic
7.	Respectful	7.	Compulsive	7.	Compulsive	7.	Compulsive
8.	Sensitive	8.	Passive–Aggressive	8A.	Passive–Aggressive	8A.	Negativistic
				8B.	Self-Defeating	8B.	Masochistic
PI.	Problem Indicator	S.	Schizotypal	S.	Schizotypal	S.	Schizotypal
		C.	Borderline	C.	Borderline	C.	Borderline
		P.	Paranoid	P.	Paranoid	P.	Paranoid

Note. The PACL PI scale measures aspects of the schizotypal, borderline, and paranoid styles, but does not directly assess these personalities.

.53 with PACL Forceful, and the MCMI-II Passive–Aggressive scale was correlated .51 with PACL Sensitive.

Factor analyses of PACL, MCMI-I, and MCMI-II personality scales have revealed very similar results. The three higher-order dimensions found in the PACL (Strack, 1987)—that is, Neuroticism, Assertiveness–Aggressiveness, and Social Extraversion–Introversion—correspond to the three factors found for the MCMI-I basic eight scales among psychiatric patients and normal adults (Retzlaff & Gibertini, 1987), and for the 13 MCMI-II personality scales with patients (Strack, Lorr, Campbell, & Lamnin, 1992). A joint factor analysis of PACL and MCMI-II basic personality scales among college students also yielded three factors (using residual scores), with corresponding PACL and MCMI-II scales loading on the same dimensions (Strack, 1991b).

We (Strack, Lorr, & Campbell, 1990) examined the circular ordering of MCMI-II personality disorder scales in a mixed group of psychiatric patients and compared results with those from the PACL among normal adults. When MCMI-II scales (using residual scores) were plotted against the orthogonally rotated first two principal components, we found a reasonably good circle that, for the most part, followed Millon's (1987, p. 20) predictions. Ordering for the PACL scales was similar, although a less complete circle was noted: Sociable, Confident, and Forceful were loaded opposite Introversive, Inhibited, and Sensitive on one dimension, while Cooperative and Respectful defined one end of a second dimension but had no opposing scales.

Millon's Personalities as Measured by the PACL

Correlational evidence shows that normal versions of Millon's basic styles are milder variants of the personalities as disorders. Unfortunately, behavioral studies and side-by-side comparisons of matched groups of normal adults and patients on the PACL and MCMI have not yet been carried out. As a result, important data are still needed to address the precise nature of similarities and differences between normal and disordered forms of Millon's personalities.

With regard to the appearance of Millon's personalities in normal form, what can be offered at this point is a portrait of each style based on Millon's theory, empirical findings from studies associating PACL scales with other measures, and clinical experience with the test. The following descriptions address (1) interpersonal style and self-presentation, (2) vocational interests and behavior, and (3) considerations for treatment when an individual presents to mental health professionals. The descriptions address normal prototypes of persons who obtain high scores on individual scales. In practice, people are seldom prototypical, instead exhibiting a mixture of traits from multiple styles. Nevertheless, the descriptions flesh out various aspects of normal personality that may not be readily grasped by extrapolating from Millon's writings on pathological character. Especially noteworthy among the normal styles are their positive dispositional features and interpersonal attitudes. Even less desirable traits are placed within a normal frame of reference.

Scale 1: Introversive

Interpersonal Style and Self-Perception

Introversive individuals prefer a quiet, retiring lifestyle that is relatively free of commotion. They are not people-oriented and tend to shun gatherings, such as parties, that require a good deal of social intercourse. Although they are not oblivious to others, they usually find social pursuits to be unrewarding and dull. Individuals with this personality style are often methodical, slow-paced, unobtrusive, and plain. They frequently blend in with their surroundings and go unnoticed by others. These individuals have little need to give or receive affection. They often blunt their feelings and rarely exhibit strong emotions. They always appear to be on an even keel and may report little internal reaction, even to major events. Introversive persons may see themselves as gentle, as easygoing, and having few needs. They may also assess themselves as having little social skill and being awkward when attention is directed their way. They may downplay their abilities in general, and appear to others as lacking in self-esteem. Those close to them may appreciate their calm demeanor and ability to stay unruffled. They may view them as reliable and steadfast, if somewhat dull and lacking in vitality. They may also feel frustrated by their lack of spontaneity and apparent inability to be moved by much of anything. They may come across as insensitive or unempathic—a result of their inability to perceive and interpret nuances of emotion.

Vocational Interests and Behavior

Individuals with an introversive personality style are frequently attracted to intellectual or mechanical occupations that allow them to be on their own. They often pursue goals that permit them to regulate the amount of information and stimulation they receive. Given a choice, they seek a stable work environment with few people and little commotion. Nevertheless, most of these individuals perform well in noisy, stimulating environments, if they are allowed to work independently at a pace they set for themselves. These individuals are usually reliable and dependable employees who are not bothered by repetitive tasks. They are quiet, slow-paced, pleasant, and nondemanding, and usually keep a calm demeanor. They do not respond well if asked to assume leadership positions or participate actively in groups. At times, coworkers may find these individuals frustrating to be with, because they often tune out those around them and may seem insensitive to their needs.

Treatment Considerations

Introversive individuals frequently break down when they have to adjust to major environmental changes and extreme shifts in their usual responsibilities. Their typical response to stress and pressure is to withdraw and shut down their feelings. In doing this, they may become insensitive and detached from themselves and others. In these circumstances, introversive individuals may present themselves for help when others goad them into it. They may not fully appreciate why others have become concerned with their well-being, or may not be aware of how their behavior has changed. In other circumstances, these individuals may experience an uncharacteristic surge of emotions. They may feel acutely tense, anxious, hypomanic, or depressed. Their distress is all the more painful, since they are not used to handling strong feelings. Some individuals may experience little change in their emotions, but an increase in somatic symptoms (they may report headaches, vague bodily pain, gastrointestinal ailments, trouble with concentration and memory, etc.).

Regardless of their presentation, introversive individuals are typically uninsightful about the problems that have led them into treatment. They tend not to be intuitive and are usually awkward in the world of feelings. They may not have the words to report their internal experiences precisely. These individuals can be expected to have difficulty in establishing a therapeutic relationship. They may expect therapy to offer a "quick fix," and will often leave treatment when they are able to resume their usual routine without undue difficulty. They are usually receptive to medical explanations for their difficulties and may welcome anxiolytic or antidepressant medication. Troubled individuals can often be helped through supportive therapy aimed at counteracting withdrawal and shoring up self-esteem. They may benefit from a careful reconstruction of the circumstances that led to their current problems. Helping these individuals learn more proactive coping skills is a frequent therapeutic goal. Behavioral techniques are especially well suited to these individuals. Group therapy is often not well tolerated, but may be useful for motivated clients who want to develop their interpersonal skills.

Scale 2: Inhibited

Interpersonal Style and Self-Perception

Inhibited individuals are shy and sensitive, prefer to keep others at arm's length, and are protective of their privacy. They tend to feel things strongly and can become overstimulated with unfamiliar people and surroundings. They try to display a positive social image and are attractive to those who appreciate their tenderness and empathic responses. However, they guard their inner selves well and will often rebuff attempts by others to get close to them. They may seem unnecessarily skittish and fearful in novel situations, appearing alert and wary of potential dangers. Although they may profess to be open to new relationships and experiences, their pervasive anxiousness and feelings of insecurity cause them to be defensive and withdrawing. These individuals typically hold a poor view of their personal abilities and social skills. For them, the world is a harsh place. They expect things to go wrong and feel that people hurt them or let them down. However, they shine in comfortable circumstances with people they know well. There they can open up, revealing their sensitive talents, cordiality, nurturance, and desire to be emotionally connected.

Vocational Interests and Behavior

Individuals with the inhibited personality style frequently seek intellectual, conventional, and artistic occupations that permit them to regulate the amount of stimulation and information they receive from their environment. They prefer stable work settings where they can operate alone or with a few close associates. They do not thrive in busy, social environments, which they frequently find too taxing of their personal resources. In a stable, safe environment, these persons are known for being kind, considerate, and loyal. They are often perceptive and tuned in to the feelings and thoughts of others. However, they are typically slow in adjusting to change and find it difficult to be assertive or active in group situations. Supervisors will do well to appreciate their sensitivity and need for interpersonal space. Since these individuals are usually not forthcoming with their feelings, it is important to request regular feedback from them about their work experiences.

Treatment Considerations

Inhibited persons are most likely to seek help when they become overwhelmed by painful feelings of anxiety, depression, inadequacy, and helplessness. They may feel fragile and unable to regulate their emotions or personal defenses. They may have experienced a failed relationship, be unable to handle interpersonal demands at home or the workplace, or become mired in anger and self-pity. They may feel that their problems are due to abuse from others or to senseless, unwarranted demands placed on them. Alternatively, these persons may turn on themselves and become overly critical and disparaging of their ability to cope with life.

When these persons are faced with stress, their usual response is to withdraw and become more distrustful. In therapy, they are likely to be wary and fearful of intrusion. It is best to employ a direct but nonthreatening approach with these individuals and to take time to build rapport. Because they are not likely to be forthcoming about how they feel, therapists will do well to seek their feedback regularly about the therapeutic relationship and proposed tasks. Even when they appear to be open, they are likely to keep their real feelings to themselves. They can be masters of disguise, appearing to be happy or pleased but actually feeling quite differently.

To begin, supportive individual or group therapy aimed at shoring up defenses and building self-esteem is recommended. Once a working alliance has been established, cognitive and interpersonal techniques may be used to develop adaptive defenses and realistic appraisals of self and others. For example, these individuals may not be aware that their sensitivity can be an asset as well as a liability. Since they feel things strongly, they are often in tune with subtle messages and responses from others. This can give them an edge in dealing with people, if they can learn to modulate their feelings and remain objective about their experience. Behavioral techniques may be useful here in controlling anxious arousal and generalized avoidance. Since these individuals have a habit of keeping others at a distance, they may have deficient interpersonal skills. Because of this, learning about people and about how to manage conflictual situations is often an important therapeutic goal.

Scale 3: Cooperative

Interpersonal Style and Self-Perception

A pleasant, agreeable, gentle demeanor is evident in cooperative people. They have a strong desire to be communal with others, and they do their best to facilitate comfortable relationships. They are typically cooperative, easygoing, thoughtful, and empathic. They prefer to let others take the lead in most circumstances. Their deferential social position is designed to secure nurturance and protection from those they view as stronger and more fit than they are. They typically see themselves as unskilled and vulnerable, and they shy away from difficult or competitive tasks. Their tendency to rely on others can keep them from learning new skills and developing a more positive self-image. They may have a superficial understanding of themselves and the world, favoring a simplistic, even rosy picture that may come across as naive and uninformed to others. This viewpoint belies their discomfort with strong emotions and interpersonal conflict. These persons dislike rocking the boat; instead, they put their effort into keeping things on an even keel. They can be skilled at smoothing over differences, absorbing conflict, and adapting themselves to changing circumstances. Those close to them appreciate these abilities and value their tender, amicable, even selfless dispositions.

Vocational Interests and Behavior

Cooperative individuals are known as team players who thrive in large, social work environments. They perform best in supportive work roles under the guidance of strong leaders. They are cordial, agreeable, and reliable, and strive to get along well with colleagues. They enjoy many conventional, social, and intellectual occupations. Their cheerful optimism helps them weather workplace stress and change relatively well. They are thoughtful of others, willing to please, and good at smoothing over conflicts and disagreements. When things are gloomy and the going gets tough, they can often find the silver lining. These individuals are usually uncomfortable being assertive and often avoid problems, rather than facing them head-on. They are followers rather than leaders, and they struggle when asked to act independently or be on their own.

Treatment Considerations

Emotional and interpersonal conflicts are often responded to by cooperative persons with denial, overconventional thinking, and feelings of helplessness, powerlessness, and failure. They may become morose, complain excessively, and cling to those they view as stronger and more capable. They may present for help with physical rather than emotional symptoms and resist psychological explanations for these difficulties. Problems often arise for these persons because their success in eliciting support from others serves to perpetuate their weak self-image and inhibits the acquisition of proactive coping skills.

These individuals are likely to seek treatment willingly and to be trustful and self-disclosing right from the start. Unfortunately, they also tend to be naïve, dependent, and resistive of therapeutic efforts that guide them toward autonomy. A nondirective approach may foster growth and independence better than more directive techniques. Helping these persons typically involves bolstering their self-worth and self-esteem, exploring problem-solving techniques, and encouraging them to try new behaviors. Cognitive techniques also may be useful in countering self-defeating thoughts and attitudes. Since these persons value communality over independence and self-assertion, it can be useful to frame therapeutic tasks as a way to increase interpersonal competence and manage conflicts before they get out of hand.

In this regard, group therapy may provide an arena for these individuals to learn better social skills, test new behaviors, and bolster their self-confidence.

Scale 4: Sociable

Interpersonal Style and Self-Perception

Sociable persons are lively, extraverted individuals who find delight in the social world. They are typically energetic, enthusiastic, and self-assured. They are socially skilled and know how to use warmth, charm, exuberance, and optimism to good effect. They prefer to be the center of attention and can be showy and ostentatious toward this end. They enjoy novel experiences and are eager to try new things. Not ones to let circumstances take their course, these persons actively manipulate others and the environment to obtain what they want. They are not happy when left on their own and may appear bored and deflated if they cannot get enough stimulation. They may also be quite mercurial when frustrated, exhibiting anger and disdain toward those who get in their way. Their social orientation and outward confidence cover insecurity about their abilities and talents. They may believe that they have to keep up a front in order to please others and secure the attention they require. Their need for stimulation and changeable emotions can be exhausting for them and those around them. Loyalty and closeness often take a back seat to their desire for something new. Others may view them as selfish, fickle, and insensitive—people who cannot be counted on unless there is something in it for them.

Vocational Interests and Behavior

Individuals with a sociable personality style often seek social, enterprising, and artistic occupations where they can exercise their need for stimulation and attention. Easily bored with repetition, they enjoy unusual duties and tasks that change frequently. They do well in large groups and seem to thrive in boisterous environments with little structure. They are extraverted, lively, and energetic. They often enjoy working with the public and make good salespersons. They are attentive to their appearance and keep a cheerful optimism, even in difficult circumstances. However, these individuals can be exasperating to some colleagues because of their quickly shifting interests and emotions. They find it difficult to stick with something once they have lost interest, and they seldom hesitate to change loyalties if an alternative gives them more of what they want. Attitudes and feelings can likewise vacillate from intense enthusiasm to disgruntled negativism in a short span of time. However, angry outbursts are just as short-lived as intense reactions in the other direction. When the air has cleared, these individuals return to their upbeat disposition as if nothing had happened.

Treatment Considerations

When presenting themselves for help, sociable persons may appear dramatically distressed, depressed, exhausted, or scattered. They may either be enraged at the people they feel have caused them trouble, or appear emotionally shut down, bored, and uninterested in life. They are typically uncomfortable with seeking treatment and may have difficulty grasping their role in a therapeutic relationship. Although they are likely to have long-standing problems with self-doubt and low self-esteem, they will probably expect a "quick fix" and may not be inclined to stay in therapy for more than a few sessions. They may come across as psychologically naïve and view the therapist as having somewhat magical powers to solve their problems quickly. They may demonstrate a superficial understanding of people and emotions, as well as a lack of insight. They are likely to resist delving into personal material and may take a dependent stance in hopes that the therapist will fix them without much effort on their own part. In this regard, they may prefer medication and behavioral techniques for managing emotions, rather than interventions that require self-focus.

Nevertheless, a direct, supportive approach that steers clear of their dependency maneuvers should be useful. Immediate goals may include reducing histrionic emotional reactivity, counteracting negative thinking, and helping them accurately assess the situations that got them into trouble. If they are inclined to go further, these persons may benefit from reexamining their perceived need for high levels of attention and stimulation, and from learning about their quickly shifting emotions as well as how to manage them. Their fickleness and boredom can be reduced by helping them see and appreciate the nuances and complexities in people and situations that they usually take for granted. Since they are used to fleeing problem situations and relationships rather than facing them, they are likely to be deficient in the mature coping skills that would allow them to manage conflicts effectively and build self-esteem. Cognitive and group therapies may prove useful with these persons in building and reinforcing interpersonal problem-solving skills.

Scale 5: Confident

Interpersonal Style and Self-Perception

Confident individuals are typically self-assured and view the world as a place of conquest where they can be on top and in charge. Their bold, competitive, ambitious interpersonal style gives the impression that they are firmly self-directed and lacking in insecurity. They use their social talents, including charm and cleverness, to obtain desired ends. They tend to believe that others should submit to their wishes and desires simply because they are entitled to them. They think highly of themselves, but often devalue others. While they expect people to deliver for them, they often do not consider others' feelings or believe in reciprocity. In this regard, they can come across as selfish, insensitive, arrogant, and overbearing. Frequently, though, they do not have to resort to egotistical brashness or overt exploitiveness to get what they want. They prefer more subtle interpersonal tactics that allow them to remain poised and unperturbed. They usually keep their feelings under wraps and are strongly defensive if others try to penetrate their personal armor. Although this helps them to succeed in difficult circumstances, it also serves to detach them from tender emotions. Hidden from all but those closest to them are a strong sensitivity to criticism and feelings of vulnerability and inadequacy.

Vocational Interests and Behavior

Confident individuals are frequently attracted to enterprising occupations that give them the status and power they seek. They are self-driven and work hard to attain their goals. They are competitive and shrewd. They do equally well on their own and in social settings, but in groups they have a need to be "one up" and will often resist roles that place them in an equal or deferential position. The self-assured, bold style of these individuals often wins them leadership positions. Colleagues frequently feel secure that these individuals will work hard to succeed and will accomplish their objectives in spite of obstacles. On the negative side, these individuals are usually more concerned with themselves than with others, and they can be insensitive and uncaring about the effects of their behavior on coworkers. Their need for success and tribute may at times take precedence over company rules, ethics, and social propriety.

Treatment Considerations

Individuals with a confident personality style frequently experience problems when they fail to achieve important goals or step on others' toes through arrogance and neglect. Unrealistic expectations and inflated self-worth may contribute to interpersonal conflicts. These individuals often harbor deep-seated feelings of guilt and inadequacy. They often doubt themselves and struggle under the heavy weight of self-imposed demands for achievement and perfection. However, even when asking for help, these individuals usually deny or downplay their turmoil and fear. They frequently blame others for their problems and can get worked into a rage when discussing the abuse they believe they have endured. They are often disdainful of seeking help and typically find it difficult to settle into a client role, which they view as passive and submissive. They may be unwilling to face personal responsibility for problems, and may even seek to outwit the therapist and sabotage treatment efforts. Not surprisingly, these individuals usually stay in therapy only long enough to restore their lost self-esteem.

Therapists will do well to take a firm yet supportive stance and to avoid power struggles. These individuals will welcome the therapist's appreciation of their suffering as well as their talents and accomplishments. By framing change techniques as methods for mastering difficult situations, therapists can ally themselves with these individuals' need to be dominant and self-directed. If amenable to more than supportive treatment, these individuals are likely to benefit from a reappraisal of their expectations for themselves and others. They may need to learn how to contain their feelings and to be less angry and judgmental. They also may need to learn to be less self-focused and more empathic toward others. Some individuals may appreciate the increased interpersonal effectiveness they will obtain from use of cooperative, prosocial methods.

Scale 6: Forceful

Interpersonal Style and Self-Perception

Active, enterprising, and socially dominant, forceful persons present themselves to others as rugged individuals who can thrive in an environment of adversity. In the dog-eat-dog world they envision, few people can be trusted. They feel that skepticism and wariness are needed to navigate safely, and they strive to maintain a superior interpersonal position that serves as a secure defense but also gives them an edge in getting what they want. Tender feelings are seldom acknowledged or expressed, and tactics of intimidation or exploitiveness are not beneath them. In this regard, others may experience these persons as brash, bullying, and unsentimental. Naturally competitive, they seek out opportunities to use their personal talents. They are typically resolute and hard-driven in pursuit of their goals, and they can be resourceful, innovative, and shrewd. They tend to be independent thinkers, risk takers, and nonconformists. They may also be impulsive and have a low tolerance for frustration. They delight in winning and may bend rules, if doing so will assist them in outfoxing an opponent. Others frequently admire their indomitable spirit and ability to succeed in difficult circumstances. They view their forthright, authoritative manner as a sign of self-confidence and leadership ability. Beyond the world of conquest, however, these persons may have trouble letting down their guard and allowing themselves to be emotional. They tend to devalue the softer side of life, which they identify with weakness. Furthermore, their tendency to be distrustful makes it difficult for them to be passively cooperative, so that others can take the lead.

Vocational Interests and Behavior

Forceful persons often aspire to mechanical and enterprising occupations that give them independence and a sense of being in control. Their strong competitive spirit gives them an edge in jobs that require a steadfast pursuit of goals in difficult circumstances. These persons are known for their hard work, toughness, and determination. Although they can tolerate group settings, these persons prefer to be outside the bounds of community rules and regulations. They are self-oriented and do not readily consider the needs of others. They can be gruff and insensitive to colleagues, and they seldom hesitate in stepping on toes, if doing so helps them achieve their ends. Their assertive, forthright style and desire to win typically earn them confidence and respect from colleagues. In many job situations, their lack of sensitivity and warmth may be overlooked because of their perseverance and ability to succeed in spite of opposition.

Treatment Considerations

When they feel overwhelmed by interpersonal and emotional difficulties, these persons are likely to exaggerate their usual methods of maintaining distance from others, becoming excessively defensive, angry, gruff, and reckless. They may also withdraw into bitterness and self-pity, or use alcohol or drugs to soothe themselves. They will typically perceive that they have been outwitted or undone by vindictive others, and will downplay or deny personal responsibility for their failures. At the core, though, they are likely to doubt themselves and to feel weak, vulnerable, and inadequate.

Because of their general distrust, disdain for the world of emotions, and awkwardness in a help-seeking role, these individuals are unlikely to enter treatment on their own. To obtain their interest and cooperation, therapists will do well to take a firm yet supportive stance. These persons are most likely to respond positively when a therapist is authoritative and allows them to be on an equal footing in the relation-ship. However, even with good rapport, these individuals are likely to be reserved and uncomfortable discussing intimate feelings. They may attempt to challenge the therapist's competence and control, especially if they feel threatened. An immediate goal is to permit venting of frustration so that they can regain their sense of self-control and competence. They may then be receptive to problem-focused treatment, including a review of their problems from a cognitive point of view. Behavioral meth-ods may be useful for anger and stress management. Getting them to change is often a matter of convincing them that doing so will increase their competence and control over harsh circumstances. If they prove amenable to long-term therapy, goals may include softening their rigid defenses and intense emotional responses, increasing their empathic regard for others, and resolving the feelings of inadequacy that lead to overcompensation. Toward these ends, these persons may respond well to modeling techniques in a one-on-one or group setting.

Scale 7: Respectful

Interpersonal Style and Self-Perception

The confidence and self-worth of respectful persons are inextricably tied to their abil-ity to meet or exceed the standards of others. They are follower of rules and conven-tions and are dedicated to pursuits that yield esteem in the eyes of those they admire. Typically pleasant and cooperative, they strive to maintain an appearance that is offensive to no one and that will not endanger their reputations. They seldom display strong emotions and may appear bland or constricted to those around them. They are usually punctual and exact. Those close to them appreciate their orderly and methodical approach to tasks, as well as their drive to get things done on time. They are loyal friends and coworkers who will go out of their way to make sure that their responsibilities are taken care of. To those who do not share their rule-bound approach to life, however, they may come across as too moralistic, strict, and unyielding. For their part, respectful individuals are not easily swayed from what they believe in. At the same time, they can be too black-and-white in their judgments. They are usually harsh on themselves and others. In trying to live up to their own expectations, they can become excessively tense and anxious. To those who are beneath their standards of propriety, they reserve open disdain and hostility. Their tendency to follow the lead of others can make them very uncomfortable in situa-tions where they have to act on their own. Furthermore, they are often so narrowly focused on a particular end that creativity loses out to convention.

Vocational Interests and Behavior

Individuals with a respectful personality style are frequently attracted to conven-tional, mechanical, and intellectual occupations that offer a structured work environ-ment and clear guidelines for performance. Given a job to accomplish, they use their organizational skills and strong work ethic to see that it gets done accurately and on time. In the workplace, they are often prized for their loyalty, conscientiousness, and willingness to persist at difficult or repetitive tasks. They take their responsibilities seriously and are motivated to please supervisors and respected colleagues. These individuals do well on their own, but they are also good team players and thrive in group settings. They are willing to cooperate and follow the lead of others. They are astute at recognizing the implicit rules of the workplace and will internalize these quickly. It is difficult for these individuals to operate successfully, if tasks and goals are not well defined and if a free-wheeling, unstructured approach is required. They are uncomfortable making decisions on their own and asserting a point of view that is not shared by others. Coworkers often value their ability to keep their nose to the grindstone and their emotions under wraps, but some of these individuals may come across as so task-oriented and constricted that they are viewed as impersonal, insensitive, and uncaring. They can be tough on subordinates, whom they hold to the same perfectionistic standards they have for themselves.

Treatment Considerations

Emotional and interpersonal problems can often be traced to respectful persons' attitudinal and behavioral rigidity. When things go wrong, their instinct is to constrict their feelings and hold fast to whatever rules apply to their situation. They may present themselves for help with anxiety, tension, and psychosomatic ailments (e.g., headaches and gastrointestinal upsets). They may also be angry and bitter at those they feel have let them down. If they perceive that their trouble is due to their own failure, they can become clinically depressed. A common thread to their symptoms is excessive criticalness: Someone or something must be blamed and punished for the problem. Although these individuals will probably be highly defended in their view of whatever trouble they are in, a sense of worry, fearfulness, and inadequacy may permeate their demeanor.

These persons are likely to view a therapist as an expert and will be superficially cooperative in an effort to obtain his or her approval. They will be punctual and carry out homework tasks with fervor. At the same time, they tend to be uncomfortable with strong emotions and are likely to resist letting down their defenses in order to explore potential shortcomings. A supportive, problem-focused approach may be useful in exploring their difficulties and restoring self-efficacy. They tend to get lost in nondirective therapy, so it is usually best to keep the level of structure fairly high. They are likely to be receptive to medication and behavioral methods for reducing anxiety, depression, tension, and stress reactivity. When their defenses are eased, these persons may benefit from a rational exploration of dysfunctional thoughts and attitudes, especially their excessive criticalness and rigid acceptance of certain standards and rules. They may also gain from learning how to be less perfectionistic and black-and-white in their judgments of themselves and others. In this regard, they may respond well to interpersonal modeling techniques in either one-on-one or group settings.

Scale 8: Sensitive

Interpersonal Style and Self-Perception

Sensitive persons are characteristically thin-skinned and moody. They stand apart from others and pursue a lifestyle unbridled by traditional rules and conventions. They are adventuresome and enjoy novel tasks and situations. They are typically spontaneous and may be valued by others as original and creative. Impatient with the status quo, these persons have trouble following accepted standards. They are wary of imposed authority and arbitrary directives, which they view as threatening their autonomy. They tend to meander through life rather than follow a beaten path. To others, they may come across as disorganized and irresponsible. They feel things strongly and find that their emotions shift quickly and unpredictably. Impulsive by nature, these individuals find it difficult to stick with a relationship or task once they have lost interest. These traits make it difficult for them to fit in and to accomplish things in a set way. In the conventional world, they may feel like square pegs trying to fit into round holes. Their self-esteem can suffer as a result, and a strong sense of ambivalence and pessimism may pervade their outlook. When frustrated, they may become mired in self-pity. They may feel unappreciated and be resentful of those they believe have an easier lot in life. Not inclined to contain negative feelings, these individuals openly express their discontent through temporary displays of anger and hostility. At their worst, they can be spoilers who are uncooperative, obstructionistic, and sour. Close acquaintances and friends expect a certain amount of negativism and emotional turbulence from them. Those who are tolerant of their idiosyncrasies often prize their sense of independence, fresh perspective, and unconventional interests. They value their resiliency and readiness to launch into new experiences at a moment's notice.

Vocational Interests and Behavior

Artistic and intellectual occupations are frequently favored by people with the sensitive personality style. They seek loosely structured work environments that allow them freedom and autonomy in interpreting task requirements. They do not respond well to strict rules and regulations. They like to determine the pace at which they work and to choose the goals they strive for. Although they appreciate stable group settings and can operate successfully within them, these persons tend to be free-thinking and not inclined to follow group norms. Their sensitive, temperamental nature requires a measure of tolerance and support from supervisors and colleagues. Since they often react quite negatively to criticism and heavy-handed authority, these should be avoided or downplayed. The talents of these persons are most likely to be realized in a workplace that is nurturing and supportive of their individuality.

Treatment Considerations

Sensitive persons may arrive in treatment displaying a plethora of emotions and negative attitudes. They may feel angry at a world they experience as arbitrary and unjust. They may feel scattered, depressed, and drained, ready to give up hope of happiness. Dependency conflicts and feelings of inadequacy are often present. In therapy, these persons are likely to shift between compliance and resistance, hope and disillusionment. Affective expression may be controlled and sensible one moment, then shift to irrationality. Therapists may feel their patience being tested by these persons, who can make even the most carefully crafted interventions seem futile and who may complain excessively about every detail of the professional relationship.

Success with these individuals entails an appreciation of their brittle egos, emotional sensitivity, quickly shifting moods, and need for clear but flexible boundaries. Initially, therapists will do well to let them vent their frustrations by being supportive and nondirective, but unsentimental. Medication and behavioral interventions may be needed to help stabilize their thoughts and feelings. Once the initial storm has cleared, it is important to obtain a rational understanding of the problem situation. This may take some time, since these individuals often have trouble separating their own view of a situation from its objective characteristics. A practical, problem-solving approach may then be useful in teaching self-control and general coping skills. Cognitive therapy may assist these persons in gaining a more realistic appraisal of themselves and the world. In addition, interpersonal and group therapy can often be employed to increase self-awareness, behavioral consistency, and social maturity.

Scale PI: Problem Indicator

As noted earlier, items for the PI scale were compiled from adjectives measuring the schizoid, cycloid, and paranoid personalities—for example, "chaotic," "fragmented," "depressed," and "suspicious." Although this scale does not define a personality style, elevated scores suggest the presence of a moderate level of personality disturbance and psychiatric symptoms. These individuals are likely to appear anxious, dysphoric, and fearful; to exhibit strong self-doubt; and to express dissatisfaction with themselves and others. They may have long-standing adjustment problems in major areas of life, such as work, school, and relationships. Those who score high on the PI scale are not likely to fit the same picture of normality as are low scorers (e.g., by exhibiting interpersonal rigidity and maladaptiveness), but further assessment is advised before any conclusions regarding the presence of a disorder are drawn.

Applications of the PACL

The PACL (Strack, 1991c, 2002) is appropriate for use with persons 16 years of age or older who read at minimally the eighth-grade level. It has been successfully applied by therapists working in counseling centers and employee assistance programs; by vocational counselors, personnel psychologists, and marriage and family counselors; by therapists doing custody and workers' compensation evaluations; and by general practitioners who work with relatively high-functioning clients. Because the PACL is quick (10 minutes) and easy to administer, it is often given during initial screening visits to assess personality style and identify persons who may have serious problems. Clinicians have found it to be useful with people who can't or won't complete questionnaire measures—for example, some medical patients, adolescents, and elderly persons. A number of clinicians use the PACL to rate their clients' personality styles, and to have spouses/partners and family members assess each other, employing the norms in the PACL manual (Strack, 1991c) for scoring (for an example, see Strack, 2005a). Although the norms are based on self-reports, they have worked remarkably well with a variety of ratings (e.g., Gould & Hyer, 2004; Plante & Boccaccini, 1997).

Counseling and Psychiatric Populations

When clinicians are using the PACL in counseling and psychiatric settings, it is important to keep in mind that the test measures *normal* trait characteristics, not personality disorder features. High scores on the PACL indicate that an individual possesses *more* of the traits of a particular normal personality style than other adults in the general population. For example, the higher an individual's score is above $T = 50$ on any particular scale, the more likely it is that he or she will fit the prototype descriptions given earlier. The test does not assess personality disorder features beyond those measured by the PI scale, and, as indicated previously, this scale should not be interpreted as suggesting the presence of personality problems unless elevated at $T \geq 60$.

Nevertheless, there are circumstances where clinicians find the PACL to be helpful with psychiatric patients: (1) assessing clients' strengths, including vocational and school interests; (2) giving feedback to clients about their personality style; and (3) obtaining personality ratings. Each of these areas is discussed in turn.

Because the MCMI-III (Millon, 2006) was designed as a diagnostic instrument and was normed on patients, base rate (BR) score elevations are associated with increased probability of psychiatric diagnosis and higher degrees of psychopathology. Furthermore, studies have not been done on the characteristics of those who obtain low BR scores on the clinical scales. Except for research studies showing that normal functioning is frequently associated with moderate scores on the MCMI-III Histrionic, Narcissistic, and Compulsive scales (Choca, 2004; Craig, 2008; McCann et al., 2001; Millon, 2006; Strack, 1993), positive personality correlates are not available for MCMI-III clinical scales. When therapists are seeking to understand the positive personality features of their clients, including goals for school and work, results of the PACL can provide valuable information, as the prototype descriptions given previously demonstrate.

The MCMI-III narrative test printouts provided by Pearson Assessments clearly indicate that they should not be disclosed to a patient and his or her family. Although trained clinicians are usually adept at communicating clinical findings to patients and families in a language they can understand, there are circumstances where the client wants to see for him- or herself what the results actually say. The interpersonal behavior and work/school sections of the PACL narrative reports were written with counseling clients in mind; because of this, these sections can be read to, or given to, a client as feedback.[1] The decision about whether to read or give the client sections of his or her narrative PACL results must be made by the clinician doing the assessment. When I provide testing feedback to my clients, I preface my remarks by explaining the strengths and limitations of self-report testing in general, along with the particular strengths and limitations of the PACL (Strack, 1991c). I indicate that the narrative test results do not take each respondent's unique circumstances into account, but that as a result of the norming process, the PACL can give a respondent a generally accurate portrait of his or her feelings, attitudes, behaviors, and interests vis-à-vis others in the general population. I tell my clients that we can discuss their feelings and reactions after they have listened to, or read, their test results, and they can let me know what fits and what doesn't fit. In my experience over many years, this feedback process is almost universally beneficial. It affords an opportunity for a transparent and collaborative interaction between a mental health provider and a client that can build trust, provides the client with limited (digestible) knowledge about psychological assessment, sets the stage for treatment planning, and helps build an expectation that self-knowledge is an important part of the assessment and treatment experience.

I have mentioned above that clinicians use the PACL to rate their clients' personality styles, and to have spouses/partners and family members assess each other. In this context, self-report data can be readily contrasted with ratings to reveal similarities and differences between self-other viewpoints. If more than one person rates an individual, scores can be combined or weighted to produce composite profiles. Of course, self-report doesn't have to be limited to one's *current* personality. Clients can be asked to describe their ideal selves, how they were as children or before a major life event, and how they imagine themselves in a variety of roles and personae (for an example, see Strack, 1997).

Case Example: Raj, the Struggling Actor

To illustrate the use of the PACL in a therapeutic context, I present the case of a college-educated, 28-year-old, single man, of mixed East Indian and non-Hispanic white heritage, who presented for mental health treatment at a veterans' outpatient clinic in southern California. Raj was the only child of his parents, who met in India, where Raj's father, an American, was stationed as an officer with the U.S. Navy. Raj's mother was born and raised near Bombay, attended college, then landed a job as a civilian interpreter for the U.S. Department of Defense. After their marriage, Raj's parents moved to the U.S. east coast. When his father retired from the Navy, his parents opened an insurance business.

Raj was raised in an ethnically mixed, affluent neighborhood. He attended both public and private schools, and reported that he was well adjusted both socially and academically. At an early age, he learned that his parents had high expectations for him. His childhood was centered on learning and academic performance. He was expected to get high marks in all of his classes, and was tutored on a daily basis at home by his mother. For extracurricular activities, Raj's parents scheduled a seemingly nonstop series of organized events that had him playing various sports; learning the piano and martial arts; and going on frequent outings to museums, concert halls, and public lectures.

The apparent goal of Raj's childhood training was for him to attend the U.S. Naval Academy. Raj was ambivalent about this during his adolescence, but he felt a strong sense of obligation to his parents, and so went along with the plan. His excellent academic and sports training made it relatively easy for him to quality for admission, and his father's contacts as a retired naval officer helped assure his commission.

Raj's naval career was not pleasant. At Annapolis, he found it very difficult to adjust to being away from home. He did not make friends easily, and by the end of his first year he found himself on academic probation, a by-product of his adjustment difficulties. He went home after his first year and begged his father to let him quit, but his father would not hear of this. Feeling no way out, Raj rallied himself and returned to the academy with determination to stick it out. He managed to graduate on time, but was in the bottom third of his class. As Raj himself did, his professors and advisors recognized that he did not have the "right stuff" to be a career officer. Accordingly, for the remainder of his commission, he was "sent to every s—thole the Navy had." He finished his career honorably, but never learned a trade that he thought would help him in the civilian world. He left the Navy as soon as possible and decided to move to Los Angeles to see whether he could make it as an actor.

Raj had always loved the performance arts and was a talented pianist. He also had dashing good looks and felt that there just might be a place for him in movies or television. Once in Los Angeles, he found an apartment and began taking acting classes. He developed a small group of friends who were also would-be actors, and eventually took jobs as a bartender and waiter to pay the bills. He worked at night because auditions were mostly held during the day. Over a period of 2 years, he managed to land a couple of modeling jobs and a part in a television commercial. He performed in a few stage plays in local theaters, but by the time he came in for treatment, he was beginning to feel that Hollywood was not particularly interested in what he had to offer.

Raj arrived at the clinic with no prior mental health treatment. He told the intake worker that he was feeling depressed about his career and wanted psychotherapy to help him figure out what to do with his life. He declined a referral to a staff psychiatrist, saying that he did not want medication.

During Raj's first appointment, he confessed that his presentation was "a favor" he had promised to his mother. Both of his parents were disappointed in his choice to become an actor, but his mother seemed nevertheless to be genuinely supportive. Raj and his mother talked on the telephone frequently. She noticed that Raj's initial enthusiasm in moving to Los Angeles had slowly degraded into "a permanent frustration."

For his part, Raj reported that he was disappointed in how slowly his career was moving. Asked what he would do if he found that acting would not become self-supporting, he replied, "I really don't know." He recognized that he was "somewhat behind" his peers in terms of developing a career identity. He chalked this up to being "stuck in the Navy for 8 years." On the positive side, Raj felt that he was happy with his choice to live on his own, and to pursue something he really loved. His stated goal for therapy was to "learn about why I'm not happy and why I'm not more successful."

Raj completed the PACL after finishing his initial counseling appointment. His test profile is given in Figure 25.1. My interpretation of the protocol follows the method outlined elsewhere (Strack, 1991c, 2008). From the information presented in Figure 25.1, it seems that Raj did not have trouble describing himself, as he checked 90 of 153 words as self-descriptive. The validity indices were all within normal range, indicating no unusual test-taking biases, so the results are likely to offer an accurate portrait of his current personality style.

To turn to the personality scales, PI is below the cutoff for significance, so it is probable that Raj has a normal-range personality style and no major personality problems. His highest three scales are Inhibited ($T = 66$), Introversive ($T = 59$), and Cooperative ($T = 58$), while his lowest scale is Forceful ($T = 32$). Each of these is used to create a portrait of Raj.

This client's highest three scale scores are fairly common in the PACL normative sample, and his lowest scale score is consistent for someone with primary traits of emotional sensitivity and introversion, as well as a cooperative/submissive interpersonal stance. The highest scales are elevated sufficiently above the normative mean of $T = 50$ to indicate that Raj has a distinct manner of interacting with the world that is readily grasped by others. His profile suggests that he is a fairly shy and polite man who makes a niche for himself by staying on the sidelines and avoiding interpersonal conflicts. On the surface, he is pleasant and cooperative and enjoys the company of a handful of people he trusts. He prefers to spend most of his free time by himself and shuns social activities, which he finds unsettling or unrewarding. He tends to view himself as being plain, awkward, and lacking in social talents. Sensitive to criticism and rejection, he vigorously guards his privacy and sidesteps situations that may pose a danger.

Individuals with this personality style are often attracted to occupations that allow them to be on their own. They prefer intellectual or mechanical pursuits that permit them to regulate the amount of information and stimulation they receive. Given a choice, they seek a stable

PERSONALITY ADJECTIVE CHECK LIST PROFILE

IDENTIFYING INFORMATION

Name: Raj W
Age: 28
Education: 16
Marital: Never Married

Sex: Male
Research code: 00000
Ethnicity: Other
Religion: Other

VALIDITY INDICES

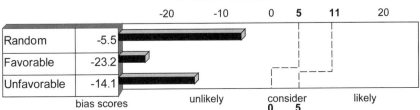

	bias scores			
Random	-5.5			
Favorable	-23.2			
Unfavorable	-14.1			

Number checked is OK [90 adjectives endorsed]
Random response set is UNLIKELY
Favorable response set is UNLIKELY
Unfavorable response set is UNLIKELY

SCALE *T* SCORES

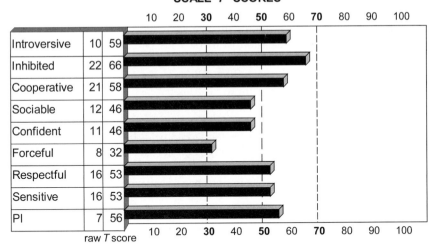

	raw	*T* score
Introversive	10	59
Inhibited	22	66
Cooperative	21	58
Sociable	12	46
Confident	11	46
Forceful	8	32
Respectful	16	53
Sensitive	16	53
PI	7	56

FIGURE 25.1. PACL test profile for case example 1 (Raj).

work environment with few people and little commotion. They do not respond well if asked to assume leadership positions or participate actively in groups.

When presenting for help, these persons are usually distrustful at first, and may need time before they feel comfortable enough to express themselves openly. The therapist will do well to go slowly at the beginning of treatment and to enlist their collaboration in planning sessions. Troubled individuals can often be helped through supportive therapy aimed at counteracting withdrawal and shoring up self-esteem. They may benefit from a careful reconstruction of the circumstances that led to their current problems. Assisting these individuals learn more proactive coping skills is a frequent therapeutic goal. Cognitive and behavioral techniques are especially well suited to these individuals. Group therapy is often not well tolerated, but may be useful for motivated clients who want to develop better interpersonal skills.

When Raj returned for his next session, we discussed the test findings in some detail. I allowed him to read a portion of the test report and asked him to tell me what fit and what didn't fit. He felt that the results accurately portrayed him. By using reflective statements, I was able to verify the elements of the test report that he agreed with. This gave me an initial map of the things he was aware of, and what he understood to be his strong and weak points. During the next two sessions, I used supportive and cognitive techniques to explore his current career and identity problems in the context of his upbringing and personal characteristics. Mindful of his emotional sensitivity, I encouraged him to be collaborative in therapy and to lead the way by bringing up topics of his choosing. I avoided offering too much information and making interpretations that might come across as intrusive or unsettling.

Being bright and relatively open, Raj came to the conclusion within a few sessions that be might not be suited to the world of acting, or at least "the scene in Hollywood." I recommended that he spend time considering alternative careers that would fit well with his personality and interests. He did his own research and, over the course of 15 sessions in 6 months, Raj decided to move back East to a community near his parents and to enroll in a university to study music and art history. The decision to be near his parents was a practical one, as he needed their help financially. Raj's father had mixed feelings about his son's decision, but, with the urging of his wife, agreed to help him as long as Raj worked part-time in the family business. Prior to Raj's move, I urged him to visit his parents and spend a few days scoping out the university and places where he might want to live, which he did. During our final sessions, we discussed the problems that were likely to crop up when he moved and began school, and we role-played situations that he felt would be difficult for him to respond to. He recognized that, among other things, he needed to counterbalance his tendency to submit and go along with his more opinionated father. In therapy he learned to be more aware of, and to trust, his instincts. He also recognized the importance of believing in himself, and to authorize himself to follow his own path in life.

A follow-up phone call 3 months after Raj left treatment found him in good spirits. He was enrolled in college classes, sharing an apartment with an old friend, and working for his parents. He acknowledged that his parents were not easy to work for and were not short of advice to give him, but he no longer felt obligated to take it. He felt that, all things considered, he could "make it work" without losing himself in the process.

Employment Screening, Fitness-for-Duty Determination, and Child Custody Evaluation

Unlike persons who voluntarily seek mental health treatment, individuals referred for evaluation to determine their fitness to perform general or specific tasks are usually motivated to present themselves in a positive light. Clients who fall into this group include military personnel; individuals seeking (or seeking to keep) jobs in a variety of areas, including law enforcement; and persons referred for child custody evaluations. To be successful, the task for these individuals is not to reveal problems, but to appear healthy and well adjusted. Although the vast majority of these clients do not know specifically how to manipulate psychological tests in order to get (or keep) a particular job, obtain custody of their children, or avoid referral for mental health treatment, they typically know not to reveal too much negative material, and to show that they possess the positive characteristics they believe are necessary for obtaining their desired outcome. Evaluators can expect these clients to present themselves in a socially desirable way on self-report measures, and to downplay their negative qualities.

As for the MMPI-2 (Butcher, 2001; Butcher et al., 2001), the majority of test items for the MCMI-III (Millon, 2006) were written to detect specific problems. Most of these are face-valid and can be readily identified by respondents (Choca, 2004; Millon, 2006). On the MMPI-2 (Butcher, 2001), job applicants usually obtain validity and standard clinical scale scores that are all within normal range. The most highly elevated among these are the Superlative (S), Correction (K), and Lie (L) scales, which are usually in the range of $T = 60$ to 70.

Large-scale job applicant studies have not been conducted with the MCMI-III. However, my colleagues and I used the MCMI-III to conduct assessments (see Strack, 2005a) of 54 men applying for jobs as armed police officers with the U.S. Department of Veterans Affairs (VA). These assessments yielded results that were consistent both with previous studies on normal samples, and with studies focusing on persons who presented themselves positively—either due to the circumstances of the screening (e.g., child custody evaluations, McCann et al., 2001), or because they were instructed to do so (e.g., Craig, Kuncel, & Olson, 1994; Daubert & Metzler, 2000; Millon, 1997). With regard to the Modifying Indices, the Disclosure (X) and Debasement (Z) scales were very low among the VA job applicants and child custody examinees (BR < 35), while the Desirability (Y) scale was elevated, on average, above BR = 75. It is significant that the X and Z scale scores of psychiatric patients asked to "fake good" (Daubert & Metzler, 2000) were more moderate (X BR $M = 55.9$, Z BR $M = 40.5$) than those of actual examinees who were motivated to present favorably.

The MCMI-III scale scores of the VA job applicants and child custody examinees (McCann et al., 2001) were universally low (BR $M < 60$) except for notable, and sometimes clinically significant, elevations on the Histrionic, Narcissistic, and Compulsive scales. The VA job applicants were most likely to have their highest elevation on the Compulsive scale (BR $M = 72.1$), followed by the Narcissistic scale (BR $M = 65.3$). Child custody examinees showed their highest elevations on the Histrionic ($M = 69.8$), Compulsive ($M = 68.4$), and Narcissistic ($M = 65.2$) scales (McCann et al., 2001, total sample). Research with non-help-seeking adults who completed a version of the MCMI using normal instructions typically showed elevations on the same three PD scales (Choca, 2004; Craig, 2008; Millon, 2006; Strack, 1993). Thus VA job applicants and child custody examinees were frequently able to appear normal on the MCMI-III.

In situations where clients are motivated to present positively on the MCMI-III, the PACL can be useful because the test provides a normal frame of reference for assessing a range of DSM (American Psychiatric Association, 2000; Sperry, 2003) personality traits. Recall that the PACL was normed on normal adults, uses *T*-scores rather than BR scores, and includes a PI scale. Because of these features, the PACL can be used to help rule out a personality disorder when an examinee obtains one or more BR score elevations above 75 on the MCMI-III. It can also be useful in fleshing out the personality profiles of persons who, on the MCMI-III, show the restricted range of scale elevations associated with "fake-good" and normal responding (i.e., elevations on Histrionic, Narcissistic, and Compulsive).

Case Example: Janice, Recovering from Drug Abuse

To demonstrate how the PACL can be used in a fitness-for-duty assessment, I offer the case of Janice, a 40-year-old, non-Hispanic white, divorced woman, who had been fired from her last job as a licensed vocational nurse (LVN) for stealing narcotic pain medication. When she was placed on leave, her license to practice was suspended. Janice came to see me with a legal document from the LVN licensing board describing the reason for the suspension and the requirements she needed to meet before she could get her license back. The document stipulated that she needed to undergo 12 months of substance abuse treatment that included random drug tests, and that when the treatment was completed, she had to receive a psychological evaluation that would verify her rehabilitation and fitness to return to work as an LVN.

During her initial visit, Janice reported that it had been 2 years since she was fired. She had completed a 12-month treatment program and felt ready to return to work. Prior to agreeing to the evaluation, I took a thorough background history, which yielded no potential red flags (e.g., history of relapse, past mental problems, convictions for criminal activities, poor employment history, history of financial problems). I explained that in order to complete the assessment, I would need to contact her treatment program, the licensing board, and her prior employer. She agreed to all of my terms.

From my interview, I learned that Janice had had no history of job problems, and no history of alcohol or drug abuse, until she injured her back in an automobile accident. She was rear-ended by a speeding driver when she slowed down to exit a local expressway. Although her insurance company paid for treatment, including surgery to repair a ruptured disk and physical therapy, she was left with chronic pain. During her rehabilitation, she came to believe that she could manage the pain with exercise and over-the-counter medication. However, as she returned to work full-time, she found that her duties caused her pain to worsen significantly. Fearing losing her job, she began using the narcotic painkillers she had been prescribed after the surgery. Gradually, she needed more and more medication to feel comfortable, but her doctors would not prescribe more. She eventually discovered that it was fairly easy to pilfer some of the medication prescribed for her patients. She continued this practice for several weeks until one of her supervisors caught her in the act. Company policy required that she be let go immediately and that the incident be reported to the licensing board.

Janice was tearful in recounting the shame of losing her job and being unable to work after her license was suspended. Without a way to make a decent living, she had to sell her home and move in with her elderly mother. She was fortunate to be able to do odd jobs, and to find a low-cost attorney to help her deal with the licensing board.

Janice reported that she knew she had a prescription drug problem long before she began taking other people's medication. However, when she lost her job, she did not immediately seek formal rehabilitation for her addiction: "Without a job I had no way to get the pain medication, but I also didn't have much pain, so I had my regular physician detox me while I was at home." By the time the licensing board told her what she would need to do to get her license back, she had been free from narcotic use for almost 6 months.

As a military veteran, Janice was able to enter a substance abuse treatment program at her local VA hospital without cost to her. She reported that she had finished the 12-month requirement several weeks before coming to see me, and was continuing to attend weekly Narcotics Anonymous (NA) meetings that were held at the VA. She said that the 12-step recovery model taught at the VA was very helpful to her in developing a more positive attitude about her pain problem, and "the courage to live my life drug-free."

Janice's counselor at the VA verified her completion of 12 months of treatment, and verified that her random drug tests had all come back "clean." In his opinion, Janice was ready to return to work, and he had already agreed to write a letter to this effect to the licensing board.

As part of a test battery, I had Janice complete the PACL along with the MCMI-III. The latter test was valid, but Janice's Modifying Indices showed the typical tendency of return-to-work candidates to respond by disclosing mostly positive material (X BR = 55, Y BR = 74, Z BR = 38). The only Axis I scale to hit clinical significance was Drug Dependence (BR = 75). On the Axis II personality scales, her highest scores were for Compulsive (BR = 72) and Depressive (BR = 68). All other Axis I and II scales were below BR = 60. At the cutoff level of BR = 75, Janice's Drug Dependence score probably reflected honesty in reporting that she had a drug problem *in the past*, as a few scale items are worded in this way. I verified this by checking all of her responses for this scale, and was happy to find that she was willing to admit to her past problems in this circumstance. I was also pleased that she did not meet test criteria for a personality disorder, and that she did not produce the stereotyped personality profile often found in people motivated to "fake good" (elevations only on Histrionic, Narcissistic, and Compulsive).

Janice's PACL profile is given in Figure 25.2. As the data in her profile indicate, she endorsed 78 of 153 adjectives as being self-descriptive and, while showing a mild tendency to present herself favorably (F = −16.0), clearly did not bias the test in this way. Her PI scale score is on the low side (T = 39), verifying results of the MCMI-III that she does not have personality problems.

Turning to the remaining scales, we note that her highest elevations are on Respectful (T = 61) and Inhibited (T = 54), and that her lowest scores are on the Confident (T = 32) and Forceful (T = 40) scales. As much as possible, her high-point scales match those from the MCMI-III (recall that the PACL does not have a Depressive scale and that this style is considered a variant of the avoidant/inhibited personality), which offers a good measure of cross-validity.

The PACL tells us that this woman's behavior is guided by a preference for solitary activity, respect for authority, and obedience to high standards of personal conduct. She tends to be introverted, slow-paced, and self-absorbed. She is often preoccupied with accomplishing the tasks that she believes determine her success and self-worth. She tends to devalue people who do not meet the guidelines she thinks are important, and she shuns activities that would detract from her pursuits. These include most social activities, which she deems frivolous and uninteresting. Tender emotions are likewise devalued, and this can make her seem dry, humorless, and uncaring.

Individuals with this personality style are frequently attracted to conventional, mechanical, or intellectual occupations that offer a structured work environment and clear guidelines for performance. Given a job to accomplish, they use their organizational skills and strong work ethic to see that it gets done accurately and on time. They take their responsibilities seriously and are motivated to please supervisors and respected colleagues. These individuals do well on their own, but they are also good team players. They are willing to cooperate and follow the lead of others. However, they are uncomfortable making decisions on their own and asserting a point of view that is not shared by others.

Emotional and interpersonal problems can often be traced to this person's attitudinal and

PERSONALITY ADJECTIVE CHECK LIST PROFILE

IDENTIFYING INFORMATION

Name: Janice
Age: 40
Education: 15
Marital: Divorced

Sex: Female
Research code: 00000
Ethnicity: Non-Hispanic White
Religion: Protestant

VALIDITY INDICES

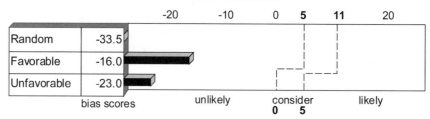

Number checked is OK [78 adjectives endorsed]
Random response set is UNLIKELY
Favorable response set is UNLIKELY
Unfavorable response set is UNLIKELY

SCALE *T* SCORES

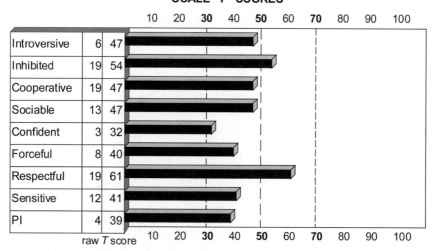

FIGURE 25.2. PACL test profile for case example 2 (Janice).

behavioral rigidity. When things go wrong, her instinct is to constrict her feelings and hold fast to whatever rules apply to her situation. Although she is typically highly defended in her view of whatever trouble she is in, a sense of worry, fearfulness, and inadequacy may permeate her demeanor. Not surprisingly, people with this personality style do well in mental health treatment and are eager to please the therapist. They work hard to complete homework tasks and will be conscientious in applying themselves to learning new behaviors.

On the basis of my complete assessment, I was comfortable giving Janice the "go-ahead" to get her license back and return to work as an LVN. I shared with her my findings, and we discussed her strengths and weaknesses. She agreed with my conclusion that she should have a probationary period when she returned to work, since neither she nor I knew whether she would be able to manage a full-time job without undue pain and stress. I recommended that as part of her return-to-work plan, she agree to continue with her NA meetings and submit to random drug screenings for a period of 6 months. As well, I strongly encouraged her to join a gym to gain strength before going back to work, and that she consider a part-time job so as not to be overwhelmed right from the start.

Janice has since reported that she got her license back on a provisional basis and was hired at a local nursing home that permitted her to start with 20 hours of work per week and go up to 40 hours when she felt ready. She said that her job was rewarding but also difficult, given her back pain. She thought that she could manage to work without hurting herself or resorting to pain medication, but also that she would be considering a switch to a job that did not require so much physical exertion.

Summary and Conclusion

This chapter has addressed the development, validation, and clinical uses of the PACL (Strack, 1987, 1991c, 2002), a unique addition to the family of assessment instruments that operationalize Theodore Millon's (e.g., Millon & Davis, 1996) model of personality and psychopathology. The PACL measures the eight basic personality styles Millon (1969) described in his earliest writings, but assesses them as normal rather than abnormal prototypes. In contrast with instruments like the MCMI-III (Millon, 2006), norms for the PACL are based on the responses of 2,507 *normal* individuals, while scale scores are transformed into *T*-scores so that administrators can gauge the extent to which respondents deviate from a normal mean. The PACL's PI scale measures traits associated with personality problems, which can be useful for those who need to screen for PDs. As an adjective check list, the PACL is distinctive among Millon instruments in being useful for obtaining observer ratings as well as self-reports. The test is frequently used by therapists who want to understand the strengths of their clients as well as their weak spots. It is used for vocational counseling, personnel selection, employee assistance, marriage and family counseling, and child custody and workers' compensation evaluations.

Acknowledgments

This chapter was prepared with support from the U.S. Department of Veterans Affairs. I thank Nadia Damm, Nicole Eberhart, Dylan Kollman, and Lisa Mitchell for their helpful comments on an earlier draft of this chapter.

Note

1. I do not recommend giving clients the entire PACL narrative report, because it contains far more technical information than they can readily interpret, and because the section focusing on treatment issues may give information that is detrimental to the client.

References

Alden, L. E., Wiggins, J. S., & Pincus, A. L. (1990). Construction of circumplex scales for the Inventory of Interpersonal Problems. *Journal of Personality Assessment, 55,* 521–536.

American Psychiatric Association. (1980). *Diagnostic and statistical manual of mental disorders* (3rd ed.). Washington, DC: Author.

American Psychiatric Association. (2000). *Diagnostic and statistical manual of mental disorders* (4th ed., text rev.). Washington, DC: Author.

Beavers, W. R., & Hampson, R. B. (1990). *Successful families: Assessment and intervention.* New York: Norton.

Blake, D. D., Weathers, F., Kaloupek, D. G., Klauminzer, G., Charney, D., & Keane, T. (1990). Prevalence of PTSD symptoms in combat veterans seeking medical treatment. *Journal of Traumatic Stress, 3,* 15–27.

Butcher, J. N. (2001). *MMPI-2 revised personnel system user's guide* (3rd ed.). Minneapolis: University of Minnesota Press.

Butcher, J. N., Graham, J. R., Ben-Porath, Y. S., Tellegen, A., Dahlstrom, W. G., & Kaemmer, B. (2001). *MMPI-2 manual for administration, scoring, and interpretation* (rev. ed.). Minneapolis: University of Minnesota Press.

Byravan, A., & Ramanaiah, N. V. (2002). On the incremental validity of MMPI-2 Psychopathology-5 scales over the revised NEO Personality Inventory scales for predicting personality disorders. *Psychological Reports, 90,* 1084–1090.

Choca, J. P. (2004). *Interpretive guide to the Millon Clinical Multiaxial Inventory* (3rd ed.). Washington, DC: American Psychological Association.

Costa, P. T., Jr., & McCrae, R. R. (1985). *The NEO Personality Inventory manual.* Odessa, FL: Psychological Assessment Resources.

Costa, P. T., Jr., & McCrae, R. R. (1992). *The Revised NEO Personality Inventory (NEO-PI-R) and the NEO Five-Factor Inventory (NEO-FFI) professional manual.* Odessa, FL: Psychological Assessment Resources.

Craig, R. J. (2008). Essentials of MCMI-III assessment. In S. Strack (Ed.), *Essentials of Millon inventories assessment* (3rd ed., pp. 1–55). Hoboken, NJ: Wiley.

Craig, R. J., Kuncel, R., & Olson, R. E. (1994). Ability of drug abusers to avoid detection of substance abuse on the MCMI-II. *Journal of Social Behavior and Personality, 9,* 95–106.

Daubert, S. D., & Metzler, A. E. (2000). The detection of fake-bad and fake-good responding on the Millon Clinical Multiaxial Inventory III. *Psychological Assessment, 12,* 418–424.

Gontag, R., & Erickson, M. T. (1996). The relationship between Millon's personality types and family system functioning. *American Journal of Family Therapy, 24,* 215–226.

Gould, S. L., & Hyer, L. A. (2004). Dementia and behavioral disturbance: Does premorbid personality really matter? *Psychological Reports, 95,* 1072–1078.

Horton, A. D., & Retzlaff, P. D. (1991). Family assessment: Toward DSM-III-R relevancy. *Journal of Clinical Psychology, 47,* 94–100.

Hyer, L., & Boyd, S. (1996). Personality scales as predictors of older combat veterans with posttraumatic stress disorder. *Psychological Reports, 79,* 1040–1042.

Loevinger, J. (1957). Objective tests as instruments of psychological theory. *Psychological Reports, 3,* 635–694.

McCann, J. T., Flens, J. R., Campagna, V., Collman, P., Lazzaro, T., & Connor, E. (2001). The MCMI-III in child custody evaluations: A normative study. *Journal of Forensic Psychology Practice, 1,* 27–44.

McHoskey, J. W., Worzel, W., & Szyarto, C. (1998). Machiavellianism and psychopathy. *Journal of Personality and Social Psychology, 74,* 192–210.

Millon, T. (1969). *Modern psychopathology.* Philadelphia: Saunders.

Millon, T. (1977). *Millon Clinical Multiaxial Inventory manual.* Minneapolis, MN: National Computer Systems.

Millon, T. (1981). *Disorders of personality: DSM-III, Axis II.* New York: Wiley.

Millon, T. (1986a). A theoretical derivation of pathological personalities. In T. Millon & G. L. Klerman (Eds.), *Contemporary directions in psychopathology: Toward the DSM-IV* (pp. 639–670). New York: Guilford Press.

Millon, T. (1986b). Personality prototypes and their diagnostic criteria. In T. Millon & G. L. Klerman (Eds.), *Contemporary directions in psychopathology: Toward the DSM-IV* (pp. 639–670). New York: Guilford Press.

Millon, T. (1987). *Millon Clinical Multiaxial Inventory–II (MCMI-II) manual.* Minneapolis, MN: National Computer Systems.

Millon, T. (1990). *Toward a new personology.* New York: Wiley.

Millon, T. (2003). *Millon Index of Personality Styles Revised manual.* Minneapolis, MN: Pearson Assessments.

Millon, T., & Davis, R. D. (1994). Millon's evolutionary model of normal and abnormal personality: Theory and measures. In S. Strack & M. Lorr (Eds.), *Differentiating normal and abnormal personality* (pp. 79–113). New York: Springer.

Millon, T., & Davis, R. D. (1996). *Disorders of personality: DSM-IV and beyond* (2nd ed.). New York: Wiley.

Millon, T., Green, C., & Meagher, R. B. (1982a). *Millon Adolescent Personality Inventory manual.* Minneapolis, MN: National Computer Systems.

Millon, T., Green, C., & Meagher, R. B. (1982b). *Millon Behavioral Health Inventory manual.* Minneapolis, MN: National Computer Systems.

Millon, T., & Grossman, S. D. (2006). Millon's evolutionary model for unifying the study of normal and abnormal personality. In S. Strack (Ed.), *Differentiating normal and abnormal personality* (2nd ed., pp. 3–49). New York: Springer.

Millon, T. (with Millon, C., & Davis, R. D.). (1997). *Millon Clinical Multiaxial Inventory–III (MCMI-III) manual* (2nd ed.). Minneapolis, MN: National Computer Systems.

Millon, T. (with Millon C., Davis, R. D., & Grossman, S.). (2006). *Millon Clinical Multiaxial Inventory–III (MCMI-III) manual* (3rd ed.). Minneapolis, MN: Pearson Assessments.

Millon, T. (with Weiss, L. G., Millon, C., & Davis, R. D.). (1994). *Millon Index of Personality Styles manual.* San Antonio, TX: Psychological Corporation.

Moos, R. H. (1974). *The Family Environment Scale.* Palo Alto, CA: Consulting Psychologists Press.

Morey, L. C., Waugh, M. H., & Blashfield, R. K. (1985). MMPI scales for DSM-III personality disorders: Their derivation and correlates. *Journal of Personality Assessment, 49,* 245–251.

Pincus, A. L., & Wiggins, J. S. (1990). Interpersonal problems and conceptions of personality disorders. *Journal of Personality Disorders, 4,* 342–352.

Plante, T. G., & Boccaccini, M. T. (1997). Personality expectations and perceptions of Roman Catholic clergy members. *Pastoral Psychology, 45,* 301–315.

Retzlaff, P. D., & Gibertini, M. (1987). Factor structure of the MCMI basic personality scales and common-item artifact. *Journal of Personality Assessment, 51,* 588–594.

Robbins, B. (1998). *WinPACL 2.0 user's guide.* South Pasadena, CA: 21st Century Assessment.

Sperry, L. (2003). *Handbook of diagnosis and treatment of DSM-IV-TR personality disorders* (2nd ed.). New York: Brunner-Routledge.

Strack, S. (1981). *Development of the Personality Adjective Check List and preliminary validation in a normal college population.* Unpublished manuscript.

Strack, S. (1987). Development and validation of an adjective check list to assess the Millon personality types in a normal population. *Journal of Personality Assessment, 51*, 572–587.

Strack, S. (1991a). *Comparison of PACL PI scale elevations in samples of psychiatric patients and normal adults.* Unpublished manuscript.

Strack, S. (1991b). Factor analysis of MCMI-II and PACL basic personality scales in a college sample. *Journal of Personality Assessment, 57*, 345–355.

Strack, S. (1991c). *Manual for the Personality Adjective Check List (PACL)* (rev. ed.). South Pasadena, CA: 21st Century Assessment.

Strack, S. (1993). Measuring Millon's personality styles in normal adults. In R. J. Craig (Ed.), *The Millon Clinical Multiaxial Inventory: A clinical research information synthesis* (pp. 253–278). Hillsdale, NJ: Erlbaum.

Strack, S. (1994). Relating Millon's basic personality styles and Holland's occupational types. *Journal of Vocational Behavior, 45*, 41–54.

Strack, S. (1997). The PACL: Gauging normal personality styles. In T. Millon (Ed.), *The Millon inventories: Clinical and personality assessment* (pp. 477–497). New York: Guilford Press.

Strack, S. (2005a). Combined use of the PACL and MCMI-III to assess normal range personality styles. In R. Craig (Ed.), *New directions in interpreting the Millon Clinical Multiaxial Inventory–III (MCMI-III)* (pp. 94–128). Hoboken, NJ: Wiley.

Strack, S. (2005b). Measuring normal personality the Millon way. In S. Strack (Ed.), *Handbook of personology and psychopathology* (pp. 372–389). Hoboken, NJ: Wiley.

Strack, S. (2008). *Essentials of Millon inventories assessment* (3rd ed.). Hoboken, NJ: Wiley.

Strack, S., & Guevara, L. F. (1999). Relating PACL measures of Millon's basic personality styles and MMPI-2 scales in patient and normal samples. *Journal of Clinical Psychology, 55*, 895–906.

Strack, S., & Lorr, M. (1990). Three approaches to interpersonal behavior and their common factors. *Journal of Personality Assessment, 54*, 782–790.

Strack, S., Lorr, M., & Campbell, L. (1989, August). *Similarities in Millon personality styles among normals and psychiatric patients.* Paper presented at the annual convention of the American Psychological Association, New Orleans, LA.

Strack, S., Lorr, M., & Campbell, L. (1990). An evaluation of Millon's circular model of personality disorders. *Journal of Personality Disorders, 4*, 353–361.

Strack, S., Lorr, M., Campbell, L., & Lamnin, A. (1992). Personality and clinical syndrome factors of MCMI-II scales. *Journal of Personality Disorders, 6*, 40–52.

Trapnell, P. D., & Wiggins, J. S. (1990). Extension of the Interpersonal Adjectives Scales to include the Big Five dimensions of personality. *Journal of Personality and Social Psychology, 59*, 781–790.

Trobst, K. K., Ayearst, L. E., & Salekin, R. T. (2004). Where is the personality in personality disorder assessment?: A comparison across four sets of personality disorder scales. *Multivariate Behavioral Research, 39*, 231–271.

Wiggins, J. S., & Pincus, A. L. (1989). Conceptions of personality disorders and dimensions of personality. *Psychological Assessment, 1*, 305–316.

CHAPTER 26

The Millon Index of Personality Styles
Revised (MIPS *Revised*)
Assessing the Dimensions of Normal Personality

Lawrence G. Weiss

The Millon Index of Personality Styles *Revised* (MIPS *Revised*; Millon, 2003) is a carefully developed, 180-item, true–false questionnaire designed as a dimensional assessment of Millon's personality domains as applied to the normal range of functioning. It is appropriate for ages 18 to 65+. Most MIPS *Revised* items require an eighth-grade education to complete, and most individuals finish it in 30 minutes or less.

The MIPS *Revised* can be administered, scored, and interpreted on a personal computer; administered in paper-and-pencil format and hand-scored; or scanned on a desktop scanner. A mail-in scoring service is also available. Computer-generated reports provide either a single-page profile (i.e., graph) of the scores, or a complete narrative interpretation of the profile pattern. The user's guide to the software includes a complete explanation of the logic that the computer program uses to analyze MIPS *Revised* profiles and to generate the interpretive reports.

The MIPS *Revised* Scales

The MIPS *Revised* consists of 24 scales grouped into 12 pairs. Each pair contains two juxtaposed scales. For example, the Asocial/Withdrawing and Gregarious/Outgoing scales are considered a pair. As shown in Table 26.1, the 12 pairs of MIPS *Revised* scales are organized into three major areas: Motivating Styles, Thinking Styles, and Behaving Styles. A brief definition of each of the 24 MIPS *Revised* scales is given in Table 26.2. The MIPS *Revised* also contains a composite of overall adjustment called

TABLE 26.1. Organization of the MIPS *Revised* Scales

Validity Indices	Motivating Styles	Thinking Guided Styles	Behaving Styles
Consistency	Pleasure-Enhancing	Externally Focused	Asocial/Withdrawing
Positive Impression	Pain-Avoiding	Internally Focused	Gregarious/Outgoing
Negative Impression	Actively Modifying	Realistic/Sensing	Anxious/Hesitating
	Passively Accommodating	Imaginative/Intuiting	Confident/Asserting
	Self-Indulging	Thought-Guided	Unconventional/Dissenting
	Other-Nurturing	Feeling-Guided	Dutiful/Conforming
		Conservation-Seeking	Submissive/Yielding
		Innovation-Seeking	Dominant/Controlling
			Dissatisfied/Complaining
			Cooperative/Agreeing

the Clinical Index, and three Validity Indices: Positive Impression, Negative Impression, and Consistency.

The Motivating Styles Scales

Three pairs of Motivating Styles scales assess the person's orientation toward obtaining reinforcement from the environment. Millonian theorists will recognize these three pairs of scales as normal-range variations of Millon's pleasure–pain, active–passive, and self–other dimensions. The first pair of scales examines the extent to which the respondent's behavior is motivated by obtaining positive reinforcement (i.e., Pleasure-Enhancing) or avoiding negative stimulation (i.e., Pain-Avoiding). The second pair assesses the extent to which the individual's activities reflect an Actively Modifying or Passively Accommodating approach toward the world. The third pair of scales focuses on the source of reinforcement, assessing the extent to which the person is primarily motivated by Self-Indulging or Other-Nurturing aims.

These three motivating aims are broad and powerful constructs that have an important history in the field of psychology. In brief, the pleasure–pain dimension is related to drive theory, the active–passive dimension to ego psychology, and the self–other dimension to self psychology and object relations theory.

The Thinking Styles Scales

Four pairs of Thinking Styles scales examine styles of information processing. The first two pairs of scales in this area, Externally or Internally Focused, and Realistic/Sensing or Imaginative/Intuiting, assess information-gathering strategies. The second two pairs—Thought-Guided or Feeling-Guided, and Conservation-Seeking or Innovation-Seeking—assess different styles of processing information once it has been gathered.

TABLE 26.2. Descriptions of MIPS *Revised* Scales

Validity Indices

Consistency. High scores indicate that a respondent was conscientious and consistent in answering test items. Low scores suggest inconsistent, careless, or confused responding.

Positive Impression. Individuals who score high on this scale answered the test by accentuating their positive characteristics. They may have biased the test by underreporting their personal difficulties.

Negative Impression. High scores indicate that a respondent answered the test by giving an unfavorable impression of his or her personal characteristics. Malingering should be considered.

Motivating Styles

Pleasure-Enhancing. High scorers on this scale tend to look for the bright side of life, are optimistic about future possibilities, find it easy to enjoy themselves, and face the ups and downs of their lives with equanimity.

Pain-Avoiding. Individuals scoring high on this scale focus on and intensify the problems of life. Perceiving the past as having been personally troubling, they always seem to be waiting for something else to go wrong, and feel that things are likely to go from bad to worse. They are easily upset by minor concerns and disappointments.

Actively Modifying. Respondents scoring high on this scale take charge of their lives and make things happen rather than waiting for them to occur. They are busily involved in modifying their environments and arranging events to suit their needs and desires.

Passively Accommodating. High scores on this scale indicate that respondents will undertake little to shape or alter their lives. They react to the passing scene, accommodating to circumstances created by others; they seem acquiescent, are unable to rouse themselves, lack initiative, and do little to generate the outcomes they desire.

Self-Indulging. Individuals scoring high on this scale are oriented toward actualizing their own needs and wishes. That is, they seek to fulfill themselves first, worry little about the impact of their behavior on others, and tend to be both independent and egocentric.

Other-Nurturing. Respondents scoring high on this scale are motivated to meet the needs of others first, and to attend to other people's welfare and desires at the expense of themselves. They are seen as nurturing and protective, taking care of others before taking care of themselves.

Thinking Styles

Externally Focused. High scorers on this scale turn to others to find stimulation and encouragement. They draw upon friends and colleagues for ideas, guidance, inspiration, and energy, as well as garnering assurances of self-worth from them and taking comfort in their presence.

Internally Focused. Respondents scoring high on this scale prefer to use their own thoughts and feelings as resources, gaining inspiration and stimulation primarily from themselves rather than from others. In contrast with externally focused individuals, these respondents experience greater serenity and comfort by distancing themselves from external sources, preferring to heed the prompting that comes from within.

Realistic/Sensing. High scorers on this scale gather their knowledge from the tangible and concrete, trusting direct experience and observable phenomena over the use of inference and abstraction. The practical and "real," the literal and factual, are what give these individuals comfort and confidence.

Imaginative/Intuiting. Individuals scoring high on this scale prefer the symbolic and unknown to the concrete and observable. They are open to the intangibles of life, and are inclined to seek out and enjoy the more mysterious experiences and speculative sources of knowledge.

Thought-Guided. High scorers on this scale prefer to process the knowledge they have by means of logic and analytic reasoning. Decisions are based on cool, impersonal, and "objective" judgments, rather than on subjective emotions.

(continued)

TABLE 26.2. *(continued)*

Feeling-Guided. Respondents scoring high on this scale form their judgments by heeding their own affective responses to circumstances, by evaluating subjectively the impact of their actions on those involved, and by following their personal values and goals.

Conservation-Seeking. High scorers on this scale are highly organized and predictable in their approach to life's experiences. They transform new knowledge in line with what is known and are careful, if not perfectionistic, in arranging even minor details. As a result, they are seen by others as orderly, conscientious, and efficient.

Innovation-Seeking. Individuals scoring high on this scale are inclined to be creative and to take risks, ready to alter and recast whatever they come upon. They seem discontented with the routine and predictable, spontaneously modifying what is given by following their hunches and seeking to effect novel, unanticipated consequences.

Behaving Styles

Asocial/Withdrawing. Individuals scoring high on this scale are characterized by their lack of affect and their social indifference. They tend to be quiet, passive, and uninvolved; they may be viewed by others as quiet and colorless, unable to make friends, as well as apathetically disengaged.

Gregarious/Outgoing. High scorers on this scale seek social stimulation, excitement, and attention. They often react dramatically to situations around them, but typically they lose interest quickly. Colorful and charming socialites, they also can be demanding and manipulative.

Anxious/Hesitating. Individuals scoring high on this scale are usually shy, timid, and nervous in social situations, strongly wanting to be liked and accepted, yet often fearing that they will be rejected. At the same time that they are sensitive and emotionally responsive, they are mistrusting, lonely, and isolated.

Confident/Asserting. Respondents scoring high on this scale tend to feel that they are more competent and gifted than the people around them. They are often ambitious and egocentric, self-assured and outspoken. Others may see them as arrogant and inconsiderate.

Unconventional/Dissenting. Respondents scoring high on this scale tend to act out in an independent and nonconforming manner. They often resist following traditional standards, displaying an audaciousness that may be seen either as reckless or as spirited and enterprising.

Dutiful/Conforming. High scorers on this scale are likely to be upstanding and self-controlled. They relate to authority in a respectful and cooperative manner, tend to behave in a formal and proper manner in social situations, and are unlikely to be self-expressive or to act spontaneously.

Submissive/Yielding. Individuals scoring high on this scale are their own worst enemies: They are accustomed to suffering rather than pleasure, are submissive, and tend to act in self-demeaning ways. Their behavior renders ineffective the efforts of others to assist them, and causes the yielders to bypass opportunities for rewards and to fail repeatedly to achieve despite possessing abilities to do so.

Dominant/Controlling. Individuals scoring high on this scale are forceful and often domineering and socially aggressive. They tend to see themselves as fearless and competitive. To them, warmth and gentleness are signs of weakness, which they avoid by being strong-willed and ambitious.

Dissatisfied/Complaining. Respondents scoring high on this scale are characterized by their tendency to be passive–aggressive, sullen, and generally dissatisfied. Their moods and behavior are highly changeable: At times, they relate to others in a sociable and friendly manner; on other occasions, they are irritable and hostile, expressing the belief that they are misunderstood and unappreciated.

Cooperative/Agreeing. High scorers on this scale tend to be highly likable socially, often relating to others in an amenable manner. They form strong loyalties and attachments to others. They cover any negative feelings, however, especially when these feelings may be viewed as objectionable by the people they wish to please.

The astute reader will observe that the Thinking Styles scales are highly consonant with the model formulated by Jung (1921/1971) and subsequently popularized in the Myers–Briggs Type Indicator (MBTI; Myers & McCaulley, 1985). The MBTI Judging and Perceiving scales have been renamed Conservation-Seeking and Innovation-Seeking in the MIPS *Revised*, to capture the original Jungian meaning more accurately. More important, however, Millon has recast these constructs in terms of their influence on one's cognitive style of dealing with the voluminous influx of information required for daily living in the information age. This is an important contribution, because cognitive differences in how individuals respond to information and the manner in which these differences are expressed in daily life have been much overlooked in generating and appraising personality traits.

The Behaving Styles Scales

Five pairs of Behaving Styles scales assess the person's style of relating to others. Millonian theorists will recognize these five pairs of scales as normal-range variations of Millon's 10 personality disorders (Millon, 1990). The MIPS *Revised* Asocial/Withdrawing and Gregarious/Outgoing interpersonal styles are the normal variants of the schizoid and histrionic personality disorders, respectively. The Anxious/Hesitating and Confident/Asserting styles are related to the avoidant and narcissistic personality disorders, respectively. The Unconventional/Dissenting and Dutiful/Conforming personality styles are consonant with the antisocial and obsessive–compulsive personality disorders, respectively in the pathological range. The Submissive/Yielding and Dominant/Controlling styles are the normal-range variants of the self-defeating/masochistic and sadistic personalities, respectively—although these are not formally recognized as disorders in the *Diagnostic and Statistical Manual of Mental Disorders*, fourth edition, text revision (DSM-IV-TR). Finally, the interpersonal styles characterized by the Dissatisfied/Complaining and Cooperative/Agreeing scales on the MIPS *Revised* are on the same continuum as the negativistic/passive–aggressive and dependent personality disorders, respectively.

As a group, the MIPS *Revised* scales have a rich theoretical foundation in a model of personality that is deeply rooted in biosocial and evolutionary theory (Millon, 1969, 1990, 1991).

Applications of the MIPS *Revised*

The MIPS *Revised* is appropriate for use with normally functioning adults. It is especially useful in organizational settings. One important application is to screen employees for general adjustment. This is particularly relevant for employees in high-risk fire and safety occupations. The MIPS *Revised* is also frequently used as an aid in identifying managerial potential, or as a source of developmental feedback to improve existing managerial talent. The MIPS *Revised* also can be used to help form work or project teams, and to improve the effectiveness with which such teams make decisions and work together. Feedback of MIPS *Revised* results can be integrated into many team-building exercises and other organizational training and development programs. Practitioners using the MIPS *Revised* in organizational settings should be aware of relevant legal and ethical issues regarding testing of job applicants.

Appropriate applications of the MIPS *Revised* also include any settings in which counselors seek to identify, understand, and assist normally functioning adults. Such settings include employee assistance programs, vocational guidance and career development programs, university counseling centers, and marriage and family counseling centers. Also appropriate are independent and group practice settings in which reasonably functional individuals seek assistance with real-life problems (divorce, child management, drinking, work stress, etc.).

The MIPS *Revised* Interpretive Reports

Interpretive reports are available with the computer version of the MIPS *Revised*. The interpretive reports carry the flare, depth, and insightful wit for which Theodore Millon's writings have become widely known. Upon reviewing these works, one has the feeling of reading carefully crafted prose rather than an automated psychological report.

More than 400 reports are built into the software. The reports differ from many computerized interpretations because the narratives do not follow a simplistic, scale-by-scale procession of scores. The reports print a description of the individual as an integrated and holistic person. Practitioners often find the reports rich with discourse on a person's style that goes beyond a simple description of behavior and fosters a new understanding of and sensitivity toward the client.

The reading level is high, and practitioners should exercise appropriate clinical judgment in deciding to give a report directly to the client. College-educated individuals easily understand the reports. Those with a high school education grasp most of the report, although parts of it will be beyond their comprehension.

It has been my experience that most normally functioning adults easily recognize themselves in these narratives and favorably receive the messages. Individuals whose interpersonal styles occasionally cause some real-life problems, however, may need to have the reports placed in an appropriate context for them. Practitioners should review each report carefully before deciding whether it is appropriate for the client to read.

Technical Characteristics of the MIPS *Revised*

The MIPS *Revised* is based on the same items, scales, and norms as the MIPS. Thus, all data-based statements in this chapter apply equally to the MIPs and the MIPS *Revised*.

Item Development

The writing of items for the MIPS *Revised* scales was guided by an explicit theory of normal personality elucidated elsewhere (Millon, 1990). Items were reviewed by content experts for correspondence with the constructs that were intended to be measured by each of the scales.

MIPS *Revised* items are scored on more than one scale. This multiple keying of items on conceptually related scales forces higher intercorrelations among some scales, but this is believed to mirror the phenomenological relatedness of these constructs in the naturally occurring world. This scale design follows a theory of prototypes in which all construct domains are assumed to be composed of a set of core or prototypal characteristics and a set of related behaviors that commonly occur but are not essential characteristics of the core trait. Core characteristics of one trait may be nonessential but related characteristics for another trait. For example, Gregarious/Outgoing behavior is one component of a Confident/Asserting style of relating to others. For each trait, the core items receive more weight in the scoring of that scale than do the supporting items. Because of this item overlap, which is common in Millon's inventories, certain statistical procedures based on scale intercorrelations may not be appropriate. For example, factor analyses should be conducted at the item level rather than on the scale intercorrelation matrix.

Representativeness of Norm Samples

After multiple pilot tests, the items were refined, and the test was then standardized on 1,000 adults in community settings in eight cities. This sample was carefully selected to closely represent the U.S. population of adults in terms of racial/ethnic group, educational level, age, gender, and region of the country. A separate set of college norms was also developed, based on a standardization sample of 1,600 students at 14 colleges and universities around the country. The student sample was carefully selected to be representative of the population of college students in terms of racial/ethnic group, age, year in school, major area of study, region of the country, and type of institution attended. We considered the representativeness of the standardization samples to be critical, because we planned to use a new norming procedure that would take into account the prevalence rates of the constructs measured in the population.

The MIPS Revised Prevalence Score System

Concept and Use

The MIPS *Revised* prevalence score (PS) system is a unique and powerful synergy of dimensional and categorical approaches to personality measurement. Categorical models sort individuals into one or another classification group. Dimensional models estimate the amount of a trait an individual possesses, or describe his or her position relative to others on some dimension of interest. To view these two approaches as inconsistent would be an unfortunate misinterpretation of the naturally occurring world, and would result in a loss of meaningful information for both the researcher and the practitioner. To accurately reflect the percentage of each of the MIPS *Revised* traits occurring in the real world, the measurement approach begins with a simple classification into trait groups based on population prevalence data and then proceeds to a more sophisticated rating of the individual's position on the underlying dimension relative to others in that particular trait group.

MIPS *Revised* PSs range from 0 to 100. The system was designed in such a way that the proportion of individuals who score at or above PS = 50 on each scale matches the prevalence of individuals in the general population who possess that trait. We accomplished this by the following procedure: For each MIPS *Revised* scale, PS = 49 was set in such a manner that the percentage of the standardization sample scoring at or above PS = 50 would correspond as closely as possible to the actuarial estimate of the prevalence rate for that trait in the general population. The population prevalence rates were estimated based on an extensive literature review of studies measuring related constructs across a wide variety of nonclinical samples, as described in the MIPS and MIPS *Revised* manuals (Millon, 1994b, 2003).

The reference point for interpretation of individual score profiles is always PS = 50. An individual who obtains scores at or above PS = 50 on any particular scale is classified as a member of the trait group defined by that scale. For example, a person scoring above PS = 50 on the Externally Focused scale is considered extraverted. Once individuals have been classified as members of particular trait groups, individual score profiles are interpreted in terms of their distance from PS = 50 on each scale. Scores higher than PS = 50 indicate higher positions within that trait group on the underlying dimension measured by the scale. Higher-scoring individuals are likely to possess the trait to a greater degree and to demonstrate the trait with greater frequency and intensity than are lower-scoring individuals within the same trait group. Simply put, two persons scoring PS = 50 and PS = 69, respectively, on the Externally Focused scale are both categorized as members of the extraverted group, but the person scoring PS = 69 is more extraverted than is the person scoring PS = 50. In fact, a score of PS = 69 on the Externally Focused scale is at the median of the extraverted group. A score of PS = 89 on the Externally Focused scale is at the 84th percentile of all members of that trait group. PSs have the same meaning across all the MIPS *Revised* scales.

Although the use of gender-based norms is required to represent empirically demonstrated gender differences in the prevalence of various personality styles in the population, referencing a person to a combined sample of men and women also may be of interest in some situations. For this reason, total group norms are provided for the general adult sample and for the general college sample.

Comment

The PS scaling procedure used for the MIPS *Revised* is preferred to both linear and normalized standard score conversions (e.g., *T*-scores), because PSs more accurately reflect differences in the prevalence of various personality traits in the population. The use of either linear or normalized *T*-score transformations with a standard psychometric cutoff score, such as one or two standard deviations above the mean, would impose an arbitrary statistical rule of thumb that bears little resemblance to the reality of population prevalence rates.

Unlike intelligence, personality variables are not necessarily distributed normally in the population. Normalized *T*-scores would, by definition, require half the population to score above 50 on all scales, which is clearly an inaccurate representation of the distribution of many personality traits in the normal population. For instance, it is simply not true that half the population is introverted and the other half extraverted, so that developing tests that result in these simplistic dichotomies is unjustified by the available actuarial data.

Linear *T*-scores would center the scale at the sample mean—that is, the average score. To describe an individual as "average" on Internally Focused, however, is meaningless, because most people are not introverted. The use of PS conversions is empirically justified by population prevalence rate data and is consistent with Millon's biosocial/evolutionary model of personology.

Reliability

The internal consistency of the MIPS *Revised* scales is quite adequate for a personality test. The median coefficient alphas are $r = .78$ for adults ($n = 1,000$) and $r = .77$ for students ($n = 1,600$). Median split-half reliabilities are $r = .82$ and $r = .80$ for the adult ($n = 1,000$) and college ($N = 1,600$) samples, respectively. The median retest reliability is $r = .85$ for adults after 2 months ($N = 50$), and $r = .84$ for students after 3 weeks ($n = 110$). Reliabilities are very comparable for females and males.

Construct Validity

The test manual for the original MIPS (Millon, 1994b) presents correlations with a wide variety of other personality tests, including the Sixteen Personality Factor Questionnaire (16PF; Cattell, Eber, & Tatsuoka, 1970), MBTI (Myers & McCaulley, 1985), California Psychological Inventory (Gough, 1987), NEO Personality Inventory (NEO-PI; Costa & McCrae, 1985), Gordon Personal Profile—Inventory (Gordon, 1978), Beck Depression Inventory (Beck & Steer, 1987), College Adjustment Scales (Anton & Reed, 1991), Minnesota Multiphasic Personality Inventory (MMPI; Hathaway & McKinley, 1967), Minnesota Multiphasic Personality Inventory–2 (MMPI-2; Butcher, Dahlstrom, Graham, Tellegen, & Kaemmer, 1989), Strong Interest Inventory (SII; Hansen & Campbell, 1985), and Jackson Personality Research Form (Jackson, 1985). These studies are strengthened by the fact that most of the subject samples were selected to be representative of working adults in the U.S. population, and were not based on samples of convenience such as college freshmen. The pattern of convergent and divergent correlations between the MIPS and these tests, obtained to demonstrate external validity, were largely consonant with expectations, based on the Millon theory of normal personology and on the item content of the respective scales. The MIPS (and MIPS *Revised*) constructs can thus be said to be well positioned within a larger nomological network of personality domains. Correlations between the original MIPS and the MMPI, MBTI, and NEO-PI have been selected for discussion in this chapter. (Please note that even in discussing research done with the original MIPS, I use the titles of individual scales in the MIPS *Revised*, for clarity in the present context.)

The MIPS was correlated with the MMPI-2 in a sample of 62 Air Force recruits referred for psychological evaluation, and with the original MMPI in a sample of 58

police officer applicants. Interestingly, the MIPS and MMPI showed a pattern of convergent validity in the clinically referred sample and a pattern of divergent validity in
the job applicant sample. In the sample of clinically referred Air Force recruits, the
MIPS scales corresponding to the MIPS *Revised* Pain-Avoiding, Passively Accommodating, Anxious/Hesitating, and Internally Focused scales correlated very highly ($r >$
.65) with several indicators of psychopathology on the MMPI-2, most notably scale
Pt (Psychasthenia), scale Sc (Schizophrenia), and scale Si (Social Introversion). By
comparison, the magnitude of the correlations between the MIPS and the MMPI in
the police applicant sample were generally quite low (Millon, 1994b). This finding
may suggest that when used with normal populations, such as job applicants, the
MIPS (and MIPS *Revised*) and MMPI measure (and MMPI-2) essentially different
domains. Although the ability of the MMPI to screen out obvious psychopathology
has been well demonstrated, the use of the MMPI to predict job performance among
normally functioning employees is less accepted (Butcher, 1979) and can be legally
problematic in many employment settings.

The MIPS Cognitive Modes (MIPS *Revised* Thinking Styles)

Relationship with the MBTI

The MIPS and the MBTI were administered to 100 adults with a median age of 40
years. Strong correlations were observed between MBTI scales and the MIPS Cognitive Modes (which correspond to the MIPS *Revised* Thinking Styles), developed to
measure similar Jungian constructs. When these data were arranged in a multitrait–
multimethod matrix using continuous bipolar scores, the correlations between the
complementary scales on the MIPS and MBTI ranged from $r = .71$ to $r = .75$.

In a separate sample of displaced executives and upper-level managers ($N = 47$),
these multitrait–multimethod correlations were also strong, ranging from $r = .67$ to r
$= .86$. The magnitude of these correlations clearly supports the hypothesis that the
MIPS Cognitive Modes and thus the MIPS *Revised* Thinking Styles scales measure
essentially the same constructs as do the MBTI.

Relationship with the Other MIPS Styles

Many other meaningful relationships were observed between certain of the MIPS
Motivating Aims and Interpersonal Behaviors (corresponding to the MIPS *Revised*
Motivating Styles and Behaving Styles) bipolarities and the MBTI scales. The MBTI
Thought Guided and Feeling Guided scales were moderately correlated with the
MIPS scales corresponding to the MIPS *Revised* Self-Indulging–Other-Nurturing
bipolarity. The direction of these correlations suggests that individuals oriented
toward obtaining reinforcement from others in their environment (Other-Nurturing
on the MIPS *Revised*) are likely to be classified as "feelers" on the MBTI, while those
oriented toward obtaining reinforcement from self (Self-Indulging on the MIPS
Revised) are more likely to be classified as "thinkers" on the MBTI. The MBTI
Thought-Guided scale was also correlated with the MIPS *Revised* Dominant/Con-
trolling scale, while the MBTI Feeling-Guided scale was correlated with the MIPS
Revised Cooperative/Agreeing scale.

Furthermore, the MIPS scales corresponding to the MIPS *Revised* Unconventional/Dissenting–Dutiful/Conforming bipolarity were moderately correlated with the MBTI Judging and Perceiving scales. The direction of these correlations suggests an important relationship between judgmental thinking and Dutiful/Conforming interpersonal behavior. Finally, the MBTI Imaginative/Intuiting scale is moderately correlated with the Innovation-Seeking scale on the MIPS *Revised*, suggesting that innovative thinking may be related to an intuiting style of processing information.

The MIPS 16 Types

There are 16 possible combinations of the four MBTI bipolar scales that are typically presented in MBTI research (Myers & McCaulley, 1985). An analogous set of 16 types has been produced using the four MIPS *Revised* Cognitive Modes bipolarities. The MIPS manual (Millon, 1994b) shows the percentages in each of these 16 MIPS types for the adult ($N = 1,000$) and college ($N = 1,600$) standardization samples, by gender and overall. The largest percentage of adult males (24%) is found in the ESTZ (Externally Focused–Realistic/Sensing–Thought-Guided–Conservation-Seeking) type. The largest percentages of adult females are found in the ENFV (Externally Focused–Imaginative/Intuiting–Feeling-Guided–Innovation-Seeking) type (15.8%) and in the ESFZ (Externally Focused–Realistic/Sensing–Feeling-Guided–Conservation-Seeking) type (14.4%). The percentages obtained can be considered representative of the general population because of the closeness of proportions of age, education level, and race/ethnicity in the samples to those in the U.S. Census data.

Shown in Table 26.3 are the percentages of the 16 typologies in specific occupational groups, including sales personnel, clerical and technical workers, upper-level managers, Air Force recruits, police applicants, and general laborers. These data are interesting because they show differences in characteristic modes of gathering and processing information across occupational groups. For example, approximately 18% of those in technical occupations were classified as ISTZ (Internally Focused–Realistic/Sensing–Thought-Guided–Conservation-Seeking, in MIPS *Revised* terms), compared with about 7% of salespersons. More than half of the police officer applicants (58%) were classified as ESTZ (Externally Focused–Realistic/Sensing–Thought-Guided–Conservation-Seeking), compared with only 24% of males in the adult standardization sample. The MIPS typologies by occupational group shown in this table should be used with caution, because these data do not imply a connection to effective job performance. Studies concerning job performance are discussed below in the section on organizational research.

Summary

The MIPS Cognitive Mode and thus the MIPS *Revised* Thinking Styles) scales operate in very similar ways to the MBTI scales, and the integration of these typologies with the MIPS Motivating Aims and Interpersonal Behaviors (corresponding to the MIPS *Revised* Motivating Styles and Behaving Styles) may provide an enriched understanding of the person taking the test.

TABLE 26.3. MIPS Percentages for Each of the 16 Styles by Occupational Group

	ISTC	ISFC	INFC	INTC
Upper management	10.1	2.3	1.5	3.2
Clerical/secretarial	8.7	9.7	1.0	1.0
Sales	7.2	4.5	1.8	0.9
Technical	18.2	1.8	1.8	3.6
General labor	10.7	10.7	0.0	0.0
Air Force recruits	9.4	3.1	3.6	1.6
Police applicants	9.2	0.3	0.3	1.4
	ISTV	ISFV	INFV	INTV
Upper management	3.9	3.1	1.5	0.7
Clerical/secretarial	2.9	1.9	7.8	1.0
Sales	0.9	1.8	9.0	6.3
Technical	9.1	0.0	1.8	7.3
General labor	1.8	8.9	10.7	7.1
Air Force recruits	1.0	4.2	8.3	3.6
Police applicants	1.7	0.3	1.4	0.0
	ESTV	ESFV	ENFV	ENTV
Upper management	12.5	0.8	7.8	13.2
Clerical/secretarial	1.0	3.9	11.7	2.9
Sales	1.8	7.2	15.3	7.2
Technical	9.1	0.0	7.3	5.5
General labor	10.7	5.4	8.9	3.6
Air Force recruits	5.2	4.2	6.8	3.1
Police applicants	5.6	2.0	1.4	3.4
	ESTC	ESFC	ENFC	ENTC
Upper management	22.0	10.2	0.8	6.2
Clerical/secretarial	16.5	18.4	10.7	1.0
Sales	20.7	7.2	2.7	5.4
Technical	20.0	7.3	0.0	7.3
General labor	10.7	7.1	3.6	0.0
Air Force recruits	21.9	7.8	8.3	7.8
Police applicants	58.0	3.6	3.4	8.1

Note. The sizes of the samples are as follows: Upper management (N = 130); Clerical/secretarial (N = 103); Sales (N = 111); Technical (N = 55); General labor (N = 56); Air Force recruits (N = 206); and Police applicants (N = 349). Key to style abbreviations, in MIPS *Revised* terminology: E, Externally Focused; I, Internally Focused; S, Realistic/Sensing; N, Imaginative/Intuiting; T, Thought-Guided; F, Feeling-Guided; C, Conservation-Seeking; V, Innovation-Seeking. Copyright 1994 by Dicandrien, Inc. All rights reserved.

Applied Organizational Research with the MIPS

I conducted six large applied research studies in various organizations and corporations around the country as part of the original MIPS prepublication research program. Results of these studies apply equally to the MIPS *Revised*. Several of these studies are summarized in this section. Interested researchers can read about the technical details of each study in the MIPS manual. (Again, the titles of individual scales in the MIPS *Revised* are used here, for clarity.)

Managerial Performance

The MIPS was administered to a sample of midlevel managers in a large telecommunications firm in the southeastern United States ($N = 51$). These were mostly white and well-educated men in the third tier of the corporation's management structure. The subjects participated in a 3-day management assessment center that included two simulated board meetings with different agendas: One meeting involved a competitive resource allocation decision, and the other involved a cooperative organizational problem-solving discussion. Other activities included an in-basket exercise; a formal presentation of a business plan to a superior, based on review of a standardized packet of information; a personnel counseling session with a disgruntled subordinate; and the preparation of a written business plan, based on the review of another standardized packet of information. Each manager's performance was rated by three trained assessors on 10 dimensions of managerial performance.

The mean MIPS profile for the managers was quite interesting. The profile suggested that these men actively sought positive reinforcement from their world by modifying surrounding circumstances and asserting themselves interpersonally in a socially confident and poised manner. The highest mean scores were on the MIPS scales corresponding to the MIPS *Revised* Pleasure-Enhancing (PS = 80.6), Confident/Asserting (PS = 72.9), Gregarious/Outgoing (PS = 70), Actively Modifying (PS = 68.5), and Externally Focused (PS = 68.5) scales. A moderate elevation was observed on the Dominant/Controlling scale (PS = 55.1). Several a priori hypotheses about the relationship of the MIPS scales to the 10 dimensions of managerial performance were supported. As predicted, oral communication was related to the MIPS scales corresponding to the MIPS *Revised* Actively Modifying, Externally Focused, Gregarious/Outgoing, and Confident/Asserting scales. Oral defense, or the ability to offer persuasive verbal responses in the face of challenges and criticism, was positively related to the Gregarious/Outgoing, Confident/Asserting, and Dominant/Controlling scales, and inversely related to the Submissive/Yielding scale. Strategic analysis was related to the Actively Modifying and Dominant/Controlling scales. Interactive problem solving was positively correlated with the Externally Focused, Gregarious/Outgoing, and Confident/Asserting scales, and negatively correlated with the Anxious/Hesitating scale. Team management was related to the Dominant/Controlling scale.

Although additional correlations were not anticipated, the MIPS scales corresponding to the MIPS *Revised* Imaginative/Intuiting and Innovation-Seeking scales were correlated significantly with several dimensions of managerial performance, including strategic analysis, interactive problem solving, oral defense, and oral communication. Because the business decisions and situations encountered at higher levels of management are both more complex and less structured, this finding may suggest that an ability to deal with novelty and ambiguity, which sensing and systematizing individuals often lack, may be helpful to effective managerial performance at the higher levels on management. Further research is needed on this topic.

Also not anticipated was a significant correlation between team management and the MIPS scales corresponding to the MIPS *Revised* Pain-Avoiding, Dissatisfied/ Complaining, and Feeling-Guided scales. Although a feeling style of cognitive processing may relate to team management because of the tendency to attend to the views of others, the positive relationship of high ability in this dimension with the Pain-Avoiding and Dissatisfied/Complaining scales is more difficult to interpret. According to MIPS *Revised* theory, the Dissatisfied/Complaining scale represents a tendency to be discontented with situations in general, and the Pain-Avoiding scale reflects a basic motivation to avoid negative reinforcement from the environment. If these findings can be replicated, they may suggest that a moderate degree of alertness to negative feedback, if appropriately channeled, can be adaptive when a person is managing a team.

These findings are consistent with definitions of leadership as a process of interpersonal influence involving persuasion rather than dominance (Hogan, Curphy, & Hogan, 1993).

Law Enforcement Performance

The relationship between the MIPS and police officer performance was studied in a predominantly Hispanic metropolitan city in the southwestern United States. The mean MIPS profile for those applicants offered admission to the training academy (*n* = 47) was noteworthy for the relatively moderate elevation on the scales corresponding to the MIPS *Revised* Dominant/Controlling (PS = 47) scale, as well as the balance of scores on the Self-Indulging (PS = 41) and Other-Nurturing (PS = 41) bipolarity. The highest scores were observed on the Thought-Guided (PS = 71), Confident/ Asserting (PS = 74), and Pleasure-Enhancing (PS = 81) scales. Also noteworthy was the mean score on the Adjustment Index (corresponding to the MIPS *Revised* Clinical Index) (*T* = 59), which was almost one full standard deviation above average.

A structured job analysis was conducted to determine the personality traits that are considered essential to effective performance as an entry-level patrol officer, with consensus ratings provided by five field training officers. The results suggested that four personality dimensions were essential to effective performance: (1) adherence to work ethic, (2) thoroughness and attentiveness to details, (3) sensitivity to the interests of others, and (4) emotional stability. The job analysis was conducted with a research version of An Inventory of General Position Requirements (IGPR; Bowling Green State University, 1992), which was developed to provide an empirical basis for matching position requirements and personality traits in specific occupations (Guion, 1991). MIPS composites were developed to measure each of the four dimensions identified in the job analysis. After 6 months of academy training, these composites were correlated with ratings on simulated tactical police exercises. The MIPS Emotional Stability composite was correlated with the use of secure police tactics during a barroom disturbance and with appropriately removing a suspect from the disturbance. Appropriate removal of the suspect was also correlated with the MIPS composites for Sensitivity to the Interests of Others and for Adherence to Work Ethic. In another exercise, the MIPS composites for Thoroughness and Attentiveness to Detail and for Adherence to Work Ethic were both correlated with properly issuing a traffic citation.

After graduation from the academy, the cadets were followed through 4 months of field training. They were rated multiple times on tasks, attitude, knowledge, and appearance. The MIPS equivalent of the MIPS *Revised* Dominant/Controlling scale showed a pattern of medium to large inverse correlations with all areas of field performance measured in this study. According to MIPS *Revised* theory, individuals with moderately high scores on the Dominant/Controlling scale demonstrate a pervasively forceful and domineering style of relating to others. Individuals with very high Dominant/Controlling scores may be chronically combative, tending toward a contentious, even hostile, tone in their relationships. In Millon's theory of personality disorders, these individuals are on the same continuum (although not as extreme) as those diagnosed with aggressive personality disorders. As written previously about these individuals, "Although many may cloak their more malicious and power-oriented tendencies in publicly approved roles and vocations, they give themselves away in their dominating, antagonistic, and frequent persecutory actions" (Millon, Millon, & Davis, 1994, pp. 12–13).

On the other hand, the polar opposite MIPS *Revised* Submissive/Yielding, was uncorrelated with field performance. This suggests a nonlinear relationship between dominance and police performance in which either too little or too much of this trait is associated with problematic performance as a law enforcement officer. This finding is also consistent with the results of the job analysis, in which the police department's field training officers indicated that sensitivity to the interests of others is essential to effective performance of police duties. Overall, these results mirror the changing conceptualization of the police officer's role from "carrying a big stick" to a highly technical position requiring considerable interpersonal skill and judgment.

Screening for Psychological Adjustment

The MIPS was administered to 297 U.S. Air Force recruits during the first week of basic training as part of a routine screening program designed to identify individuals who are psychologically incapable of adjusting to military service. MIPS results were not available to the psychologists making these decisions. One hundred and sixty-nine recruits passed the initial mass screening, based on their responses to a structured life history questionnaire. Ninety-five recruits were referred for further testing, but were then cleared for duty based on the test results. Thirty-three recruits were recommended for discharge from the military after a complete psychological evaluation.

The mean MIPS profiles for these groups (again, presented here with MIPS *Revised* scale names) were dramatically different. Whereas the group that passed the initial screening was reasonably balanced on the pleasure–pain bipolarity, for example, the group found unfit for duty scored extremely high on pain (Pain-Avoiding PS = 98) and extremely low on pleasure (Pleasure-Enhancing PS = 1).

A Clinical Index (again, the MIPS *Revised* equivalent of the MIPS Adjustment Index) was developed, based on a composite of scales. The following six MIPS *Revised* PS values were placed on the positive side of the Clinical Index: Pleasure-Enhancing, Gregarious/Outgoing, Confident/Asserting, Dutiful/Conforming, Dominant/Controlling, and Cooperative/Agreeing. The Pleasure-Enhancing scale was weighted twice as heavily as the other five scales. The following six MIPS *Revised* PS values entered the negative side of the equation for the Clinical Index: Pain-Avoiding, Asocial/Withdrawing, Anxious/Hesitating, Unconventional/Dissenting, Submissive/Yielding, and Dissatisfied/Complaining. The Pain-Avoiding scale was weighted twice as heavily as the other five scales. This Clinical Index was then converted to a *T*-score, using the mean and *SD* of the standardization sample.

The unfit-for-duty group scored more than two and a half standard deviations below average on the Clinical Index (T = 23). A *T*-score less than or equal to 35 points on the Clinical Index was identified as a cutoff score, because it correctly classified 100% of recruits in the unfit for duty group while misclassifying fewer than 20% of recruits who were actually fit for duty. The correlation of the Clinical Index with fit versus unfit designations was at the upper limit of the statistic. This study suggested that use of the Clinical Index in the screening program could have significantly reduced the caseload of the examining psychologists.

Although the cutoff score should be cross-validated in an independent sample, the MIPS *Revised* Clinical Index holds considerable promise in a wide variety of organizational settings in which screening for overall adjustment is considered job relevant, such as safety-sensitive positions or positions working with children or the elderly. Individuals who score below T = 35 on this index should be administered a clinical-range instrument such as the Millon Clinical Multiaxial Inventory–III (MCMI-III; Millon, 1994a) to assess for psychopathology.

Absenteeism and Disciplinary Personnel Actions

The MIPS was administered to a sample of hourly workers employed by a medium-sized municipal government in the southeastern United States (N = 41), and absenteeism and disciplinary records were obtained. These employees were predominantly laborers working in the city maintenance, landscape, and sanitation departments. The sample was largely male (76%) and African American (56%), with a high school education or less (70%). The median age was 35 years.

The mean MIPS Behaving Styles scales for this sample were characterized by high scores on the Dutiful/Conforming (PS = 60) and Cooperative/Agreeing (PS = 61) scales. These employees tended to use more Realistic/Sensing (PS = 63) modes of gathering information and Conservation-Seeking (PS = 55) strategies for processing information. In general, this sample of laborers was considerably more introversing, asocial/withdrawing, and submissive/yielding, as well as less enhancing and modifying, than were samples of managers and executives.

MIPS scores were correlated with personnel records for the preceding 12 months. The MIPS *Revised* Dominant/Controlling scale was inversely correlated with both disciplinary personnel action taken against an employee (r = –.35, p < .01) and absenteeism (r = –.33, p < .01). In addition, the MIPS *Revised* Anxious/Hesitating scale was positively related to absenteeism (r = .32, p < .01). Thus, we can speculate that employees with high scores on the Dominant/Controlling scale and low scores on the Anxious/Hesitating scale will have better attendance records than other employees. According to MIPS *Revised* theory, individuals who score high on the Dominant/Controlling scale seek to arrange and control the events in their lives to meet their schedules, needs, and priorities. In addition, individuals scoring low on the Anxious/Hesitating scale tend to feel more secure about their personal worth and to be more decisive about taking action than those who score higher. Perhaps these employees take better command of potential conflict between their personal and work schedules than those who are absent more often.

Career Decision Making

Two studies examined the use of the MIPS in career decision making. In the first study, the MIPS was administered to 70 clients participating in career management counseling at a large, nationally based firm that specializes in executive outplacement and management consulting to Fortune 500 companies. The sample consisted of all upper-level managers who had been displaced during corporate downsizing. The mean MIPS *Revised* profile for this sample suggested that, on average, these managers were people who actively sought positive reinforcement from the environment and who were assertive and gregarious/outgoing in interpersonal relations. Their preferred information-gathering styles were extraverted and realistic, while their preferred information-processing styles were thought-guided and conservation-seeking.

Correlations with the SII (Hansen & Campbell, 1985) show that a conservation-seeking style of processing information is significantly correlated with conventional occupations involving methodical, organized, or clerical tasks. The polar opposite MIPS *Revised* scale, Innovation-Seeking, is correlated with interest in enterprising activities, which require entrepreneurial, persuasive, and political behaviors. The SII Enterprising scale is also significantly correlated with the MIPS *Revised* Actively Modifying, Externally Focused, Gregarious/Outgoing, Confident/Asserting, and Dominant/Controlling scales.

An interest in business management on the SII was positively correlated with the MIPS *Revised* Dominant/Controlling and Confident/Asserting scales, and negatively correlated with the Passively Accommodating scale. By contrast, an interest in office practices on the SII was correlated with systematizing style of processing information and with the MIPS *Revised* Dutiful/Conforming and Cooperative/Agreeing scales. Furthermore, the Gregarious/Outgoing MIPS *Revised* scale was correlated with an interest in both sales and merchandising as expressed on the SII.

In the second study, the MIPS and the SII were administered to a sample of 100 community college students identified as expressing uncertainty about their career goals and describing their uncertainty as troublesome and an unresolved issue for them. A canonical analysis yielded three distinct patterns of relationships between MIPS *Revised* and SII scales, labeled the "retreator," the "feeler," and the "conscientious conformer." Retreators were characterized by the Anxious/Hesitating and Cooperative/Agreeing scales on the MIPS *Revised*. They did not trust others or take risks easily. They preferred disconnection from the world of work and might develop interpersonally defensive career intentions. For the retreators, career indecision might reflect a lack of receptivity to the social relations that are part of most work settings.

There was a hint at some compatibility with highly structured subordinate/follower roles in work.

The feelers were characterized by the Other-Nurturing, Feeling-Guided, and Cooperative/Agreeing scales on the MIPS *Revised*. Although retreators and feelers both tended to have high Cooperative/Agreeing scores, they differed in their approach toward others. Retreators might use cooperative/agreeing behavior as a way of avoiding more meaningful and, perhaps, threatening interpersonal communication; feelers, on the other hand, were socially open, and their Cooperative/Agreeing behavior lacked the defensive quality shown by retreators. Feelers showed a pattern of being people-oriented, and avoiding activities that were highly regulated and that involved calculation or the use of standardized procedures to find solutions.

The conscientious conformer was characterized by the MIPS *Revised* Dutiful/Conforming, Realistic/Sensing, and Conservation-Seeking scales. This variant was very similar to the pattern of MIPS *Revised* scales found to correlate with the Conscientiousness factor of the NEO-PI (see below). These students tended to express interest in office practice, domestic activities, social service, and religious activities.

General negative affectivity—that is, the propensity to focus on and experience painful emotional states—may provide a framework for understanding chronic career indecision. Perhaps the strong need for systems that characterizes the conscientious conformer, and the willingness to defer to the wishes of others that characterizes both the retreator and feeler, represent two methods of avoiding possible negative stimulation from the work environment. Students who exhibit pervasive career indecision present unique challenges for counselors in traditional vocational guidance programs. The often-used career counseling techniques of exploration, job shadowing, and placement assistance may be inadequate for these clients. To remediate chronic career indecision, counselors may need to address the underlying personality issues (Super, 1983; Tango & Dziuban, 1984).

Summary

The studies reviewed in this section provide empirical support for many of the applications of the MIPS *Revised* suggested earlier in this chapter.

Factor Structure of the MIPS

Results of Factor Analysis

We studied the factor structure of the original MIPS, using a principal-components analysis at the item level in a sample of 2,600 subjects (Weiss & Lowther, 1995). Results apply equally to the MIPS *Revised*. This study suggested five factors that were consistent with the five-factor model of personality and which accounted for 24.8% of the total variance. Subjects with high scores on the first factor were likely to endorse items such as "I often feel on edge, waiting for something to happen." The first factor was interpreted as measuring Maladaptation. The second dimension was interpreted as representing Extraversion or Surgency. It was marked by items such as "I have great confidence in my social abilities." The third factor, termed Conscientiousness, was defined by items such as "I plan ahead and then act decisively to make my plans happen." The fourth dimension, interpreted as Disagreeableness, contained items such as "I look out for myself first, and then think of others." The fifth factor was marked by items such as "I am a realistic person who does not like to speculate about things." This factor was interpreted as representing the opposite pole of openness to experience—namely, Closed-Mindedness. These findings were consonant with the five-factor model of personality (Goldberg, 1993), except that we obtained the reverse poles of the Agreeableness and Openness to Experience Factors—namely, Disagreeableness and Closed-Mindedness.

Relation to the Five-Factor Model of Personality

We (Weiss & Lowther, 1995) correlated the MIPS factors with several measures of the five-factor model of personality, including the NEO-PT (Costa & McCrae, 1985), the Goldberg Adjective Checklist (Goldberg, 1992), and the second-order factors of the 16PF (Cattell et al., 1970). The pattern of correlations was consistent with expectations. For example, the MIPS Maladaptation, Surgency, Conscientiousness, Disagreeableness, and Closed-mindedness factors correlated $r = .81$, $r = .70$, $r = .72$, $r = -.43$, and $r = -.33$, respectively, with the NEO Neuroticism, Extraversion, Conscientiousness, Agreeableness, and Openness scales in a sample of 61 adults.

Factor Patterns by Occupational Group

Mean MIPS *T*-scores for the five factors were examined in several occupational samples (Weiss & Lowther, 1995), and some very interesting patterns emerged. Among the five occupational groups studied, the police officers ($N = 354$) had the highest Conscientiousness score ($X = 56$) and the lowest Maladaptation score ($X = 39$). Midlevel managers ($N = 83$) had the highest mean scores on the Surgency factor ($X = 54$) and the lowest mean scores on the Closed-Mindedness factor ($X = 45$). Conversely, a sample of hourly municipal employees ($N = 41$) had the lowest scores on the Surgency factor ($X = 46$) and the highest score on the Closed-Mindedness factor ($X = 57$). Air Force recruits ($N = 288$) also had high Closed-Mindedness scores ($X = 54$). Perhaps most interestingly, the sample of displaced executives ($N = 72$) had the highest Disagreeableness score ($X = 55$).

Factor Scores by Gender and Age

T-score means for the factor scores were also examined by gender for the adult norm sample ($n = 500$ males and $n = 500$ females) and the college norm sample ($n = 800$ females and $n = 800$ males). The mean scores for the Closed-Mindedness and Conscientiousness factors were higher in the adult than in the college samples, while the college samples presented higher mean scores on Maladaptation. Most intuitive of all, however, was the finding that the highest mean score for males was Disagreeableness, while the lowest mean score for females was Disagreeableness. This was true for both adults and college students.

Using the Factor-Based Scales

Researchers and practitioners can calculate the appropriate *T*-score for each factor by using the information contained in Table 26.4 and applying the following formula:

$$\frac{RS - M}{SD} \times 10 + 50$$

where *RS* is the sum of the items in the factor, *M* is the raw score mean, and *SD* is the raw score standard deviation. For each of the five factors, this procedure will yield a linear *T*-score. Note that *T*-scores have a mean of 50 and a standard deviation of 10. A person scoring *T* = 60 on Maladaptation, for example, would be one standard deviation above the mean on this trait. Note that using the *M* and *SD* of the combined sample (*N* = 2,600) allows natural age and gender differences to emerge in the transformed scores.

Theoretical Implications of the Five-Factor Model

The five-factor model has emerged as an important force in the investigation of personality structure (Digman, 1990). The MIPS and MIPS *Revised* appear to factor into five dimensions that are consistent with the five-factor model of personality. This finding is important because of the parallels between the theoretically derived MIPS/MIPS *Revised* scales and the empirically derived five-factor model. The MIPS/MIPS *Revised* scales have a rich theoretical foundation in a model of personality that is deeply rooted in biosocial and evolutionary theory (Millon, 1969, 1981, 1990). The five-factor model, on the other hand, is largely devoid of theory, having its roots

TABLE 26.4. MIPS (and MIPS *Revised*) Items That Define the Five Factors, and the Raw Score Mean (*M*) and Standard Deviation (*SD*) for Each Factor

Maladaptation (*M* = 13.61, *SD* = 8.82)
   True: 11,13,17,18,25,27,34,38,39,40,45,49,52,54,56,57,60,62,63,68,69,72,82,85,86,87,95,100,105,
      111,122,126,139,148,155
   False: 58,81,94,106

Surgency (*M* = 13.07, *SD* = 4.63)
   True: 3,28,41,47,65,73,123,132,149,158,162,166,167,170,172,174,180
   False: 20,91,142,143

Conscientiousness (*M* = 13.95, *SD* = 5.28)
   True: 4,33,48,59,67,79,84,112,119,137,153,157,159,163,168,171,173,177,179
   False: 42,107,135

Disagreeableness (*M* = 6.76, *SD* = 4.02)
   True: 43,75,83,89,96,108,113,116,118,133,147,150
   False: 71,80,92,99,121,127,144

Close Mindedness (*M* = 6.87, *SD* = 3.06)
   True: 16,21,29,37,46,64,78,88,90,102,114,117,125,130

Note. To obtain the raw score for each factor, count 1 point for each item endorsed in the keyed direction.

in the statistical analysis of lists of adjectives used by ordinary people to describe others (Goldberg, 1993). The parallels between the Millonian taxonomy and the five-factor model observed in this study could launch a theoretical effort to "bootstrap" the five-factor model into two well-established and accepted theoretical frameworks of personology, the beginnings of which are outlined below.

The first factor, termed Maladaptation or Neuroticism, is marked by several items from the MIPS *Revised* Pleasure-Enhancing and Pain-Avoiding bipolarity. According to the theory, persons scoring high on this factor are likely to show a significant tendency to focus attention on potential threats to their emotional and physical security. Their expectation of and heightened alertness to the signs of potential negative feedback can lead them to disengage from everyday relationships and pleasurable experiences. Those scoring low on Maladaptation are likely to be motivated more by pleasure than pain; to possess attitudes and behaviors designed to foster and enrich life; and to generate joy, pleasure, contentment, and fulfillment, and thereby strengthen their capacity to remain competent physically and mentally. The Maladaptation factor also contains several items from the MIPS *Revised* Dissatisfied/Complaining and Anxious/Hesitating scales, which are the normal-range variants of the avoidant and negativistic disorders.

The second factor, termed Extraversion or Surgency, contains items from the MIPS *Revised* Externally Focused and Internally Focused scales. These scales are derived from the work of Jung (1921/1971) and reflect the direction of the individual's attentions and interests. High scorers on this factor look to the external environment for sources of information and cognitive inspiration (Millon, 1994b). In terms of interpersonal behaviors, the Surgency factor also contains items from the MIPS *Revised* Gregarious/Outgoing and Dominant/Controlling scales, which are the normal-range variants of the histrionic and sadistic personalities.

The Conscientiousness factor is marked by items from the MIPS *Revised* Actively Modifying and Passively Accommodating scales, as well as from the Conservation-Seeking scale. The Actively Modifying and Passively Accommodating bipolarity corresponds to the active–passive dimension of Millon's theory. Those who score high on Conscientiousness are instrumental in actively seeking to modify their lives and to intrude on passing events by energetically and busily shaping their circumstances. In the cognitive sphere, they exhibit a conservation-seeking style of processing information, akin to the judgment preference abstracted from Jung's notions (Myers, 1962). Disposed to operate within established perspectives, conservation seekers assimilate new information to previous points of view, exhibiting thereby a high degree of dependability and consistency, if not rigidity, in their functioning. It is noteworthy that only two of the items from the MIPS *Revised* Dutiful/Conforming and Unconventional/Dissenting bipolarity load on this factor. This is important, in light of Loevinger's (1994) criticism of the operationalization of the conscientiousness construct in the five-factor model as merely measuring interpersonal conformity. The current formulation of Conscientiousness appears to be more cognitive than interpersonal.

The Disagreeableness factor is marked by items from the MIPS *Revised* Self-Indulging and Other-Nurturing bipolarity based on Millon's taxonomy, as well as from the Thought-Guided and Feeling-Guided bipolarity based on Jungian theory. Self-focused, those scoring high on the Self-Indulging scale tend to make up their own minds and reach their own decisions without perceiving the need to seek input or gain approval from others. At best, they are self-starting and self-actualizing. At times, however, they may become self-absorbed, caring little about the needs and priorities of others and focusing largely on their own interests. Persons scoring high on Disagreeableness also present a style of thinking and processing information in which experiences are interpreted in light of reason and logic, and decisions are made based on tangible and impersonal facts, with less consideration for the feelings or interests of others.

The Closed-Mindedness factor is marked by items from the MIPS *Revised* Realistic/Sensing scale based on Jungian typology, as well as from the Dutiful/Conforming and Cooperative/Agreeing scales based on the Millonian taxonomy. Realistic/Sensing high scorers are inclined toward information-gathering strategies based on tangible facts and decision-making strategies based on realistic options. They are less inclined to consider the possibilities of intangible, unstructured, or ambiguous situations. Items from the Dutiful/Conforming and Cooperative/Agreeing scales represent the normal-range variants of the obsessive–compulsive and dependent personality disorders, respectively. Conformers are notably respectful of tradition and authority and do their best to uphold conventional rules and standards. Cooperative/Agreeing high scorers are noted for their dependence on safe and supportive relationships, and for their lack of openness to new and unusual experiences that may threaten their emotional security.

Summary

This section has expanded the five-factor model by showing the empirical relationships of those five dimensions with the theoretical works of Millon and Jung. Future research on the five-factor model should seek to place that model into the larger nomological network of established personality theories to further our understanding of the structure of normal personality.

Expanding the Dimensions of Normality

Millon's model is perhaps one of the most thorough and coherent theories of personality offered by the field's great thinkers. Nonetheless, the model may still have room for expansion. Recall that Millon's taxonomy as originally proposed was based on a 2×4 matrix in which the active and passive domains were crossed with self, other, self–other ambivalence, and pain to produce his original eight personality types. The model was subsequently extended by Millon into a 2×5 matrix in which active and passive were also crossed with pain–pleasure discordance for a total of 10 personality types. Millon further extended his thinking about normal-range personality by incorporating the Jungian-like cognitive styles of information gathering and processing into the MIPS and MIPS *Revised*.

I have begun to consider an extension of Millon's matrix in which the active and passive dimensions are crossed with pleasure. These crossings were excluded in Millon's earlier taxonomies, because they were judged to have little relevance for the elucidation of psychopathological personality types (T. Millon, 1993, personal communication). However, the concept of pleasure may relate meaningfully to healthy personality functioning.

Many forms of psychopathology have been related to forces that either impede or confuse one's strivings for pleasure. Paul Meehl (1987) challenged the classic analytic view that anhedonia (i.e., the inability to experience pleasure) is always a function of some impedance in one's pleasure strivings, often due to guilt or anxiety. He asserted that some individuals simply have low capacity to experience pleasure. This opens the door to viewing hedonic capacity on a continuum from high to low ability to experience pleasure, or strong to weak responsivity to rewards. Observing that some individuals seem to experience pleasure in almost any situation, Meehl (1987, p. 37) wrote, "I conjecture that these people are the lucky ones at the high end of the hedonic capacity continuum, i.e., they were "born three drinks ahead."

Individuals with a normal capacity to experience pleasure are also subject to many of the same life stresses as are those with anhedonia. Their experience of stress is buffered, however, by an ability to feel a sense of enjoyment in life's occasional rewards. This ability to experience pleasure may provide them with a prophylactic against depressogenic cognitions and reduce susceptibility to various forms of psychopathology.

Responsiveness to pleasure is a spectrum phenomenon. The ability to experience pleasure reaches broadly into every aspect of personality. The experience of pleasure provides motivation for a host of appropriate social, occupational, and recreational behaviors that are essential for the maintenance of self-esteem, if not for personal growth and self-actualization. Any formulation of healthy personality functioning should therefore include a discussion of pleasure and the various means by which individuals seek to obtain pleasure in their daily lives. Perhaps the two most basic variants of the pleasure-seeking orientation are the active and passive pleasure styles.

The Active Pleasure Style

The active pleasure style is characterized by a normal predisposition to experience reinforcement from positive events (as opposed to the absence of pain), combined with a tendency to arrange and actively modify the circumstances of one's life to obtain the desired reinforcement. Individuals with this style differ to the extent that they find positive reinforcement in diverse stimuli. Some find pleasure in the usual rewards of successful careers and energetically pursue this course in either a gregarious and confident, or sometimes a dominant or controlling, manner.

Others are more inclined toward recreational pleasures. They frequently seek to combine work with play and look for opportunities to have fun while conducting business. They are likable colleagues, workmates, and bosses who set a tone of enjoying work. In the extreme, they are somewhat ill disposed to attend to the mundane details of responsible adult life, choosing to focus their attentions in that regard only when the demands of the situation are forced upon them, and then only with sufficient effort to remove the immediate threat of negative environmental stimuli and return their attentions to the active pursuit of pleasure. They are adventurous, fun-loving, enjoyable companions, who are often viewed by significant others as less responsible and mature than most people of their age and station in life. At times, their behavior may result in some minor inefficiencies in daily living, and perhaps major life problems as well. The data show that this personality style is common. Approximately 37% of adults and 34% of college students could reasonably be classified as presenting an active pleasure style.[1]

Following Millon's (1981) format for elaborating personality types, I have characterized the active pleasure type in terms of five functional processes and three structural attributes. In terms of functional processes, the behavioral presentation of these individuals is characterized as energetic, and their interpersonal style is best described as catalytic. That is, they are often the catalysts in interpersonal relations who make things happen. Their cognitive style is characterized as enriched, active, and lively; they are always thinking of how best to modify their environments to suit their needs and desires. Their expressed mood is best characterized as happy; they usually enjoy what they are doing. When events go wrong, they respond with appropriate affect and then quickly return to their usual mood. The dominant unconscious mechanism for dealing with intrapsychic conflict is rationalization. This is a second-line defense, however, as these individuals are usually confrontive; they attempt to deal forcefully yet appropriately with the progenitor of any inner turmoil. Only when this is not possible or successful are they likely to resort to rationalization, often devaluing that reinforcement which they could not achieve.

In terms of structural attributes, the self-image of the active pleasure type is characterized by a sense of competence; these individuals see themselves as tough and able to influence, if not dominate, others, but always in a socially skilled manner. Because of their high energy and drive, they often see themselves as competitive as well as competent. Their internalized content is best described as ambitiousness; inner representations are characterized by a strong drive to achieve that which they find reinforcing or pleasurable. Impulses to take advantage of others in the service of these drives are modulated by choosing socially acceptable goals and methods of influence. Intrapsychic organization is integrated, consisting of holistic, well-formed, stable mechanisms of internal regulation adequately modulating controls, defenses, and expressive channels.

The Passive Pleasure Style

The passive pleasure style is also noted for a normal orientation toward enjoying positive reinforcement, but this is combined with a general tendency to wait passively for such reinforcement. These individuals expect good things to happen to them without any real effort on their part. They are likable because of their easygoing style and positive outlook, but are sometimes prone to be anxious/hesitating and submissive/yielding in their interpersonal relations. They are self-indulgent and optimistic about future events, although they lack the exaggerated self-worth and sense of entitlement of those who lean toward being narcissistic. Their optimism often seems unwarranted in the view of significant others who know their circumstances and history. They are unlikely to be proactive in dealing with life, often waiting for situations to force them to move off a dead-center position. They may see no need, for example, to look for another apartment or a better job even when circumstances might suggest otherwise, assuming that things will work out in their own time and in their own way. Things do work themselves out often enough to maintain their behavior and avoid serious troubles.

When pervasive, however, this style can begin to cause significant inefficiencies in daily living. Those with this style seem to ignore the genuine life difficulties their behavior may create and are not appropriately distressed by these circumstances. In some cases, they may be brought to counseling by significant others who view them as lacking motivation to better themselves. Their behavior may have a dependent quality in the view of those who care for them, but the behavior is not motivated by dependence strivings or attachment needs. In today's vernacular, a person with the passive pleasure style might well be referred to as a "couch potato" (i.e., someone whose idea of pleasure is to lie on a comfortable couch eating snacks and watching television).

The data show that although the passive pleasure style is not overly rare, it is much less common than the active pleasure style. About 1 in every 12 people may show this pattern. In terms of percentages, approximately 8% of adults and 8% of college students present a passive pleasure style.[2]

In terms of functional processes, the behavioral presentation of these individuals is best characterized as hedonic, and their interpersonal style can be summarized as easygoing or "laid back." They readily experience pleasures that are laid on their plate, but are not motivated to pursue such rewards. Their cognitive style is marked by optimism, and expressed mood is untroubled. These individuals seem unphased by most daily stresses. The primary unconsciousness mechanism is suppression. Conflicts that cannot be reframed with a positive outlook are simply put out of mind. In terms of structural attributes, the passive pleasure type maintains a self-image characterized as lucky, or perhaps blessed. Their internalized content may be best characterized as relaxed; they have few strong drives or impulses and their inner representations revolve around finding ways to remove themselves from normal daily stresses. Finally, their intrapsychic organization is naive; few things bother them, so there is little need for strong mechanisms of internal regulation and control; nor are there strong impulses and drives toward change or self-actualization. Internal structures are not well formed, but are adequate to modulate the diluted affect that does occur, and there is a high threshold for impulse discharge.

Summary

The ability to experience pleasure is important to the understanding of healthy personality functioning. Both the active and passive pleasure styles have adequate hedonic capacity. A person with the passive pleasure style can enjoy the rewards that come his or her way, but does not anticipate pleasure and is not motivated to pursue it. A person with the active pleasure style plans to obtain rewards and works to bring them to fruition.

Much work, both theoretical and empirical, remains to be done to integrate the concept of pleasure more fully into our understanding of normal personality functioning. For example, do the active and passive pleasure styles take on different forms if an individual is also high on the self or other dimension of Millon's theory? Only time will tell whether these two personality styles will stand the test of clinical experience. However, elaboration on the concept of pleasure is an important step in viewing healthy personality functioning as more than the absence of psychopathology.

Future Research with the MIPS *Revised*

There are many areas of fruitful research for the MIPS *Revised*—especially differentiating normal from abnormal personality styles, expanding our understanding of normality, and further validating organizational applications. Perhaps the most obvious research study that has not yet been conducted is examining the relationship between the MIPS *Revised* and the other Millon inventories, most importantly the MCMI-III. How do the personality disorder scales on the MCMI-III relate to the personality styles measured by the MIPS *Revised*? Where is the line between normality and abnormality? A joint item-level factor analysis of responses from both personality-disordered and nonclinical samples would allow one to establish a cutoff point to determine whether treatment has moved the client into the functional distribution (see Jacobson & Truax, 1991, for appropriate formulas). In this way, we may more clearly draw the elusive line between clinical and nonclinical populations, which is so important in gauging the dimensions of normality.

The applications of the MIPS described above were largely in organizational settings. Thus numerous research projects on industrial personnel and on organizational training and development are appropriate. The MIPS *Revised* Clinical Index cutoff score of $T = 35$, described above, needs to be cross-validated in an independent sample. The importance of the MIPS *Revised* Imaginative/Intuiting and Innovation-Seeking scales for effective information processing among higher-level managers, suggested above, needs to be explored further. Also as suggested above, the possible effect of the MIPS *Revised* Pain-Avoiding and Dissatisfied/Complaining styles in managing teams needs further research. The role of the MIPS *Revised* in the initial formation of work teams should also be explored. Further exploration of the use of the MIPS *Revised* in vocational counseling and career development is appropriate.

When one is studying job performance, it is critical to begin with a job analysis. The IGPR (Bowling Green State University, 1992) is the only job analysis instrument that was developed to provide an empirical basis for matching job requirements and personality traits in specific occupations (Guion, 1991). The relationship between the MIPS *Revised* personality styles and the IGPR dimensions is an important area for future researchers. This would allow practitioners to make empirically supported hypotheses about connections between job requirements and personality styles, thus selecting job candidates based on defensible scientific principles rather than on professional opinion alone. Such research would represent an important scientific advance in an era when the use of personality tests for personnel selection is under intense legal and professional scrutiny.

Areas of research that have not yet been touched are applications in the marriage and family arena, as well as the use of the MIPS *Revised* to assist in making classification and placement decisions with prison inmates.

On the theoretical front, the active pleasure and passive pleasure styles I have described above need serious research attention. How can these styles be operationalized, what are the correlates of these types with other personality styles, and how are individuals with these styles perceived by significant others?

On the treatment front, Beck, Freeman, and Associates (1990) have proposed an elaborate schema of typical core cognitive beliefs held by individuals with each of the personality types. They suggest that these beliefs are at the core of individuals' uncomfortable emotions and inefficient behaviors, and they offer well-articulated cognitive treatment strategies targeting these beliefs. The relationship between these core cognitive belief structures and particular personalities needs to be explored empirically. Do individuals with different personality types endorse these belief sets differently? Do individuals with nonpathological personality styles endorse the relevant belief sets with less intensity than do those with personality disorders, or do they have a different set or beliefs? Do these sets of beliefs have implications for helping normal individuals understand and improve themselves?

Notes

1. For this analysis, individuals in the MIPS *Revised* adult (N = 1,000) and college (n = 1,600) standardization samples were classified as active pleasure types if their MIPS *Revised* PS values met both of the following conditions: (1) Actively Modifying PS > Passively Accommodating PS, and Actively Modifying PS > 59; and (2) Pleasure-Enhancing PS > Pain-Avoiding PS, and Pleasure-Enhancing PS > 59.

2. For this analysis, individuals in the MIPS *Revised* adult (N = 1,000) and college (N = 1,600) standardization samples were classified as passive pleasure types if their MIPS *Revised* PS values met both of the following conditions: (1) Passively Accommodating PS > Actively Modifying PS, and Passively Accommodating PS > 59; and (2) Pleasure-Enhancing PS > Pain-Avoiding PS, and Pleasure-Enhancing PS > 59.

References

Anton, W. D., & Reed, J. R. (1991). *College Adjustment Scales: Professional manual*. Odessa, FL: Psychological Assessment Resources.

Beck, A. T., Freeman, A., & Associates. (1990). *Cognitive therapy of personality disorders*. New York: Guilford Press.

Beck, A. T., & Steer, R. A. (1987). *Manual for the revised Beck Depression Inventory*. San Antonio, TX: Psychological Corporation.

Butcher, J. N. (Ed.). (1979). *New developments in the use of the MMPI*. Minneapolis: University of Minnesota Press.

Butcher, J. N., Dahlstrom, W. G., Graham, J. R., Tellegen, A., & Kaemmer, B. (1989). *Minnesota Multiphasic Personality Inventory–2: Manual for administration and scoring*. Minneapolis: University of Minnesota Press.

Bowling Green State University. (1992). *An inventory of general position requirements*. Bowling Green, OH: Author.

Cattell, R. B., Eber, H. W., & Tatsuoka, M. M. (1970). *Handbook for the Sixteen Personality Factor Questionnaire (16 PF)*. Champaign, IL: Institute for Personality and Ability Testing.

Costa, P. T., & McCrae, R. R. (1985). *The NEO Personality Inventory manual*. Odessa, FL: Psychological Assessment Resources.

Digman, J. M. (1990). Personality structure: Emergence of the five-factor model. *Annual Review of Psychology, 41*, 417–440.

Goldberg, L. R. (1992). The development of markers for the Big-Five factor structure. *Psychological Assessment, 4*(1), 26–42.

Goldberg, L. R. (1993). The structure of phenotypic personality traits. *American Psychologist, 48*, 26–34.

Gordon, L. V. (1978). *Gordon Personal Profile—Inventory manual* (rev. ed.). New York: Psychological Corporation.

Gough, H. G. (1987). *California Psychological Inventory: Administrator's guide*. Palo Alto, CA: Consulting Psychologists Press.

Guion, R. M. (1991, May). *Matching position requirements and personality traits*. Paper presented at the annual convention of the Society of Industrial and Organizational Psychology, Montréal.

Hansen, J. C., & Campbell, D. P. (1985). *Manual for the Strong Interest Inventory* (4th ed.). Palo Alto, CA: Consulting Psychologists.

Hathaway, S. R., & McKinley, J. C. (1967). *Minnesota Multiphasic Personality Inventory manual*. New York: Psychological Corporation.

Hogan, R., Curphy, G. J., & Hogan, J. (1993, April). *What we know about leadership: Effectiveness and personality*. Paper presented at the annual convention of the Society for Industrial and Organizational Psychology, San Francisco.

Jackson, D. N. (1985). *Personality Research Form manual* (3rd ed.). Port Huron, MI: Research Psychologists Press.

Jacobson, N. S., & Truax, P. (1991). Clinical significance: A statistical approach to defining meaningful change in psychotherapy research. *Journal of Consulting and Clinical Psychology, 59*(1), 12–19.

Jung, C. G. (1971). *The collected works of C. G. Jung: Vol. 6. Psychological types* (H. G. Baynes, Trans., rev. by R. F. C. Hull). Princeton, NJ: Princeton University Press. (Original work published 1921)

Loevinger, J. (1994). Has psychology lost its conscience? *Journal of Personality Assessment, 62*(1), 2–8.

Meehl, P. E. (1987). Hedonic capacity: Some conjectures. In D. C. Clark & J. Fawcett (Eds.), *Anhedonia and affect deficit states* (pp. 33–50). New York: PMA.

Millon, T. (1969). *Modern psychopathology: A biosocial approach to maladaptive learning and functioning*. Philadelphia: Saunders.

Millon, T. (1981). *Disorders of personality: DSM-III, Axis II*. New York: Wiley.

Millon, T. (1990). *Toward a new personology: An evolutionary model*. New York: Wiley.

Millon, T. (1991). Normality: What may we learn from evolutionary theory? In D. Offer & M. Sabshin (Eds.), *The diversity of normal behavior* (pp. 100–150). New York: Basic Books.

Millon, T. (2003). *Millon Index of Personality Styles Revised manual*. Minneapolis, MN: Pearson Assessments.

Millon, T. (with Millon, C., & Davis, R.). (1994a). *Millon Clinical Multiaxial Inventory–III manual*. Minneapolis, MN: National Computer Systems.

Millon, T. (with Weiss, L. G., Millon, C., & Davis, R.). (1994b). *Millon Index of Personality Styles manual*. San Antonio, TX: Psychological Corporation.

Myers, I. B. (1962). *The Myers–Briggs Type Indicator*. Palo Alto, CA: Consulting Psychologist Press.

Myers, I. B., & McCaulley, M. H. (1985). *Manual: A guide to the development and use of the Myers–Briggs Type Indicator*. Palo Alto, CA: Consulting Psychologists Press.

Super, D. E. (1983). Assessment in career guidance: Toward truly developmental counseling. *Personnel and Guidance, 61*(9), 555–562.

Tango, R. A., & Dziuban, C. D. (1984). The use of personality components in the interpretation of career indecision. *Journal of College Student Personnel, 25*(6), 509–512.

Weiss, L. G., & Lowther, J. (1995, March). *The factor structure of the Millon Index of Personality Styles*. Paper presented at the annual convention of the Society for Personality Assessment, Atlanta.

CHAPTER 27

A Brief MIPS *Revised* Case Study

Caryl Bloom

The Millon Index of Personality Styles *Revised* (MIPS *Revised*) is designed to measure the personality styles of normally functioning adults. As a theory-based inventory, the MIPS *Revised* has trait scales that are not generated empirically, but consist of conceptually generated polarities that represent its theoretical elements. These scales have a rich theoretical foundation in a model of personality that is deeply rooted in biosocial and evolutionary theory. When these representations are valid, they can generate personality characterizations and research hypotheses by pointing to phenomena beyond those employed in their original development. The MIPS *Revised* test personality style scores can serve as a foundation, a basic framework of attributes and inclinations—to assist the clinician in developing a fuller understanding of other features, interests, symptoms, or values of the person being assessed.

The following case was selected for its ability to illustrate clinically useful interpretive strategies of a woman pursuing a career change. The results provide us with information as to her motivating, thinking, and behaving styles.

J. is a 31-year-old single female with an MBA in marketing management. For 5 years, she has been engaged in the sales division of a Swiss company, selling high-end timepieces to upscale stores. A model employee owing to her upbeat nature, ambitiousness, and self-confidence, she has devoted her energies and arranged her life in pursuit of her advancement in the company. Though she has achieved success in her career, it has been at the cost of a less than fulfilling personal life. Coworkers admire her professionalism, but describe her as strong-willed and sometimes arrogant.

The present MIPS *Revised* evaluation was prompted by an opportunity to increase both her salary and status as vice president of the marketing division of a Fortune 500 company. This position will present new challenges, as well as responsibilities for a large staff to oversee, direct and supervise. J. has always been very goal-oriented, and advancing her career has been her sole focus since college days. This position would be a large step toward fulfilling her career goals.

During college she joined a sorority, but soon stopped going to meetings. She states that the lack of structure and conflicting values among members of the group did not fit her personal style. Although she remained friends with some of the members, and would occasionally party with them, social camaraderie for her was short-lived. She focused on her studies and graduated with high honors from both her undergraduate and her graduate programs.

J. is presently living alone. She has never had a long-term relationship. According to her, relationships end because men found her to be too controlling, self-centered, and "cold." She has a few women friends, none of whom are particularly close. As in college, she gets bored with her friends, since their priorities in life are very different than hers. J. says that she would like a long-term relationship—possibly even marriage and a family—but she is not willing to sacrifice her career at this point in her life.

Both J.'s parents were alcoholics, and her mother committed suicide when J. was 13. She and an older sister essentially raised themselves, owing to her father's continued excessive drinking; rarely at home after her mother died, he frequented local bars all evening after work. Both girls began to work part-time in their teens to earn and save enough money for college. This was when J. said she developed her work ethic, ambitiousness, and organizational skills.

In line with the new firm's general policy, all potential candidates for executive positions were asked to take the MIPS-R. Figure 27.1 presents J.'s MIPS *Revised* Profile and Interpretive Report.

MILLON™ INDEX OF PERSONALITY STYLES *REVISED*

Profile of Prevalence Scores   **Norm Group: Adult Female**

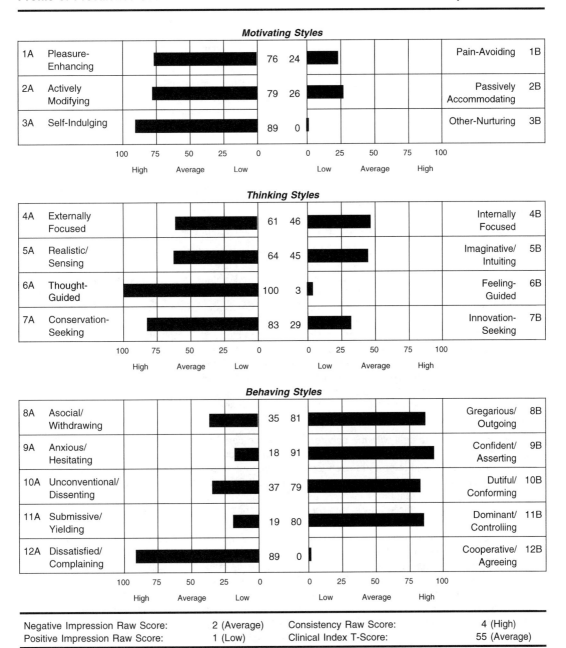

| Negative Impression Raw Score: | 2 (Average) | Consistency Raw Score: | 4 (High) |
| Positive Impression Raw Score: | 1 (Low) | Clinical Index T-Score: | 55 (Average) |

FIGURE 27.1. MIPS *Revised* Profile and Interpretive Report for J *(p. 1 of 3).*

INTERPRETIVE SUMMARY

Positively oriented motivations moderately influence the respondent's outlook. Inclined to seek rewarding experiences in whatever environment she finds herself, she aims toward achieving that which she finds satisfying and fulfilling in life. Her social and intellectual energies are stimulated by and organized around this pursuit. Generally optimistic about her chances of success, she believes that good things are likely to come her way. Typically pleased with the world she has created for herself, she looks favorably on those around her, anticipating satisfactory relationships and positive outcomes from most interactions and endeavors.

She leans moderately toward taking charge of her life, making things happen rather than waiting for them to occur, modifying her environment and relationships, and arranging events to suit her needs and desires. Actively pursuing the favorable things in life, she takes the initiative and intervenes in the affairs of others. Continually and substantially transforming her environment, she is stimulus-seeking, life-engaging, and confidently buoyant, viewing her experiences as being determined by her own actions rather than by forces beyond her control.

Very oriented toward fulfilling her own needs and priorities before those of others, she usually makes her own decisions with little formal advice from others. Neither does she tend to be overly concerned about pleasing others, preferring to do things her own way and taking the consequences of doing so. Comfortable with herself as well as with the world she has created by virtue of her energy and will, she is able to function as an optimistic and self-directed person.

Logical, organized, practical, and concerned with the tangible and the present, the respondent seeks to impose a clear structure upon her life, to operate efficiently, and to make impersonal, objective decisions and judgments. Assuming a take-charge attitude, she attempts as well to be systematic, consistent, and conscientious in her dealings with others. Firmly avoiding indecisiveness or vacillation, she is also self-assured and confident of the correctness of her opinions. Perhaps overly assertive and power-oriented at times, she is nevertheless likely to be a good organizer of others in the work environment, an administrator who can blend task orientation with effective leadership. This effectiveness is apparent in her knowing when and how to be affable and accommodating, and when and how to supervise and direct. Strongly inclined to reason things through, she seeks to ensure that her own behaviors and those of others conform with carefully considered rules and principles. Enjoying the authoritative role of leader or executive, she often acts in a crisp and decisive manner, especially when faced with situations that are characterized by ambiguity or uncertainty.

She strongly prefers to deal with the concrete, that which can be appraised through the senses, and readily attends to the observable and factual. She also prefers activities and tasks that have visible, quick results and to perform such tasks herself, thus ensuring that they are done effectively and with dispatch. Her self-confidence often wins respect from others. In achieving goals, she will organize the steps and resources involved as well as apply the logic and analysis required for success. Owing to her efficient style, she prefers to undertake jobs that are well structured and to work with people who are as energetic and strongly task-oriented as she is. Setting priorities is important to her style in both work and social relationships. For the most part, the achievement of a goal is more important than the needs and habits of those involved. Inefficiency or laziness can cause her to be demanding and perhaps even overbearing. On the other hand, she can usually prevent such problems by preparing the groundwork well in advance and by using well-developed social skills. Nevertheless, she might fail to listen to views contrary to her own and exhibit a lapse in sensitivity to the feelings and wishes of those with whom she lives and works. These possible tendencies could cause difficulties that she could have averted by more carefully attending to those around her. Though she is normally easy to get along with when difficult decisions are to be made, she prefers to be surrounded by compliant people. She is likely to adhere strongly to the values

FIGURE 27.1. *(p. 2 of 3)*

and procedures she has become accustomed to, resisting innovations and alternatives that could eventually prove more effective or lead to greater social harmony.

For the most part, the respondent exhibits an air of general imperturbability, appearing most often as self-absorbed, coolly unimpressionable, yet buoyantly optimistic. Possessing a sense of high self-worth, she acts in a confident and assured manner. Transcending the constraints of ordinary thinking, she possesses sufficient social talent and presumption to take bold and risky actions to advance her aspirations. Adept in dealing with others, she can be quite persuasive in attracting them to causes she espouses. Also present is an empowering ambition that drives her not only to be successful, but also to be among the best in her field of endeavor. Her belief that she is special is matched by her expectation that others will view her in a similar fashion and will consequently treat her well. Competitive and astute in her dealings with others, able to clearly visualize her future goals, and able to take full advantage of her strengths and talents, she can effectively marshal these capabilities to achieve what she has set out to accomplish. Believing in herself, she is prepared to work hard for long periods to obtain what she believes she deserves. Potentially problematic in all this, however, is the feeling of being entitled, an assumption that she deserves special favors without the need to reciprocate. Also troublesome may be a proclivity toward taking family and colleagues for granted, at times putting her personal or professional interests ahead of their best interests. Willing at times to disregard conventional standards of social conduct and devising plausible reasons to justify behaviors that might be socially overpowering and lacking in sensitivity, she can sometimes deceive herself as much as those around her. Nonetheless, her boldness and ambition often do make good things happen, benefiting not only herself but also the lives of others.

RAW SCORES

100 Percent of items answered

Pleasure-Enhancing (1 A)	31	Conservation-Seeking (7 A)	51
Pain-Avoiding (I B)	9	Innovation-Seeking (7B)	22
Actively Modifying (2A)	39	Asocial/Withdrawing (SA)	14
Passively Accommodating (2B)	12	Gregarious/Outgoing (8B)	45
Self-Indulging (3A)	27	Anxious/Hesitating (9A)	4
Other-Nurturing (3B)	17	Confident/Asserting (9B)	50
Externally Focused (4A)	31	Unconventional/Dissenting (IOA)	17
Internally Focused (4B)	11	Dutiful/Conforming (1 OB)	52
Realistic/Sensing (5A)	21	Submissive/Yielding (11 A)	11
Imaginative/Intuiting (5 B)	21	Dominant/Controlling (11 B)	28
Thought-Guided (6A)	38	Dissatisfied/Complaining (12A)	34
Feeling-Guided (6B)	15	Cooperative/Agreeing (12B)	16

Clinical Index Raw Score   39.3

FIGURE 27.1. *(p. 3 of 3)*

PART V

EPILOGUE

CHAPTER 28

Future of the Millon Inventories and Their Scientific Base

Theodore Millon
Caryl Bloom

As noted at the beginning of this volume, the Millon inventories were intended to be evolving assessment tools, to be refined periodically to reflect substantive progress. This second edition of the book marks the implementation of one of the "future objectives" discussed in the first edition—namely, the new Facet Scales for the Axis II scales. In this chapter, we review two additional areas in which developments are currently proceeding.

Proposals for Further Developments of the Millon Inventories

All of the Millon inventories have been refined and strengthened on a regular basis by both theoretical logic and research data. These efforts will continue. The Millon Clinical Multiaxial Inventory–III (MCMI-III) has been coordinated with the most recent official diagnostic schema, the *Diagnostic and Statistical Manual of Mental Disorders*, fourth edition, text revision (DSM-IV-TR; American Psychiatric Association, 2000), in an even more explicit way than before. Although the publication of the first version of the MCMI (Millon, 1977) preceded the publication of the DSM-III (American Psychiatric Association, 1980), Millon played a major role in formulating the official manual's personality disorders, contributing thereby to their conceptual correspondence. The DSM-III-R (American Psychiatric Association, 1987) was subsequently published in the same year as the MCMI-II; the inventory was modified in its final stages to make it as consonant as possible with the conceptual changes introduced in the then-forthcoming classification. The MCMI-III (Millon, 1994a) strengthened these correspondences further by drawing on many of the criteria of the DSM-IV (American Psychiatric Association, 1994) as the basis for drafting its items. This chapter reports on a select set of theoretical and empirical developments that are being carefully weighed for inclusion in future Millon inventories, or as guides in the refinement process for future inventories in the Millon family of instruments. Although we refer mainly to the MCMI, the developments are broad enough to apply to all the Millon instruments.

There has been a steady growth of interest in personality and its disorders since the late 1970s. The founding of the *Journal of Personality Disorders*; the creation of the International Society for the Study of Personality Disorders; and a surge of clinical, theoretical, and research literature all reflect this renaissance in personality theory and assessment (Millon, 1984, 1990; Millon & Davis, 1996). Much of this knowledge has been incorporated into the DSM and contributes to an increasingly solid base for refined diagnostic decisions. In addition, Millon's work has led him to articulate an expanding base of diagnostic criteria and personality concepts (e.g., Millon, 1990, 1994b; Millon & Davis, 1996), much more extensive than those of earlier DSMs. This growing body of clinical literature has provided much of the knowledge base for the MCMI-III. To the extent that DSM-IV(-TR) also reflects these advances, its correspondence with the MCMI-III has been further strengthened. Numerous cross-validation and cross-generalization studies have been and continue to be executed with the goal of evaluating and improving all of the elements embodied in the MCMI-III and other Millon instruments—their items, scales, scoring procedures, algorithms, and interpretive text (see Choca, 2004; Craig, 1993, 2005; Marvish, 1994, 2002). These ongoing investigations will continue to provide an empirical grounding for further work on each of these instruments.

Assessment of Personality Subtypes

Personality disorders are best thought of as prototypes. Within each prototype, however, lie numerous variations. There is no one single schizoid or avoidant or depressive or histrionic type; instead, there are several variations—different forms in which each core or prototypal personality expresses itself. With the publication of *Disorders of Personality: DSM-IV and Beyond*, Millon and Davis (1996) elaborated a series of personality subtypes for each of the major prototypes deduced from Millon's (1990) evolutionary theory. These subtypes essentially represent readings of the modern and historical literature in convergence with clinical wisdom, cultural myth, and empirical fact. Often they are simply mixtures of major types. The deficient conscience, fraudulent dealings, and arrogant attitude of the "unprincipled" narcissistic individual, for example, is reminiscent of the con artist or charlatan, a cultural stereotype incarnating a kind of antisocial narcissism. Likewise, the "nomadic" antisocial individual, represented as a gypsylike roamer or vagrant existing as a scavenger at the margins of society, essentially reflects a mixture of the schizoid and antisocial types.

In other cases, the subtypes exist at the confluence of Millon's evolutionary theory and other organizing principles. Psychodynamic thinkers, for example, have described the "compensating" narcissistic individual, who counteracts deep feelings of inferiority and lack of self-esteem by creating the illusion of being superior and exceptional. Similarly, the "hypersensitive" avoidant person represents a more manifestly cognitive variant of a major type, being intensely wary and suspicious—alternately panicky, terrified, edgy, and timorous, and then thin-skinned, high-strung, petulant, and prickly.

Beside the obvious relationship of each subtype to its cousins, all the subtypes share an important feature: Each is a statement of particular truth about the nature of the personological landscape—a claim that the world contains such-and-such a personality in it, more by historical accident than by ontological necessity. Each is a specific manifestation of a major type in the context of our particular times and culture, and if history or culture were different, then the subtypes would probably be different also. The major prototypes, on the other hand, are in a sense required by the theory, just as existence, adaptation, and replication are required by the laws of evolution. Although the subtypes lack the deductive inevitability of major prototypes, they nevertheless bring the major types down to a level of unparalleled descriptive specificity and, it is hoped, proportionately increased clinical utility.

However, it is precisely because the subtypes are not inevitable products of the evolutionary theory that they bear a greater burden of validational evidence than do the major types, and they also present a greater challenge for reliable and valid assessment. In particular, the issue of base rates (BRs), the prevalence of the various subtypes, is of particular importance. Because the BRs for some of the major types (e.g., the schizoid and sadistic types) are quite low, many of the subtypes are likely to be quite rare. A particular clinician, in fact, might go years between seeing individuals with a particular subtype, making such validational research almost impossible in any one clinical setting. Moreover, some subtypes may be seen quite frequently, while others will hardly ever be observed. All of the problems associated with the prediction of low-BR phenomena, such as suicide or murder, are also problems here.

Nevertheless, several directions could be pursued in order to advance the assessment utility of the Millon inventories in relation to the subtypes. Millon and Davis (1996), for example, presented MCMI-III code types for each personality disorder subtype. Thus, on theoretical grounds, it is expected that an "unprincipled" narcissistic individual will appear as a 5–6A, while a "compensating" narcissistic person is more likely to appear as a 5–8A or a 5–2A. Such a code type approach would seem to be the most straightforward, especially where these subtypes exist predominately as a mixture of two or more major types. In the coming years, as clinicians already skilled in Millon's theory become well enough acquainted with these subtypes to provide useful external validity ratings, studies that examine the diagnostic efficiency of these MCMI-III profile patterns will become possible. Not all persons with 5–8A code types, for example, may be deemed to exhibit "compensating" narcissism. Conversely, some individuals who do seem to demonstrate "compensating" narcissism may produce profiles other than the 5–8A. Eventually, the items most directly responsible for each subtype profile will be identified and examined against the content of the subtypes, and a feedback process will begin through which the item content of the inventories and the content of the subtypes themselves are mutually refined. Items for future Millon inventories will be written with accurate classification of these subtypes in mind.

How an emphasis on personality subtypes will affect the length of future instruments, and how it will influence their exact item compositions, are of course open questions at this time. The answers in part are dependent upon the nature of the empirical problems encountered. Certainly, it would seem difficult to provide an accurate assessment of over 60 subtypes with tests of less than 200 items. Even if all of the MCMI-III items were oriented toward Axis II, for example, that would still leave fewer than three unique items per subtype—far too few to protect discriminant validity. Fortunately, the BRs of some the major personality patterns (i.e., the antisocial and borderline types) make their subtypes more important than those of the schizoid pattern, for example. Where compromises in inventory length must be made, then, they will favor the assessment of those subtypes that are most clinically relevant, at least for pencil-and-paper forms. Future computer-administered versions of the Millon tests, programmed to optimize the selection of items based on a patient's pattern of prior responses, need not administer an entire item bank and are thus much more likely to yield highly specific, subtype-relevant information.

Trait Subscales

There are four levels of clinical interpretation within an inventory—item level, trait level, scale level, and profile configuration. Trait subscales are clinically useful. Recall that each personality syndrome is viewed in the prototypal model as a covariant attribute structure whose features, taken one by one, are neither necessary nor sufficient for the diagnosis of the syndrome. Although theoretically the most prototypal member of a syndrome possesses all its features, most individuals will not. As astute clinicians know, no two narcissistic personalities are exactly alike, no two antisocial personalities are exactly alike, and so on. In the DSM-IV(-TR), nine criteria are listed for borderline personality disorder, of which five are required for diagnosis. Conceivably, then, two individuals might both be diagnosed with the disorder while having only one feature or criterion in common, allowing for considerable trait or criterion heterogeneity within any personality type. The specific personality traits that an individual possesses are of interest when we want to know what kind of schizoid personality an individual exhibits, what kind of dependent, and so on—a fact that is obviously relevant to the identification of adult subtypes described above. However, an individual may also receive specific disorder subscale elevations in the absence of a diagnosis. These correspond to problematic trait characteristics that deserve attention but are not so pervasively expressed as to constitute full-fledged personality disorders (Millon, 1994b). The DSM-IV(-TR) allows problematic traits to be noted on Axis II, but apparently this possibility is rarely used in clinical practice, perhaps because the DSM is criterion- rather than trait-oriented.

The existence of personality traits as a legitimate level of organization in human personality, and their utility in clinical interpretation, argue that they should be represented in any inventory of personality disorders. Because of its relative brevity, traits have not yet been explicitly represented in the MCMI. Instead, the structure of the inventory at levels before that of syndrome or disorder has drawn upon an item-weighting system informed by the strength of each item's validational data, the intrinsic interrelatedness of the personality disorders, and the prototypal structure of mental disorders generally. An item-weighting system ranging from 1 to 3 points was introduced in the MCMI-II. In the MCMI-III, prototypal items are given a weight of 2 points; all others are weighted at 1 point only. Because the prototypal items demonstrate substantive, structural, and external validation (Loevinger, 1957) on their "home" scale, they are given a heavier weight than are subsidiary items selected on the basis of external validation alone. Prototypal items represent features of their respective disorders and are doubly weighted. Nonprototypal items represent features that, while not central, are nevertheless relevant to their respective disorders. Thus an item such as "I like to be the center of attention when I'm in a group," might be weighted 2 points on the Histrionic scale and 1 point on the Narcissistic scale.

Such multiple assignments have caused some to express concern regarding the discriminant validity of the MCMI scales. For example, exploratory studies with the Millon Adolescent Clinical Inventory (MACI), designed according to the 3–2–1 weighting system, show that factoring the items assigned to each personality scale separately results in brief subscales that often share over half their items. Similar results would have been likely to emerge for the MCMI-II. In contrast, the MCMI-III personality scales were designed to be shorter, using a 2–1 weighting system. Factor studies currently underway reveal, not unexpectedly, that the item overlap of the resulting MCMI-III factor traits is substantially more favorable to clinical use. The results of these inductive or "bottom-up" studies must, of course, be examined in conjunction with theoretical or "top-down" considerations to appraise their value. Trait subscales need not be designed for every Axis II disorder, but might instead be constructed only for those disorders of greater clinical relevance frequently seen in clinical settings—certainly the antisocial, borderline, and paranoid, and perhaps the narcissistic and dependent, but not, for example, the schizoid or sadistic disorders.

Refinement across Diverse Data Sources

One of the fundamental principles in instrument construction is that validity should be built into an instrument from the beginning. Loevinger (1957), Jackson (1970), and Skinner (1986) have discussed test construction as an iterative three-stage process. In the first, rational stage, the content of each construct to be measured is defined as precisely as possible. Items may be written and refined by multiple so-called experts in the theory of the construct, sorted according to their discriminative characteristics, ranked in terms of difficulty level, and so on, all before being put to actual subjects. In the second, internal stage, the items are given to real individuals. Various statistics are then calculated to ensure that the items tap a single dimension. Items with strong relationships to scales for which they were not intended may be deleted or reassigned. In addition, a correlation matrix of the instrument's scales may be examined for anomalies, and items may be reassigned or dropped to bring this pattern in line with theoretical expectations. In the third, external stage, the newly developed scales are assessed against other instruments of established reputation. Items that pass through all three stages are said to have been validated theoretically, statistically, and empirically. The Millon inventories have been constructed according to this tripartite logic.

Although inventories should be constructed to mirror our expectations regarding relationships between constructs both internal and external to the instrument as precisely as possible, they should also possess a generative value. That is, an inventory should assist in the accumulation of new knowledge. If our test is intended to assess personality disorders, we might expect, for example, that individuals classified with dependent personalities will also be classified as experiencing depressive episodes more often than, say, antisocial individuals, simply because dependent persons are likely to feel helpless and hopeless more often than are antisocial persons, who take the initiative in changing their external world (albeit usually in a destructive fashion). These internal–internal and internal–external expectations form a set of constraints that our inventory must be constructed to satisfy. Each such constraint is an additional point through which the instrument's predictions are triangulated with reality as it is assumed to exist. The larger this set of constraints, the better, for if the inventory can satisfy many such constraints at the beginning, then we can have greater confidence that it will meet future challenges.

Sometimes, for example, after an instrument has been constructed, certain variables about which we had no preformed ideas show a significant relationship. Perhaps in the beginning we believed that those with antisocial personalities should also report high family distress and a high incidence of alcoholism. Perhaps we also believed that those with dependent personalities should report overprotective parents and an inability to end relationships, and these expectations were built into the instrument. About the relationship between dependent personality and the incidence of alcoholism, however, we may have no expectations at all—so that the magnitude of this second relationship is "free to vary," simply because we do not know much about it, how it should be evaluated, or whether it should even exist at all. How do we evaluate this observed, but unexpected, relationship? Having constructed our instrument to satisfy multiple constraints in the form of theoretically driven expectations, we are no longer working with just any item pool. The more our test satisfies many different constraints, the greater our expectations of the generalizability of the entire system of instrumentation. Demonstrated validity in diverse areas of the nomological network becomes a promissory note that observed relationships between intervening variables elsewhere is not peculiar to their particular mode of operationalization, but is instead representative of nature's structure and thus worthy of genuine scientific interest. In general, the more constraints an instrument satisfies at the outset, the more confidence we can have in the validity of relationships that are unanticipated.

At the current time, most psychological instruments are developed within a single data source—be it self-report, clinical ratings, observer ratings, or projective testing observations—and then validated against instruments of already established utility within that same data source. Validation against instruments from other data sources, while important, is usually secondary. Thus a new self-report scale to measure dependence finds evidence for its validity first against other self-report dependence scales, and then against observer ratings and projectives, and so on. Lower correlations between self-report forms and observer-rated forms are attributed to method considerations, and often rightfully so. Unfortunately, this rather haphazard style of instrument development often leads to confusing results when such instruments are paired against each other in a multitrait–multimethod matrix. The Narcissistic scale of a self-report instrument may correlate more highly with the Histrionic rating scale, and so on. Many such mismatches are likely to be found for any given set of personality instruments—a fact that has undermined confidence in the valid assessment of personality disorders.

A much better method blurs the distinction between internal and external by viewing test construction as a system of relations or constraints to be satisfied across multiple data sources. Here, the goal is to build an entire suite of instruments that inform each other across the entire construction process. The more data sources that can be involved, the better. For example, a self-report inventory for the personality disorders, an observer-rated version of the same inventory, and a clinical checklist would be constructed simultaneously, not one at a time. Correlation matrices between all instruments would be inspected at every stage. Thus, if during development it was found that the observer-rated Narcissistic scale correlated more highly with the self-report Histrionic scale than with its parallel self-report Narcissistic scale, indicating a lack of convergent validity, the items from both pools would be examined—not only with regard to their content characteristics and correlation to their assigned scale, but also in terms of their cross-method correlations. Violations of multitrait–multimethod considerations would be tracked to particular items, and these would be reassigned, dropped, or rewritten. Thus, rather than being examined post hoc, multitrait–multimethod considerations become a fundamental part of the item selection process from the beginning, allowing each instrument to strengthen the others. Validity is built into an entire system of instrumentation, and not simply into a single instrument. Future versions of some Millon inventories may be constructed in this fashion.

What are the requirements for the construction of such a test suite? The first is essentially practical, reflecting a much larger investment on the part of participants and the need for more iterations in the development process. Both patients and their clinicians must be subjected to the agonies of providing data for a large item pool. The second is theoretical, and is the more difficult of the two, requiring expert clinical judgment concerning the constructs the test seeks to embrace. The test developers begin this construction process knowing that correlations between similar scales across diverse data sources will be less than unity, and that this reflects measurement error as much as it does the informational biases of the respective sources. Persons can be expected to differ in terms of their levels of self-knowledge and the extent to which they distort objective information. The egocentricity of the narcissistic individual, and his or her tendency to construe reality in self-favoring ways, make him or her less likely than the pessimistic and self-focused depressive person to provide valid self-report information. We might conjecture, then, that the correlation between self-reported and clinician-rated narcissistic personality is likely to be less than that between self-reported and clinician-rated depressive personality. This is the problem the theorist faces. Knowing that the multitrait–multimethod matrix reflects informational biases as well as measurement error, the theorist must provide a substantive framework within which to evaluate the direction and magnitude of its correlations, and to determine the path in which the results are best refined. In turn, this involves knowing (1) those traits or characteristics for which individuals with each personality pattern can typically be expected to provide valid self-report information; (2) those traits or characteristics for which individuals with each personality pattern cannot be expected to provide such information; (3) those traits or characteristics for which clinicians can typically be expected to provide valid ratings; and (4) those traits or characteristics that, for whatever reason, clinicians will not easily be able to rate reliably.

Unfortunately, the DSM's Axis II, deliberately formulated to be atheoretical and thus to exist at a descriptive rather than an explanatory level, cannot provide the substantive framework necessary to guide such research. Rather than providing a coherent deductive foundation within which to ask questions about the various personalities, Axis II is best viewed as a body of descriptive material collated across several perspectives but not really coordinated with any of them. Whereas the periodic table of the elements is the unique province of chemistry, the problematic behaviors that are to be "carved up" into diagnostic categories are often given to psychopathologists by parties whose standards are extrinsic to psychopathology as a science. Perhaps we live in a more enlightened age—but it was not so long ago that Sullivan, a founder of the interpersonal school, proposed the "homosexual personality," that the "masochistic personality" came under fire as reflecting biases against women. Philosophers of science agree that the system of kinds undergirding any domain of inquiry must itself be answerable to the question that forms the very point of departure for the scientific enterprise: Why does nature take this particular form rather than some other? Why these particular diagnostic groups rather than others? One cannot merely accept any list of kinds or dimensions as given. Committee consensus is not science. Instead, a taxonomic scheme must be justified, and to be justified scientifically, it must be justified theoretically. Taxonomy and theory are intimately linked.

Item writers involved in attempts to construct a coordinated suite of multi-method instruments—such as future versions of the MCMI, the Millon Index of Personality Styles *Revised* (MIPS *Revised*; Millon, 2003), and the Millon–Grossman Personality Domain Checklist (MG-PDC; see Grossman, Tringone, & Millon, Chapter 24, this volume)—require a strong theoretical basis on which the various personality patterns can be compared and contrasted for their manifestations across different data sources. Relevant example questions are "What traits does the narcissistic individual possess about which he or she is likely to have self-knowledge and will admit to?" and "What traits does the narcissistic person possess about which he or she is unlikely to have self-knowledge?" For us, this basis is Millon's evolutionary theory (Millon, 1990). Although a detailed exposition is beyond the scope of this chapter, the theory essentially seeks to explicate the structure and styles of personality with reference to deficient, imbalanced, or conflicted modes of ecological adaptation and reproductive strategy. As noted in earlier chapters, the four phases in which evolutionary principles are demonstrated are labeled "existence," "adaptation," "replication," and "abstraction." The first relates the serendipitous transformation of random or less organized states into those possessing distinct structures of greater organization; the second refers to homeostatic processes employed to sustain survival in open ecosystems; the third pertains to reproductive styles that maximize the diversification and selection of ecologically effective attributes; and the fourth concerns the emergence of competencies that foster anticipatory planning and reasoned decision making. Polarities derived from the first three phases—pleasure–pain, passive–active, and other–self, respectively—are used to form "traits" (as in the MIPS *Revised*), as well as to construct a theoretically embedded classification system of personality disorders (as in the MCMI-III). Personalities we have termed "deficient" lack the capacity to experience or to enact certain aspects of the three polarities (e.g., the schizoid individual has a faulty substrate for both pleasure and pain); those spoken of as "imbalanced" lean strongly toward one or another extreme of a polarity (e.g., the dependent individual is oriented almost exclusively to receiving the support and nurturance of others); and those we judge "conflicted" struggle with ambivalence toward opposing ends of a bipolarity (e.g., the passive–aggressive individual vacillates between adhering to the expectations of others and enacting what is wished for the self). These polarities lend the model a holistic, cohesive structure that facilitates the comparison and contrast of groups along fundamental axes—sharpening the meanings of the derived constructs, preventing their definitions from being coopted by one perspective or school to the exclusion of others, and "fixing" them against construct drift.

In addition to providing a polarity model from which to derive the entire constellation of personality disorders, Millon and his associates have also stressed that personality is an intrinsically multioperational construct. That is, personality disorders are not simply about behavior, or about cognition, or about unconscious conflicts; rather, as disorders of the entire matrix of the person, they embrace all of these data domains. Millon and associates have set forth comprehensive (exhaustive of the major domains of personality) and comparable (existing at approximately equal levels of abstraction) attributes for eight functional and structural domains of the personality (Grossman et al., Chapter 24, this volume). Each cell of the resulting 8×15, domain-by-personality-pattern circumplex contains the diagnostic attribute that, in our judgment, best captures the expression of each personality style within that particular domain.

In contrast, the criteria of the DSM-IV(-TR) are both noncomprehensive (no real scheme for the meaningful distribution of personality attributes has been developed) and noncomparable (the criteria run the gamut from very broad to very narrow). Noncomprehensive criteria lead to redundancies and omissions; noncomparable criteria lead to a mixture of levels. Consider, for example, the DSM-IV-TR criteria for dependent personality disorder (American Psychiatric Association, 2000, p. 725). Criterion 1 states, "Has difficulty making everyday decisions without an excessive amount of advice and reassurance from others." Criterion 2, however, says almost the same: "Needs others to assume responsibility for most major areas of his or her life." In fact, five of the eight dependent personality criteria seem oriented toward the interpersonal conduct domain; two seem oriented toward the self-image domain; and only one is concerned with cognitive style. The domains of regulatory mechanisms, object representations, morphological organization, mood/temperament, and expressive behaviors are completely unaddressed. Or consider the DSM-IV-TR criteria for obsessive–compulsive personality disorder (American Psychiatric Association, 2000, p. 729). Criterion 5 is relatively narrow and behavioral: "Is unable to discard worn-out or worthless objects even when they have no sentimental value." In contrast, criterion 8 requires more inference: "Shows rigidity and stubbornness." In fact, the inability to discard worthless objects could well be considered simply a behavioral manifestation of the trait of rigidity. Failure to multioperationalize the personality disorders via comprehensive and comparable attributes almost certainly contributes to diagnostic inefficiency and invalidity, and provides an important critique of the content validity of the DSM-IV(-TR) criteria sets. Even more problematic, because the DSM-IV(-TR) is usually taken as the "gold standard" by which other measures of personality disorder are judged, and because most modern measures seek to conform to the DSM in some way, the degree to which these criteria sets distort the practice of modern clinical science is an open question: There is no gold standard for the gold standard. Because most test authors consider it necessary to construct their instruments in accordance with the diagnoses and criteria of the DSM-IV(-TR), we can conclude that almost every extant instrument emphasizing the DSM is to an unknown extent contaminated by this problem—a consideration that argues strongly for the role of theory as a guide in selecting attributes, criteria, or items with which to operationalize personality disorders.

Obviously, its atheoretical shortcomings, together with its noncomprehensive and noncomparable format, make the DSM difficult to regard even now as a gold standard for the MCMI-III (which actually features many items as rephrases of the official criteria) or MG-PDC. Because of their theoretical anchoring, the MCMI-III and MG-PDC are perhaps best regarded as measures of the DSM-IV(-TR) constructs, but more—the "more" being the surplus meaning provided by the theory. However, as the theory continues to evolve along the lines necessary to construct a coordinated suite of instruments (of which the MCMI will be only one essential component), the relationship between future MCMIs and future DSMs will require close consideration and perhaps even a reevaluation. That an atheoretical, but official, classification should serve as the standard against which a theoretically grounded system is judged can only be described as a paradox—one faced not only by integrative theorists, but by interpersonal and psychodynamic thinkers as well.

Proposals for a Clinical Science of Personology

Let us now summarize a number of themes derived from our professional careers. They compose a framework or scaffold devised some years ago by Millon (1999a), in an attempt to build a structure for a clinical science of personality.

An effort should be made to coordinate the separate realms that constitute our field—namely, its relation to the universal laws of nature, its subject domain theories, its derivable classification schemas, its diagnostic assessment tools, and its therapeutic techniques. As noted in earlier chapters, a truly mature clinical science—one that is designed to create a synergistic bond among its elements—will explicitly embody the following five elements, rather than leaving them to develop independently and to stand as autonomous and largely unconnected functions:

1. *Universal scientific principles* grounded in ubiquitous laws of nature. Despite varied forms of expression (e.g., in physics, chemistry, and psychology), these principles should provide an undergirding framework for guiding and constructing subject-oriented theories.

2. *Subject-oriented theories*, or explanatory and heuristic conceptual schemas of nature's expression in what we call "personality" and "psychopathology." These theories should be consistent with established knowledge in both its own and related sciences (e.g., biology, sociology), and from which reasonably accurate propositions concerning clinical conditions can be both deduced and understood, enabling thereby the development of a formal classification system.

3. *Classification of personality styles and disorders*, or a taxonomic nosology derived logically from the personological theory. This classification should provide a cohesive organization within which its major categories can readily be grouped and differentiated, permitting thereby the development of relevant and coordinated assessment instruments.

4. *Clinical and personality assessment instruments*, or tools that are empirically grounded and quantitatively sensitive. These should enable the theory's propositions and hypotheses to be adequately investigated and evaluated, and the categories constituting its nosology to be readily identified (diagnosed) and measured (dimensionalized), thus specifying target areas for interventions.

5. *Integrated therapeutic interventions*, or planful strategies and modalities of treatment; these should be designed in accord with the theory and oriented to modify problematic clinical characteristics, consonant with professional standards and social responsibilities.

The coordination of these elements (i.e., making them reciprocally enhancing and mutually reinforcing) constitutes the essence of a clinical science. Working together, these clinical components will produce integrated knowledge that is greater than the sum of its individual constituent parts. What is aspired to is the synthesis of clinical elements that have been disconnected and pursued independently in the 20th century. Just as each person is an intrinsic unity, each component of a clinical science of personology should not remain a separate element of a potpourri of unconnected parts. Rather, each facet of our clinical work should be integrated into a gestalt, a coupled and synergistic unity in which the whole will become more informative and useful than its individual parts.

As was the case with its DSM-III and III-R forerunners, not only was the DSM-IV(-TR) classification derived intentionally in an atheoretical manner, but no coherent theoretical system was seriously explored to provide a consistent framework for coordinating the various syndromes. Such a conceptual schema would be helpful, even if the established nosology were reliably anchored to empirical research, which it is not. If all of the principal clinical syndromes or personality disorders could be logically derived from a systematic theoretical foundation, this would greatly facilitate an understanding of psychopathology, organize this knowledge in an orderly and consistent fashion, and connect the data it provides to other realms of psychological theory and research, where they could then be subjected to empirical verification or falsification. Especially promising in this regard are a number of dimensional schemas, such as those proposed by Cloninger, Benjamin, Millon, Costa, and Tellegen. From such sources, psychopathology might advance much in the way that physics has. In describing the features that have given physics much of its success as a scientific discipline, Meehl (1978) has noted that "The physicist's scientific power comes from . . . the immense deductive fertility of the formalism" (p. 825).

A proposal that will be congenial to our psychological confreres—though perhaps less so to our more medically oriented colleagues—is specifically that personality "disorders" *not* be conceived of as discrete disease entities, as are many medical syndromes (e.g., measles, smallpox). We should be adamant about the need to explicitly recognize the intrinsic heterogeneity of each of the DSM-IV(-TR) Axis II personality disorders; this argues for the wisdom of formalizing a paradigm shift from a "disease-entity-based" to a "prototypal" diagnostic model. We must move in the direction of what Cronbach and Meehl (1955) termed "bandwidth fidelity" decades ago. Here a balance was struck between conceptual breadth and identification precision. Cantor, Smith, French, and Mezzich (1980) addressed the prototypal model over two decades ago, as follows:

The recent revisions in the standard diagnostic manual have brought the system even closer to the prototype view than before. Diagnostic criteria are now presented as prototypes—larger sets of correlated features rather than selected defining ones; guidelines for diagnosis also emphasize the potential heterogeneity of the symptoms of like-diagnosed patients. Moreover, a potential for overlap in clinical features across different diagnostic categories is underscored. . . . They help to emphasize, rather than obscure, the probabilistic nature of diagnostic categorization. The recent changes . . . represent a shift in beliefs similar to ones occurring in other domains, away from the classical view of categorization systems and towards the prototype view. (pp. 191–192)

Westen and his colleagues (Westen & Arkowitz-Westen, 1998; Westen & Shedler, 1999, 2000) have articulated a compelling argument favoring a prototypal model for DSM's personality categories. Their solutions may, in our judgment, strengthen the observation that most personality disorders show a "natural" measure of commonality—that is, repetitive patterns of psychic cohesion, rather than an "anarchy" of unique or random trait dynamics. Prototypal patterns derived from their Shedler–Westen Assessment Procedure–200 (SWAP-200) technique are highly similar to those obtained with the MPDC and MG-PDC (see Tringone, 1997; Grossman et al., Chapter 24, this volume).

A further proposal is that we replace the Axis I–Axis II distinction with a three-part continuum demarcated by three prototypal groupings: "personality patterns," "complex syndromes," and "simple reactions." Among the most important steps taken in forming the DSM-III multiaxial system was the partition of the personality disorders from the main body of clinical syndromes and their placement in a separate axis. Clinicians in the past were often faced with the task of deciding whether a patient was best diagnosed as possessing a personality or a symptom syndrome; that choice was no longer necessary. Henceforth, clinicians could record not only the current clinical picture, but also those characteristics that made the patient vulnerable and typified his or her behaviors over extended periods, both prior to and concurrent with the presenting Axis I complaint. The differentiated multiaxial format enabled practitioners to place the clinical syndromes of Axis I within the context of the individual's susceptibilities and pervasive style of functioning.

As noted in an earlier chapter (see Millon, Boice, & Sinsabaugh, Chapter 2), this two-part distinction is, in our judgment, no longer as significant as Millon thought when he proposed it at the DSM-III Task Force meetings in 1975. Given space limitations, we cannot elaborate as fully as we would like the alternative we are now suggesting (see Millon, 1999a). Essentially, this proposal is designed to construct a three-point continuum of pathological complexity: simple reactions, or clinical symptoms that are relatively free of "contaminating" personality traits; complex syndromes, or distinct symptom constellations that are enmeshed within a complex network of problematic personality traits and vulnerabilities; and personality patterns, or configurations of relatively cohesive personality traits and dispositions. Personality patterns should be further differentiated into personality "styles," which signify relatively distinctive arrangements of traits that facilitate normal or healthy adaptive functioning, and personality "pathologies" (not "disorders"), which signify relatively distinctive configurations of traits that foster periodic adaptive failures in normal psychosocial life.

Let us elaborate briefly. Simple reactions, complex syndromes, and personality patterns (styles/pathologies) may demarcate points on a continuum. At one end would be simple reactions, which are conceived of as fairly simple and singular clinical symptoms, essentially unconnected to personality characteristics of which the person as a whole is composed. At the other end of the continuum would be personality styles and pathologies (the latter of varying levels of severity); these are composed of sets of long-standing and interrelated cognitive attitudes, interpersonal styles, biological temperaments, and intrapsychic processes. Complex syndromes would lie between the other two points on the complexity continuum—manifestly akin to simple reactions in their symptom picture, but interwoven with and mediated by problematic personality traits and vulnerabilities. This formulation was first presented in Millon's (1969) now "ancient" *Modern Psychopathology* text as "behavior reactions," "symptom disorders," and "pathological personalities."

Clinical signs in personality pathologies reflect the operation of deeply embedded characteristics of problematic functioning—that is, constellations of maladaptive traits that manifest themselves automatically and color many facets of individuals' everyday lives. By contrast, simple reactions are relatively discrete clinical responses that derive from specific neurochemical dysfunctions or are prompted by distinct, yet rather ordinary stimulus experiences (e.g., an innocuous garden snake). As noted, such simple reactions operate independently of a patient's personality makeup; their form and content are determined largely by the character of a biological vulnerability (e.g., neurochemical susceptibility to depression) or the specifics of an external precipitant (e.g., a modestly judgmental older adult); and they are not contaminated by the intrusion of unusual or intervening psychic forces. Simple reactions are best understood, then, *not* as consequences of the intricate interactions among intrapsychic mechanisms, interpersonal dynamics, cognitive misperceptions, and the like, but as simple and straightforward responses to an endogenous liability or to adverse and circumscribed stimulus conditions.

The overt clinical features of simple reactions and complex syndromes are often indistinguishable; moreover, both may be prompted *in part* by specific internal vulnerabilities or external precipitants. Complex syndromes, however, are also connected to sets of problematic personality traits, whereas simple reactions are not. A complex syndrome arises when a patient's personality vulnerability has been triggered—that is, when the personality's equilibrium has been upset or "disordered." At that point, a complex of psychically troublesome coping efforts comes into play as the patient seeks to reestablish a modicum of stability. Unfortunately, as is often seen in medical diseases, the reparative effort may itself become problematic, creating additional stressors and malfunctions. In such cases, therapy must alter not only the symptomatic reaction to the precipitating source of the difficulty, but also the upsurge of the many "secondary" complications that stem from the patient's complex of mediating processes.

Given our definitional distinctions, a complex syndrome arises in response to what may objectively be seen as an ordinarily insignificant or innocuous event; despite the usually trivial character of the precipitant, however, the patient will manifest a mix of complicating responses that are not typical of how "normal" persons respond in these circumstances. Thus a complex syndrome may not "make sense" in terms of actual realities. It signifies an unusual vulnerability and an overreaction on the part of the patient—that is, a tendency for objectively neutral stimuli to touch off and activate cognitive misperceptions, unconscious memories, and pathological interpersonal responses. Complex syndromes signify the stirring of traits that constitute troublesome facets of patients' personality patterns; they are seen only in individuals who are encumbered with the residues of adverse earlier life experiences that have led to the acquisition of maladaptive intrapsychic defenses, cognitive beliefs, and interpersonal habits. The precipitating stimuli stir up a wide array of intervening emotions and thoughts, which "take over" as determinants of patients' responses; the stimuli serve merely as catalysts, setting in motion a chain of complex intermediary processes that transform what would otherwise have been fairly simple and straightforward responses in "normal" individuals. Because of the contaminating intrusion of these transformations, complex syndromes may acquire an irrational and often "symbolic" quality. For example, in a complex phobic syndrome, the object that is feared may come to represent something else; thus a phobia of elevators may symbolize a more generalized and unconscious anxiety about being closed in and trapped by others.

Intrusions of this complex nature do not occur in what we have defined as simple reactions. Here, the responses stem from neither deep psychic vulnerabilities nor widespread misperceptions, but from a delimited class of biological frailties or environmental precipitants. These symptomatic responses do not "pass through" a chain of complicating and circuitous intrapsychic and cognitive transformations before they emerge in manifest form. In addition to the restricted number of agents that give rise to them, simple reactions are distinguished from complex syndromes by the more or less direct route through which they are channeled and expressed clinically.

Elaborating on Grossman et al. (Chapter 24, this volume), we should like to record the personological utility of expanding the range and comparability of routinely appraised clinical domains. Although it may be difficult to identify and "carve" those "joints" that meaningfully divide the raw behaviors and traits constituting personality, we should, at the very least, utilize similar descriptive clinical domains throughout our assessment work. Inconsistencies in the clinical phenomena that are tapped by our diagnostic tools, as well as in those that embody the diagnostic criteria of the DSM, result in a lack of comparability and parallelism. Clinical domain commonalities should be routinely addressed to ensure that different instruments of personality appraisal can be compared and evaluated. Although the domains included to assess personality patterns with various projective and objective techniques include a wide range of useful clinical indices, it would make good scientific and practical sense if certain specific realms were consistently addressed—for example, mood/affect, cognitive style, interpersonal conduct, and self-image.

The notion of "domains" arises from the observation that personality has been viewed from many different perspectives. Classical Rorschach theorists, for example, hold that their instrument can assess the habitual structure of percepts or the vicissitudes of drives, whereas self-report test theorists hold that interpersonal attitudes and self-image beliefs are central. The problem with attempting to coordinate such diverse perspectives on personality is how to do so in a logical way that is consonant with the intrinsic organismic integrity of personality itself.

As noted previously, perhaps the best way to organize the domains of personality draws on a distinction made in the biological sciences between "structure" and "function." The basic science of anatomy investigates embedded and essentially permanent structures that serve, for example, as substrates for mood and memory; physiology examines underlying functions that regulate internal dynamics and external transactions. As an integrated totality, personality must depend on structural and functional domains, just as does any organic system. In most cases, these domains parallel major approaches to the field. Nothing is really new here, except the fact that these domains are presented in juxtaposition as a means of obtaining as a complete a representation of personality patterns as possible—one that would eschew past dogmatisms of personality theory, just as psychotherapists have sought to break free of their school-oriented past. For example, an expressive behaviors domain would represent the behavioral legacy of Thorndike, Skinner, and Hull, whereas an interpersonal conduct domain would represent the relational tradition, as originated by Sullivan and expressed more recently by Benjamin, Kiesler, Wiggins, and others. A cognitive style or content domain would represent the growing cognitive tradition, of which Beck and Ellis are the most notable clinical exponents; the regulatory mechanisms and object representations domains would parallel the ego defenses and object relations orientations, respectively, of the psychodynamic school. All of these are legitimate approaches to assessing personality, and their combined existence can encompass the diverse empirical data for personality pathologies encompassing the full scope of individuals' makeup.

Unless future assessors wish to return to a dogmatic, school-oriented past, we must be prepared to incorporate all these perspectives as legitimate content facets of personality. The alternative is a reduction of the personality matrix to a narrow or singular perspective (be it behavioral, cognitive, psychodynamic, or some other)—in other words, to treat a part as if it was the whole.

One step toward the goal of sharpening diagnostic assessments is to spell out a distinctive clinical feature for every diagnostically relevant clinical domain aligned with every personality prototype, as done by Grossman et al. in Chapter 24. For example, if the attribute "interpersonal conduct" is deemed a valuable clinical domain in assessing personality, then *each* assessment tool should be examined to see how that clinical characteristic can be recognized for *each* personality style or disorder. When an assessment program includes all relevant clinical domains (e.g., behaviors, affects, cognitions) and specifies a distinguishing feature on every attribute for each style or pathology of personality, assessment tools will both become fully comprehensive in their clinical scope, and possess parallel and directly comparable clinical indices for all Axis II categories.

Developing or refining instruments in the preceding fashion will not only furnish logic and symmetry to all clinical assessments, but will enable investigators to be systematic in determining the relative diagnostic efficiency (e.g., sensitivity, positive predictive power) of comparable assessment tools and their presumed domain variates. Moreover, clinicians will be able to assess comprehensively both typical and unusual personality patterns, as well as to establish the coherence, if not the "validity," of classically established clinical prototypes.

A similar argument can be made with regard to the DSM diagnostic criteria. Most of the criteria, even in the data-based DSM-IV(-TR), lack both adequate empirical support or clinical comprehensiveness. Some criteria are insufficiently explicit or, conversely, are overly concrete in their operational referents. Many are redundant both within their own diagnostic class and with other classes. All are insufficiently comprehensive in syndromal scope or display a lack of parallelism and symmetry among corresponding personality categories.

The final proposal we would like to make relates to the fact that the prototypes constituting the body of DSM Axis II represent derivations based essentially on a series of "ideal" or "pure" textbook conceptions of each ostensibly discrete and boundaried disorder. There are, however, numerous variations of the "textbook" Axis II disorders—divergences from the published prototypes that reflect both the results of empirical research and the observations of everyday clinical work.

Given the philosophical and multidimensional complexities of any personality construct, we must resist the ever-present linguistic compulsion to simplify and separate constructs from their objective reality, and then to treat them as if these clinical constructions were fixed "disease entities." Constructs (e.g., personality prototypes) should be used heuristically, as guidelines to be reformulated or replaced as necessary; only the unique ways in which the constructs are seen in specific patients should be of primary clinical interest. The DSM Axis II disorders are "nomothetic," in that they comprise hypothetical or abstract taxons (Meehl, 1995) derived from historical, clinical, or statistical sources (biochemical, intrapsychic). Given the "fixed" nature in which each of these constructs is promulgated in the DSM, would it not be wise to generate a range of personality *subtypes* to represent trait constellation variants that come close to corresponding to the distinctive or "idiosyncratic" character of our actual patients? Here again, Westen and Shedler's (1999, 2000) productive empirical work is well worth reviewing, as are Millon's own more clinically based efforts with Davis (Millon & Davis, 1996, 2000).

Not only is Axis II of DSM *not* an exhaustive listing of the personality configurations we see in many of our patients, but it does not begin to scratch the surface of human individuality and variability. A DSM-IV(-TR) diagnosis alone, unsupplemented by information from additional descriptive domains, constitutes an insufficient basis for articulating the distinctive, complex, and often conflictual trait dynamics of a person. Nomothetic propositions and diagnostic labels are superficialities to be overcome as understanding is gained. They constitute a crude first step, but they are not sufficient for useful clinical work; in fact, if left as they are, they should be regarded as prescientific.

As we have stated previously, and as all experienced clinicians know, there is no single schizoid (or avoidant, or depressive, or histrionic) personality pattern. Rather, there are innumerable variations—different forms in which the prototypal personality expresses itself. Life experience subsequently influences and reshapes constitutional dispositions in a variety of ways, taking divergent turns and producing shadings composed of meaningfully discriminable psychological features. The course and character of each person's life experiences are, at the very least, marginally different from all others, producing influences with sequential effects that may generate *recombinant mixtures* of personality. Some of those result in contrasting inclinations within the same person, such as those stemming from parents who are strikingly different in their child-rearing behaviors—one rearing pattern conducive to the formation of an avoidant style in the child, the other to an obsessive–compulsive one. Internal schisms of character, so well understood by our analytic colleagues, are quite common, as are the discrepancies we see between overt and covert characteristics in many of our patients.

As we've stated elsewhere, the inexact fit between a patient and his or her diagnostic label is a nagging and noisome reminder of the individuality of personality; it reflects the "idiographic" as contrasted with the "nomothetic" approach to psychological assessment. This incessant conceptual trouble has fueled the development of modern multiaxial taxonomies, but these are at best only preliminary steps in what might come to be the right direction. (Parenthetically, we should note the absurdities these taxonomies can create in what are termed "comorbidities"; see Carson, 1996.)

Ideally, a diagnosis alone should be both necessary and sufficient to begin treatment—all a clinician needs to know. Were ideals realities, individuals would fit their diagnostic categories perfectly, with pristinely prototypal presentation. Yet such a thing seldom occurs. The monotypic categories of the DSM are but a crude and global beginning in a march toward specification and the accommodation of a taxonomy of individuality. Although the initial phases of a diagnostic taxonomy must consist of categories of broad bandwidth and little specificity, DSM diagnostic categories provide gross distinctions, if not invalid ones. As clinical knowledge and empirical studies accrue, the manifestation of classification groupings must become more sharply delineated; that is, broad diagnostic taxons should be broken down into multiple, narrow taxons of greater specificity and individually descriptive value, as we have begun to do in formulating personality category "subtypes." All we ask is that such personality subtypes reflect the individualities of human nature and pathology. Clinicians and students must learn not only DSM textbook personalities, but subtype mixtures that are seen in clinical reality. In several of recent books (Millon, 1999b; Millon & Davis, 1996, 2000), Millon and his colleagues have sought to describe a number of these early stage variations.

References

American Psychiatric Association. (1980). *Diagnostic and statistical manual of mental disorders* (3rd ed.). Washington, DC: Author.

American Psychiatric Association. (1987). *Diagnostic and statistical manual of mental disorders* (3rd ed., rev.). Washington, DC: Author.

American Psychiatric Association. (1994). *Diagnostic and statistical manual of mental disorders* (4th ed.). Washington, DC: Author.

American Psychiatric Association. (2000). *Diagnostic and statistical manual of mental disorders* (4th ed., text rev.). Washington, DC: Author.

Cantor, N., Smith, E. E., French, R. D., & Mezzich, J. (1980). Psychiatric diagnosis as prototype categorization. *Journal of Abnormal Psychology, 89,* 181–193.

Carson, R. C. (1996) Seamlessness in personality and its derangements. *Journal of Personality Assessment, 66,* 240–247.

Choca, J. (2004). *Interpretive guide to the Millon Clinical Multiaxial Inventory* (3rd ed.). Washington, DC: American Psychological Association.

Craig, R. J. (Ed.). (1993). *The Millon Clinical Multiaxial Inventory: A clinical research information synthesis.* Hillsdale, NJ: Erlbaum.

Craig, R. J. (Ed.). (2005). *New directions in interpreting the MCMI-III.* Hoboken, NJ: Wiley.

Cronbach, L. J., & Meehl, P. E. (1955). Construct validity in psychological tests. *Psychological Bulletin 52,* 281–302.

Jackson, D. N. (1970). A sequential system for personality scale development. In C. D. Spielberger (Ed.), *Current topics in clinical and community psychology* (Vol. 2, pp. 61–92). New York: Academic Press.

Loevinger, J. (1957). Objective tests as instruments of psychological theory. *Psychological Reports, 3,* 635–694.

Marvish, M. (Ed.). (1994). *The use of psychological testing for treatment planning and outcome assessment.* Hillsdale, NJ: Erlbaum.

Marvish, M. (Ed.). (2002). *The use of psychological testing for treatment planning and outcome assessment* (3rd ed.). Hillsdale, NJ: Erlbaum.

Meehl, P. E. (1978). Theoretical risks and tabular asterisks: Sir Karl, Sir Ronald, and the slow progress of soft psychology. *Journal of Consulting and Clinical Psychology 46,* 806–834.

Meehl, P. E. (1995). Bootstraps taxometrics: Solving the classification problem in psychopathology. *American Psychologist, 50,* 266–275.

Millon, T. (1969). *Modern psychopathology.* Philadelphia: Saunders.

Millon, T. (1977). *Manual for the Millon Clinical Multiaxial Inventory (MCMI).* Minneapolis, MN: National Computer Systems.

Millon, T. (1984). On the renaissance of personality assessment and personality theory. *Journal of Personality Assessment, 48,* 450–466.

Millon, T. (1990). *Toward a new personology.* New York: Wiley.

Millon, T. (1999a). Reflections on psychosynergy: A model for integrating science, theory, classification, assessment, and therapy. *Journal of Personality Assessment, 72,* 437–456.

Millon, T. (2003). *Millon Index of Personality Styles Revised.* Minneapolis, MN: Pearson Assessments.

Millon, T., & Davis, R. D. (1996). *Disorders of personality: DSM-IV and beyond.* New York: Wiley.

Millon, T., & Davis, R. D. (2000). *Personality disorders in modern life.* New York: Wiley.

Millon, T. (with Grossman, S., Meagher, S., Millon, C., & Everly, G.). (1999b). *Personality-guided therapy.* New York: Wiley.

Millon, T. (with Millon, C., & Davis, R. D.). (1994a). *Millon Clinical Multiaxial Inventory–III manual.* Minneapolis: National Computer Systems.

Millon, T. (with Weiss, L. G., Millon, C., & Davis, R. D.). (1994b). *Millon Index of Personality Styles (MIPS) manual.* San Antonio, TX: Psychological Corporation.

Skinner, H. A. (1986). Construct validation approach to psychiatric classification. In T. Millon & G. L. Klerman (Eds.), *Contemporary directions in psychopathology: Toward the DSM-IV* (pp. 307–330). New York: Guilford Press.

Tringone, R. F. (1997). The MPDC: Composition and clinical application. In T. Millon (Ed.), *The Millon inventories: Clinical and personality assessment* (pp. 449–474). New York: Guilford Press.

Westen, D., & Arkowitz-Westen, L. (1998). Limitations of Axis II in diagnosing personality pathology in clinical practice. *American Journal of Psychiatry, 155,* 1767–1771.

Westen, D., & Shedler, J. (1999). Revising and assessing Axis II: I. Developing a clinically and empirically valid method. *American Journal of Psychiatry, 156,* 258–272.

Westen, D., & Shedler, J. (2000). A prototype matching approach to diagnosing personality disorders: Toward DSM-V. *Journal of Personality Disorders 14,* 109–126.

Author Index

Abbott, P. J., 276
Aberson, C. L., 550
Abrams, R. C., 300, 301, 302–303, 303
Ackerman, A., 450–451
Acklin, M. W., 88
Agronin, M., 301
Agronin, M. E., 304, 313, 314
Aiduk, R., 116
Aiken, L., 454
Alagna, S. W., 436
Alberts, M., 458
Alden, L. E., 613
Alexopoulos, G. S., 310
Alferi, S., 442
Allport, G. W., 51, 52, 55, 57
Alterman, A. I., 282
Altice, F. L., 468
Alyman, C. A., 248, 251
Ames, A., 299, 300
Andersen, B. L., 443–444, 447
Andersen, T. J., 136
Anderson, D., 257
Anderson, K. O., 439
Anderson, R., 458
Anderson, R. E., 124
Andrews, G., 444
Anglin, M. D., 277
Anisman, H., 439
Anthony, V. L., 517

Anton, W. D., 651
Antoni, M. H., 76, 162, 164, 166, 169, 171, 172, 173, 306, 314, 434, 435, 437, 438, 439, 440, 441, 442, 443, 444, 445, 445–446, 446, 447, 455, 458, 460, 464, 468, 470, 554
Archer, R, P., 116, 135, 136, 136–137
Arean, P., 310
Arena, P., 442
Arkowitz, H., 6–7
Arkowitz-Westen, L., 690
Arpin, K., 451
Ash, E., 517
Aspinwall, L. G., 434, 439, 440, 441
Assal, J. P., 454
Ayearst, L. E., 613

B

Baert, H., 371
Bagby, M. R., 265
Bagby, R., 351
Bagby, R. M., 306
Bahr, G. R., 276
Ball, S. A., 270, 271, 272, 274, 278, 280, 281, 282, 283, 284, 285, 286, 291
Bandura, A., 39, 438
Bangsberg, D. R., 467

Barchas, J., 438
Barefoot, J., 444
Barlow, D. H., 16, 328
Barnum, R., 516
Baron, J. R., 446
Barrios, F. X., 116
Barron, J. W., 15
Barroso, J., 445
Barrow, J. C., 550
Barry, D. T., 510, 512, 516
Barsky, A., 450
Barthlow, D. L., 116
Bassett, 469
Baty, B., 437
Bauchowitz, A. U., 469
Baucom, D., 350
Baum, A., 162, 437, 438, 446, 447
Baum, J. D., 446
Baumeister, D., 208
Beach, S., 347, 349
Beals, J., 446
Beavers, W. R., 613
Beck, A. T., 31, 40, 129, 279, 280, 281, 291, 315, 457, 458, 557, 651, 668, 693
Becker, M. H., 436
Beebe, B., 330, 331
Beekman, A. T. F., 297
Belin, T. R., 310
Bell, C., 347
Belter, R. W., 83
Ben-Abdallah, A. B., 275, 278
Benjamin, L. S., 13, 40, 307, 313, 689, 693
Bennet, A. D., 517
Ben-Porath, Y. S., 61, 116, 117, 377, 401–402, 415
Benton, D., 445
Benton, S. A., 550
Benton, S. L., 550
Bergner, M., 480
Berndt, E. R., 450
Bernstein, I. H., 378
Berry, D. T. R., 136
Beutler, L. E., 309
Bhate, S. R., 516
Biederman, J., 256
Binder, R. L., 374
Birchler, G., 349
Bivens, A., 271, 372, 420
Black, W. C., 124
Blake, D. D., 614
Blalock, S., 445
Blashfield, R. K., 116, 377, 415, 613
Blatt, S. J., 17

Bleuler, E., 138
Bloch, S., 446
Bloom, C, 17–18, 56
Bloom, J. R., 447
Blum, N., 307
Blumenthal, J., 445
Bobbitt, R. A., 480
Boccaccini, M. T., 614, 629
Bockian, N., 516
Boeke, S., 450
Boice, 62, 600, 690
Bonavida, B., 445
Boone, D. E., 116
Booth-Kewley, S., 439
Bornstein, R. F., 88, 136
Botkin, J., 437
Bouchard, T. J., 401
Bowen, M., 332
Bowles, C., 162, 438
Bradley, L., 469
Bradley, L. A., 439
Bradley, P. E., 73
Brand, A. H., 438
Brandenburg, N. A., 417, 426
Brandwin, M., 458
Brasfield, T. R., 276
Brazil, P. J., 248
Breckenridge, J. S., 309
Bremer, B., 440
Briggs, R. S., 396
Brislin, R. W., 391
Broadhead, W., 451
Brockington, I. F., 378
Brodie, L. A., 190
Brolin, R., 469
Bronfenbrenner, U., 331
Brooner, R. K., 284, 285
Brown, 438
Brown, G., 443
Brown, G. K., 557
Brown, J., 258, 443
Brown, M. Z., 276
Brown, R. S., 265
Brown, S., 446
Brown, S. A., 446
Browne, G., 451
Brownell, K. D., 281, 446
Brunell-Neuleib, S., 136
Burgess, C., 441
Burisch, M., 71, 72, 118, 119, 310
Burnett, R., 444
Burns, K., 445
Busby, R. M., 117

Bushman, B., 208
Buss, A., 70
Buss, D., 68
Butcher, J. N., 61, 83, 116, 117, 158, 160, 190, 251, 306, 376, 635, 651, 652
Byravan, A., 613
Byrnes, D., 438, 460

C

Cacciola, J. S., 282
Calhoun, G. B., 117, 517
Calsyn, D. A., 275, 284
Calsyn, R. J., 442
Cameron, L., 437
Campbell, B. K., 271, 273
Campbell, C. A., 266, 267
Campbell, D. P., 651, 659
Campbell, D. T., 72, 77, 583
Campbell, L., 612, 617
Campbell, L. F., 117
Campbell, W. K., 208
Cantor, N., 73, 581, 582, 689
Caporaso, N., 436
Carey, K. B., 276
Carey, M. P., 276, 310
Caricco, A., 438
Carl, M., 446
Carney, R., 445, 451
Carrico, A., 441, 447
Carrieri, M. P., 468
Carroll, J., 159
Carroll, K. M., 270, 282
Carson, R. C., 20, 695
Carstensen, L. L., 310
Carter, W. B., 480
Carver, C. S., 438, 440, 441, 442, 461
Casey, D. A., 300, 301
Caspi, A., 297, 302
Castner, N. M., 441
Cattell, R. B., 73, 75, 118, 124, 400, 423, 424, 651, 661
Caudill, M., 453
Cauffman, E., 516
Chacko, R. C., 468
Chaisson, R. E., 467
Chambers, D., 443
Chambers, W. N., 446
Charlebois, E. D., 467
Chase, H., 445
Chatterjee, A., 303
Cheek, J. M., 396

Chen, E. Y., 276
Chesney, M., 444, 467
Chesney, M. A., 443
Chitwood, R. P., 252, 253, 267
Choca, J., 680
Choca, J. P., 83, 84, 85, 89, 90, 92–93, 114, 117, 122, 159, 160, 370, 372, 411, 414, 415, 417, 418, 419, 420, 630, 635
Christensen, A. J., 468
Christman, N. J., 440
Clara, R., 371
Clark, L. A., 118, 307
Clarkin, J., 337
Clarkin, J. F., 582
Cleckley, H., 201
Clifford, M., 458
Cloninger, 689
Cloninger, C. R., 70
Cloninger, R., 13
Clouse, R. E., 441
Coates, A., 309
Coates, T. J., 442
Coffman, G. A., 300
Coffman, K., 458
Coffman, S. G., 267
Cohen, B. J., 299
Cohen, S., 437–438, 438, 442, 455
Coleman, J. C., 494
Compton, W. M., 275, 278
Conway, T., 442
Conwell, Y., 447
Cook, V., 436
Coolidge, F. L., 299, 300, 301, 304, 306
Coon, D. W., 311
Cooney, N. L., 284
Cooper, A. M., 87
Corbisiero, J.R., 271, 272
Corbitt, E. M., 307
Corea, S., 301
Corey, P., 451
Cornell, D. G., 513, 514, 516, 517
Cornes, C., 310
Cornish, J. A. E., 550
Corr, M. J., 468
Corrigan, S. A., 277
Costa, P. R., Jr., 438
Costa, P. T., 61, 118, 423, 651, 661
Costa, P. T., Jr., 297, 306, 580, 613, 689
Cottler, L. B., 275, 278
Coyne, J., 349
Coyne, J. C., 442
Craig, R., 351, 353

Craig, R. J., 78, 79, 83, 84, 89, 252, 271,
    273, 372, 373, 377, 411, 415, 417, 419,
    420, 630, 635, 680
Craighead, L. W., 38, 39
Craighead, W. E., 38, 39
Cronbach, L. J., 114, 119, 412, 583, 689
Cronkite, R., 450
Crowley, T. J., 275
Croyle, R., 437
Crues, D., 438
Cruess, D., 443, 445, 468
Cruess, S., 438, 443, 444, 468
Cuddihee, R. M., 442
Cuerdon, T., 453
Culver, J., 442
Cummings, N. A., 437, 452
Curphy, G. J., 656
Curtis, J., 309
Cushman, L. A., 450
Cuthbert, B., 347
Cutrona, C., 442

D

Dahlstrom, L. E., 164
Dahlstrom, W. G., 74, 83, 160, 164, 166,
    169, 171, 306, 651
Dam, H., 136
D'Angelo, T., 446
Darwin, C., 68, 69
Daubert, S. D., 636
Davidson, J. K., 453, 468
Davidson, R., 278, 279, 280
Davis, D. D., 31, 129
Davis, R. D., 21, 25, 26, 61, 64, 69, 70, 97–
    98, 99, 113, 114, 117, 118–119, 119, 120,
    121–122, 124, 126, 127, 128, 192, 211,
    251, 257, 266, 276, 281, 305, 308, 348,
    351, 352, 353, 354, 366, 366–367, 406,
    407, 409, 410, 411, 414–415, 417, 418,
    419, 420, 421, 422, 425, 426, 463, 495,
    497, 499, 529, 535, 548, 550, 552, 553,
    554, 555, 556, 557, 563, 570, 571, 572,
    580, 582, 583, 584, 598, 610, 611, 615,
    639, 657, 680, 681, 694, 695
Davison, G. C., 39
Dawes, R. M., 79, 374
Dawson, K. S., 271
de Graeff, A., 455
de Groot, M. H., 274
de May, H. R. A., 370, 375
De Vellis, B., 436, 445
De Vellis, R. F., 436

de Vries, M., 439
Dean, J., 298
Deeg, 297
Deeks, S. G., 467
DeGruy, F., 451
del Rio, C., 120, 411, 418, 420
DeLaCruz, M., 310
Deleon, H., 300
Delin, C. R., 469
Delmonico, R. L., 310
DelVecchio, W. F., 136
DeMarco, G., 310
Dembroski, T. M., 438
Derksen, J., 122
Derksen, J. J. L., 369, 370, 373, 375, 402
Desai, A., 303
Dévieux, J., 513, 516
Devine, E. C., 454
Dick, L. P., 312
Diesenhaus, H., 65
Digman, J. M., 122, 124, 297, 662
Dimond, M., 446
Dimsdale, J. E., 438
Dixon, R. A., 297
Dobson, K. S., 309
Docherty, J. P., 78
Doering, S., 455
Donat, D. C., 271, 272
Dorken, H., 437
Dornbrand, L., 310
Dorr, D., 114, 135, 136
Doughtie, E. B., 73
Drachman, R., 436
Draper, M. R., 550
Drogin, E. Y., 182
Dubbert, P., 446
Duberstein, P. R., 447
Duivenvoorden, H., 445
Duker, J., 163
Dunkel-Schetter, C., 442
Dunn, T., 85, 87, 415, 417
Dunsmore, J., 444
Duran, R., 442
Dutton, D., 208
Dyce, J. A., 419
Dyer, F. J., 180, 192, 194, 496
Dziuban, C. D., 660

E

Eagan, D., 270
Eber, H. W., 118, 651
Edwards, J. R., 438

Efantis-Potter, J., 437
Eisen, E., 448, 450
Eisen, S., 445
Eldridge, N., 41
Elkins, D. E., 116
Ell, K., 446
Ellis, A., 31, 40
Ellis, C. G., 307, 693
Emmelkamp, P., 443
Enders, C., 278
Epstein, L. H., 447
Epstein, N., 350
Epstein, S., 77
Erdur-Baker, O., 550
Erickson, M. T., 613
Essa, M., 300
Esterling, B., 438
Esterling, B. A., 438
Evans, D., 442
Everly, G., Jr., 201, 231
Exner, J. E. Jr., 59, 135, 152
Eysenck, H., 423
Eysenck, H. J., 70, 73

F

Fabrega, H., 300
Faddis, S., 310
Fals-Steward, W., 270, 271, 273, 278, 280, 291, 349
Farabee, D., 270
Farvolden, P., 306
Fawzy, F. I., 444, 445, 447
Feinglos, M. N., 439
Felling, J., 257
Felton, B. J., 441
Fiel, A., 265
Finch, J. F., 378
Finkel, S. I., 303
Finkelstein, S. N., 450
Finn, S. E., 371
First, M. B., 307, 347
Fiske, 72
Fiske, D. W., 77, 583
Fitch, M., 451
Fitzpatrick, R., 442
Flaherty, J. A., 438
Fleming, C., 275, 284
Fletcher, K. E., 516
Fletcher, M. A., 438, 445
Flum, D., 469
Foa, E. B., 309
Fogel, B. S., 301

Fogel, F., 302
Folkman, S., 438, 442, 443
Ford, A., 443
Foster, F. M., 557
Fowler, K. A., 330
Fox, B. H., 439, 445–446
Frances, A., 308, 337, 581, 582, 583
Frank, B., 468
Frank, E., 310
Franken, I. H. A., 274
Frankenburg, F. R., 307
Frasure-Smith, N., 439, 447, 451
Fredrickson, B. L., 366
Freedland, K., 445, 451
Freeman, A., 31, 129, 281, 668
Freeman, D., 446
French, R., 581
French, R. D., 73, 689
Frenzel, M. P., 438
Freud, S., 67–68, 69
Freyhan, F.A., 36
Friedland, G. H., 468
Friedman, H. S., 439
Friedman, M., 310
Friedman, S. H., 310
Fritz, H. L., 438
Fuller, G., 159
Fulop, G., 451
Funch, D. P., 442

G

Gafni, A., 451
Gallagher, D., 309, 310
Gallagher, T., 275
Gallagher-Thompson, D., 309, 311, 312
Ganellen, R. J., 137
Gantz, 310
Garb, H. N., 135, 246
Garetz, F. K., 301
Garfield, S., 581
Garske, G. G., 310
Gass, C. S., 247
Gatchel, R., 458
Gatz, M., 309
Geer, J., 216
Genero, N., 582
Gerber, P. D., 446
Gerson, R., 351
Gerson, S., 310
Getter, H., 284
Gibbon, M., 307
Gibertini, M., 417, 419, 420, 426, 617

Gill, K., 275
Gillen, D., 469
Gilligan, C., 70
Gillis, J. R., 256, 265
Gilmore, M., 582
Gilson, B. S., 480
Giordino, K., 445
Glanz, L., 436, 437
Glaser, B. A., 117, 517
Glaser, R., 437, 438, 447, 455
Glasgow, R., 444
Glasgow, R. E., 438, 439
Glass, D. R., 78
Glass, G. V., 453, 454
Glavin, Y., 300
Gleick, J., 331
Gliberstadt, H., 163
Glickhauf-Hughes, C., 85
Glynn, T., 437
Godel, K., 70
Gold, J. R., 584
Goldberg, J., 256, 265
Goldberg, L. R., 72, 118, 122, 124, 423, 661, 663
Golden, C. J., 257
Goldfried, M.R., 39
Goldstein, D., 438, 441, 445, 458
Goldstein, J., 453
Goldstein, K., 37, 257
Gonik, U. L., 453
Gontag, R., 613
Gonzalez, J. S., 442, 468
Goodkin, K., 438, 439, 443, 445, 445–446, 455, 458, 459, 460
Gordillo, V., 468
Gordon, L. V., 651
Gotay, C., 437
Gottesman, I. I., 401
Gottheil, E., 447
Gottlieb, M., 354
Gough, H. G., 75, 651
Gould, S., 41
Gould, S. L., 303, 614, 629
Grady, K., 438, 445
Graham, F., 516
Graham, J. R., 61, 83, 116, 117, 160, 164, 166, 169, 171, 306, 651
Graham, M. A., 450
Gray, J. A., 70
Greco, F. A., 310
Green, A., 469
Green, C., 435, 437, 458, 610
Green, C. J., 78, 162

Green, P., 445
Green, S. M., 528
Greenberg, P. E., 450
Greenblatt, R. L., 370
Greene, R. L., 159
Greer, S., 445
Gregoire, T. K., 277
Grella, C. E., 277
Griffin, R., 116
Griffith, L. S., 441
Grillo, J., 265
Grilo, C. M., 510, 512, 516
Grisso, T., 516
Gronnerod, C., 136
Gross, J. J., 298
Grossberg, G., 303
Grossman, S. D., 4, 6, 19, 25, 61, 62, 64, 76, 84, 112, 113, 114, 120, 124, 128, 129, 192, 306, 314, 352, 406, 407, 411, 418, 420, 422, 424, 425, 435, 528, 531, 554, 598, 599, 603, 609, 686
Groth-Marnat, G., 84, 85
Grove, J., 437
Grove, W. M., 424
Gruen, W., 444
Grünbaum, A., 18
Grunberg, N., 447
Grunberg, N. E., 447
Gueldner, S. H., 298
Guevara, L. F., 612, 613–614
Guion, R. M., 656, 668
Gupta, M., 349
Gurian, B., 302
Gurman, A. S., 40
Gurtman, M. B., 420
Guzman, A., 192, 251

H

Haddy, C., 372, 415, 420
Haefner, D., 436
Hair, J. F., 124
Haller, D. L., 271, 273
Hambleton, R., 369, 388
Hamer, R., 451
Hammer, J., 451
Hamovitch, M., 446
Hampson, R. B., 613
Hampson, S., 439
Handler, L., 136
Hanley-Peterson, P., 309, 310
Hansen, J. C., 651, 659

Hanser, 310
Hanson, A., 309
Harder, D. W., 370
Hare, R. D., 201, 516
Hargreaves, W., 451
Harker, J., 445
Harkness, A., 449
Harkness, A. R., 401–402, 423
Harlow, L., 443
Harper, R. G., 468
Harrington, H., 302
Harris, R. E., 60, 113, 115, 116, 117, 125
Hart, S., 208
Hartnett, S., 438
Harvey, M., 516
Hase, H. E., 72
Hathaway, S. R., 74, 115, 651
Hauben, C., 374, 376–377, 415, 417
Havlir, D. V., 467
Haybittle, J., 445
Hayflick, L., 296
Hays, R. B., 442
Heberman, R., 446
Hecht, F. M., 467
Hehlbach, S., 451
Heijnen, C., 455
Heiland, W. F., 301
Heinrichs, R. W., 248–249, 251
Helgeson, V. S., 438, 442
Hellenbosch, G., 375
Hellman, C. J. C., 452
Helson, R., 297
Hempel, C., 55–56, 60, 66
Hempel, C. G., 20
Henderson, M. C., 550
Hendriks, V. M., 274
Henke, C., 451
Henke, C. J., 437
Henricks, T., 454
Henry, S. B., 469
Herbert, T., 438
Herrmann, C., 444
Hersen, M., 302, 304
Hershberger, P. J., 468
Herzog, C., 297
Hess, A. K., 190
Heyman, R., 347
Hiatt, M. D., 513, 514, 516
Hiller, J. B., 136
Hilsabeck, R., 265
Hilsenroth, M. J., 136
Hilton, N., 310
Hinrichsen, G., 310, 441

Hirsch, D., 440
Hirschfeld, R. M., 78
Hoffman, J., 116, 270
Hoffman, V., 277
Hoffschmidt, S. J., 517
Hogan, J., 656
Hogan, R., 656
Holahan, C. J., 441
Holland, J. C., 439, 450
Holzemer, W. L., 469
Hook, J. N., 299
Hooker, K., 298
Horn, J. L., 557
Horney, K., 26
Horowitz, L. M., 73
Horowitz, S. V., 300, 301, 302–303, 303
Horton, A. D., 613
Houck, P. R., 310
House, J. A., 442
House, J. S., 438, 446
Houts, P. S., 310
Howieson, D. B., 245
Hser, Y. I., 277
Hsu, L. K. G., 469
Hsu, L. M., 374, 417, 418, 426
Hughes, C., 437
Hull, 693
Hultsch, D. F., 297
Hume, A., 271
Hurewitz, A., 454
Hurt, S. W., 582
Huxley, T. H., 69
Hyer, L., 89
Hyer, L. A., 303, 309, 310, 614, 629
Hyler, S. E., 306

I

Ironson, G., 434, 437, 440, 445, 446, 447
Ivey, G., 87

J

Jackson, B., 443
Jackson, D. N., 71, 118, 535, 583, 585, 651, 683
Jacobs, D., 450, 453
Jacobs, J. L., 278
Jacobson, N. S., 40, 668
Jacobson, P., 440

Jaffe, A., 451
Jaffe, M., 443
James, S. A., 438
Jamison, C., 310
Jamison, K., 442
Jang, K. L., 401
Janigian, A. S., 450
Jankowski, D., 83
Janzen, H. L., 419
Jarvik, L., 310
Jarvis, G., 446
Jaynes, G., 117
Jenkins, J. B., 210, 237
Jenkins, S. A., 310
Jennings, J., 439
Jennings, T. E., 270
Jeste, D. V., 302
Jewell, J. J., 415
John, O. P., 297
Johnson, J., 459
Johnson, J. H., 438
Johnson, M. D., 302
Johnson, R. S., 310
Johnson, S. B., 438
Johnston, C., 546
Jones, C., 297
Jones, C. J., 297
Jordan, J. V., 327
Jorgensen, K., 136
Jung, C., 67, 68
Jung, C. G., 647, 663, 664

K

Kadden, R. M., 284, 285
Kaell, A., 454
Kaemmer, B., 83, 306, 651
Kaiser, H. F., 124
Kalarchian, M., 469
Kalichman, S.C., 276
Kalsbeek, W. D., 438
Kamarck, T., 439
Kamphaus, R. W., 536
Kaplan, B., 451
Kaplan, G. A., 439
Karel, M. C., 310
Kaslow, N., 347
Katz, C., 458
Katz, I. R., 309
Katz, S., 443
Kauffman, R. H., 445
Kaufman, A., 310

Kazdin, A. E., 38, 39
Kazi, A., 444
Keefe, F., 444
Keith, S., 309
Kelly, A., 270–271, 272, 276, 280, 291
Kelly, C., 163
Kelly, T. P., 516
Kemeny, M. E., 445
Kemmer, B., 160
Kemper, T. S., 517
Kendell, R. E., 378
Kerkhof, A. J. F. M., 297
Kernberg, 34
Kernberg, O. F., 89
Kiani, R., 438
Kidorf, M., 284
Kiecolt-Glaser, J., 437, 438, 447, 455
Kiesler, D. J., 29, 40, 41, 693
Kilgore, R. B., 87
Kimmerling, R., 450
King, G. D., 163
King, J., 446
King, V. L., 284
Kirscht, J., 436
Kistner, J. A., 517
Kleban, M. H., 298
Kleinsasser, D., 199, 213
Klerman, G., 450
Klerman, G. L., 279, 280, 581
Kling, D., 440
Kniskern, K., 40
Knoblauch, S., 330
Koenigh, H., 442
Kolitz, S., 437, 458, 459
Kominars, K. D., 550
Kopans, B., 450
Kopper, B. A., 116
Korchin, S. J., 158
Kotila, M., 450
Kouzekanani, K., 271, 272, 276, 280, 291
Kovacs, M., 536
Kraemer, H. C., 447
Kraepelin, Emil, 22
Kraft, I. A., 73
Krantz, D. S., 438, 447
Krishnamurthy, R., 135, 136–137
Krozely, M. G., 310
Krueger, R. F., 401, 423
Kumar, M., 438
Kuncel, R., 635
Kunik, M., 468
Kunik, M. E., 300, 301
Kupfer, D. J., 309

Kvaal, S. A., 84
Kwan, V. S. Y., 297

L

Laaksonen, R., 450
Lahey, B. B., 528
Lam, J. N., 374
Lamb, R., 442
Lamnin, A., 617
Landis, K. R., 438
Lantinga, L., 458
Lapidos, S., 310
Larrea, M. A., 517
Lauderdale, D., 469
Lawton, M. P., 298, 309
Lazarus, A. A., 20
Lazarus, R. S., 438, 442
Le Marchand, L., 437
Lee, D. J., 420
Lee, J., 446
Lees-Haley, P. R., 265
Lefkowitz, R., 309
LeMont, D., 469
Lenzenweger, M. F., 302
Lerman, C., 436, 437
Leserman, J., 442, 444, 446
Lesperance, F., 439, 451
Levenson, J., 451, 452
Leventhal, E., 437
Leventhal, H., 437
Levin, J., 438, 446
Levine, D., 160
Levine, J., 160, 162, 164, 171, 173
Levine, M. N., 441
Levy, K. N., 17, 40
Levy, S., 446, 447
Lew, R., 436
Lewin, D., 468
Lewin, K., 20
Lewis, S. J., 370
Lezak, M. D., 245, 246, 247
Li, L., 277
Lichstein, K. L., 310
Lichtenstein, E., 281
Lichtman, R. R., 438, 443
Liles, D., 311
Lilienfeld, S., 449
Lilienfeld, S. O., 135, 328, 330
Linehan, M. M., 236, 276, 340
Lingoes, J. C., 60, 113, 115, 116, 117, 125

Lippman, M., 446
Litt, M. D., 284
Livesley, W. J., 118, 304, 401, 422, 423, 424, 585
Lo, T. T. Y., 276
Locke, K. D., 271
Loeber, R., 528, 546
Loevinger, J., 20, 71, 72, 73, 75, 79, 118, 387, 535, 537, 538, 540, 583, 609, 611, 663, 683
Logsdon, R. G., 310
Loney, B. R., 517
Longabaugh, R., 284
Loper, A. B., 517
Loranger, A. W., 307
Lord, F M., 75
Lorig, K., 454
Loring, D. W., 245
Lorr, M., 612, 617
Losada, M. F., 366
Lovallo, W., 446
Lowenstein, E., 73
Lowther, J., 660, 661
Lucas, G. M., 467
Lustman, P., 468
Lustman, P. J., 441
Lutgendorf, S., 437, 438, 439, 441, 443, 445, 460
Lynch, T. R., 310
Lyons, J., 451, 458

M

MacAndrew, C., 116
MacFarlane, M., 347, 348, 366
Magnavita, J., 347
Magnavita, J. J., 34, 328, 329, 331, 332, 334, 337, 348, 355, 366
Magni, G., 446
Mahoney, M. J., 38, 39
Maier, S. F., 216
Maiman, L., 436
Malarkey, W., 455
Maletta, G., 301
Malow, R. M., 270, 277
Mangine, S., 307
Manheimer, E., 446
Manson, S., 446
Mantell, J., 446
Margo, J. L., 301
Marguilles, S., 438
Markert, R. J., 468

Markon, K. E., 401, 423
Marlatt, G., 446
Marlatt, G. A., 281
Marmion, J., 300, 301
Marshall, M., 351
Marteau, T. M., 446
Marucha, P., 455
Marvish, M., 680
Matano, R. A., 271
Matarazzo, J. D., 248
Matheson, S., 89
Matt, D. A., 310
McAdams, D., 298, 319–320
McCaffrey, R. J., 116
McCann, B., 436
McCann, J. T., 160, 180, 191, 192, 194, 495,
    496, 499, 501, 502, 504, 509, 511, 514,
    630, 635
McCarthy, D. M., 378
McCarthy, P. R., 309
McCaul, K. D., 438
McCaulley, M. H., 647, 651, 653
McCleary, J., 458
McClelland, D. C., 138
McCracken, L., 444
McCrae, R. R., 61, 118, 297, 306, 423, 580,
    613, 651, 661
McCullough, 310
McCurry, S. M., 309, 310
McDaniel, L. K., 439
McElreath, L., 309
McGill, J., 468
McGoldrick, M., 351
McGregor, B. A., 444, 455
McHoskey, J. W., 614
McIntosh, S., 550
McKinley, J. C., 74, 115, 651
McKinnon, W., 162, 438
McMahan, R. C., 270, 270–271, 271, 272,
    274, 276, 278, 279, 280, 281, 284, 291
McNiel, D. E., 374
McNulty, J. L., 116, 401–402, 423
McReynolds, C. J., 310
Meager, R., 435, 468
Meager, R. B., 609, 610
Meagher, R., 458
Meagher, S., 84, 128, 554
Mediansky, L., 446
Meehl, P. E., 72–73, 73, 79, 114, 118, 119,
    412, 415, 583, 665, 689, 694
Mefford, I., 438
Meichenbaum, D., 436
Mendelson, T., 310

Menninger, K., 423
Mercado, A., 455
Mercer, D. E., 291
Meredith, W., 297
Merrell, K. W., 529
Mertens, J., 371
Messich, J. E., 301
Messina, N., 270, 271, 272, 274, 280, 282,
    283, 284, 285
Metcalfe, W. E., 420
Mettlin, C., 442
Metzler, A. E., 636
Meyer, G. J., 136
Meyerowitz, B. E., 441
Mezzich, J., 73, 581, 689
Mezzich, J. E., 300
Michels, R., 87
Mihura, J. L., 136
Miles, D. R., 271, 273
Miller, H. R., 160
Miller, K. B., 190
Miller, L. V., 453
Miller, M. D., 310
Miller, P., 365
Miller, S., 365
Miller, W. R., 301
Millikan, C. P., 248, 251
Millon, C., 76, 84, 128, 306, 314, 434, 528,
    531, 554, 657, 695
Millon, T., 4, 6, 9, 10, 16, 17–18, 19, 20, 21,
    25, 26, 28, 32, 34, 37, 38, 40, 43, 49, 56,
    61, 62, 63, 64, 64–65, 66, 69, 70, 71, 73,
    76, 83, 84, 85, 88, 96, 97–98, 99, 112,
    113, 114, 115, 117, 118–119, 120, 121–
    122, 124, 126, 127, 128, 129, 135, 139,
    159, 162, 167, 168, 170, 172, 173, 180,
    181, 185, 192, 196, 197, 198, 201, 202,
    203, 205, 206, 211, 213, 214, 216, 217,
    218, 219, 221–222, 223, 225, 227, 230,
    231, 236, 240, 249, 262, 271, 276, 278–
    279, 281, 283, 284, 296, 297, 305, 306,
    308, 312, 314, 328, 329, 333, 348, 351,
    352, 353, 354, 366, 366–367, 370, 371,
    373, 374, 375, 376, 378, 379, 380, 387,
    387–388, 388, 397, 405, 406, 407, 408,
    409, 410, 411, 414, 414–415, 415, 416,
    417, 418, 419, 420, 421, 422, 424, 425,
    426, 434, 435, 457, 458, 461, 463, 464,
    468, 470, 476, 495, 496, 497, 498, 499,
    501, 502, 503, 528, 529, 530, 531, 532,
    533, 535, 538, 544, 545, 548, 550, 551,
    552, 553, 554, 555, 556, 557, 558, 559–
    560, 561, 563, 570, 571, 572, 578, 580,

581, 582, 583, 584, 585, 586, 588, 598,
599, 600, 603, 610, 611, 612, 614, 615,
616, 617, 630, 635, 639, 643, 644, 647,
648, 649, 650, 651, 652, 653, 657, 658,
662, 663, 664, 666, 667, 679, 680, 681,
682, 686, 687, 688, 689, 690, 691, 694,
695
Milne, B. J., 302
Minor, S., 76, 306, 314, 435
Mintz, J., 310
Miramontes, H., 469
Miranda, J., 451
Modzierz, G. J., 370
Moffitt, T. E., 302
Molinari, V., 299, 300, 301
Monahan, J., 374
Montaner, J. S. G., 467
Moore, F. D., 452
Moore, R. D., 467
Moorehead, M., 469
Moos, R., 450
Moos, R. H., 441, 613
Moreland, K. L., 79
Morey, L. C., 83, 116, 160, 377, 415, 582,
613
Morris, T., 441, 445
Morrisey, E., 443
Morse, J. Q., 310
Mortensen, E. L., 391
Moskowitz, R., 443
Moss, A., 467
Mostashari, F., 468
Mott, M., 446
Motta, R. W., 260
Mouton, A., 117
Mowbray, C. T., 548, 550
Mroczek, D. K., 297
Muhlhauser, I., 454
Mulder, C. L., 439, 445
Mulder, N., 455
Mumford, E., 453, 454
Munley, P. H., 117
Munoz, R., 451
Muran, E. M., 260
Murphy, D. A., 276
Murphy, E., 443
Murphy, T. J., 370
Murray, C., 546
Murray, E. J., 7
Murray, H. A., 52
Murrie, D. C., 516, 517
Myers, I. B., 647, 651, 653, 663
Myers, M. G., 446

N

Narrow, W. E., 450
Nash, J., 437
Neal, A. V., 437, 446
Nemes, S., 270
Neugarten, B., 298
Newcomb, M., 443
Newman, S., 442
Newton, F. B., 550
Nezu, A. M., 310
Nezu, C. M., 310
Nezworski, M. T., 135
Nicassio, P. M., 441
Nich, C., 270
Niederehe, G., 309
Nielsen, J., 442
Niemi, M. L., 450
Nishimoto, R., 446
Nomilal, D., 275
Norcross, J. C., 350
Norman, W., 423
Norman, W. T., 72
Northcott, H., 446
Northouse, A., 442
Nunberg, H. G., 374
Nunnally, J., 414
Nunnally, J. C., 378
Nurse, A. R., 347, 354
Nussbaum, P., 303

O

O'Connor, B. P., 419
Oden, A., 446
Oden, T. M., 249, 251
O'Donohue, W. T., 328, 330
O'Farrell, T., 349
Ofman, P., 89
Ohnishi, H., 420
Oldenberg, B., 444, 447
O'Leary, A., 438
Olson, R., 353
Olson, R. E., 252, 271, 273, 419, 635
Onstad, J. A., 79
Ornish, D., 447
Ortega, A., 116
Osman, A., 116
Osman, D. C., 257
Osman, J. R., 116
O'Sullivan, M. J., 437
Ouimette, P., 450

Overholser, J. C., 252
Owen, P. L., 158
Oxman, T., 446

P

Page, S., 462
Pakula, A., 77
Palav, A., 116
Pallak, M. S., 437, 452
Panounen, S. V., 423
Parad, H. W., 73
Pargament, K., 442
Paris, J., 304
Parish, M., 469
Parkins, S. Y., 419
Parry, J., 182
Pascale, L., 450–451
Pasnau, R., 442
Patrick, C., 453
Patrick, J., 159
Patterson, M. J., 411, 418
Paul, A. M., 327, 328
Paykel, E., 443
Penedo, F. J., 270, 444
Pennebaker, J. W., 438
Pepper, S. P., 10–12, 96, 97, 99
Pereira, D., 437, 438
Perez-Stable, E., 451
Perkins, D., 442
Perkins, K. A., 447
Perkins, R., 444
Perry, S., 87, 337, 440
Persons, J. B., 314
Petersen, A. C., 494
Peterson, C., 438
Peterson, C. A., 370
Petrocelli, J. V., 117
Pettingale, K., 445
Pettingale, K. W., 441
Peuschold, D., 516
Pfohl, B., 307
Piersma, H. L., 370, 420
Pilkonis, P. A., 78
Pincus, A. L., 29, 613, 616
Pine, F., 93
Pinsoneault, T. B., 503
Pinto, M., 510, 516
Piotrowski, C., 83
Plante, T. G., 614, 629
Plomin, R., 70
Polakoff, D., 267

Pope, K. S., 77, 251
Porter, L., 451
Portillo, C. J., 469
Posluszny, D., 437
Powers, D., 311
Powers, P. S., 469
Price, J. R., 265
Prince, R., 447

Q

Quine, W. V. O., 20, 67

R

Rae, D. S., 450
Rajagopal, D., 298
Ramanaiah, N. V., 613
Ramnath, R., 84, 128
Rapp, R. C., 277
Raue, P., 310
Rawson, R., 270
Ray, P. B., 312
Razin, A., 444
Reed, G. M., 445
Reed, J. R., 651
Regier, D., 434, 448, 449
Regier, D. A., 450
Reiser, M. F., 446
Reiss, D., 348
Reitan, R. M., 246, 247–248
Reizes, J. M., 450
Reto, C., 469
Retzlaff, P., 412
Retzlaff, P. D., 83, 85, 87, 89, 117, 192, 199,
    213, 265, 415, 417, 419, 420, 426, 613,
    617
Revenson, T. A., 441
Reynolds, C., 162, 438
Reynolds, C. F., 309, 310
Reynolds, C. R., 536
Reynolds, P., 439
Reznikoff, M., 271, 272
Rich, M., 451
Richards, S. K., 274
Richardson, G., 516
Richmond, B. O., 536
Richter, S., 446, 458
Rickard, H. C., 309
Rimer, B., 437
Ritz, S., 469

Riva, M. T., 550
Robbins, B., 615
Roberts, B. W., 136, 297
Robertson, E. K., 446
Robertson, J. M., 550
Robertson, K. B., 468
Robins, C. J., 310
Robinson, J. R., 301
Rock, C., 436
Rogers, C. R., 32
Rogers, R., 192, 194, 265
Romm, S., 516
Rorer, L. G., 79
Rorschach, H., 59–60, 138
Rosch, E., 73, 425
Rosen, A., 79, 415
Rosenstock, I. M., 436
Rosenthal, R., 136
Rosowsky, E., 300, 301, 302
Rossi, G., 370–371, 371, 372, 373, 374, 375, 376–377, 377, 402, 415, 417
Rossiter, L., 451
Roth, A. J., 450
Roth, L., 302
Rounsavill, B. J., 270
Rubinstein, R. L., 309
Ruegg, R., 308
Rushton, J. P., 70
Russell, D., 442
Russell, E. W., 247, 249, 251, 257, 267
Russell, J. A., 70
Russell, S. L. K., 247
Rustin, J., 330
Rutherford, M. J., 282
Ruttan, L. A., 248–249, 251
Rybarczyk, B., 310

S

Saab, P., 434
Sacks, A., 310
Sadavoy, J., 302, 304, 312
Salekin, R. T., 192, 517, 613
Sandberg, M. L., 79
Sanne, H., 446
Santry, H., 469
Sarason, I., 459
Saxon, A. J., 275, 284
Schaefer, C., 442
Schafer, L. C., 438
Scheier, M., 446
Scheier, M. F., 438

Schinka, J. A., 274
Schlesinger, H. J., 453, 454
Schneider, C. J., 452
Schneiderman, N., 434, 438, 444, 447
Schnurr, P. P., 400, 446
Schram, L., 278, 279, 280
Schrodt, C. J., 300
Schroeder, M. L., 118, 585
Schroll, M., 444
Schuckit, M., 278
Schuckitt, M., 443
Schuldberg, D., 158
Schwartz, K., 271
Schwartz, L. S., 438, 446
Scogin, F., 309, 310
Seelen, J., 251
Segal, D. L., 299, 300, 301, 302, 304
Seligman, M., 366
Seligman, M. E. P., 216, 438
Seung-Hui, C., 99
Sevin, B., 439, 445, 460
Sewell, K. W., 192
Shanley, L. A., 89, 159, 370
Sharfstein, S., 453
Shchrodt, C, J., 301
Shea, M. T., 78, 584
Shedler, J., 307, 690, 694
Sheehan, E., 265
Sheier, M., 461
Shellenberger, S., 351
Sherwood, N. E., 116
Shiner, R. L., 297
Shipley, M., 442
Sickel, A. E., 307
Siegal, B. R., 442
Siegal, H. A., 277
Siegel, J., 443
Silberman, C. S., 302
Silverman, K., 284, 285
Silvestro, A., 446
Simon, T., 437
Simonsen, E., 391, 402, 423
Singh, N., 468
Sinsabaugh, 62, 600, 690
Skinner, H. A., 77, 582, 683, 693
Sklar, L. W., 439
Slavson, S. R., 30
Sloore, H., 122
Sloore, H. V., 369, 370, 371, 372, 373, 374, 375, 376–377, 402, 415, 417
Small, B. J., 297
Smith, A. P., 437–438
Smith, B. L., 136

Smith, D., 159
Smith, E. E., 73, 581, 689
Smith, G. T., 378
Smith, K., 437
Smith, T. W., 468
Smyth, J., 454
Smyth, K., 303
Snively, C. A., 277
Snow, L., 311
Snow-Turek, A. L., 300
Snyder, S. L., 310
Sobel, D., 434
Sobolew-Shubin, A., 450
Solano, L., 445
Solomon, G., 445, 446
Solomon, G. F., 445
Somwaru, D. P., 377, 415
Song, V., 436
Sorenson, J. L., 277
Sorter, D., 330
Spencer, H., 69
Sperry, L., 636
Spiegel, D., 439, 447
Spiegel, J., 459
Spielberger, C. D., 557
Spiro, A., III, 297
Spitzer, R. L., 307
Spitznagel, E. L., 275, 278
Spotts, E., 347
Springer, J., 438
Stafford, E., 517
Stanton, M., 349
Stark, M. J., 271, 273
Starkey, 249
Starr, K., 461
Steer, R. A., 557, 651
Steffen, A., 310, 311
Stefurak, T., 517
Stein, M. J., 441
Stern, M. J., 450–451
Sternhall, P. S., 468
Steunenberg, B., 297
Stiglin, L. E., 450
Stivers, M., 445
Stoller, K., 284
Stone, A., 451, 454
Stone, M. H., 148, 211
Stoner, J., 199, 213
Strack, S., 83, 117, 306, 372, 406, 415, 416,
    418, 419, 420, 421, 422, 423, 425, 548,
    550, 560, 609, 610, 611, 612, 613–614,
    615, 616, 617, 629, 630, 631, 632, 635,
    639

Strain, J., 451, 455
Strauss, M., 303
Streiner, D. L., 160
Stricker, G., 584
Stronks, D., 450
Stump, J., 309
Suinn, R. M., 446
Sullivan, 693
Super, D. E., 660
Surwit, R. S., 439
Swanson, G., 309
Sweet, J. J., 257
Swets, J. A., 374
Swirsky-Sacchetti, T., 266
Szyarto, C., 614

T

Tackett, J. L., 401
Talajic, M., 439, 451
Tamiello, M., 446
Tango, R. A., 660
Tanzer, N., 370
Tatham, R. L., 124
Tatsuoka, M. M., 118, 651
Taylor, C. B., 438
Taylor, J., 517
Taylor, S. E., 434, 438, 439, 440, 441, 442,
    443, 445
Teeter, R. B., 301
Tellegen, A., 70, 83, 160, 306, 424, 651,
    689
Temoshok, L., 442
Teri, L., 309, 310
Terracciano, A., 297
Theorell, T., 446
Thoits, P.A., 442
Thomas, G. V., 307
Thomas, R. W., 257
Thompson, G. J., 210, 237
Thompson, K. E., 277
Thompson, L., 309, 310
Thompson, L. W., 301, 309, 310, 311, 312
Thompson, S. C., 450
Thorndike, 693
Tilley, B. C., 437
Tischer, P., 162, 164, 166, 173
Tobac, A., 376–377, 415
Toner, B. B., 256, 265
Toobert, D., 439
Topol, E., 458
Tourian, K., 276

Tracey, T. J., 312
Tracy, H., 458
Trapnell, P. D., 613
Trijsburg, R. W., 444
Trimakas, K., 370
Trimble, J., 446
Trimboli, F., 87
Tringone, R., 4, 61, 528, 531, 582, 583, 584, 586, 603, 686, 690
Trobst, K. K., 613
Trosten-Bloom, A., 366
Truax, P., 668
Trull, T. J., 580, 581, 583
Tseng, W., 550
Turk, D., 436
Turner, H. A., 442
Turpin, J. O., 310
Twenge, J., 208
Twisk, J. W. R., 297
Tyrell, D. A., 437–438
Tyson, D., 271, 278, 279

U

Uhlenhuth, E., 443
Ulvenstam, G., 446
Umberson, D., 438
Uomoto, J., 310

V

Vaillant, G. E., 446
Valdez, L., 467
Valliant, G. E., 438
Van de Vijver, F., 370
Van den Bos, G. R., 452
Van den Brande, I., 370, 374, 376–377, 415, 417
Van Denburg, E., 85, 89, 159, 370
van der Ark, L. A., 372, 402
van der Meer, C. W., 274
van der Pompe, G., 439, 447, 455
Van Hasselt, V. B., 302
Vanderpool, H., 446
Vasterling, J. J., 310
Vehage, F., 450
Vernon, P. A., 401
Vernon, S. W., 437
Vickery, D. M., 452
Viglione, D. J., 136
Vincent, K. R., 163

Visscher, B. R., 445
Vita, J., 451
von Bertalanffy, L., 331

W

Wachtel, P. L, 26
Wadden, T., 469
Wadden, T. A., 446
Wakefield, J. A., 73
Wakefield, J. C., 330
Walker, S. R., 276
Wallston, B. S., 436
Wallston, K. A., 310, 441, 442
Walters, J., 271
Waltimo, O., 450
Wamboldt, M., 347
Wanberg, K. W., 557
Wang, H. J., 445
Watkins, J., 78
Watson, C. G., 257
Watson, D., 423
Watts, J. M., 469
Waugh, M. H., 116, 377, 613
Weaver, K., 468
Webb, L. M., 261, 264
Webb, W. W., 415
Weinberg, D., 373
Weinberger, J., 585
Weiner, I. B., 137, 139
Weintraub, J., 461
Weisberg, M., 462
Weiss, E., 159, 160, 161
Weiss, L. G., 660, 661
Weiss, S., 442
Weisse, C., 162, 438
Weissman, H. N., 264
Weissman, M., 450
Weissman, M. M., 279, 280, 329
Weller, S. B., 276
Wellisch, D., 442
Wells, E. A., 275, 284
Wells, M., 85
Welsh, D., 309
Welsh, G. S., 164
Wenger, A., 192, 251
West, S. G., 378
Westen, D., 307, 585, 690, 694
Westlake, R., 301
Weston, D., 17
Wetzler, S., 159
Whisman, M., 358

Whitehouse, P., 303
Whitney, D., 366
Widiger, T. A., 118, 307, 402, 420, 423, 580, 581, 582, 583
Wiedenfield, S., 438
Wiens, A. N., 248
Wiggins, J. S., 29, 60, 78, 116, 613, 616, 693
Wiklund, I., 446
Wilcoxin, M., 458, 462
Wilhelmsson, C., 446
Wilhemsen, L., 446
Willett, J. B., 302
Williams, C. L., 61, 116
Williams, J. B., 307
Williams, R. B., 444, 447
Williams, S., 438
Williams, W., 300
Wills, T. A., 281, 282, 438, 442
Wilson, E. O., 69, 70
Wilson, G., 469
Wilson, G. T., 281
Wilson, J., 309
Wilson, S., 454
Wilson, W., 436, 439, 454
Wimberly, S., 444
Wise, C. M., 439
Wish, E., 270, 283
Wittgenstein, L., 581
Wolfson, D., 246, 247–248
Wood, J. M., 135
Wood, J. V., 438, 443
Woods, T., 440, 442, 446
Woody, G. E., 291

Woolf, S., 435
Wortman, C., 442
Worzel, W., 614
Wright, J. C., 73
Wyshak, G., 450

Y

Yalom, I. D., 40
Yeates, E., 447
Yong, L., 307
Young, J., 468
Young, J. E., 129
Young, L. D., 439, 441

Z

Zachariah, P., 443
Zachary, R. A., 77
Zanarini, M. C., 307
Zanesco, L., 446
Zarski, J., 458
Zeiss, A. M., 310
Zeiss, R. A., 310, 311
Zich, J., 442
Ziegler, T. A., 517
Zimmerman, M., 307
Zook, A., 458
Zook, C. J., 452
Zuckerman, M., 438, 440, 442, 446
Zwaveling, A., 450
Zweig, R. A., 304, 313, 314

Subject Index

Abnormality, 409–410

Abstraction phase, 69–71, 552*t*, 553

Abuse, childhood, 109*f*, 511–512

Abusive Experiences scale, 567*t*

Academic Concerns scale, 567*t*

Acceptance, diagnosis and treatment of disease and, 441

Active orientation
  Millon College Counseling Inventory (MCCI) and, 555*t*
  overview, 551–552
  personality polarity model and, 70
  temperament and, 22

Active-dependent personality style, 531

Actively Modifying scale, 645*t*, 663

Active-passive (adaptation) polarity, 69–71, 114, 353, 552*t*, 553

Addictive disorders. *see also* Substance abuse
  case example of, 286–292, 287*t*
  couples treatment and, 349
  depressive personality and, 278–283
  employment functioning and, 277–278
  HIV risk behavior and, 275–277
  MCMI subgroup membership and, 271–272
  overview, 270–271, 292
  psychosocial interventions and, 449
  relapse and, 280–283
  treatment outcomes and, 274–275, 283–286
  treatment retention and, 272–274

Adolescent period, 494–495. *see also* Millon Adolescent Clinical Inventory (MACI)

Affect cluster, 145, 152

Affective conditions, organically based, 252–256

Affective examination, 245–252, 257

Aggressive pattern of personality, 197–198, 198*t*, 200–213, 202*t*, 203*t*, 206*t*, 207*t*, 209*t*, 210*t*, 212*t*

Aggressive personality. *see* Sadistic personality

Aging. *see also* Older adults
  assessment and, 303–305, 304*t*, 305*t*
  dementia and, 302–303
  overview, 296–297, 319–320
  personality theory and, 305–309, 306*t*–307*t*, 309*t*

Alcohol Abuse scale, 569*t*. *see also* Addictive disorders

Alcohol addiction, 272, 280–283. *see also* Addictive disorders

Alcohol Dependence scale. *see also* Addictive disorders
  couples treatment and, 349
  Danish MCMI-I and, 395*t*, 397*t*, 398*t*–399*t*, 400–402, 401*t*
  MCMI-III and, 87

Alcohol Use Inventory (AUI), 557. *see also* Addictive disorders

Alzheimer's dementia, 254–255

Ambivalent personality patterns, 531–532, 551

American Psychiatric Association, 425n

Anger Dyscontrol scale, 569t

Anger scale, 116

Antisocial personality. *see also* Antisocial personality disorder; Antisocial scale
  addictive disorders and, 284–286
  case example of, 187
  correctional settings and, 197–198, 198t, 199f, 200f
  couples treatment and, 352–354
  functional-structural domain and, 123t
  interpersonal style of, 29
  overview, 200–201
  temperament and, 22

Antisocial personality disorder. *see also* Antisocial personality; Antisocial scale
  correctional settings and, 201–205, 202t, 203t
  HIV risk behavior and, 275–277
  sadistic personality disorder and, 205–206
  Unruly scale and, 507

Antisocial personality scale, 88–89

Antisocial scale. *see also* Antisocial personality; Antisocial personality disorder
  borderline personality disorder and, 235
  correlations between the MMPI and the MCMI and, 160
  Danish MCMI-I and, 395t, 397t, 398t–399t, 400–402, 401t
  dependent personality disorder and, 225–226
  depressive personality disorder and, 216–217
  gender differences and, 238–239, 238f
  histrionic personality disorder and, 230–231
  masochistic personality disorder and, 228
  schizoid personality disorder and, 219
  sensitivity of, 417–418, 418t

Anxiety. *see also* Anxiety scale
  case example of, 92
  dependent personality disorder and, 225
  diagnosis and treatment of disease and, 440–441
  Dutch translation project and, 376
  treatment planning and, 334–335, 335f

Anxiety disorders, 22–23

Anxiety scale. *see also* Anxiety
  case example of, 183
  Danish MCMI-I and, 395t, 397t, 398t–399t, 400–402, 401t
  Dutch translation project and, 376

Anxiety/Fears scale, 533

Anxiety/Tension scale, 568t

Anxious Feelings scale, 513

Anxious/Hesitating scale, 646t

Appraisals
  diagnosis and treatment of disease and, 440, 445–446
  risk behaviors and, 439
  stress-related symptoms and, 438

Arthritis, rheumatoid, 441, 454

Artificial theoretical synthesis, 6–8

Asocial/Withdrawing scale, 646t

Assessment in general
  challenge of conceptualizing personality and, 330–332
  clinical science and, 53–55
  domain-oriented, 27–36
  expert testimony and, 179
  Facet Scales and, 127–128
  instrument construction and, 58–61
  managed care and, 158–161
  of medical patients, 456–477, 457f, 465t, 471f–475f
  older adults and, 303–305, 304t, 305t
  personology and, 688–695
  role of MCMI in the history of, 64–76
  theory and, 55–58, 329–330
  therapeutic planning and, 62–64
  understanding the level of, 332–333, 333f

Asthma, 454

Attachment, psychopathology and, 329–330

Attention Deficits scale, 533, 569t

Attention-deficit/hyperactivity disorder (ADHD), 256, 533

Attitudes, diagnosis and treatment of disease and, 445–446

Authentic self-realization, 32

Avoidance, diagnosis and treatment of disease and, 441

Avoidant personality. *see also* Avoidant personality disorder; Avoidant scale
  addictive disorders and, 279–280, 281–282
  compared to shyness, 410
  correctional settings and, 197–198, 198t, 199f, 200f
  couples treatment and, 352–354
  depressive personality and, 278, 279–280
  functional-structural domain and, 123t
  HIV risk behavior and, 276–277
  interpersonal style of, 29
  levels of interpretation with the MCMI-III and, 99
  older adults and, 308–309, 309t
  treatment planning and, 334–335, 335f

Avoidant personality disorder, 213–215, 214t, 215t, 505. *see also* Avoidant personality; Avoidant scale
Avoidant scale. *see also* Avoidant personality; Avoidant personality disorder
  antisocial personality disorder and, 202–203
  borderline personality disorder and, 235
  Danish MCMI-I and, 395t, 397t, 398t–399t, 400–402, 401t
  dependent personality disorder and, 225
  depressive personality disorder and, 216
  gender differences and, 238–239, 238f
  negativistic personality disorder and, 211
  overview, 88–89, 142
  schizoid personality disorder and, 219
  sensitivity of, 417–418, 418t
  treatment planning and, 334
Avoidant-Dependent personality style, 90, 92
Axis I clinical syndromes, case example of, 107f–108f, 109f–110f

B

Bariatric surgery, 469–470, 470–476, 471f–475f, 476–477
Base rate scores. *see* BR scores
Beck Depression Inventory-II (BDI-II), 557
Behaving Styles scales, 644t, 646t, 647
Behavioral activation, older adults and, 310
Behavioral assessment domain, 28
Belgian BR scores, 373–375, 382. *see also* Dutch translation project
Big Five Interpersonal Adjective Scales (IAS-B5), 613
Biological factors, 52
Biology, personality polarity model and, 69
Biosocial-learning theory, personality theory as, 113
Bipolar: Manic scale
  case example of, 150
  Danish MCMI-I and, 394, 395t, 397t, 398t–399t, 400–402, 401t
Bizarre Mentation (BIZ) scale, 116–117
Board of Trustees of the Society of Personality Assessment, 135–136
Body Disapproval scale, 510
Borderline personality. *see also* Borderline personality disorder; Borderline scale
  attachment and, 330
  correctional settings and, 199f
  couples treatment and, 354
  dimensional model and, 410

functional-structural domain and, 123t
interpersonal style of, 29
overview, 566t
treatment planning and, 335, 335–336
Borderline personality disorder. *see also* Borderline personality; Borderline scale
  Borderline tendency scale and, 509
  case example of, 142, 153
  correctional settings and, 197–198, 233–236
Borderline scale. *see also* Borderline personality; Borderline personality disorder
  case example of, 140, 142, 148, 183
  correlations between the MMPI and the MCMI and, 160–161
  Danish MCMI-I and, 395t, 397t, 398t–399t, 400–402, 401t
  levels of interpretation with the MCMI-III and, 100
  sensitivity of, 417–418, 418t
Borderline tendency scale, 500t, 509
BR scores
  Belgian BR scores and, 373–375, 382
  cross-examination traps and, 191
  Dutch translation project and, 370
  Facet Scales and, 124–125, 127
  Grossman Facet Scales and, 192–193
  MCMI-III and, 85–86
  Millon Adolescent Clinical Inventory (MACI) and, 497–498, 501
  overview, 97, 406, 681
  validity and, 412–413
Brain damage. *see also* Neuropsychological evaluation
  affective examination and, 245–252
  effects of on MCMI-II and MCMI-III results, 252–253
  emotional reactions to head trauma and, 259–260
  intentional deception and, 263–266
  organically based affective conditions and, 252–256
  rehabilitation and, 266
  schizophrenia and, 257–259

C

California Psychological Inventory (CPI), 75
Cancer, 439, 441, 450
Capacity for Control and Tolerance for Stress cluster, 144–145, 150–151

Career Confusion scale, 567t
Case conceptualization
  moving from theory to, 56
  multidimensional assessment and, 158
  older adults and, 312–314, 313t
  overview, 60–61
Catalytic sequences, 37–38, 41, 62
Categorical model, 23, 327, 422–425
Chaos theory, 331–332
Child custody evaluations, 191, 634–639, 638f
Child protective service consultation, 186–188
Childhood abuse, 109f
Childhood Abuse scale, 511–512
Classical test theory, 139
Classification system, 24–25, 66–67
Clinical judgment, 89, 245–246, 261
Clinical observation, instrument construction
  and, 61
Clinical pathways, 54
Clinical Personality Patterns
  case example of, 142, 148, 183, 187, 189
  cross-examination traps and, 191–192
  Grossman Facet Scales and, 193
  levels of interpretation with the MCMI-III
    and, 99–100
Clinical science, 53–55
Clinical Signs scales
  Millon College Counseling Inventory
    (MCCI) and, 555–556, 571
  overview, 549t, 550, 568t–569t
Clinical Syndrome scales
  case example of, 189
  cross-examination traps and, 191–192
  Dutch translation project and, 376
  MCMI-III and, 87, 138–139
  Millon Adolescent Clinical Inventory
    (MACI) and, 512–514
  overview, 124
  treatment planning and, 334
Clinical syndromes, 22–23, 157–158
Clinician-Administered PTSD Scale (CAPS),
  614–615
Closed-Mindedness factor, 664
Coding, profile validity of the MCMI-III and,
  86–87
Cognitive assessment domain, 30
Cognitive behavioral therapy (CBT), 309–312
Cognitive functioning, neuropsychological
  evaluation and, 251
Cognitive Mediation cluster, 144, 150
Cognitive modes, 30–31
Cognitive restructuring, diagnosis and
  treatment of disease and, 441

Cognitive style
  Millon Index of Personality Styles *Revised*
    (MIPS) and, 652–653, 654t
  overview, 114
  personality pattern attributes and, 123t
Cognitive Style/Content domain of the MG-
  PDC, 590f, 602
Cognitive therapies, 31
Cognitively Pessimistic scale, 124
Comorbid personality patterns
  antisocial personality disorder, 202–203,
    202t
  assessment and, 334
  avoidant personality disorder and, 213–214,
    214t
  compulsive personality disorder, 222–223, 223t
  dependent personality disorder, 225–226,
    225t
  depressive personality disorder, 216–217,
    216t
  histrionic personality disorder, 230–231, 230t
  masochistic personality disorder, 228, 228t
  narcissistic personality disorder, 209, 209t
  negativistic personality disorder, 212t
  older adults and, 301–302
  sadistic personality disorder, 205–206, 206t
  schizoid personality disorder, 218–219, 219t
Complex case consultation, 340–344, 343f
Complex syndromes, treatment goals and, 26–
  27
Compliant pattern of personality, 197–198,
  198t, 221–231, 223t, 224t, 225t, 227t,
  228t, 230t, 231t
Compulsive personality. see also Compulsive
  scale
  case example of, 382
  correctional settings and, 197–198, 198t,
    199f, 200f
  couples treatment and, 348, 353–354, 356
  depressive personality and, 278–279
  functional-structural domain and, 123t
  interpersonal style of, 29
  narcissistic personality disorder and, 209
Compulsive personality disorder, 221–224,
  223t, 224t
Compulsive personality scale, 88–89
Compulsive scale. see also Compulsive
  personality
  Belgian BR scores and, 375
  compulsive personality disorder and, 222
  correlations between the MMPI and the
    MCMI and, 160
  cross-examination traps and, 191–192

Danish MCMI-I and, 394, 395*t*, 397*t*, 398*t*–399*t*, 400–402, 401*t*

Dutch translation project and, 377–381, 379*t*, 380*t*, 381*t*

gender differences and, 238–240, 238*f*

histrionic personality disorder and, 230

sensitivity of, 417–418, 418*t*

Computer systems, guidelines for the use of the MCMI-III, 77–79

Conduct Problems scale, 533

Confident personality, 565*t*, 623–624

Confident scale, 531

Confident/Asserting scale, 646*t*

Confirmatory factor-analytic (CFA) methods, 122

Conforming scale, 500*t*, 508, 531–532

Conscientious personality, 565*t*–566*t*, 663

Conservation-Seeking scale, 646*t*

Construct validity. *see also* Validity

instrument and scale development and, 118–119

Millon Index of Personality Styles *Revised* (MIPS) and, 651–652

Millon Personality Diagnostic Checklist (MPDC) and, 583–584

overview, 412

Constructs, 115

Content scales in general, 114–117, 117–119, 119–126, 123*t*, 125*t*

Content validity, 194–195, 584. *see also* Validity

Contextual factors, 52

Conversion disorder, compared to malingering, 264

Coolidge Axis II Inventory (CATI), 306*t*

Cooperative personality, 620–622

Cooperative/Agreeing scale, 646*t*, 664

Coping skills

diagnosis and treatment of disease and, 439–447, 441–442

personality and, 445, 451

personality theory and, 551

psychosocial interventions and, 443–444

risk behaviors and, 439

social support and, 442

Coronary artery disease, 438

Correctional officers, personality and, 197–198, 198*t*

Correctional settings

aggressive pattern of personality and, 200–213, 202*t*, 203*t*, 206*t*, 207*t*, 209*t*, 210*t*, 212*t*

Colorado study of the MCMI-III in, 198–200, 199*f*, 200*f*

compliant pattern of personality and, 221–231, 223*t*, 224*t*, 225*t*, 227*t*, 228*t*, 230*t*, 231*t*

gender differences and, 237–241, 238*f*, 240*f*, 241*f*, 242*f*

personality and, 196–197, 197–198, 198*t*, 241–242

reserved pattern of personality and, 213–221, 214*t*, 215*t*, 216*t*, 217*t*, 219*t*, 221*t*

severe personality disorders and, 231–237

Couples treatment

case example of, 358–366, 359*f*, 361*f*, 362*f*, 363*f*

MCMI and, 350–355, 354–355

overview, 347–350, 366–367

therapeutic process and, 355–358

Criterion-related validity, 194–195

Cross-cultural considerations, 389, 402–403. *see also* Dutch translation project; Translation of the MCMI

Cross-examination traps, 190–192

Current Clinical Signs scales, 533–535

D

Danish MCMI-I. *see also* Dutch translation project; Translation of the MCMI

cross-cultural issues and, 402–403

factor analysis of, 400–402, 401*t*

psychometric properties of, 391–400, 392*t*, 393*t*, 394*t*, 395*t*, 396*t*, 397*t*, 398*t*–399*t*

Debasement scale

case example of, 90, 96–100, 102*f*–111*f*, 148, 187

Danish MCMI-I and, 394, 395*t*, 397*t*, 398*t*–399*t*, 400–402, 401*t*

Millon Adolescent Clinical Inventory (MACI) and, 504

Millon Behavioral Medicine Diagnostic (MBMD) and, 463

overview, 562–563

profile validity of the MCMI-III and, 87

Deception, intentional, 263–266

Deductive (rational, theoretical) method of construction, 118–119, 121

Defensive mechanisms, 40–41, 52

Dejected personality, 564*t*

Delinquent Predisposition scale, 513

Delusional Disorder scale

case example of, 93

Danish MCMI-I and, 395*t*, 397*t*, 398*t*–399*t*, 400–402, 401*t*

Dementia, 254–255, 302–303

Demographic factors, guidelines for the use of the MCMI-III, 77–78

Denial, diagnosis and treatment of disease and, 441

Denigrated personality, 566t

Dependent personality. see also Dependent personality disorder; Dependent scale
addictive disorders and, 282
case example of, 358–366, 359f, 361f, 362f, 363f
correctional settings and, 197–198, 198t, 199f, 200f
couples treatment and, 352–354
depression and, 5
functional-structural domain and, 123t
interpersonal style of, 29
overview, 551

Dependent personality disorder, 224–226, 225t, 227t, 506. see also Dependent personality; Dependent scale

Dependent scale. see also Dependent personality; Dependent personality disorder
case example of, 183, 185
correlations between the MMPI and the MCMI and, 160–161
Danish MCMI-I and, 394, 395t, 397t, 398t–399t, 400–402, 401t
gender differences and, 238–239, 238f
overview, 88–89, 142
sensitivity of, 417–418, 418t

Depression. see also Depressive personality; Depressive scale
case example of, 92
dementia vs., 254–255
dependent personality disorder and, 225
diagnosis and treatment of disease and, 440–441, 450–451
older adults and, 301, 309–310
personality domains and, 5

Depressive Affect scale, 513–514

Depressive Moods scale, 533–534

Depressive Outlook scale, 568t

Depressive personality. see also Depression; Depressive personality disorder; Depressive scale
addictive disorders and, 278–283
case example of, 142, 358–366, 359f, 361f, 362f, 363f
correctional settings and, 197–198, 198t, 199f, 200f
functional-structural domain and, 123t

Depressive personality disorder. see also Depression; Depressive personality; Depressive scale
correctional settings and, 215–218, 216t, 217t
Doleful scale and, 505–506
masochistic personality disorder and, 228

Depressive scale. see also Depression; Depressive personality; Depressive personality disorder
borderline personality disorder and, 235
case example of, 148
Danish MCMI-I and, 395t, 397t, 398t–399t, 400–402, 401t
dependent personality disorder and, 225
gender differences and, 238–239, 238f
masochistic personality disorder and, 228
overview, 92, 116–117, 124
sensitivity of, 417–418, 418t

Desirability scale
case example of, 187
Danish MCMI-I and, 394, 395t, 397t, 398t–399t, 400–402, 401t
Millon Adolescent Clinical Inventory (MACI) and, 503–504
Millon Behavioral Medicine Diagnostic (MBMD) and, 463
Millon College Counseling Inventory (MCCI) and, 562
profile validity of the MCMI-III and, 87

Detached personality, 551

Detached/ambivalent personality, 280, 281–282

Determinism, 51

Developmental framework, 552t

Diabetes
cognitive restructuring and, 441
Millon Behavioral Medicine Diagnostic (MBMD) and, 468–469
psychosocial factors in, 439
treatment success and recovery and, 453–454

Diagnosis
American Psychiatric Association and, 425n
case example of, 107f–108f, 109f–110f, 145, 337–340, 339f
couples treatment and, 349–350
criteria of, 22–23
Diagnostic and Statistical Manual of Mental Disorders (DSM), 36, 687–688
dimensional versus categorical debate and, 422–423

of disease, 439–447
expert testimony and, 180
Facet Scales and, 127–128
factorial structure and, 412
forensic evaluations and, 194–195
guidelines for the use of the MCMI-III, 78–79
idiographic tradition and, 57–58
instrument construction and, 61
integration of the MCMI with the MMPI and, 163–173, 174
interpretation with the MCMI-III and, 84–85, 97–99
issues regarding, 15–19
managed care and, 158–161, 174
MCMI and, 417–418, 418t
Millon Adolescent Clinical Inventory (MACI) and, 495, 497–498
Millon Personality Diagnostic Checklist (MPDC) and, 583–585
Millon-Grossman Personality Domains Checklist (MG-PDC) and, 582
older adults and, 304–305, 305t
overview, 157–158, 689–690, 693–695
personalized assessment and, 23–25, 36–43
Rorschach Comprehensive System and, 137–138
schizophrenia and, 257–259
therapeutic planning and, 63–64
treatment planning and, 336–337
Diagnostic and Statistical Manual of Mental Disorders (DSM)
Axis I of, 5
Belgian BR scores and, 373–374
case example of, 109f–110f
clinical science and, 53–54
couples treatment and, 349–350
depressive personality disorder and, 215–216
diagnosis and, 36, 687–688
Dutch translation project and, 380–381
evolutionary theory and, 22–23
expert testimony and, 180
Facet Scales and, 127–128
forensic evaluations and, 194–195
Grossman Facet Scales and, 113
guidelines for the use of the MCMI-III and, 84–85
history of the MCMI and, 67
idiographic tradition and, 57
instrument and scale development and, 60, 119
issues regarding, 15–19

levels of interpretation with the MCMI-III and, 97–98
managed care and, 159–160
Millon Adolescent Clinical Inventory (MACI) and, 495, 497–498
Millon College Counseling Inventory (MCCI) and, 571
Millon Pre-Adolescent Clinical Inventory (M-PACI) and, 530
negativistic personality disorder, 210–211
neuropsychological evaluation and, 263–266
older adults and, 305–309, 309t
overview, 157–158, 405–406, 679–680, 687–688, 689–690, 693–695
Personality Adjective Check List (PACL) and, 609
personality disorders and, 196–197
personality traits and, 682–683
personalized assessment and, 8, 23–25
posttraumatic stress disorder, 259
sadistic personality disorder, 205
therapeutic planning and, 63–64
Diagnostic Interview for DSM-IV Personality Disorders (DIPD-IV), 307t
Dialectical behavior therapy, older adults and, 310
Dimensional model
MCMI model and, 422–425
overview, 406–411, 407f, 408f, 409f, 410t
personalized assessment and, 23
Dimensional personality classification, 327
"Diminished capacity" defense, 182
Disagreeableness factor, 663–664
Disclosure scale
case example of, 187
Danish MCMI-I and, 395t, 397t, 398t–399t, 400–402, 401t
Millon Adolescent Clinical Inventory (MACI) and, 503
Millon Behavioral Medicine Diagnostic (MBMD) and, 463
Millon College Counseling Inventory (MCCI) and, 561–562
overview, 87, 90
Discordant personality, 551
Discriminant analysis, addictive disorders and, 272–273
Disease
complications and, 455
course of, 444–447
diagnosis of, 439–447
psychosocial interventions and, 443–444
treatment success and recovery and, 453–455

Disruptive Behaviors scale, 533

Dissatisfied/Complaining scale, 646*t*

Distribution of a test score, 414–415

Doleful scale, 500*t*, 505–506

Domain-oriented assessment and treatment, 27–36

Dominance versus Submissiveness, 420

Dominant/Controlling scale, 646*t*, 663

Dramatizing scale, 500*t*, 506

Drug Abuse scale, 569*t*

Drug addiction, 272, 280–283. *see also* Addictive disorders

Drug Dependence scale
  couples treatment and, 349
  Danish MCMI-I and, 395*t*, 397*t*, 398*t*–399*t*, 400–402, 401*t*
  MCMI-III and, 87

Dustbowl empiricism, 118

Dutch translation project. *see also* Danish MCMI-I; Translation of the MCMI
  Belgian BR scores and, 373–375
  case example of, 382–384
  construct equivalence with the original MCMI-III, 371–373, 372*t*
  convergent validity and, 375–377, 376*t*, 377*t*
  overview, 369–371

Dutiful/Conforming scale, 646*t*, 663, 664

Dysthymia clinical scale
  case example of, 92
  Danish MCMI-I and, 395*t*, 397*t*, 398*t*–399*t*, 400–402, 401*t*
  Dutch translation project and, 376
  overview, 124

E

Eating disorder, 109*f*

Eating Disorders scale, 568*t*–569*t*

Eating Dysfunctions scale, 512

Eclecticism, 20

Ecological-motivational theory, 113–114, 331–332

Economic resources, risk behaviors and, 439

Education, professional, 77, 84–85

Egocentricity index, 152–153

Egotistic scale, 500*t*, 506–507

Emerging Personality Patterns scales, 530–533, 531*f*

Emotional functioning, 109*f*, 168, 170–171, 172–173, 251

Emotionality, lifespan perspective of, 297–298

Emotionality versus Restraint dimension, 420

Empathy, couples treatment and, 356

Employment functioning, 277–278, 655–660

Employment screening, 634–639, 638*f*, 655–660

Evolutionary theory
  Facet Scales and, 127
  history of the MCMI and, 67–69
  Millon College Counseling Inventory (MCCI) and, 552–553, 552*t*
  Millon-Grossman Personality Domains Checklist (MG-PDC) and, 580
  overview, 20–23, 406, 686–687
  personality and, 63, 69–71, 114
  personalized psychotherapy and, 25–26
  therapeutic planning and, 64

Existence phase, 69–71, 552*t*, 553

Expert testimony
  case example of, 181–190, 184*f*
  cross-examination traps and, 190–192
  Grossman Facet Scales and, 192–194
  overview, 177–181

Expressed Concerns scales
  Millon Adolescent Clinical Inventory (MACI) and, 509–512
  Millon College Counseling Inventory (MCCI) and, 555–556, 570–571
  overview, 549*t*, 550, 567*t*–568*t*

Expressive Behavior domain of the MG-PDC, 588*f*, 597–598, 602

Expressive behaviors, 28, 114, 123*t*

External (criterion group) method of construction, 118–119

External/criterion validation
  Millon Pre-Adolescent Clinical Inventory (M-PACI) and, 540–543, 540*t*, 542*t*
  overview, 71–72, 74–76, 684–685

Externally Focused scale, 645*t*, 663

Extraversion factor, 663

F

Facet Scales. *see* Grossman Facet Scales

Factitious disorder, neuropsychological evaluation and, 263–264

Factor analysis
  of the Danish MCMI-I, 400–402, 401*t*
  Facet Scales and, 122, 124
  nomothetic tradition and, 51

Factorial structure
  of the Millon Index of Personality Styles *Revised* (MIPS), 660–664, 662*t*
  overview, 117, 411–422, 416*f*, 418*t*, 421*t*

Familial resources, risk behaviors and, 439
Family Discord scale, 115, 511
Family Disquiet scale, 567t
Family dysfunction, content scales and, 115
Family systems, 334, 351
Feedback mechanisms, challenge of
    conceptualizing personality and, 331–332
Feeling-Guided scale, 646t, 663–664
Financial Burdens scale, 568t
Fitness-for-duty determination, 634–639, 638f,
    657–658
Five-factor model of personality
    instrument and scale development and, 118
    Millon Index of Personality Styles *Revised*
        (MIPS) and, 661, 662–664
    overview, 580
    Personality Adjective Check List (PACL)
        and, 613
Forceful personality, 624–626
Forceful scale, 500t, 507–508
Forensic psychology
    case example of, 181–190, 184f
    content validity and, 194–195
    cross-examination traps and, 190–192
    Grossman Facet Scales and, 192–194
    overview, 177–181
Functional domains of personality, 410t
Functional-structural domain, personality
    pattern attributes by, 123t

G

Gender differences
    addictive disorders and, 279
    correctional settings and, 237–241, 238f,
        240f, 241f, 242f
    depressive personality and, 279
    Millon Behavioral Medicine Diagnostic
        (MBMD) and, 466
    Millon Index of Personality Styles *Revised*
        (MIPS) and, 661
Genetic traits, 68–69
Glasgow Coma Scale, 253–254
Glucose control, 438, 468–469
Gregarious/Outgoing scale, 646t, 663
Grossman Facet Scales
    assessment and, 127–128
    case example of, 129–131, 360, 361f, 363f
    couples treatment and, 352
    deductive methodology and, 113–114
    development of, 119–126, 123t, 125t
    factorial structure and, 117

in forensic cases, 192–194
instrument and scale development and,
    117–119
Millon Adolescent Clinical Inventory
    (MACI) and, 498–499, 504–509
overview, 112–113, 125t, 126–127, 131,
    192–193, 418–419, 420–421, 421t, 500t
procedural considerations and, 119–126,
    123t, 125t
treatment planning and intervention and,
    128–131
Grossman Personality Facet Scales, 107f
Guidelines for MCMI-III use, 76–79

H

Halstead-Reitan Battery (HRB), 248
Halstead-Russell Neuropsychological
    Evaluation System-Revised (HRNES-R),
    249
Harris-Lingoes subscales, 115–116
Health care, 433–434, 433–456, 447–456. *see
    also* Managed care
Health preoccupation, 108f–109f
Health psychology, 434
Helplessness, diagnosis and treatment of
    disease and, 441–442
Help-seeking behaviors, psychosocial factors
    in, 437
Heterogeneity, therapeutic planning and, 63
Historical traditions, in personology, 50–53
History of the MCMI, 64–76, 113–114, 114–
    117
Histrionic personality. *see also* Histrionic
    personality disorder; Histrionic scale
    correctional settings and, 197–198, 198t,
        199f, 200f
    couples treatment and, 354, 356
    depressive personality and, 278–279
    functional-structural domain and, 123t
    interpersonal style of, 29
    neuropsychological evaluation and, 261
    overview, 122
Histrionic personality disorder, 229–231,
    230t, 231t, 506. *see also* Histrionic
    personality; Histrionic scale
Histrionic scale. *see also* Histrionic personality;
    Histrionic personality disorder
    avoidant personality disorder and, 214
    compulsive personality disorder and, 222–223
    correlations between the MMPI and the
        MCMI and, 160–161

Histrionic scale *(cont.)*
  cross-examination traps and, 191–192
  Danish MCMI-I and, 394, 395*t*, 397*t*,
    398*t*–399*t*, 400–402, 401*t*
  depressive personality disorder and, 217
  gender differences and, 238–239, 238*f*
  overview, 88–89
  sensitivity of, 417–418, 418*t*
HIV infection, 460–461, 466–468
HIV risk behavior, 275–277
Hospitalization, managed care and, 159
HPV infection, 459–460
Hypertension, 438, 441

I

Ideation cluster, 150
Identity Diffusion scale, 510
Identity Quandaries scale, 567*t*
Idiographic tradition
  assessment of the individual and, 57–58
  instrument construction and, 61
  nomothetic tradition and, 53
  overview, 50, 52–53
  therapeutic planning and, 63–64
Imaginative/Intuiting scale, 645*t*
Immature Representations subscale
    (Dependent), 194
Immune system functioning, psychosocial
    factors in, 438
Impulses, 52, 533
Impulsive Propensity scale, 513
Independent personality, 551
Individuality, 51, 52–53, 57
Inductive (internal consistency or itemic)
    method of construction, 118–119
Information Processing cluster, 144, 150
Inhibited personality, 564*t*, 619–620
Inhibited scale, 500*t*, 505, 532
Innovation-Seeking scale, 646*t*
Insanity defense, 182
Instrumentation
  construction of, 58–61, 117–119, 683–
    688
  overview, 9, 679–688
  understanding the level of, 332–333, 333*f*
Insurance, diagnosis and, 158–161
Integrated science, 54–55
Integrative model
  evolutionary theory and, 26
  integrating the MMPI and the MCMI and,
    161–163

Millon Personality Diagnostic Checklist
    (MPDC) and, 586–587
Millon-Grossman Personality Domains
    Checklist (MG-PDC) and, 598–600
  overview, 6–8
  philosophical issues with, 8–10
Interaction, system transactions and, 40–42
Internal consistency, 73, 414, 684–685
Internally Focused scale, 645*t*, 663
Internal/structural validation, 71
International Association of Cross-Cultural
    Psychology, 388–389
International Personality Disorder
    Examination (IPDE), 307*t*
International Test Commission, 388–389
International Union of Psychological Science,
    388–389
Interpersonal alienation, 109*f*
Interpersonal assessment domain, 29–30
Interpersonal behavior, 28–30, 166–168, 169–
    170, 172
Interpersonal conduct, 114, 123*t*
Interpersonal Conduct domain of the MG-
    PDC, 589*f*, 602
Interpersonal Perception cluster, 145, 146,
    153
Interpersonal theory, 13, 29–30
Interpersonal therapies, 29, 29–30, 310
Interpretation of assessment results
  case example of, 100–101, 102*f*–111*f*
  errors in, 97
  guidelines for the use of the MCMI-III, 77–
    79
  idiographic tradition and, 58
  levels of interpretation with the MCMI-III
    and, 96–100
  Millon Index of Personality Styles *Revised*
    (MIPS) and, 648
Interventions. *see also* Psychosocial
    interventions; Treatment planning
  case example of, 129–131
  clinical science and, 53–55
  Facet Scales and, 128–131
  Millon-Grossman Personality Domains
    Checklist (MG-PDC) and, 598–600
  overview, 9–10, 689, 691
Intrapsychic assessment domains, 33–34
Intrapsychic Content domain of the MG-PDC,
    594*f*, 602
Intrapsychic Mechanisms domain of the MG-
    PDC, 593*f*, 602
Intrapsychic objects, mechanisms, and
    morphology, 32–35

Intrapsychic Structure domain of the MG-
PDC, 595*f*, 602
Intrapsychic therapies, 34–35
Introversion scale, 500*t*, 505
Introversion versus Extraversion dimension, 420
Introverted personality, 564*t*, 618–619
Inventory of General Position Requirements
(IGPR), 656–657
Inventory of Interpersonal Problems, 613
IQ testing, brain damage and, 249

K

Klecksographie game, 138

L

Learning disabilities, neuropsychological
evaluation and, 256
Lifespan psychology, 297–298, 298–302, 299*t*.
see also Older adults
Lifestyle behaviors, diagnosis and treatment of
disease and, 446–447, 452
Living Arrangement Problems scale, 568*t*
Logical positivism, 60

M

MACI. *see* Millon Adolescent Clinical
Inventory (MACI)
Major Depression clinical scale. *see also*
Depressive scale
case example of, 92
Danish MCMI-I and, 394, 395*t*, 397*t*,
398*t*–399*t*, 400–402, 401*t*
Dutch translation project and, 376
Maladaptation factor, 663
Malingering, neuropsychological evaluation
and, 261, 264–266
Managed care, 158–161, 174, 434, 447–456.
see also Health care
Marital therapy. *see* Couples treatment
Masochistic personality. *see also* Masochistic
personality disorder; Masochistic scale
correctional settings and, 197–198, 198*t*,
199*f*, 200*f*
functional-structural domain and, 123*t*
Masochistic personality disorder, 227–229,
228*t*, 508–509. *see also* Masochistic
personality; Masochistic scale

Masochistic scale. *see also* Masochistic
personality; Masochistic personality
disorder
case example of, 148
Danish MCMI-I and, 394, 395*t*, 397*t*,
398*t*–399*t*, 400–402, 401*t*
gender differences and, 238–240, 238*f*
sensitivity of, 417–418, 418*t*
MCCI Interpretive Report, 571–572
MCMI. *see also* MCMI-III
addictive disorders and, 274–275
administration of, 350–351
affective examination and, 248–249
compared to the PACL, 615–617, 616*t*
correlations between the MMPI scales and,
159–161
couples treatment and, 350–355
diagnosis and, 158–161
dimensional versus categorical debate and,
422–425
factorial structure and, 117
integration of with the MMPI, 161–163,
163–173
interpretation of results from, 351–355
overview, 158
Rorschach Comprehensive System and,
136–137
MCMI-II, factorial structure and, 117
MCMI-III. *see also* Grossman Facet Scales;
individual scales; MCMI
affective examination and, 248–252
case example of, 90–93, 91*t*, 100–101,
102*f*–111*f*, 139–154, 141*f*, 143*f*, 149*f*,
151*f*
clinical syndrome scales, 87
compared to the PACL, 616*t*
couples treatment and, 350–355
deductive methodology and, 113–114
expert testimony and, 180–181
Facet Scales and, 119–126, 123*t*, 125–126,
125*t*
factorial structure and, 117
guidelines for the use of, 76–79, 83–85
instrument and scale development and,
117–119
integration of with the Rorschach, 135–139,
139–154, 141*t*, 143*t*, 149*t*, 151*t*, 154
interpretation of, 83–85
levels of interpretation with, 96–100
nature and purpose of, 137–139
neuropsychological evaluation and, 251–266
overview, 85–86, 112–113, 306*t*, 405–406
profile validity of, 86–87

MCMI-III *(cont.)*
  psychometric properties of, 135–136
  Rorschach Comprehensive System and,
    136–137
  scales for personality styles/disorders, 87–89
  treatment planning and, 333–337, 335*f*
MCMI-III interpretation model, 83–85
MCMI-MMPI battery, 161–163, 163–173,
  173–174
Medical illnesses, personality disorders and,
  98
Medical model, 42–43
Mental Health Upset scale, 567*t*
Mental state, expert testimony and, 181–186,
  184*f*
Millon Adolescent Clinical Inventory (MACI).
  see also Grossman Facet Scales
  administration and scoring of, 499–501,
    500*t*
  applications and limitations of, 495–497
  case example of, 520–521, 522*f*–527*f*
  Clinical Syndrome Scales and, 512–514
  deductive methodology and, 113–114
  development of, 497–499
  Expressed Concerns scales, 509–512
  Facet Scales and, 119–126, 123*t*, 125*t*,
    126–127, 126*t*
  factorial structure and, 117
  integrating the profile from, 514–515
  interpretation of, 501–502, 515–516
  Modifying Indices and response styles of,
    502–504
  overview, 76, 112–113, 494–495, 517, 683
  Personality Pattern scales, 504–509
  research regarding, 516–517
Millon Behavioral Medicine Diagnostic
  (MBMD)
  case example of, 470–476, 471*f*–475*f*
  development of, 463
  overview, 76, 306*t*, 456–477, 457*f*, 465*t*,
    471*f*–475*f*, 477–478
  psychosocial factors in health preservation
    and health care delivery, 433–456
  research regarding, 463–470, 465*t*
  secondary prevention and, 461–462
  use of in assessing adjustment to disease,
    461–462
  use of in health preservation, 458–461
  use of with medical patients, 458
Millon Clinical Multiaxial Inventory. *see*
  MCMI; MCMI-III
Millon Clinical Multiaxial Inventory - III,
  103*f*–105*f*, 679–688

Millon College Counseling Inventory (MCCI)
  administration and scoring of, 558–559
  case example of, 572–577, 574*f*, 576*f*
  construction and validation of, 556–557
  development of, 550
  interpretation of, 559–572, 564*t*–569*t*
  overview, 548–550, 549*t*, 578
  recommendations for the use of, 558
  theory and, 550–556, 552*t*, 555*t*
Millon Index of Personality Styles *Revised*
  (MIPS)
  applications of, 647–648
  case example of, 671–675, 673*f*–675*f*
  cognitive modes, 652–653, 654*t*
  couples treatment and, 366–367
  dimensions of normality and, 664–667
  factorial structure of, 660–664, 662*t*
  future research regarding, 668–669
  interpretative reports from, 648
  organizational research and, 655–660
  overview, 76, 306*t*, 643, 686–687
  personality style scales and, 643–647, 644*t*,
    645*t*–646*t*
  technical characteristics of, 648–652
Millon Personality Diagnostic Checklist
  (MPDC), 583–585
Millon Pre-Adolescent Clinical Inventory (M-
  PACI)
  case example of, 543–545, 544*f*
  Current Clinical Signs scales and, 533–535
  development and validation of, 535–543,
    538*t*, 539*t*, 540*t*, 542*t*
  Emerging Personality Patterns scales and,
    530–533, 531*f*
  overview, 528–530, 529*t*, 545–547
Millon-Grossman Personality Domains
  Checklist (MG-PDC), 588*f*–596*f*
  case example of, 600–602
  development of, 585–587
  domain/tactical therapeutic options and,
    598–600
  history of, 581–585
  Millon Personality Diagnostic Checklist
    (MPDC) and, 583–585
  overview, 580–581, 587–588, 588*f*–596*f*, 603
  use of, 587–588, 588*f*–596*f*
Millon-Illinois Self-Report Inventory (MI-SRI), 65
Minnesota Multiphasic Personality Inventory
  (MMPI)
  content scales and, 115–116
  correlations between the MCMI scales and,
    159–161
  criticism of, 247

diagnosis and, 158–161
instrument construction and, 59–61, 118
integration of with the MCMI, 161–163,
    163–173
overview, 61, 158, 387
Personality Adjective Check List (PACL)
    and, 613
profile validity of the MCMI-III and, 87
Rorschach Comprehensive System and,
    136–137
schizoid personality and, 99
subscales for, 113
Minnesota Multiphasic Personality Inventory-
    2 (MMPI-2)
    compared to the MCMI-III, 139
    content scales and subscales, 115
    criticism of, 247
    Dutch translation project and, 375–376
    overview, 306t
    Rorschach Comprehensive System and,
        136–137
MMPI. *see* Minnesota Multiphasic Personality
    Inventory (MMPI)
MMPI DSM-III personality disorder scales,
    116
MMPI-2. *see* Minnesota Multiphasic
    Personality Inventory-2 (MMPI-2)
Moderate Personality Disorder Scales/Clinical
    Personality Patterns
    levels of interpretation with the MCMI-III
        and, 96
    MCMI-III and, 87–89
    personality style scales and, 89
Modifying Indices, 189, 502–504
Mood, 35–36
Mood assessment domain, 35
Mood disorder, organic, 253–254
Mood therapies, 35–36
Mood/Affect domain of the MG-PDC, 592f,
    602
Mood/temperament, 114, 123t
Morbidity of certain diseases, psychosocial
    factors and, 444–447
Morphological organization
    case example of, 140, 142
    overview, 33–34, 114
    personality pattern attributes and, 123t
Mortality of certain diseases, psychosocial
    factors and, 444–447
Motivating Styles scales, 644, 644t, 645t
M-PACI. *see* Millon Pre-Adolescent Clinical
    Inventory (M-PACI)
Multimodal therapy, 20

N

Narcissistic personality. *see also* Narcissistic
    personality disorder; Narcissistic scale
    addictive disorders and, 284–286
    case example of, 152–153, 187
    correctional settings and, 197–198, 198t,
        199f, 200f
    couples treatment and, 352–354
    depression and, 5, 278–279
    functional-structural domain and, 123t
    interpersonal style of, 29
    overview, 200–201
    temperament and, 21–22
Narcissistic personality disorder. *see also*
    Narcissistic personality; Narcissistic
    scale
    correctional settings and, 207–210, 209t,
        210t
    Egotistic scale and, 506–507
    sadistic personality disorder and, 206
Narcissistic scale. *see also* Narcissistic
    personality; Narcissistic personality
    disorder
    antisocial personality disorder and, 202
    avoidant personality disorder and, 214
    compulsive personality disorder and, 223
    correlations between the MMPI and the
        MCMI and, 160–161
    cross-examination traps and, 191–192
    Danish MCMI-I and, 394, 395t, 397t,
        398t–399t, 400–402, 401t
    dependent personality disorder and, 226
    gender differences and, 238–239, 238f
    histrionic personality disorder and, 230
    levels of interpretation with the MCMI-III
        and, 100
    overview, 88–89
    sensitivity of, 417–418, 418t
National Comprehensive Cancer Network
    (NCCN), 450
Natural theoretical synthesis, 6–8
Needy personality, 564t–565t
Negativistic personality. *see also* Negativistic
    personality disorder; Negativistic scale;
    Passive-aggressive personality
    correctional settings and, 197–198, 198t,
        199f, 200f
    couples treatment and, 354
    functional-structural domain and, 123t
    interpersonal style of, 29
    overview, 200–201
    sadistic personality disorder and, 206

Negativistic personality disorder, 210–213,
    212t, 508. see also Negativistic
    personality; Negativistic scale
Negativistic scale. see also Negativistic
    personality; Negativistic personality disorder
  borderline personality disorder and, 235
  case example of, 148
  Danish MCMI-I and, 395t, 397t, 398t–
    399t, 400–402, 401t
  depressive personality disorder and, 217
  gender differences and, 238–240, 238f
  negativistic personality disorder and, 211
  overview, 88–89
  sensitivity of, 417–418, 418t
NEO Personality Inventory-Revised (NEO-PI-R)
  compared to the MCMI-III, 139
  overview, 61, 306t
  Personality Adjective Check List (PACL)
    and, 613
Neoplastic changes in tissue, psychosocial
    factors in, 438
Neurobiological model, 13
Neuropsychological evaluation
  affective examination and, 245–252
  future research regarding, 266–267
  intentional deception and, 263–266
  MCMI-III and, 251–266
  organically based affective conditions and,
    252–256
  purposes of, 244–245
  rehabilitation and, 266
  schizophrenia and, 257–259
  somatic symptoms and, 260–263
Neuroticism factor, 663
Nomothetic tradition
  assessment of the individual and, 55–57
  idiographic tradition and, 53
  instrument construction and, 59–61
  overview, 50, 51–52
  therapeutic planning and, 62–63
Normality, 409–410, 553–554, 610–611, 664–
    667
Nosology, 9, 61

O

Object relations, 33
Object representations, 114, 123t
Objective tests, affective examination and,
    246–247
Objectivity, history of the MCMI and, 67
Oblique rotation method, 124

Observation, clinical, 61
Obsessions/Compulsions scale, 533, 569t
Obsessive-compulsive personality disorder,
    508, 533. see also Compulsive personality
    disorder
Office training program, 197–198, 198t
Older adults. see also Aging
  assessment and, 303–305, 304t, 305t
  case example of, 314–319, 317t, 318f
  comorbidities and, 301–302
  dementia and, 302–303
  overview, 296–297, 319–320
  personality disorders and, 298–302, 299t
  personality theory and, 297–298, 305–309,
    306t–307t, 309t
  treatment and, 309–312, 311t, 312–314,
    313t, 315t–316t
Oppositional personality, 566t
Oppositional scale, 500t, 508
Organically based affective conditions, 252–256
Organicism, 10–12
Organizational research, 655–660
Other-Nurturing scale, 645t, 663–664
Outgoing scale, 531

P

Pain-Avoiding scale, 645t, 663
Pain-pleasure (survival) polarity, 114. see also
    Survival phase
Parallel behavior therapies, 28
Parallel cognitive therapies, 31
Parallel interpersonal therapies, 29–30
Parallel intrapsychic therapies, 34–35
Parallel mood/temperament therapies, 35–36
Parallel self-image therapies, 32
Paranoid personality. see also Paranoid
    personality disorder; Paranoid scale
  correctional settings and, 199f
  dimensional model and, 410
  functional-structural domain and, 123t
  interpersonal style of, 29
  levels of interpretation with the MCMI-III
    and, 99
Paranoid personality disorder, 197–198, 236–
    237. see also Paranoid personality;
    Paranoid scale
Paranoid scale. see also Paranoid personality;
    Paranoid personality disorder
  case example of, 140, 142, 183
  correlations between the MMPI and the
    MCMI and, 160

Danish MCMI-I and, 394, 395*t*, 397*t*, 398*t*–399*t*, 400–402, 401*t*
    levels of interpretation with the MCMI-III and, 100
    sensitivity of, 417–418, 418*t*
Parasuicide behavior, borderline personality disorder and, 234
Part functions, nomothetic tradition and, 51
Passive orientation
    Millon College Counseling Inventory (MCCI) and, 555*t*
    overview, 551–552
    personality polarity model and, 70
    temperament and, 21–22
Passive pleasure style, 666–667
Passive-aggressive personality. *see also* Negativistic personality; Passive-Aggressive scale
    addictive disorders and, 279–280
    case example of, 148
    depressive personality and, 279–280
    interpersonal style of, 29
Passive-Aggressive scale, 160–161. *see also* Passive-aggressive personality
Passive-ambivalent personality style, 531–532
Passive-independent personality style, 531
Passively Accommodating scale, 645*t*, 663
Pathogenic processes, 26–27
Pathology. *see* Psychopathology in general
Pearson Assessments, 76, 86–87, 89
Peer Alienation scale, 567*t*
Peer Insecurity scale, 511
Perceptual Thinking Index (PTI), 142, 144
Personality Adjective Check List (PACL)
    applications of, 629–639, 633*f*, 638*f*
    case example of, 631–634, 633*f*, 636–639, 638*f*
    compared to the MCMI, 615–617, 616*t*
    development of, 611–612
    linking normality and pathology with, 610–611
    overview, 306*t*, 609, 639
    personality styles and, 617–629
    research regarding, 612–615
    theoretical foundation of, 610
    T-scores and, 615
Personality Diagnostic Questionnaire-Fourth Edition Plus (PDQ-4+), 306*t*
Personality Disorder Interview-IV (PDI-IV), 307*t*
Personality disorders. *see also specific personality disorders*
    assessment of, 680–682
    case example of, 110*f*, 153

comorbid psychiatric conditions and, 301–302
correctional settings and, 196–197, 231–237
couples treatment and, 348, 354
epidemiology of, 299–301
expert testimony and, 180, 181–186, 184*f*
gender differences and, 237–241, 238*f*, 240*f*, 241*f*, 242*f*
HIV risk behavior and, 275–277
integration of the MCMI with the MMPI and, 162
lifespan perspective of, 298–302, 299*t*
MCMI-III and, 68, 78, 84, 87–89, 97–98
Millon Personality Diagnostic Checklist (MPDC) and, 584–585
neuropsychological evaluation and, 251
nomothetic tradition and, 56
overview, 157–158
personality polarity model and, 69–71
therapeutic planning and, 62–64
treatment and, 312–314, 313*t*, 315*t*–316*t*
Personality domains, 4–5, 27–36, 64
Personality in general
    assessment and, 6, 12–13, 55, 334–336, 335*f*
    challenge of conceptualizing, 330–332
    clinical science and, 53–55
    coping style and, 441–442, 445, 451
    correctional settings and, 196–197
    evolutionary theory and, 406
    gender differences and, 237–241, 238*f*, 240*f*, 241*f*, 242*f*
    history of the MCMI and, 50–53, 68
    lifespan perspective of, 297–298
    MCMI-III and, 139
    overview, 62
    personology and, 688–695
    theory and, 329–330
    treatment planning and, 62–63, 334–336, 335*f*
Personality Pattern scales, 504–509
Personality patterns, 106*f*–107*f*, 123*t*. *see also* Comorbid personality patterns; Personality styles
Personality polarity model, 69–71
Personality prototypes, 23–25, 426*n*
Personality psychology, aging and, 297–298
Personality styles. *see also specific styles*
    addictive disorders and, 272–274
    evolutionary theory and, 22–23
    Facet Scales and, 121–122
    integration of the MCMI with the MMPI and, 162

Personality styles *(cont.)*
  lifespan perspective of, 297–298
  MCMI-III scales for, 87–89
  Millon College Counseling Inventory
      (MCCI) and, 554–555, 555*t*, 563–570,
      564*t*–569*t*
  Millon Index of Personality Styles *Revised*
      (MIPS) and, 643–647, 644*t*, 645*t*–646*t*
  neuropsychological evaluation and, 251
  overview, 564*t*–569*t*
  Personality Adjective Check List (PACL)
      and, 617–629
Personality Styles scales
  case example of, 90–93, 91*t*
  overview, 88–89, 548, 549*t*, 564*t*–569*t*
Personality subtypes. *see also specific subtypes*
  addictive disorders and, 271–272
  assessment of, 680–682
  evolutionary theory and, 22
  overview, 426*n*
Personality system, system transactions and,
      40–41
Personality taxonomy, dimensional model and,
      406–411, 407*f*, 408*f*, 409*f*, 410*t*
Personality theory
  history of, 113–114
  integration of the MCMI with the MMPI
      and, 162–163
  Millon College Counseling Inventory
      (MCCI) and, 551–552, 552*t*
  Millon Pre-Adolescent Clinical Inventory
      (M-PACI) and, 535
  older adults and, 305–309, 306*t*–307*t*, 309*t*
  overview, 196, 688–695
Personality-guided therapy, 328–329, 348–349
Personalized assessment, 23–25, 36–43
Personalized psychotherapy. *see also*
      Treatment
  case example of, 129–131
  clinical constructs and, 25–26
  evolutionary theory and, 25–26
  Facet Scales and, 129
  overview, 19, 43
  theory and, 20–25, 329–330
Person-focused systems model, 41
Personological bifurcations, 21–22
Personology
  Facet Scales and, 121–122
  historical traditions in, 50–53
  Millon-Grossman Personality Domains
      Checklist (MG-PDC) and, 581
  overview, 52–53, 688–695
  treatment planning and, 327–329

Pharmacotherapy, 35–36, 310
Philosophical issues, 8–10
Planning, therapeutic. *see* Therapeutic
      planning
Pleasure-Enhancing scale, 645*t*, 663
Pleasure-pain polarity, 70
Polarity model, 21, 39, 114, 353–354, 687
Polythetic structural model, 73–74
Positive predictive power, 417
Positive reframing, diagnosis and treatment of
      disease and, 441
Postconcussive syndrome, 253
Posttraumatic stress disorder, 259–260, 614–
      615
Post-Traumatic Stress disorder scale
  Belgian BR scores and, 375
  case example of, 93
  Danish MCMI-I and, 394, 395*t*, 397*t*,
      398*t*–399*t*, 400–402, 401*t*
  Dutch translation project and, 376, 381
  MCMI-III and, 87
  neuropsychological evaluation and, 251
  overview, 568*t*
Posttraumatic symptoms, 383–384
Potential parings, 38, 41
Pragmatic model, external/criterion validation
      and, 75–76
Prevention, 435–447, 461–462
Primary prevention, 435–447
Prison personalities, 197–198, 198*t*
Problem Indicator scale, 629
Process of assessment, 9–13
Professional boards, evaluations for, 188–
      190
Professional training/background, 77, 84–85
Profile Report, examples of, 141*f*, 148, 149*f*,
      184*f*, 339*f*, 343*f*, 359*f*, 362*f*, 471*f*–475*f*,
      522*f*–527*f*, 544*f*, 574*t*, 576*f*, 673*f*–675*f*
Projective assessment, 328
Projective drawings, expert testimony and,
      179
Prototypal model, 23, 327
Psychiatric labels, diagnostic system and, 16–
      17
Psychic DNA, 4
Psychodynamic Character Inventory, 85
Psychodynamic foundation, 54
Psychological adjustment, 657–658
Psychological theory, 69–70
Psychometric properties, 135–136
Psychometric testing, expert testimony and,
      179–180
Psychopathic Deviate scale, 115

Psychopathology in general
clinical science and, 53–54
evolutionary theory and, 406
MCMI-III and, 139
neuropsychological evaluation and, 251
overview, 6, 553–554, 610–611
personalized assessment and, 12–13, 26, 36–43
personalized psychotherapy and, 19
theory and, 20–25, 329–330
Psychosis, Rorschach Comprehensive System and, 138
Psychosocial interventions, 443–444, 447, 452. *see also* Interventions
Psychotherapy, theory and, 329–330. *see also* Treatment

R

Realistic/Sensing scale, 645*t*, 664
Reality Distortions scale, 535
Receiver operating characteristics (ROC) curve analyses, 374–375
Regulatory mechanisms, 33, 114, 123*t*
Rehabilitation, neuropsychological evaluation and, 266
Relapse, substance use, 280–283
Relational conduct, 28–30
Relational matrix, 366
Relational personality classification, 327
Relationships, 29–30, 331–332
Reliability
Millon Index of Personality Styles *Revised* (MIPS) and, 651
Millon Pre-Adolescent Clinical Inventory (M-PACI) and, 538–539, 538*t*
overview, 411–422, 416*f*, 418*t*, 421*t*
Reliability scale, 502–503
Religiosity, diagnosis and treatment of disease and, 442, 446
Replication phase, 69–71, 114, 552*t*, 553. *see also* Self-other polarity
Report writing, 84–85
Reports, clinical, 76–77, 102*f*–111*f*
Reserved pattern of personality, 197–198, 198*t*, 213–221, 214*t*, 215*t*, 216*t*, 217*t*, 219*t*, 221*t*
Resistance, defensive mechanisms and, 40–41
Respectful personality, 626–627
Response style, 106*f*, 560–563, 612
Response Tendencies scales, 549*t*, 557
Rheumatoid arthritis, 441, 454

Risk assessment, 186–190
Risk behaviors, 275–277, 436–437, 439
Risk factors, stress-related symptoms and, 437–438
ROC curve analyses. *see* Receiver operating characteristics (ROC) curve analyses
Romantic Distress scale, 567*t*
Rorschach Comprehensive System
case example of, 139–154, 141*f*, 143*f*, 149*f*, 151*f*
clinical science and, 54
expert testimony and, 179
instrument construction and, 59–60
integration of with MCMI-III, 135–139, 139–154, 141*t*, 143*t*, 149*t*, 151*t*, 154
multidimensional assessment and, 158
nature and purpose of, 137–139
overview, 137–138
psychometric properties of, 135–136
relationship of the Millon inventories and the MMPI to, 136–137

S

Sadistic personality. *see also* Sadistic personality disorder; Sadistic scale
correctional settings and, 197–198, 198*t*, 199*f*, 200*f*
couples treatment and, 354
functional-structural domain and, 123*t*
overview, 200–201
Sadistic personality disorder, 205–207, 206*t*, 207*t*, 507–508. *see also* Sadistic personality; Sadistic scale
Sadistic scale. *see also* Sadistic personality; Sadistic personality disorder
antisocial personality disorder and, 202
case example of, 148
Danish MCMI-I and, 394, 395*t*, 397*t*, 398*t*–399*t*, 400–402, 401*t*
dependent personality disorder and, 226
gender differences and, 238–240, 238*f*
sensitivity of, 417–418, 418*t*
Schedule for Nonadaptive and Adaptive Personality (SNAP), 307*t*
Schemas, 31, 41, 51
Schizoid personality. *see also* Schizoid personality disorder; Schizoid scale
case example of, 187
correctional settings and, 197–198, 198*t*, 199*f*, 200*f*
Schizoid personality *(cont.)*

couples treatment and, 354, 356
functional-structural domain and, 123*t*
interpersonal style of, 29
levels of interpretation with the MCMI-III and, 98, 99
overview, 98
Schizoid personality disorder. *see also* Schizoid personality; Schizoid scale
case example of, 185
correctional settings and, 218–221, 219*t*, 221*t*
Introversion scale and, 505
Schizoid scale. *see also* Schizoid personality; Schizoid personality disorder
antisocial personality disorder and, 202–203
avoidant personality disorder and, 214
case example of, 183, 185, 189, 190
compulsive personality disorder and, 223
Danish MCMI-I and, 394, 395*t*, 397*t*, 398*t*–399*t*, 400–402, 401*t*
gender differences and, 238–239, 238*f*
masochistic personality disorder and, 228
overview, 88–89, 99
schizoid personality disorder and, 219
sensitivity of, 417–418, 418*t*
Schizophrenia. *see also* Schizotypal personality; Schizotypal scale
brain injury and, 257–259
Minnesota Multiphasic Personality Inventory (MMPI) and, 247
neuropsychological evaluation and, 257–259
Rorschach Comprehensive System and, 138
Schizophrenic spectrum disorders, 117, 138
Schizotypal personality. *see also* Schizophrenia; Schizotypal scale
correctional settings and, 199*f*
dimensional model and, 410
functional-structural domain and, 123*t*
interpersonal style of, 29
Schizotypal personality disorder, 197–198, 232–233
Schizotypal scale. *see also* Schizophrenia; Schizotypal personality
case example of, 92, 183
Danish MCMI-I and, 395*t*, 397*t*, 398*t*–399*t*, 400–402, 401*t*
levels of interpretation with the MCMI-III and, 100
sensitivity of, 417–418, 418*t*
Science, 51–52, 53–55
Scoring, 77–79, 86–87, 392
Screening, correctional settings and, 196–197
Secondary prevention, 461–462

Self-actualization, 32
Self-care behavior, risk behaviors and, 439
Self-defeating personality disorder. *see* Masochistic personality disorder
Self-demeaning scale, 500*t*, 508–509
Self-destructive potential, 109*f*
Self-Devaluation scale, 510
Self-esteem, 5, 216, 224–225
Self-image, 31–32, 114, 123*t*
Self-image assessment domain, 31–32, 591*f*, 602
Self-image therapies, 32
Self-Indulging scale, 645*t*, 663–664
Self-injury risk, borderline personality disorder and, 234
Self-other polarity, 70, 114. *see also* Replication phase
Self-Perception cluster, 145, 152–153
Self-propagating strategy, 70
Self-schemas, 51
Self-worth, risk behaviors and, 439
Semistructured interviews, 307*t*
Sensitive personality, 627–629
Sensitivity, 417–418
Sensorimotor/autonomy stage, 70
Severe Personality Pathology Scales
case example of, 140, 142, 148, 183, 189
cross-examination traps and, 191–192
Grossman Facet Scales and, 193
levels of interpretation with the MCMI-III and, 96, 100
Sexual Discomfort scale, 510–511
Shedler-Westen Assessment Procedure-200 (SWAP-200), 307*t*
Shyness, compared to avoidant personality, 410
Sixteen Personality Factor Questionnaire (16PF), 65, 118
Sociable personality, 565*t*, 622–623
Social Insensitivity scale, 511
Social support, 439, 442, 446
Sociobiology, personality polarity model and, 69
Somatic symptoms, neuropsychological evaluation and, 260–263
Somatoform disorders, neuropsychological evaluation and, 260–263
Somatoform scale
case example of, 92–93
Danish MCMI-I and, 395*t*, 397*t*, 398*t*–399*t*, 400–402, 401*t*
Dutch translation project and, 376
MCMI-III and, 87
Spiritual Doubts scale, 568*t*

Spiritual resources, 439, 442, 446
Standardization, cross-examination traps and,
    190–192
Standardized Psychiatric Examination, 299
State v. Galloway (1993), 182
State-Trait Anxiety Inventory (STAI), 557
Strategies, 40
Stress
    addictive disorders and, 282
    Capacity for Control and Tolerance for
        Stress cluster and, 144–145, 150–151
    dependent personality disorder and, 225
    diagnosis and treatment of disease and,
        442–443
    integration of the MCMI with the MMPI
        and, 166–168
    risk behaviors and, 439
Stress-coping model, 162
Stress-related symptoms, psychosocial factors
    in, 437–438
Strong Vocational Blank, 75
Structural domains of personality, 410*t*
Structural Interview for Disorders of
    Personality-Revised (SIDP-R), 299–302
Structural personality classification, 327
Structured Clinical Interview for DSM-IV Axis
    II Personality Disorders (SCID-II), 307*t*
Structured Interview for DSM-IV Personality
    (SIDP-IV), 307*t*
Structured interviews, 307*t*
Subject-oriented theories, 688
Submissive scale, 500*t*, 506, 532
Submissive/Yielding scale, 646*t*
Subscales in general, 114–117, 117–119. *see*
    also specific scales
Substance abuse. *see also* Addictive disorders
    couples treatment and, 349
    HIV risk behavior and, 275–277
    neuropsychological evaluation and, 255
    relapse and, 280–283
Substance Abuse Proneness scale, 512
Suicidal Tendency scale, 514, 568*t*
Suicide, 116–117, 234
Surgency factor, 663
Surgery, treatment success and recovery and,
    454–455
Survival phase, 114. *see also* Pain-pleasure
    (survival) polarity
Symptoms, evolutionary theory and, 22–23
Synergistic therapy, 36–43, 41, 43
System transactions, 40–42
Systems theory, 331–332

T

Tactics, 40
Taxonomy
    assessment of the individual and, 57
    clinical science and, 53–55
    history of the MCMI and, 66–69
    instrument construction and, 61
    overview, 688
Technology, guidelines for the use of the
    MCMI-III, 77–79
Temperament, 21–22, 35–36
Temperament assessment domain, 35
Temperament therapies, 35–36
Temperamentally Woeful scale, 124
Tertiary prevention, 462
Test-retest reliability, 414
Thematic Apperception Test (TAT), 54, 158
Theoretical/substansive validation, 71, 72–73
Theory
    assessment of the individual and, 55–58
    clinical science and, 53–55
    content scales and, 114–115
    deductive methodology and, 113–114
    evolution and, 20–23
    Facet Scales and, 121–122
    history of the MCMI and, 50–53, 66–69
    instrument construction and, 58–61
    MCMI-III and, 139
    Millon Pre-Adolescent Clinical Inventory
        (M-PACI), 529–530
    overview, 9
    from philosophy to, 20–25
Therapeutic context, personalized assessment
    in, 36–43
Therapeutic planning. *see also* Treatment
    planning
    assessment and, 62–64
    Millon-Grossman Personality Domains
        Checklist (MG-PDC) and, 598–600
    Personality Adjective Check List (PACL)
        and, 630–634, 633*f*
Therapist, role of, 29–30
Thinking Styles scales, 644, 644*t*, 645*t*–646*t*,
    647
Thought disorder, 144
Thought Disorder scale
    case example of, 93
    Danish MCMI-I and, 395*t*, 397*t*, 398*t*–
        399*t*, 400–402, 401*t*
    Dutch translation project and, 376
Thought-Guided scale, 645*t*, 663–664
Three-stage validation model, 387

Training, professional, 77, 84–85

Transactions, system transactions and, 40–42

Translation of the MCMI. *see also* Dutch translation project
cross-cultural issues and, 402–403
factor analysis of the Danish MCMI-I and, 400–402, 401*t*
guidelines for, 388–389
issues regarding, 389–390
linguistic procedures for, 390–391
overview, 387–388
psychometric properties of, 391–400, 392*t*, 393*t*, 394*t*, 395*t*, 396*t*, 397*t*, 398*t*–399*t*

Treatment. *see also* Interventions; Personalized psychotherapy; Treatment goals; Treatment planning
older adults and, 309–314, 311*t*, 313*t*, 315*t*–316*t*
outcomes of, 272–275, 283–286, 309–312, 311*t*
overview, 27–36, 439–447
theory and, 329–330
treatment planning and, 337

Treatment goals. *see also* Treatment planning
case example of, 110*f*–111*f*
complex syndromes and, 26–27
Millon-Grossman Personality Domains Checklist (MG-PDC) and, 599–600

Treatment outcomes
addictive disorders and, 272–275, 283–286
older adults and, 309–312, 311*t*

Treatment planning. *see also* Therapeutic planning
case example of, 129–131, 337–344, 339*f*, 343*f*, 573, 575, 577
Facet Scales and, 128–131
MCMI-III and, 333–337, 335*f*
Millon-Grossman Personality Domains Checklist (MG-PDC) and, 598–600
overview, 345
personality styles and, 617–629

Treatment-refractory cases, treatment planning and, 336

Triangulation, schizophrenia and, 257–259

True Response Inconsistency scale, 502–503

T-scores
cross-examination traps and, 191
expert testimony and, 180–181
Millon Index of Personality Styles *Revised* (MIPS) and, 661

overview, 97

Personality Adjective Check List (PACL) and, 615

Tyrannical subtype of sadistic personality, 211

U

Uncertain Self-Image subscale (Borderline), 194

Unconventional/Dissenting scale, 646*t*, 663

Unruly personality, 565*t*

Unruly scale, 500*t*, 507, 532–533

Unstable scale, 533

V

Validity
content scales and subscales, 115
Dutch translation project and, 375–377, 376*t*, 377*t*
Millon Behavioral Medicine Diagnostic (MBMD) and, 464–469, 465*t*
Millon College Counseling Inventory (MCCI) and, 556–557, 560
Millon Index of Personality Styles *Revised* (MIPS) and, 644*t*, 645*t*, 651–652
Millon Personality Diagnostic Checklist (MPDC) and, 583–584
Millon Pre-Adolescent Clinical Inventory (M-PACI) and, 535–543, 538*t*, 539*t*, 540*t*, 542*t*
overview, 71–76, 411–422, 416*f*, 418*t*, 421*t*, 684–685
translation of the MCMI and, 390

Validity Index, 90

Validity scales, 86–87

Variable Response Inconsistency scale, 502–503

Vulnerability, stress-related symptoms and, 437–438

W

Wechsler Adult Intelligence Scale-Revised (WAIS-R), 249

World hypotheses, 10–12